Springer

Berlin
Heidelberg
New York
Barcelona
Hong Kong
London
Milan
Paris
Singapore
Tokyo

Anisah el Helou

Atlas of Diagnostic Nuclear Medicine

Foreword by H. Kriegel

With 368 Figures,
91 in Color,
in More Than 2000 Separate Illustrations

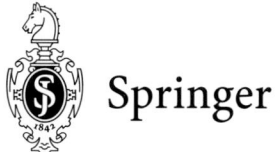

Springer

Dr. med. Anisah el Helou
Postfach 102046
69010 Heidelberg
Germany

Translation:
Terry C. Telger, 6112 Waco Way, Forth Worth, TX 76133, USA

Library of Congress Cataloging-in-Publication Data
El Helou, Anisah, 1938-Atlas of diagnostic nuclear medicine / Anisah el Helou ; Foreword by Heinz
Kriegel. p. ; cm.
    Includes bibliographical references and index.
    ISBN 3-540-65175-6 (hardcover : alk. paper)
1. Radioisotope scanning–Atlases. I. Title.
[DNLM: 1. Radionuclide Imaging–Atlases. WN 17 E41a 2000]
RC78.7.R4 E436 2000
616.07'575–dc21

ISBN 3-540-65175-6 Springer-Verlag Berlin Heidelberg New York

Springer-Verlag Berlin Heidelberg New York
a member of BertelsmannSpringer Science+Business Media GmbH

© Springer-Verlag Berlin Heidelberg 2001
Printed in Germany

Production: PRO EDIT GmbH, 69126 Heidelberg, Germany
Cover design: design + production GmbH, Heidelberg, Germany
Typesetting and Reproduction of the figures: AM-productions GmbH, 69168 Wiesloch, Germany
Printing and binding: Stürz AG, Universitätsdruckerei, 97017 Würzburg, Germany

Printed on acid-free paper   SPIN: 10675815   21/3135/ML   5 4 3 2 1 0

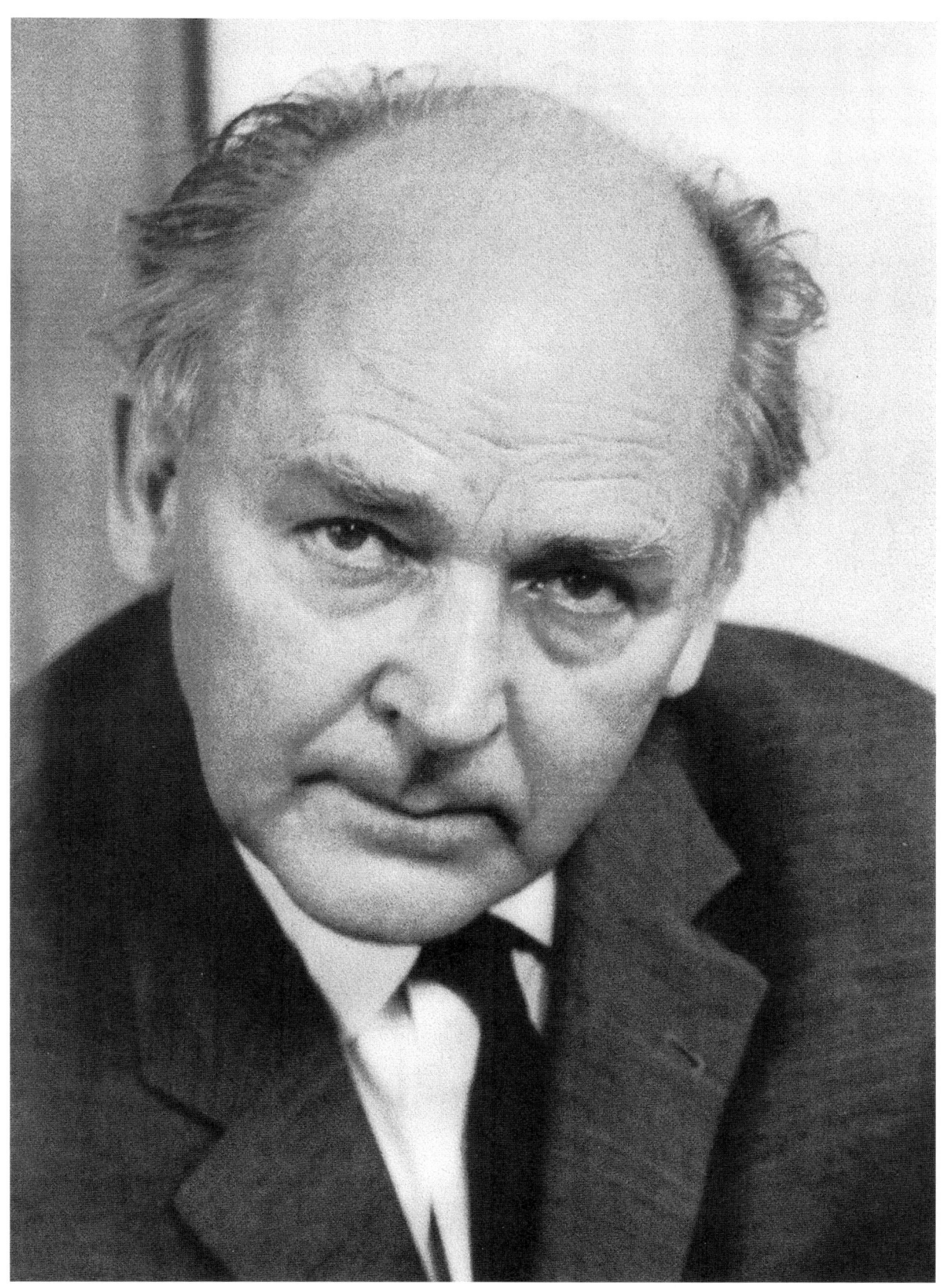

Fritz Straßmann
* 22.02.1902 in Boppard   † 22.04.1980 in Mainz

Foreword

Today nuclear medicine must be considered an established specialty, an essential tool in medical diagnosis and treatment, and an important component of medical education. The use of „open radionuclides" has provided the key to visualizing changes in biologic structures as well as detecting pathophysiologic and space-occupying processes within the body.

During the many years in which nuclear medicine has evolved, numerous radiopharmaceuticals have been tested both for the quality of their diagnostic yield and for the safety of their radioactive emissions. Meanwhile, the sensitivity and diagnostic capabilities of nuclear imaging equipment at hospitals, offices, and institutions have been substantially improved, and quality standards for nuclear medicine protocols and examinations have been established on the basis of intensive research.

While a great many comprehensive reference works have been published on the principles and practices of radiology, there has been a dearth of works dealing with „classic" nuclear medicine. Thus, an atlas portraying the results of nuclear medicine examinations is a welcome addition to the radiologic literature.

In compiling the images, the author has drawn materials from the files of her own nuclear medicine practice. Her selection of diagnostic images vividly illustrates the range of applications of radionuclide imaging. The atlas also includes an historical overview outlining the evolution of nuclear medicine.

It is hoped that this atlas will advance the understanding of nuclear medicine methods and examinations in allied specialties and among students of medical imaging.

Munich, Spring 2000

Heinz Kriegel

Preface

Nuclear medicine is a relatively young medical discipline. Serious work with medical radioisotopes began at German universities in 1950. Before the first production facilities were established in Europe, radioisotopes had to be flown into Germany from the United States. As a result, radionuclide studies could not be performed during inclement weather. The German Roentgenographic Society was the first professional society to recognize the importance of nuclear medicine as a specialty and founded the Association for the Study of Radioisotopes (RIAG). Next came the Association for the Study of Radioisotopes in Internal Medicine (ARIGIM), whose first large symposium, held in Freiburg in 1962, had an attendance of approximately 100. On February 22, 1963, the director of the former Czerny Hospital in Heidelberg, Prof. Becker, ended the rivalry between the two societies by persuading Prof. von Hevesy, a Nobel Prize winner, to serve as the first joint chairman. Shortly thereafter, the Society of Nuclear Medicine was founded at the request of small groups of European specialists. By its tenth annual meeting, the Society had a roster of 600 members from 22 countries.

There is scarcely any other specialty in which the natural sciences, technology, physiology, and the various clinical disciplines are so closely united as in nuclear medicine. As a result, nuclear medicine relies to a unique degree on interdisciplinary cooperation for its effectiveness and continued development.

This atlas provides an ideal supplement to existing textbooks of nuclear medicine. By emphasizing images over written text, the *Atlas of Nuclear Medicine* can provide physicians, medical students, and other interested readers with an overview of the capabilities and limitations of radionuclide imaging. Advances in equipment technology and radiopharmaceuticals have been so rapid that some of the chapters may not reflect cutting-edge methodology. It should be kept in mind, however, that innovations are not always good and that time is needed to establish the validity of new techniques.

I dedicate this atlas to my esteemed teacher, Prof. Fritz Strassmann, and hope that it will advance his wish that nuclear medicine be used for positive and peaceful purposes. I am grateful to his wife, Irmgard Strassmann, for providing me with his photograph. I also express thanks and appreciation to all my colleagues who worked tirelessly and in great detail, going beyond their regular duties. Without them, this book would not have been possible.

Heidelberg, Spring 2000

A. el Helou

Contents

Abbreviations

AP, PA, LPO, etc.	Projections (anteroposterior, posteroanterior, left posterior oblique, etc.)
ATP	Adenosine triphosphate
BBB	Blood-brain barrier
Bq	Becquerel (1 Bq = 1 disintegration/s)
CCK	Cholecystokinin
CHD	Coronary heart disease
Ci	Curie (1 Ci = 3.7×10^{10} Bq)
CNS	Central nervous system
CT	Computed tomography
DMSA	Dimercaptosuccinic acid
DTPA	Diethylene triamine penta-acetic acid
EANM	European Association of Nuclear Medicine
ECAT	Emission computed axial tomography
ECG	Electrocardiography
EDTA	Ethylene diamine tetra-acetic acid
EF	Ejection fraction
EHDP	Ethylhydroxydiphosphonate
ERCP	Endoscopic retrograde cholangiopancreatography
HDA	Heptadecanic acid
HIDA	See IDA
HMPAO	Hexamethylpropylene amine oxime
HL	Half-life
HSA	Human serum albumin
HVL	Half-value layer
I	Iodine
IBZM	Iodobenzamide
ICDR	Iododeoxycytidine
IDA	Iminodiacetic acid
L	Lumbar vertebra (L1, L2, etc.)
LAD	Left anterior descending coronary artery
LCA	Left coronary artery
LCX	Left circumflex artery (circumflex branch of the left coronary artery)
MAA	Macroaggregated albumin
MAG3	Mercaptoacetyltriglycine
MDP	Methylene diphosphonate
MI	Myocardial infarction
MIBG	Meta-iodobenzylguanidine
MIBI	Methoxyisobutylisonitrile
MRI	Magnetic resonance imaging
OIF	Octaiodofluorescein
p.i.	Postinjection
RA	Rheumatoid arthritis
PET	Positron emission tomography (positron ECAT)

PRIND	Prolonged reversible ischemic neurologic deficit
PTD	Percutaneous transluminal dilatation
PTH	Parathyroid hormone
PVP	Polyvinylpyrrolidone
RBC	Red blood cells
RCA	Right coronary artery
RES	Reticuloendothelial system
RFS	Renal function scanning
RIN	Radioisotope nephrography
ROI	Region of interest
RUQ	Right upper quadrant of the abdomen
SPECT	Single-photon emission computed tomography
T	Thoracic vertebra (T1, T2, etc.)
TIA	Transient ischemic attack
$\mathbf{T_{max}}$, **TTP**	Time to peak activity
$\mathbf{T_{1/2}}$	Fall of time-activity curve to one-half peak
V/Q	Ventilation-perfusion ratio

Projections in Radionuclide Imaging

Body

Anterior (= AP view)
Posterior (= PA view)
Left lateral (LL)
Right lateral (RL)

Head

Frontal
Occipital
Vertex

R anterior L (R Ant L)
L posterior R (L Pos R)
Anterior L posterior (Ant L Pos)
Posterior R anterior (Pos R Ant)
Right posterior oblique (RPO)
Right anterior oblique (RAO)
Left posterior oblique (LPO)
Left anterior oblique (LAO)

1 **Head and Neck**

1.1
Brain

Radionuclide imaging of the brain is based on the tendency of lesions of the brain and meninges to accumulate radiopharmaceuticals, while almost all other intracerebral areas show an undetectable degree of uptake. The mechanisms of radionuclide uptake in the brain are not yet fully understood but presumably involve the following factors:

▌ Local breakdown or functional abnormality of the blood-brain barrier
▌ Circumscribed intracerebral location of tissue foreign to the brain
▌ Localized increase or decrease in circulating cerebral blood volume
▌ Use of lipophilic or physiologic radiolabeled compounds

1.1.1
Cerebrovascular Disease

Little is known for certain about the mechanisms responsible for increased radiotracer uptake in regions of brain infarction. There is considerable evidence that transient insults produce only microinfarcts that are not detectable by radionuclide imaging. A well-developed collateral circulation prevents increased uptake in the irreversibly damaged cellular tissue, but images acquired during the repair stage of neovascularization and macrophage infiltration show intense uptake in the infarcted area.

The following classification of cardiovascular events is employed in nuclear medicine:

▌ Transient ischemic attack (TIA): a reversible neurologic deficit that persists for less than 24 h.
▌ Prolonged reversible ischemic neurologic deficit (PRIND): an event that lasts for more than 24 hours and resolves completely.
▌ Completed stroke: a completed cerebral infarction associated with acute and protracted symptoms and tissue necrosis. There may or may not be complete resolution of the deficits.

1.1.2
Brain Tumors

Radiotracer is mostly concentrated in the extracellular space of a tumor. Very little uptake occurs in the tumor cells themselves, and consequently the uptake is tumor-nonspecific. Tumors whose capillaries still have roughly the same structure as normal brain capillaries show at most a trace amount of radionuclide uptake that is only occasionally detectable.

1.1.3
Sensitivity of Radionuclide
Imaging in Cerebral Diagnosis

The sensitivity results presented below are based on a statistical review of a total of 17,074 radionuclide examinations including 12,197 tumors, 4279 cerebrovascular lesions, and 296 inflammatory lesions (see Tables 1.1–1.5).

Table 1.1. Sensitivity comparison of radionuclide imaging and computed tomography (based on collective statistical analysis)

Type of disease	Radionuclide imaging		Computed tomography		Both modalities	
	No. of patients	Sensitivity (%)	No. of patients	Sensitivity (%)	No. of patients	Sensitivity (%)
Infarction	343	76	339	70	180	95
TIA	69	88	65	28		
PRIND	75	74	75	69	75	87

Table 1.2. Sensitivity of radionuclide imaging: dependence on tumor location (after el Helou et al., 1980)

Location of brain tumor	No. of patients	Sensitivity (%)
Supratentorial	566	83
Frontal	67	96
Parietal	47	94
Temporal	41	90
Occipital	14	93
Basal and sellar	26	65
Infratentorial	113	65
Cerebellar	33	82
Brain stem	10	40
Cerebellopontine angle	10	100

Table 1.3. Sensitivity of radionuclide imaging: dependence on tumor type (after el Helou et al., 1980)

Tumor type	No. of patients	Sensitivity (%)
Astrocytoma (grade I–II)	63	66
Oligodendroglioma	58	74
Glioblastoma multiforme (grade III–IV astrocytoma)	234	96
Meningioma	308	94
Metastases	576	91
Subdural hematoma	43	88
Brain abscess	143	94

Table 1.4. Sensitivity comparison of radionuclide imaging and computed tomography in the detection of brain tumors (after el Helou et al., 1980)

Tumor type	Radionuclide imaging		Computed tomography	
	No. of patients	Sensitivity (%)	No. of patients	Sensitivity (%)
Mixed tumors	536	84	537	94
Gliomas				
Grade I–II	32	82	38	97
Grade III–IV	99	100	100	100
Meningioma	146	97	148	97
Metastases	211	83	230	95

Table 1.5. Sensitivity of cerebral angiography and radionuclide brain imaging (after el Helou et al., 1980)

Tumor type	Sensitivity of angiography (%)	Sensitivity of radionuclide imaging (%)	No. of patients
Overall			
Pre-1968	82.3	82.7	3954
Post-1968	87	79	750
Glioblastoma	88	84	147
Meningioma	92	94	214
Metastases	73	84	122
Astrocytoma	84	69	151

Tumors. In a review of 1060 patients with brain tumors, the sensitivity of radionuclide imaging was 63% for the detection of grade I–II astrocytomas, 96% for grade III-IV astrocytomas, 79% for oligodendrogliomas, 94% for meningiomas, 91% for metastases, and 83% for subdural hematomas. In a review of 2184 patients, the sensitivity of tumor detection depended on the radiopharmaceutical used. Only ^{99m}Tc pertechnetate and ^{99m}DTPA provided a sensitivity higher than 90%. The sensitivities obtained with ^{99m}gluconate, ^{67}citrate, ^{99m}Tc-labeled phosphate complexes, ^{113m}indium-DTPA/EDPA, and ^{99m}Co-bleomycin ranged from 82% to 87%.

The sensitivity of sequential imaging depends on the grade of tumor malignancy. A sensitivity of 60–69% was found for gliomas, 85% for glioblastomas, 82% for meningiomas, and 79–84% for metastases. Comparing the sensitivities of computed tomography (CT) and radionuclide imaging (RI) in 352 patients with grade I–IV gliomas, we found a mean sensitivity of 84% with RI versus 98% with CT. In other studies we compared the sensitivities for supratentorial tumors and tumors located in the posterior fossa. CT and RI were equally sensitive in detecting supratentorial lesions (93%), but CT was more sensitive than RI in detecting posterior fossa tumors (81% vs. 76%). Combining both modalities improved the yield slightly but not to a statistically significant degree. Sensitivity comparisons in 163 patients showed a definite dependence on tumor grade. CT was markedly superior to RI in detecting grade I–II gliomas (CT 98%, RI 59%) but was comparable in the detection of grade III-IV gliomas (CT 100%, RI 99%). Comparing the sensitivity of emission computed tomography (ECAT) with that of conventional CT in 119 patients who underwent both examinations, ECAT was 93% sensitive in detecting tumors while CT showed a sensitivity of 96%.

A comparative study of cerebral angiography and radionuclide brain imaging was subdivided into two parts based on stages of technical development:

▌ In 3954 patients examined prior to 1968, radionuclide brain scans showed a sensitivity of 82.7% in tumor detection compared with 82.3% for angiography.
▌ In 750 patients examined since 1968, the overall sensitivity of radionuclide brain scans was 79% versus 87% with angiography.

Radionuclide imaging was more sensitive in detecting meningiomas and metastases, while angiography was superior in detecting astrocytomas. Both modalities showed comparable sensitivities in the detection of glioblastomas.

With regard to rates of accurate tumor localization, radionuclide imaging was superior for glioblastomas and meningiomas while angiography was better for astrocytomas and oligodendrogliomas. Results varied in the localization of metastases and sarcomas.

Cerebrovascular Disease. In a statistical review of 1250 examinations, RI showed an overall sensitivity of 52% in the detection of cerebrovascular disease. Dynamic scanning increased the detection rate by 21% in 405 examinations. Dynamic imaging increased sensitivity by 33% in the diagnosis of TIAs (297 patients) and by 19% in the diagnosis of completed stroke (389 patients). A comparative study of CT and RI showed that RI was superior in detecting cerebral infarction, TIA, and PRIND while CT was superior for intracranial hemorrhages.

In a comparison of ECAT and planar imaging, ECAT was superior in the diagnosis of cerebral infarction. The superiority of CT over ECAT in the detection of cerebrovascular abnormalities was documented in 107 patients (CT 88%, ECAT 76%).

Inflammatory Disease. Radionuclide imaging showed a sensitivity of 94% for brain abscess (152 patients), 75% for encephalitis (112 patients), and 75% for meningitis (32 patients). Follow-up imaging during chemotherapy demonstrated the superiority of RI in the relatively small case numbers available.

When we consider on the one hand the excellent patient tolerance for sequential scanning, and on the other that encephalitis has a mortality rate of 10–20% and that there were 102,796 deaths from cerebrovascular disease in Germany in 1979, we can appreciate the potential value of nuclear medicine imaging as a routine primary study. This is especially true when we consider the increase in sensitivity provided by positron-emission tomography (PET) and magnetic resonance imaging (MRI).

1.2
Parotid Gland

Radionuclide imaging of the parotid gland is based on radiotracer uptake in the glandular tissue or in the remnant left by surgical resection. Differences in uptake intensity and the time-activity curve yield information on parotid function and support the suspicion of postirradiation changes in a patient who has received radiation to the neck. The detection of parotid tumors is of secondary importance, especially since benign tumors are not specific in their uptake of $^{99m}TcO4$. Radionuclide imaging can still be useful, however, for demonstrating residual healthy tissue and helping the surgeon determine the extent of the operation.

When inflammation is present, the hyperemic condition of the gland can produce an initial upstroke in the time-activity curve, but clearance of the radiotracer is delayed during the washout phase and after stimulation, presumably due to luminal narrowing of the excretory ducts. As in all glandular tissues, secretion is decreased in the presence of chronic recurring inflammation.

Radionuclide scanning is of little help in diagnosing ductal stenoses or fistulae, which are better evaluated by contrast sialography.

For these reasons, parotid scintigraphy has not gained an established role as a routine clinical study.

1.3
Thyroid Gland

The diagnosis of thyroid disease is still a somewhat confusing issue owing to the many diagnostic options that are available and to continual refinements and further differentiation of the diagnostic spectrum. The cutoff point at which diagnostic efforts become exorbitant relative to the expected gain is becoming increasingly difficult to define. This emphasizes the importance of an intensive interdisciplinary approach to save costs and benefit the patient.

Today more than 60 separate types of thyroid disease have been identified. In dealing with the very large number of patients who seek treatment for goiter, the physician's task is to differentiate benign conditions from a malignant process that may present as a "nodular goiter" and to exhaust all diagnostic options to ensure that carcinoma is not missed and that unnecessary therapeutic measures are avoided.

The indications for thyroid scanning have changed considerably as a result of new technical advances such as ultrasonography. Today radionuclide scanning should be used selectively as a modality that can provide both qualitative and quantitative information.

▌ *Qualitative* scanning is useful for the subjective evaluation of thyroid function and for distinguishing between hot and cold nodules.

▌ *Quantitative* scanning yields information on global or regional thyroid metabolism per unit time and can document this information in the form of quantitative data.

Radionuclide scanning also has a significant role in screening for metastases in patients with a thyroid malignancy. It is the only satisfactory modality that can provide the physician with a whole-body survey.

1.4
Parathyroid Gland

Imaging of the parathyroids is very difficult because of their anatomic location and the lack of organ-specific radiopharmaceuticals. Given the fact that large parathyroid adenomas may contain necrotic foci, there is justification for the claim that large adenomas are more difficult to visualize than small hormone-producing adenomas. Despite these difficulties, radionuclide scanning can be used adjunctively with ultrasound as an effective aid to surgical localization. The scanning protocol requires a quiet, recumbent patient, since only double-tracer subtraction imaging of the thyroid and parathyroids can provide accurate localization.

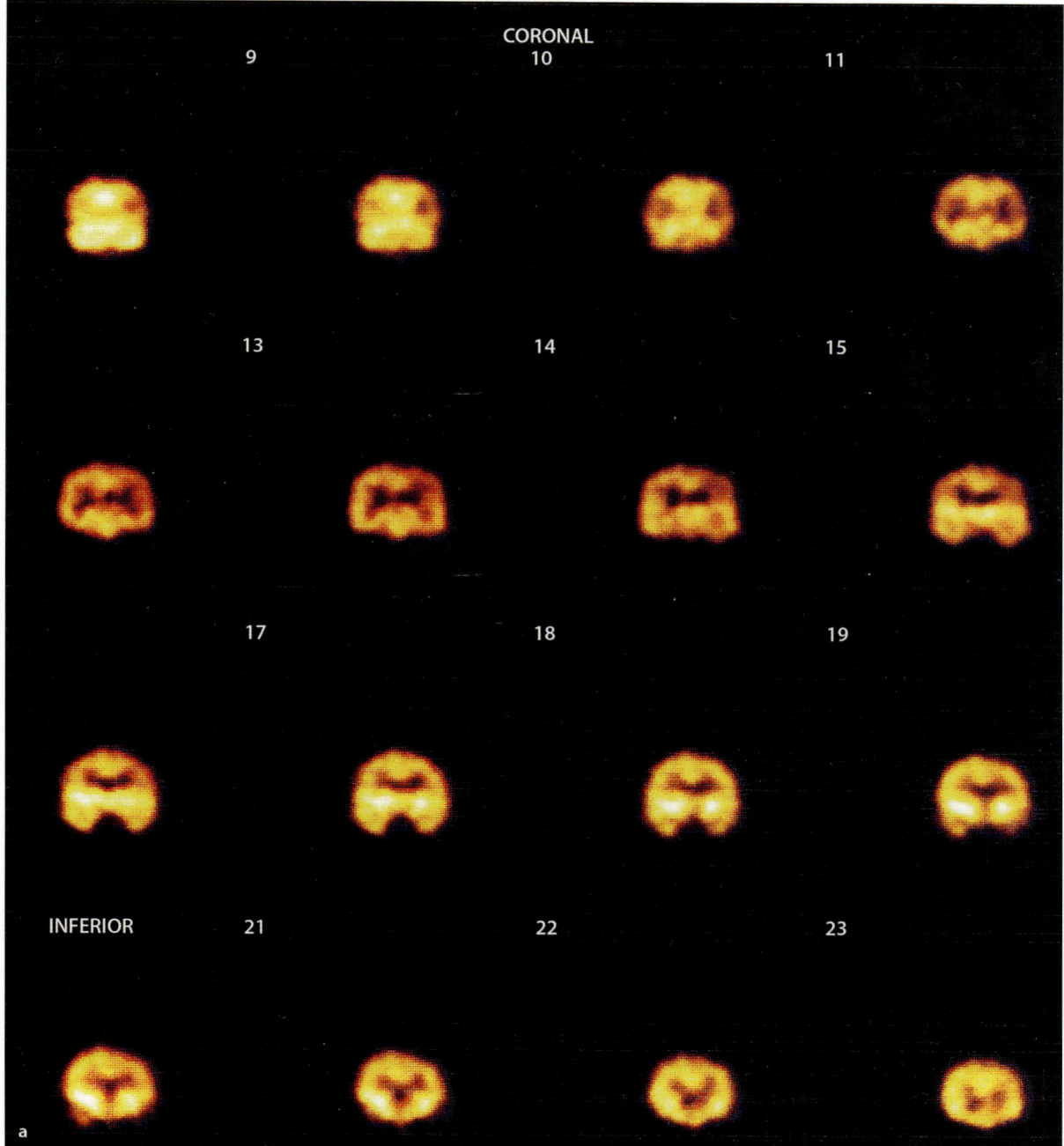

Fig. 1.1 a. Brain scan in a 54-year-old woman shows a significant perfusion defect in the left frontal area, moderate hypoperfusion on the right side, and a nonhomogeneous distribution of activity in the right occipital and temporoparietal areas. This pattern is suggestive of brain atrophy, but incipient Alzheimer's disease can also produce these features

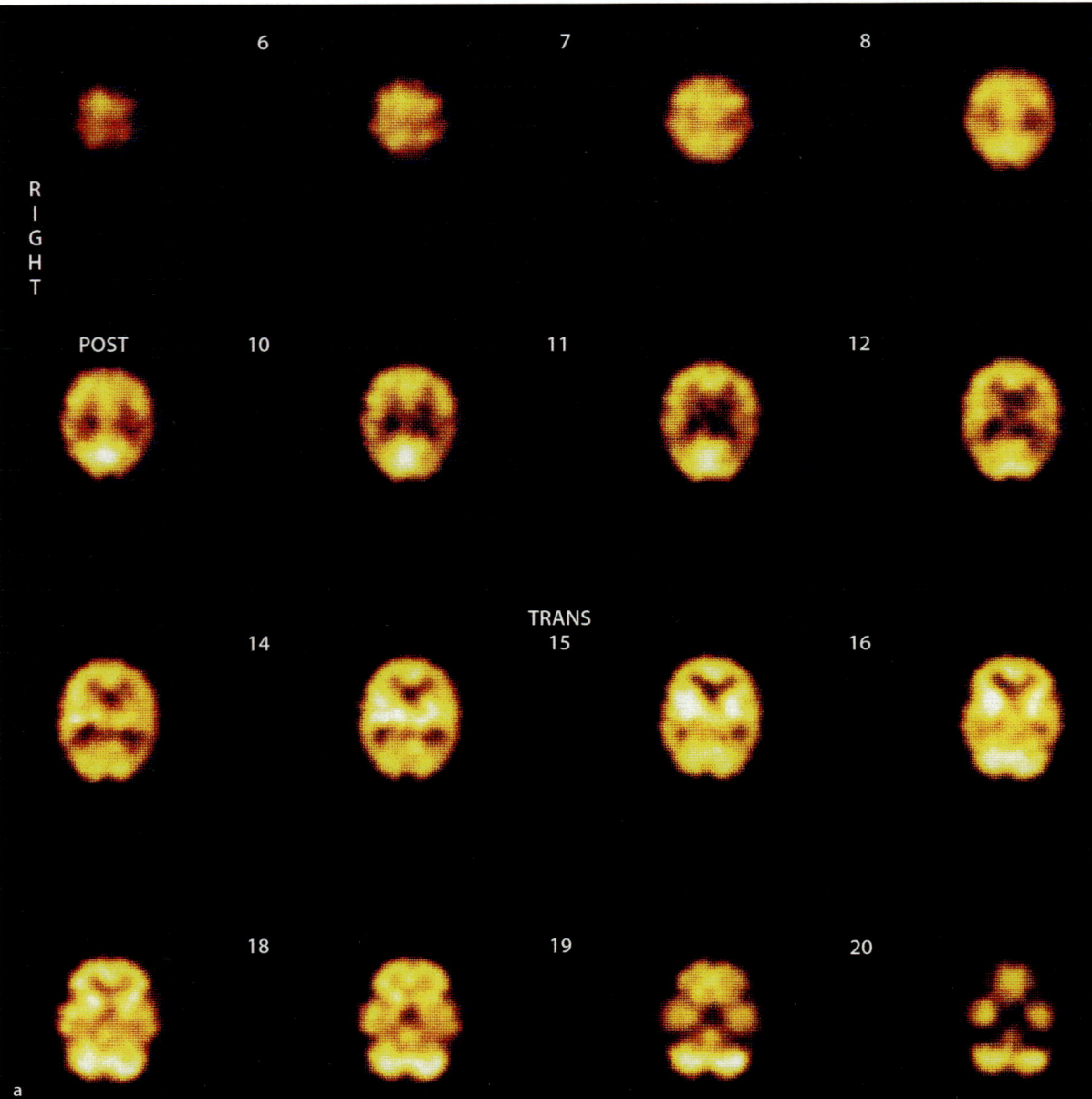

Fig. 1.1 a. *Continued*

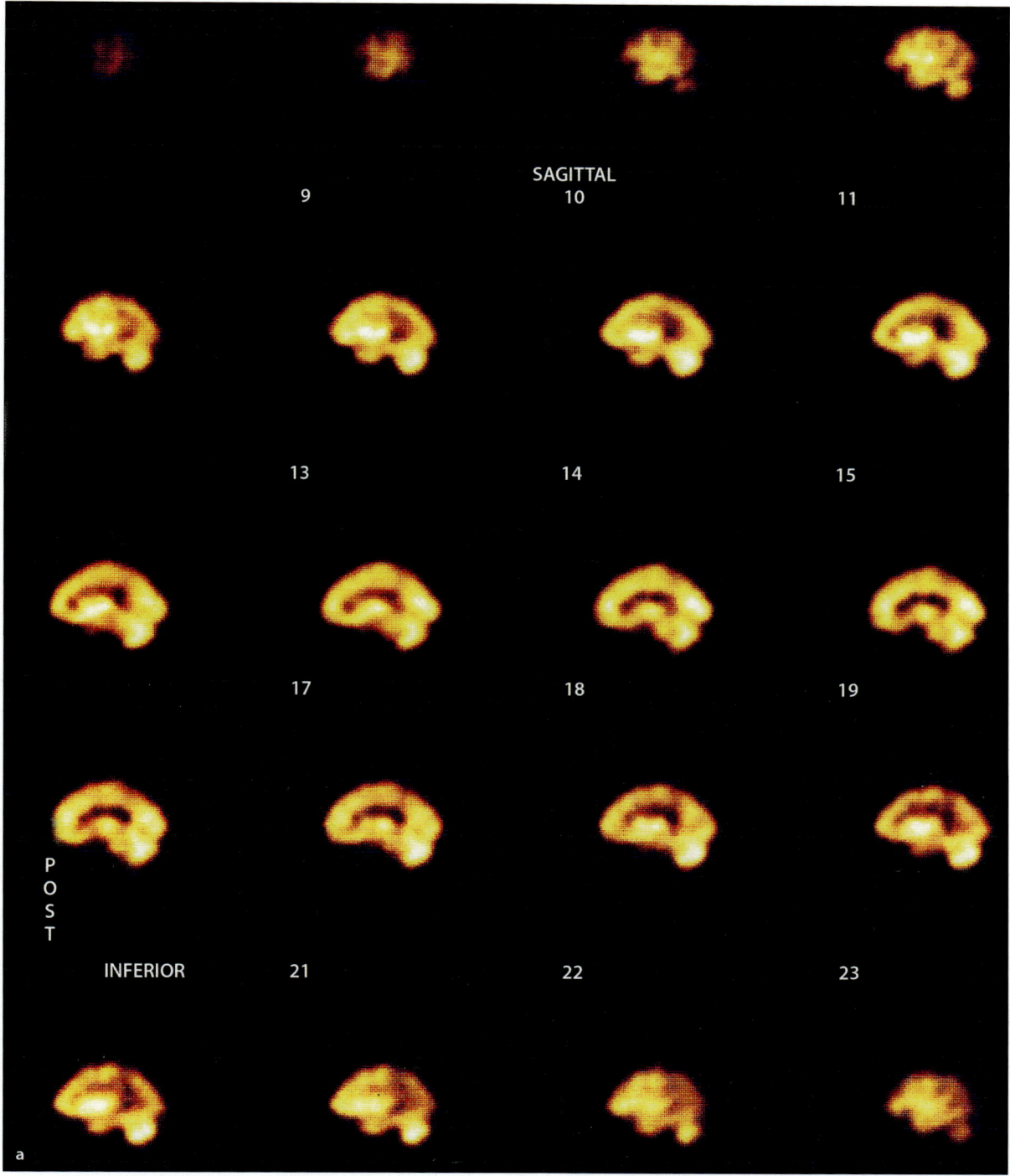

Fig. 1.1 a. Brain scan in a 54-year-old woman shows a significant perfusion defect in the left frontal area, moderate hypoperfusion on the right side, and a nonhomogeneous distribution of activity in the right occipital and temporoparietal areas. This pattern is suggestive of brain atrophy, but incipient Alzheimer's disease can also produce these features

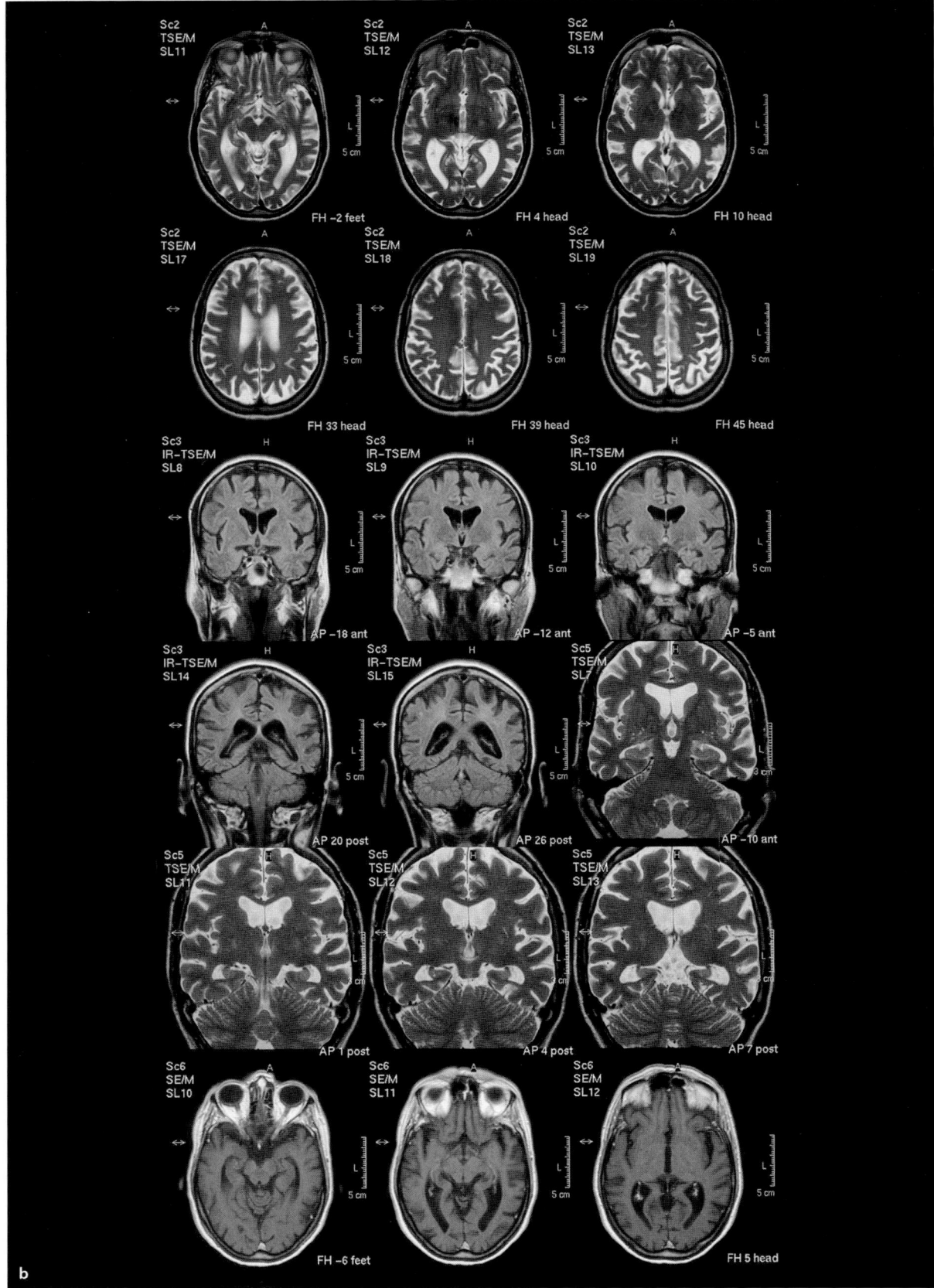

Fig. 1.1 b. CT and MRI do not advance the differential diagnosis, showing only brain atrophy consistent with a neurodegenerative disease

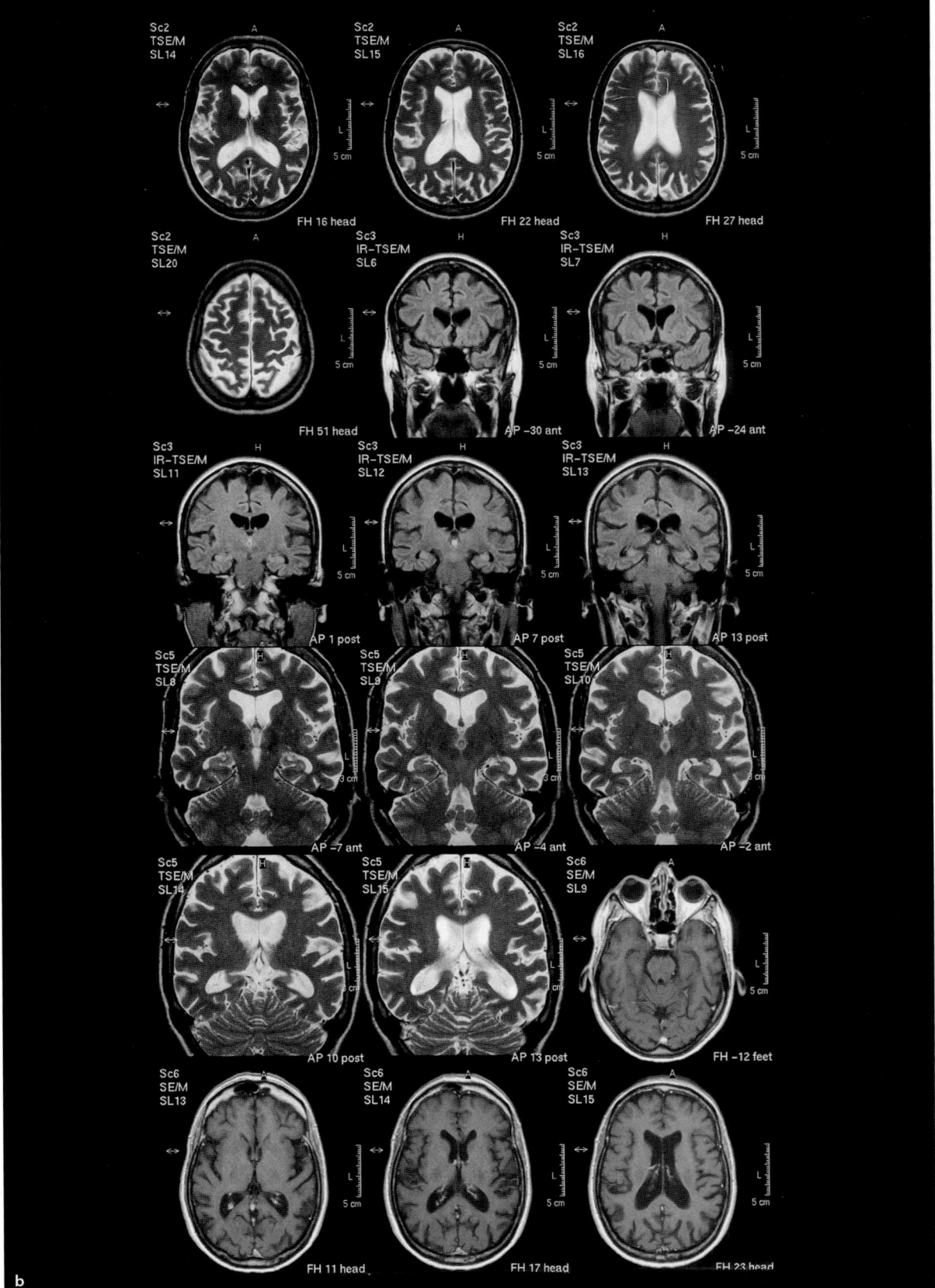

Fig. 1.1 b. *Continued*

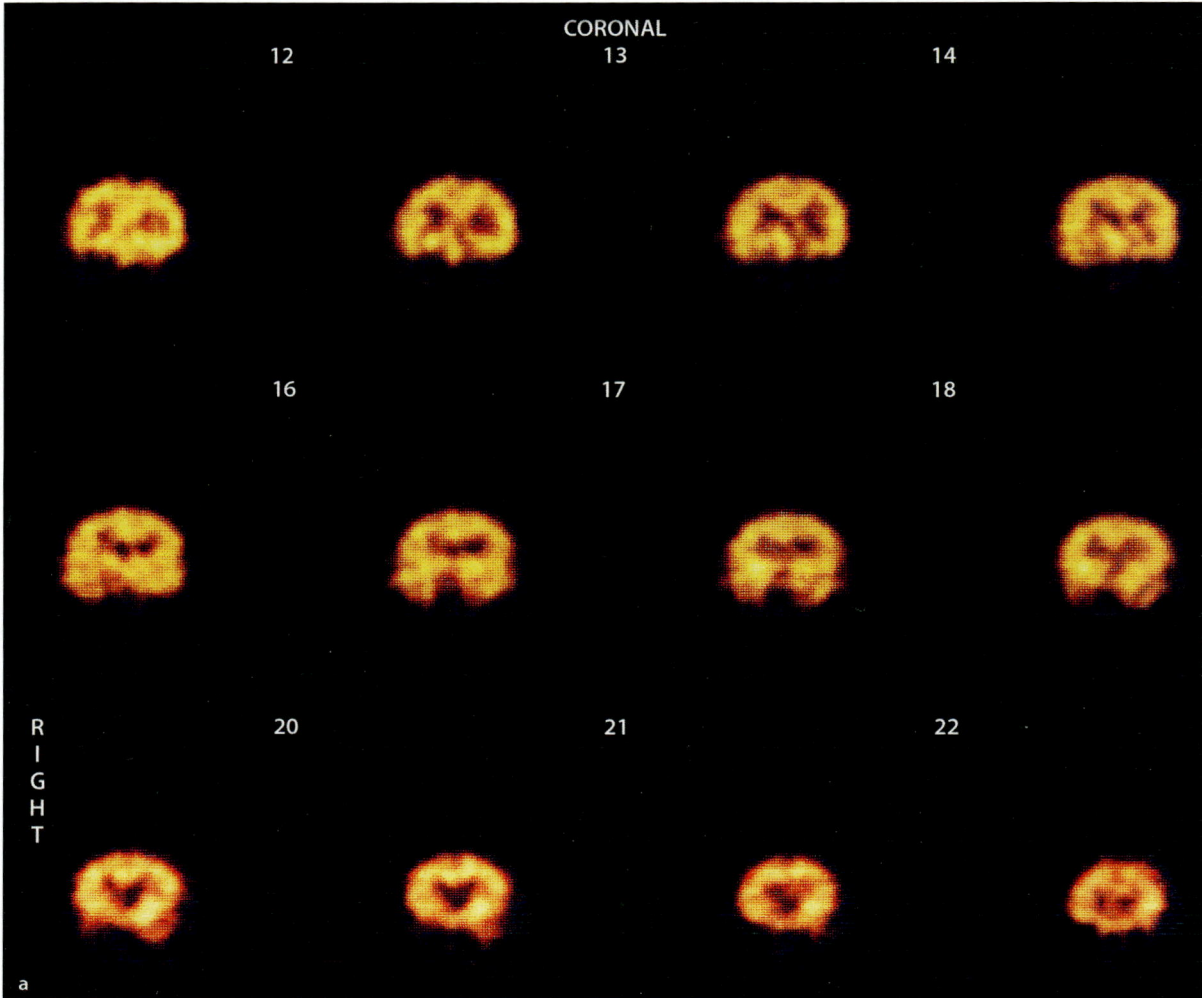

Fig. 1.2 a,b. Brain scan in a 67-year-old woman with vertiginous symptoms and known plaque formation in extracranial vessels shows mild, disseminated hypoperfusion with no evidence of a recent or old infarct. The changes are potentiated after diamox administration, indicating a disseminated disturbance of cerebral blood flow in which the cerebrovascular reserve is still reasonably intact

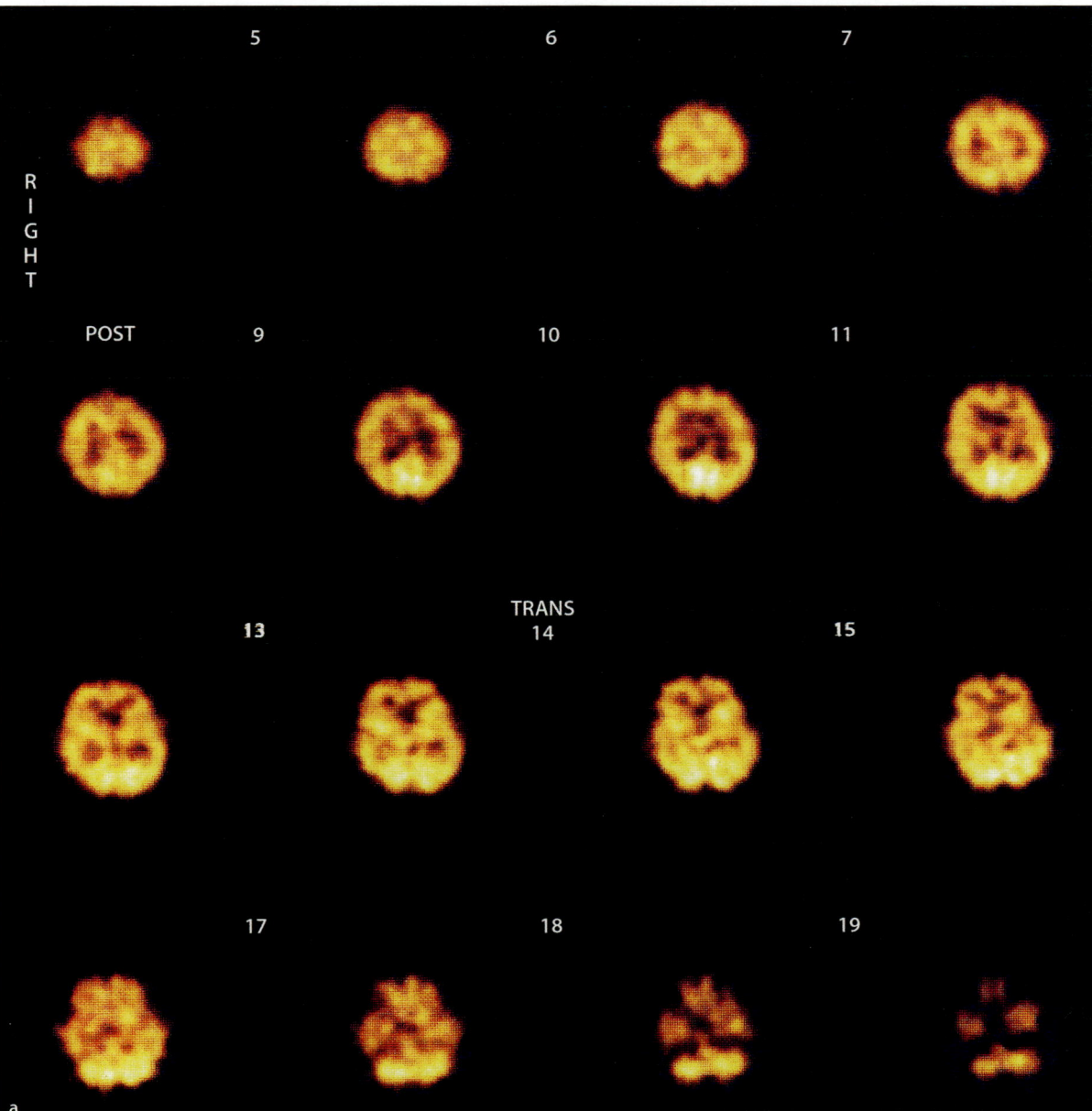

Fig. 1.2 a. *Continued*

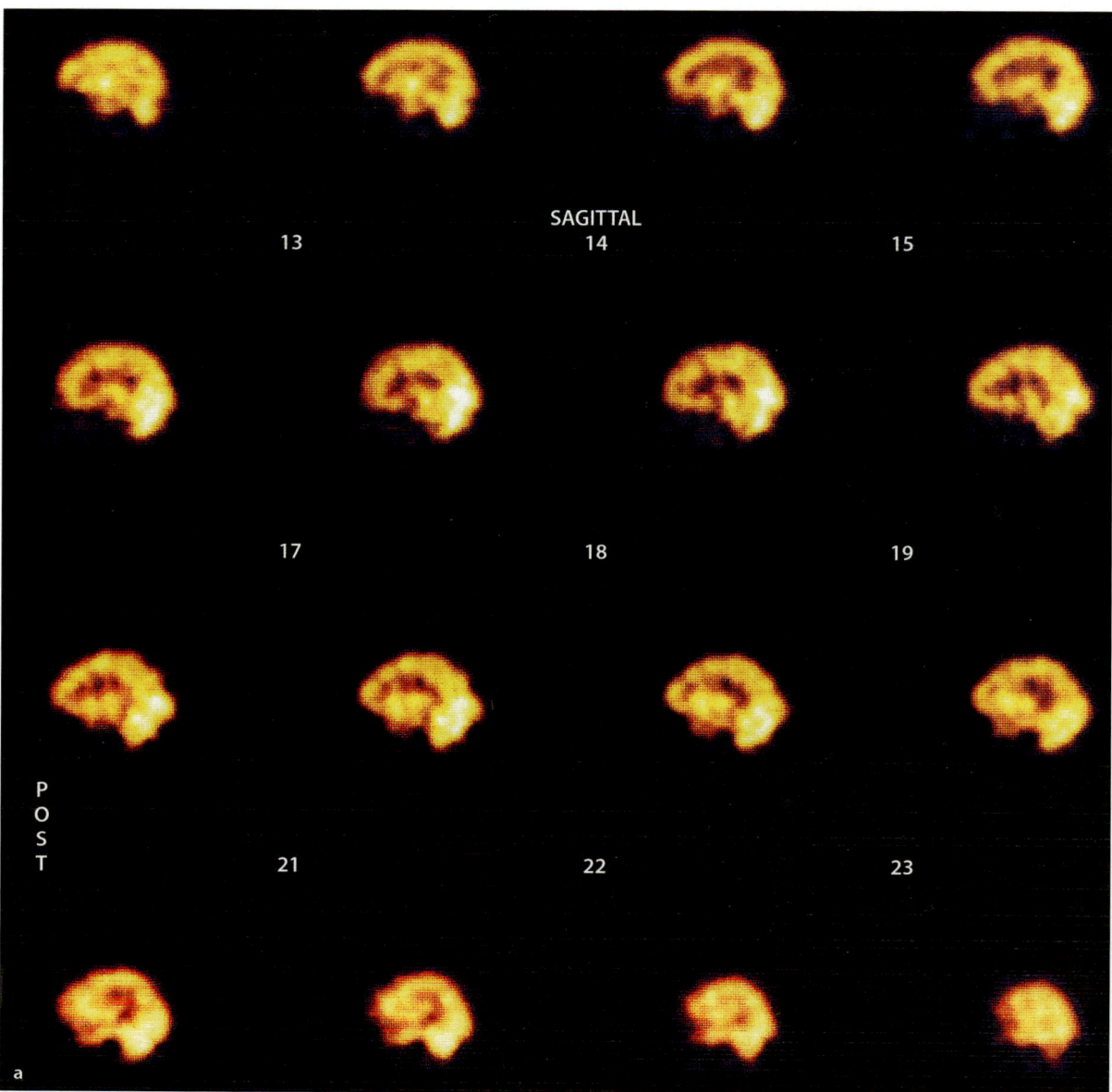

SAGITTAL

13   14   15

17   18   19

P
O
S
T   21   22   23

a

Fig. 1.2 a. *Continued*

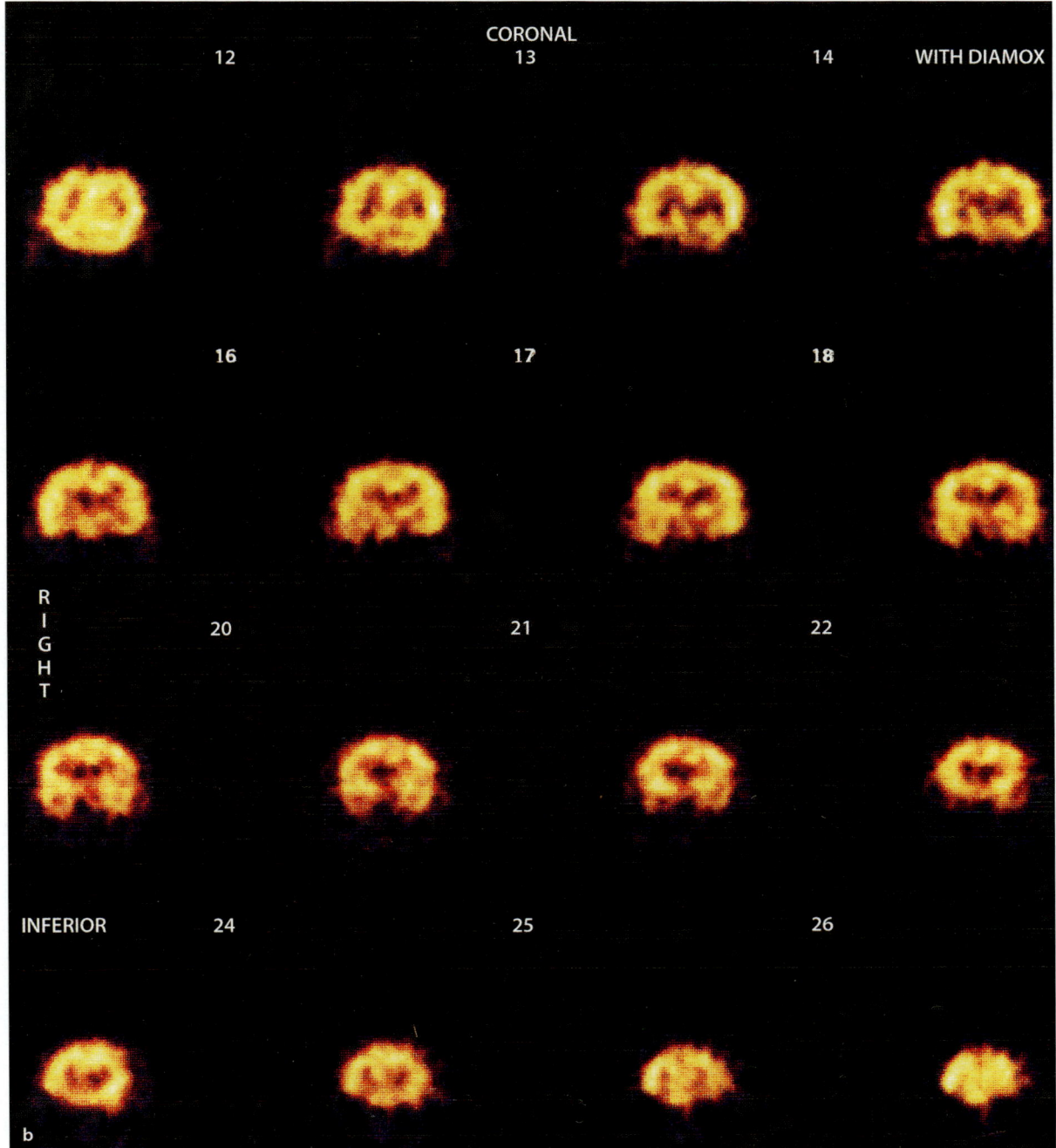

Fig. 1.2 a,b. Brain scan in a 67-year-old woman with vertiginous symptoms and known plaque formation in extracranial vessels shows mild, disseminated hypoperfusion with no evidence of a recent or old infarct. The changes are potentiated after diamox administration, indicating a disseminated disturbance of cerebral blood flow in which the cerebrovascular reserve is still reasonably intact

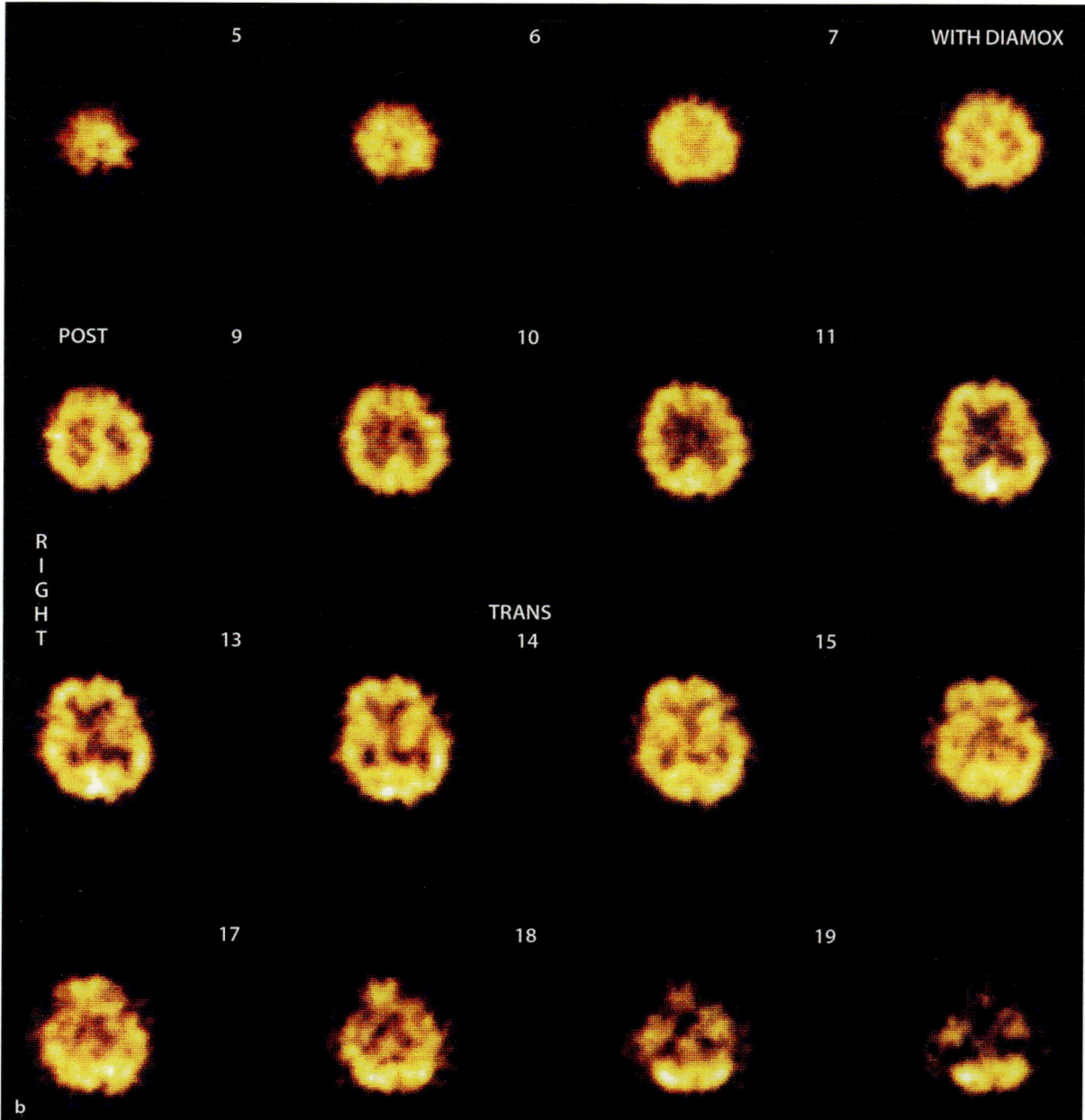

Fig. 1.2 b. *Continued*

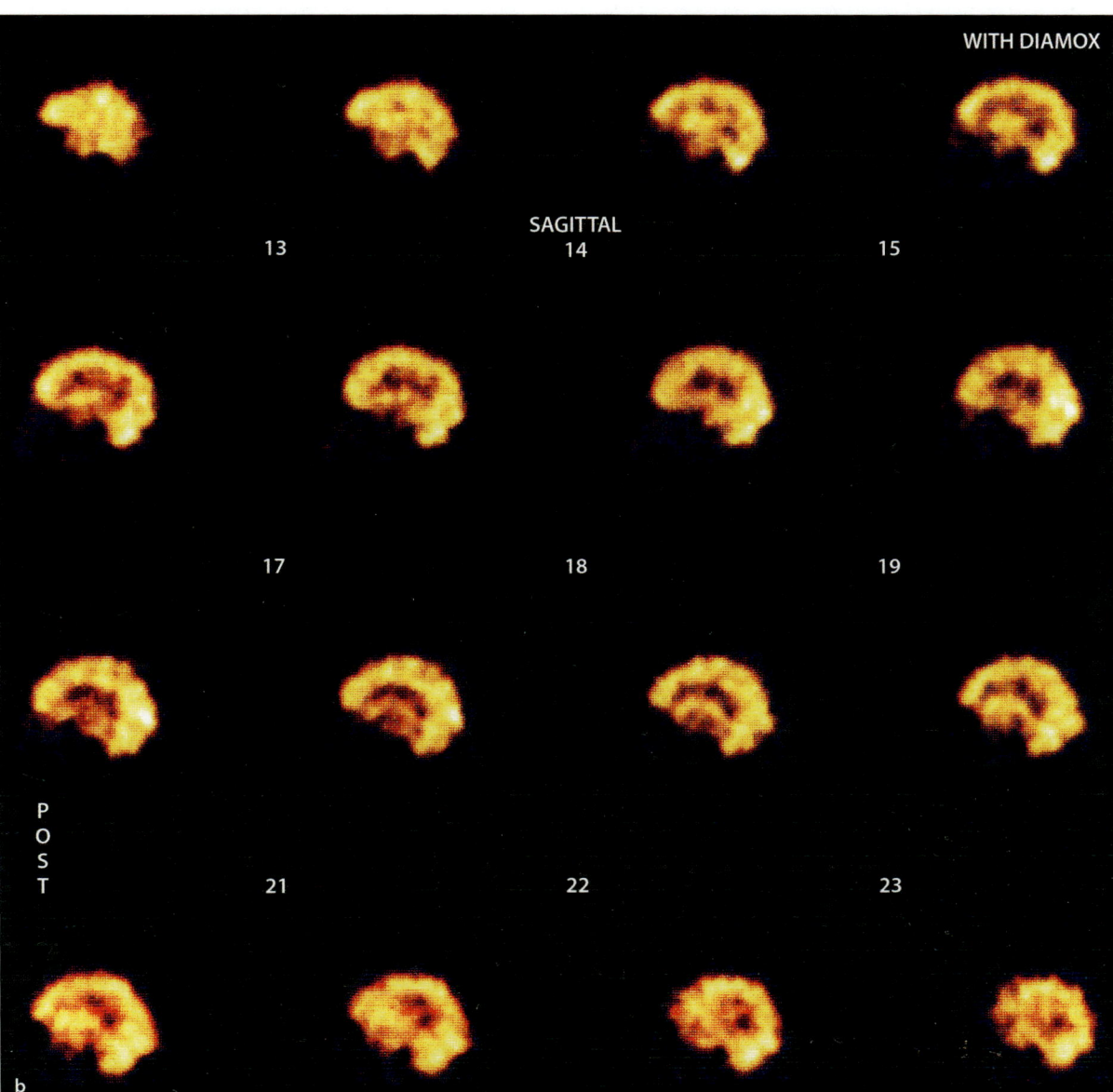

Fig. 1.2 b. *Continued*

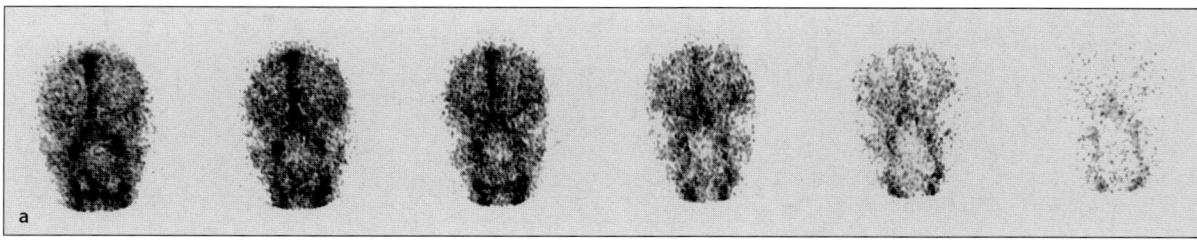

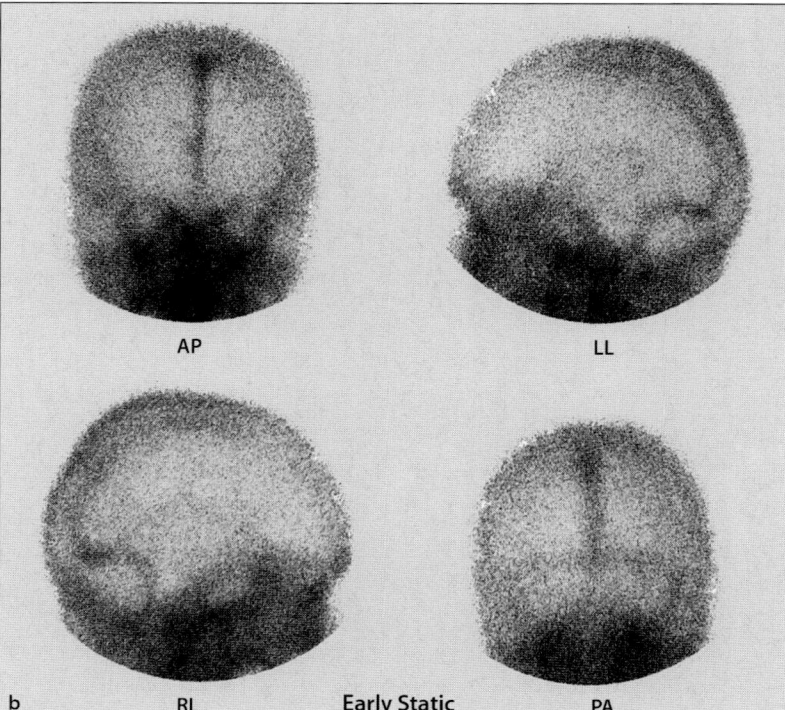

AP   LL

RL   **Early Static**   PA

Fig. 1.3 a–c. This patient complained of pressure behind the eyes spreading to the forehead. Sequential perfusion scans (**a**) show a ringlike mass with a nonhomogeneous activity distribution in the right parasagittal and basal region. This mass is not seen in the early (**b**) or delayed (**c**) static images. The findings are suspicious for an aneurysm, which was confirmed by angiography

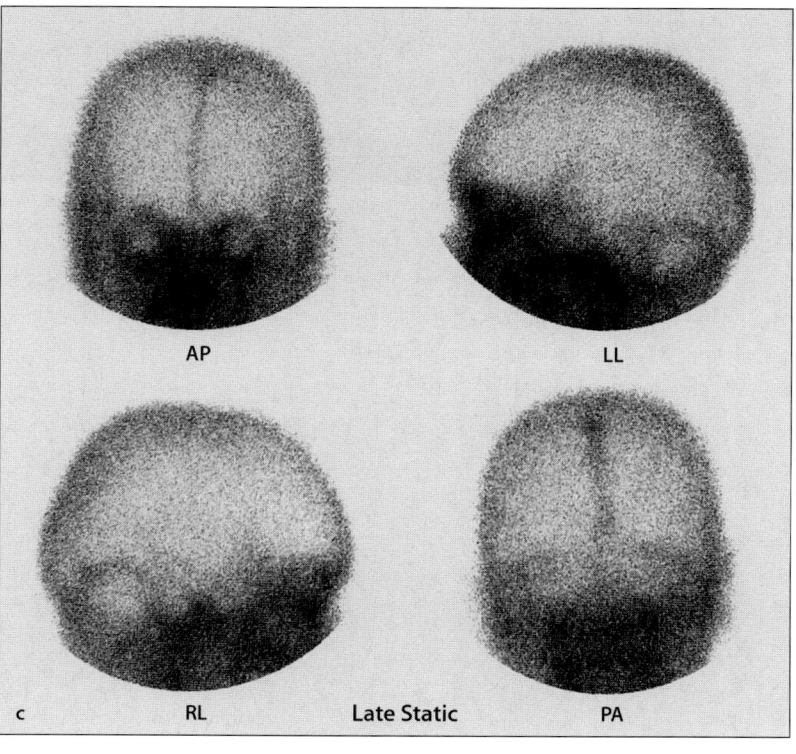

AP   LL

RL   **Late Static**   PA

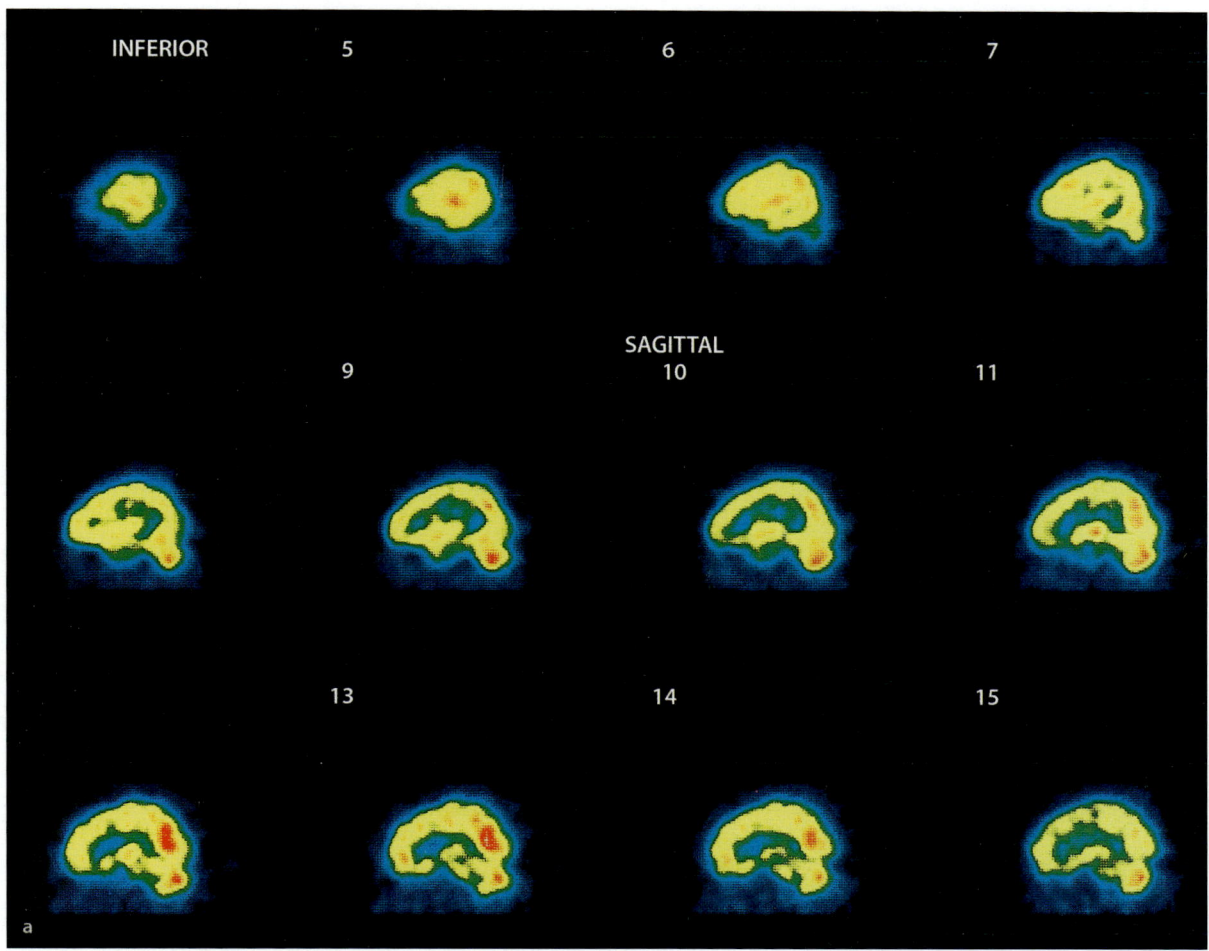

Fig. 1.4 a,b. Brain scan in a 68-year-old woman with gait abnormalities and headache of increasing severity shows a perfusion defect in the middle cerebral artery territory, with likely partial involvement of the left posterior cerebral artery. The scan also shows disseminated, nonhomogeneous increased uptake throughout the brain. This pattern is consistent with a left-sided infarct accompanied by multiple angiopathic microlesions, and this was confirmed by MRI

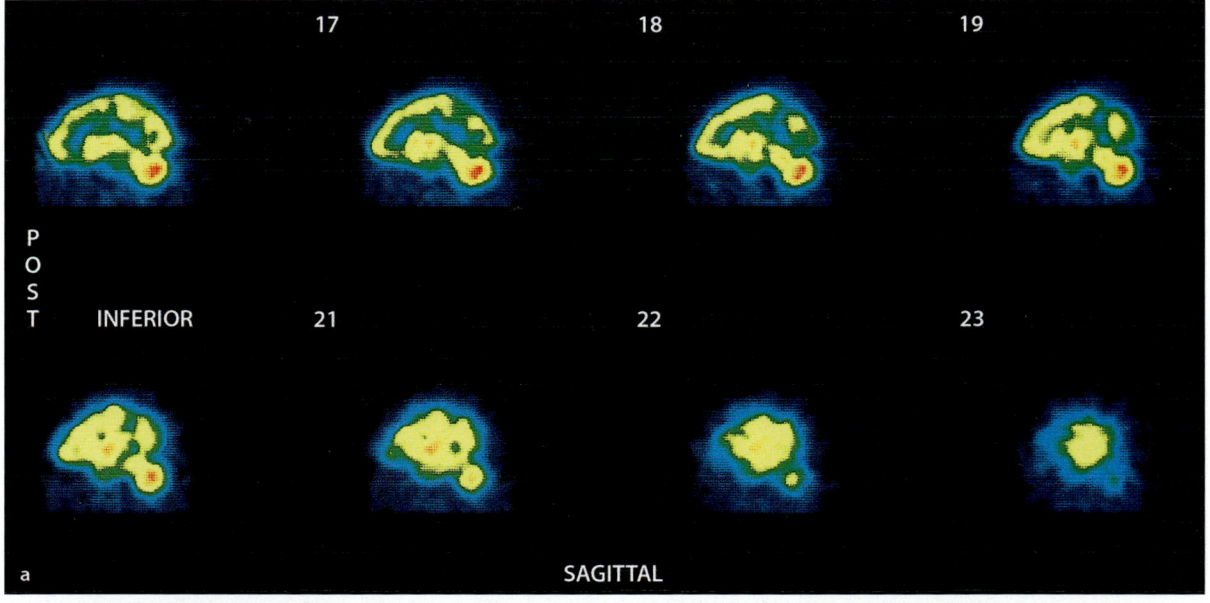

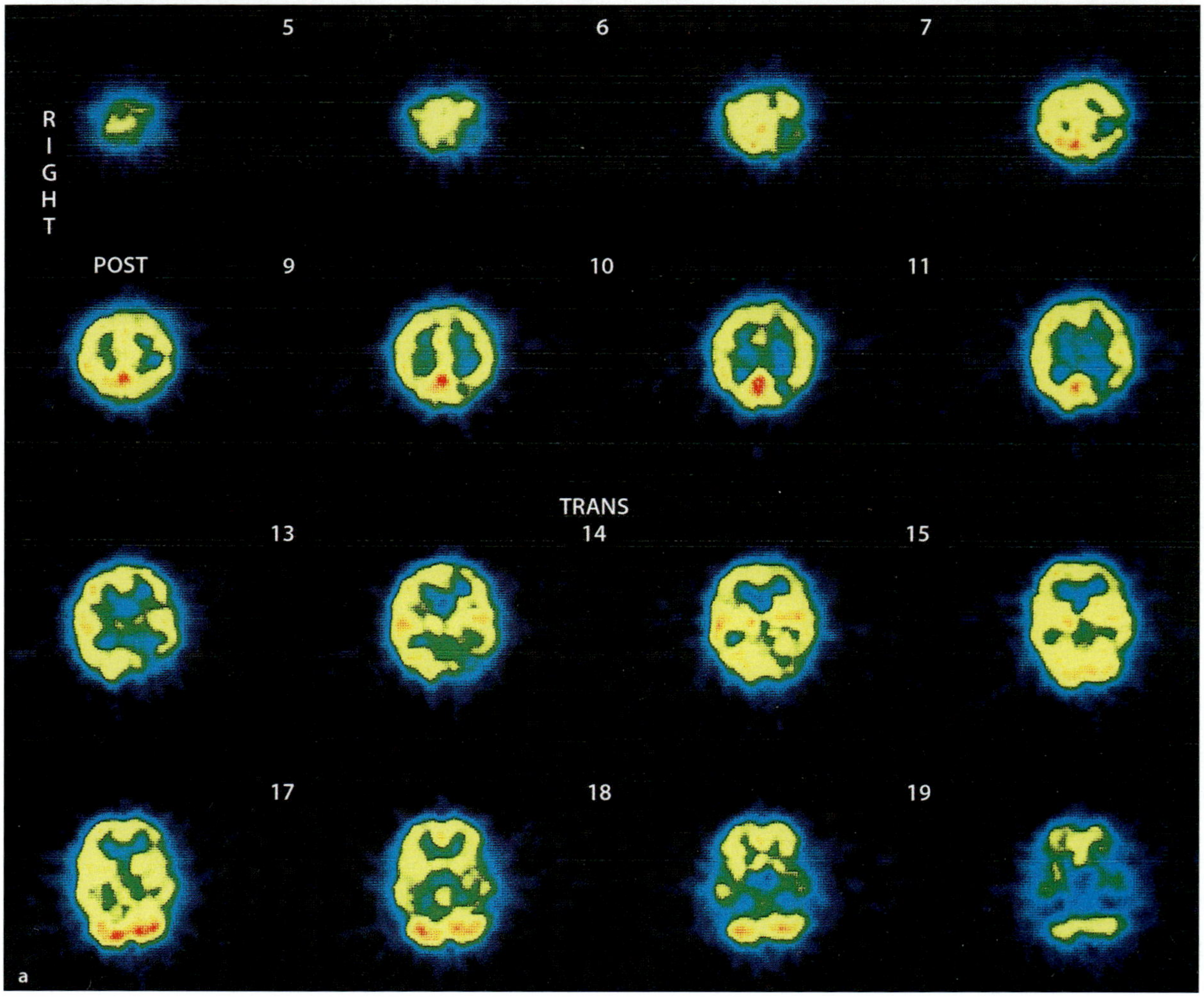

Fig. 1.4 a. *Continued*

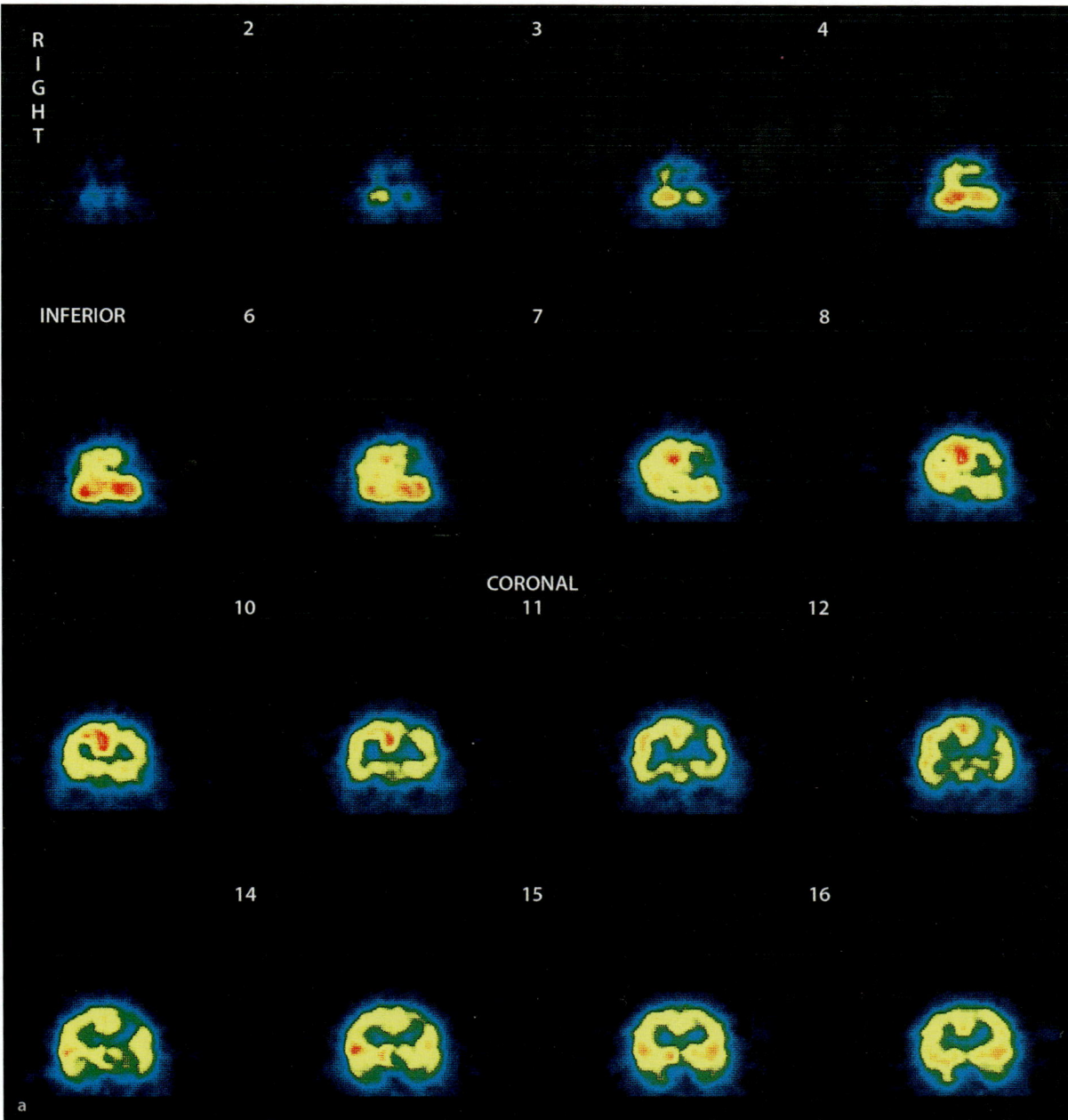

Fig. 1.4 a,b. Brain scan in a 68-year-old woman with gait abnormalities and headache of increasing severity shows a perfusion defect in the middle cerebral artery territory, with likely partial involvement of the left posterior cerebral artery. The scan also shows disseminated, nonhomogeneous increased uptake throughout the brain. This pattern is consistent with a left-sided infarct accompanied by multiple angiopathic microlesions, and this was confirmed by MRI

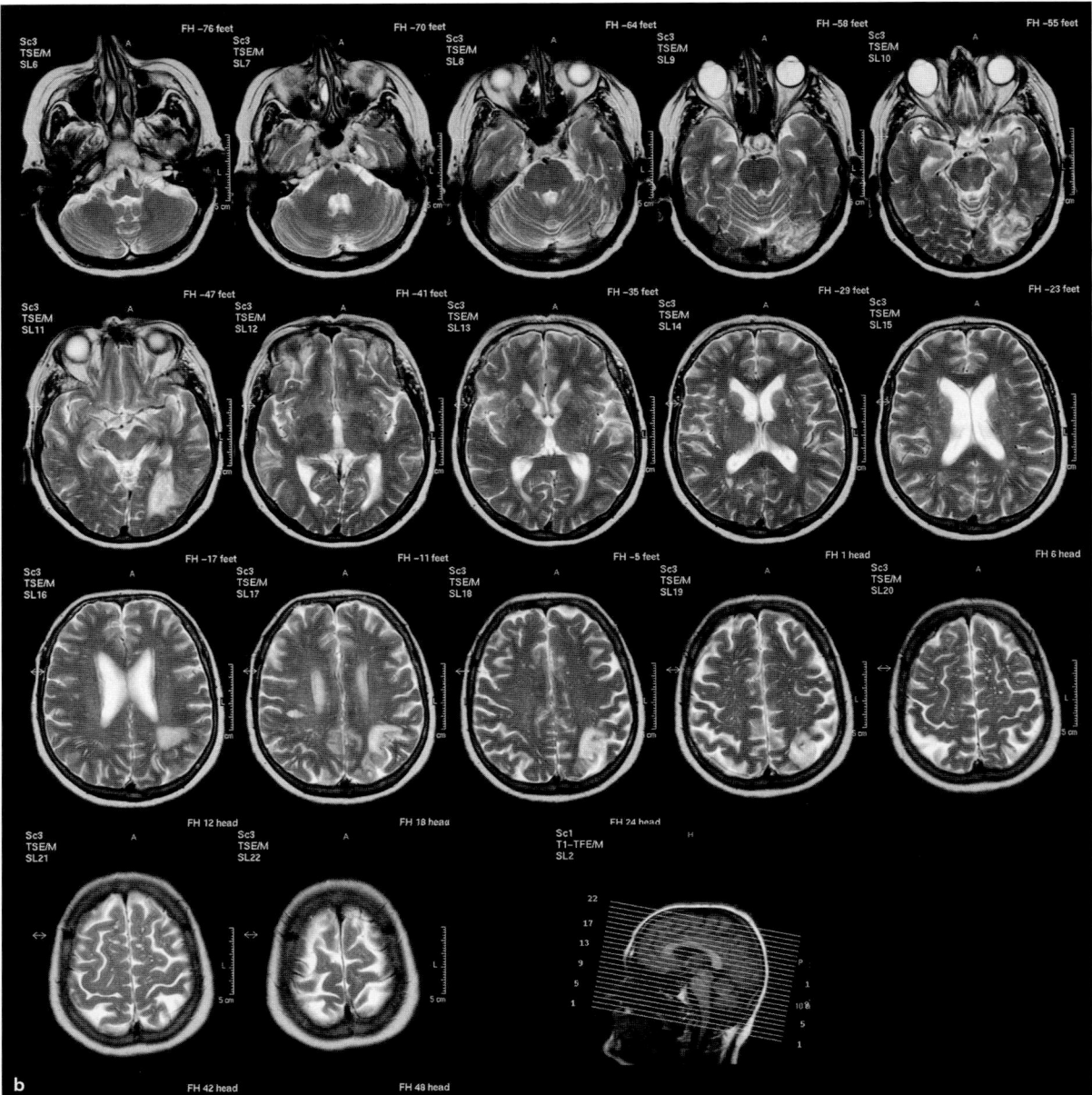

Fig. 1.4 a,b. Brain scan in a 68-year-old woman with gait abnormalities and headache of increasing severity shows a perfusion defect in the middle cerebral artery territory, with likely partial involvement of the left posterior cerebral artery. The scan also shows disseminated, nonhomogeneous increased uptake throughout the brain. This pattern is consistent with a left-sided infarct accompanied by multiple angiopathic microlesions, and this was confirmed by MRI

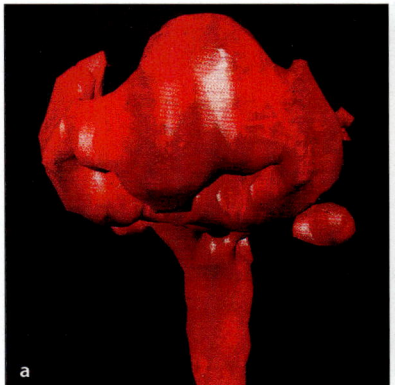
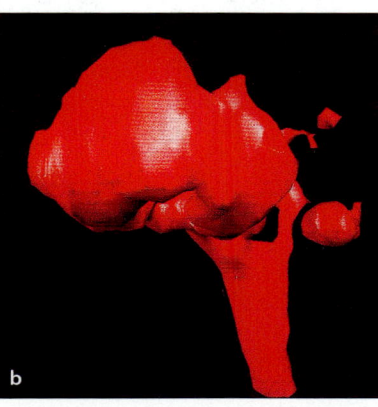

Fig. 1.5 a–c. Cerebrospinal fluid (CSF) imaging was done to investigate right-sided otorrhea in a 52-year-old woman. At 3 hours after radiotracer instillation, the basal cisterns and fourth ventricle appear normal. Image at 24 hours shows a collection of CSF projected over the mastoid process and lateral petrous pyramid. Image at 48 hours shows persistence of the collection in the mastoid process area with almost no residual tracer in the spinal canal. Most CSF is absorbed through the pacchionian granulations, but a communication between the left mastoid process or a cyst and the CSF pathways delays absorption. The decreased uptake in the left parietal region results from local cicatricial changes in the CSF spaces

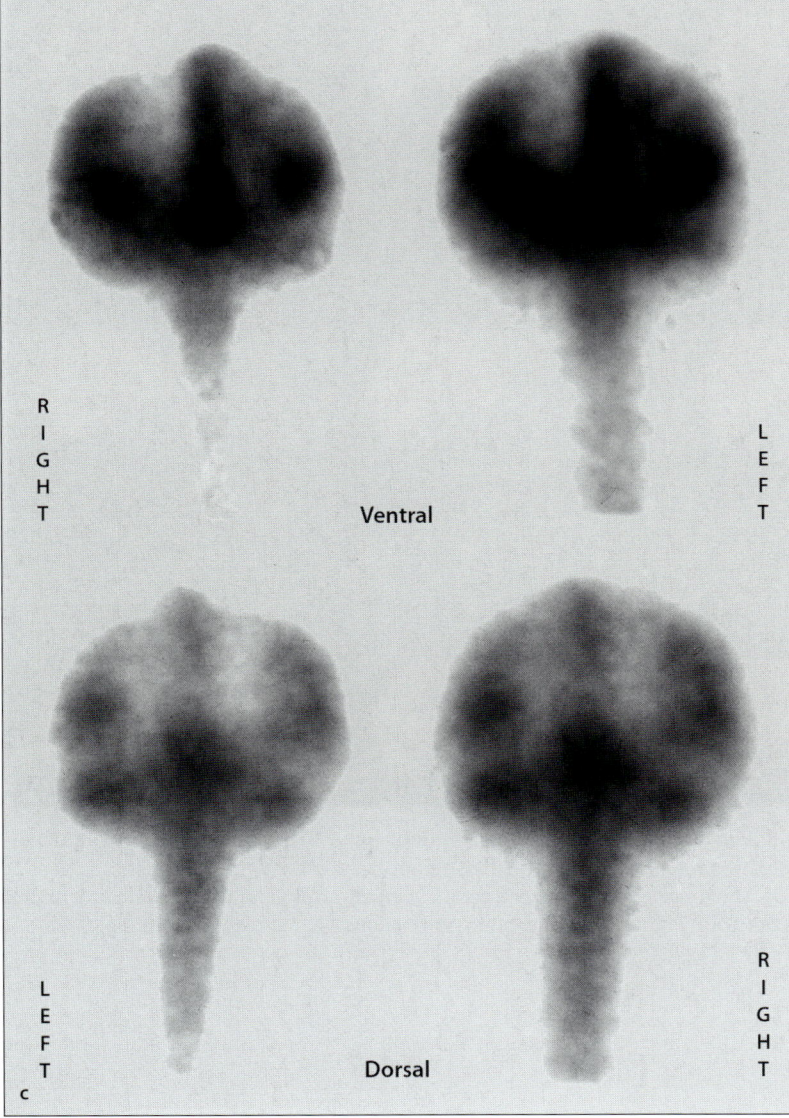

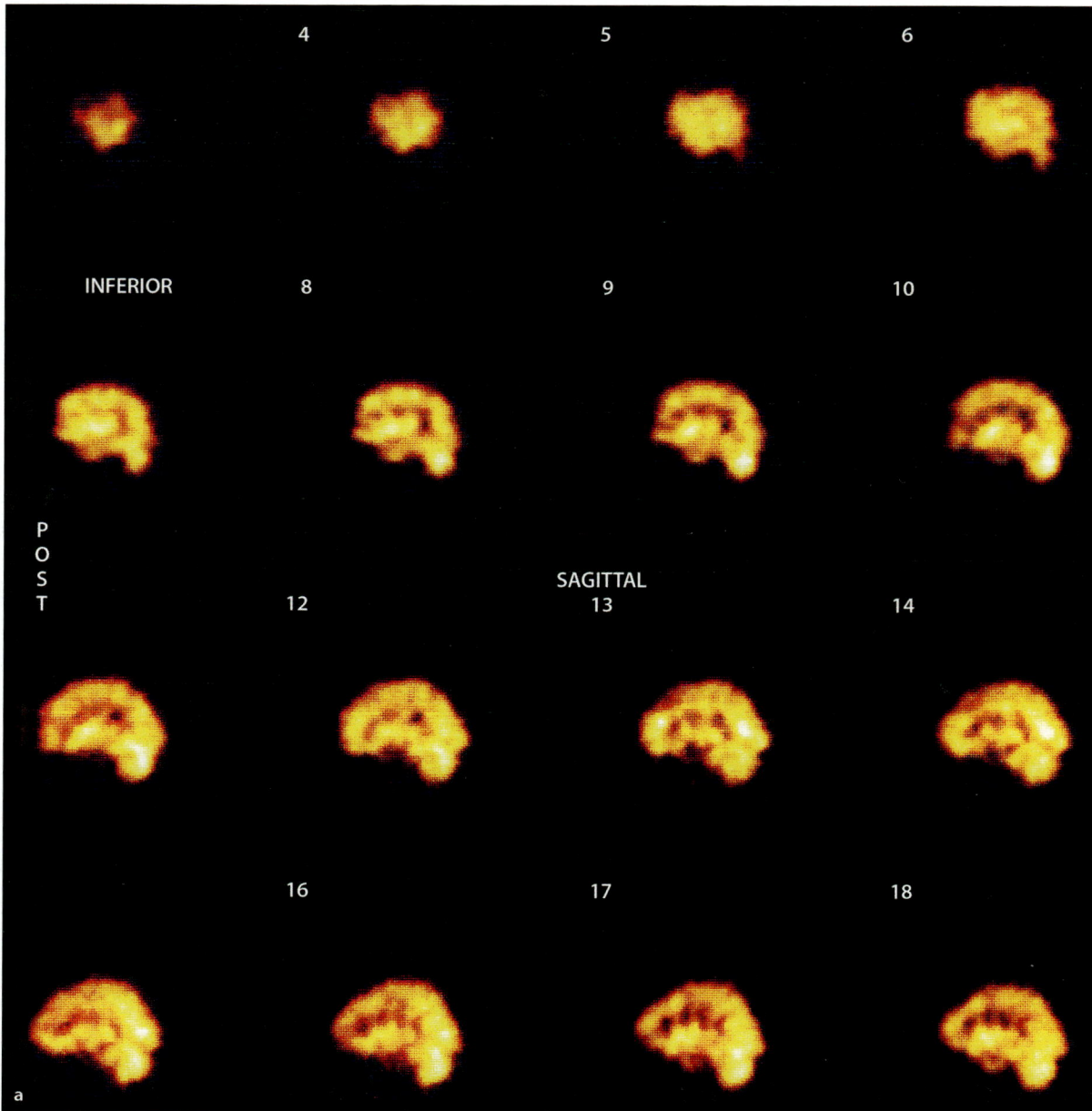

Fig. 1.6 a–d. Brain scan before (**a**) and after diamox (**b**) in a 39-year-old man complaining of headache shows a perfusion defect in the right frontal area with relatively high tracer uptake at the lesion periphery. This pattern suggests an avascular mass compressing the surrounding tissue. The lesion was identified by MRI (**c, d**) and postoperatively as an arachnoid cyst causing indentation and secondary hypertrophy of the adjacent brain parenchyma

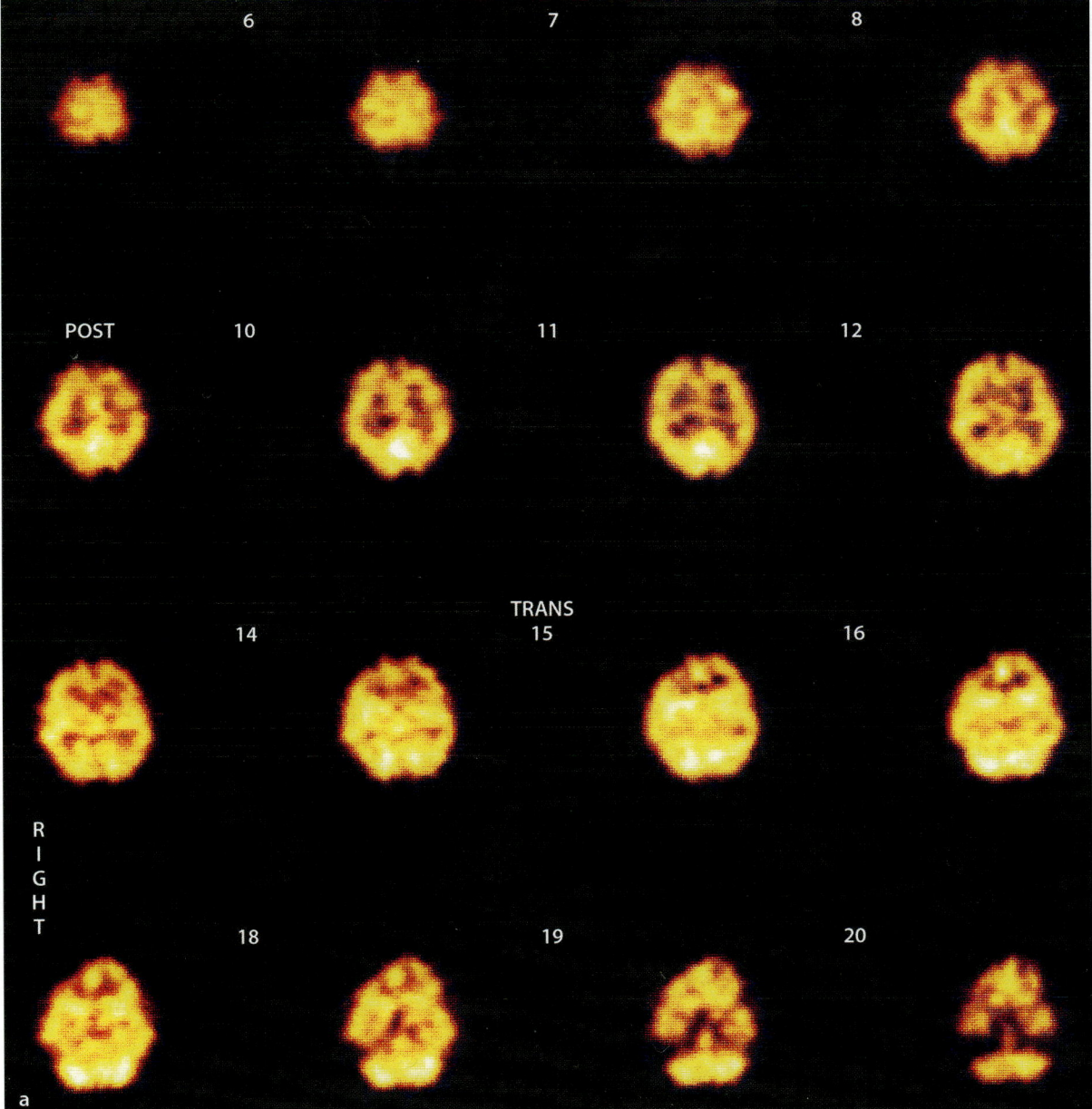

Fig. 1.6 a. *Continued*

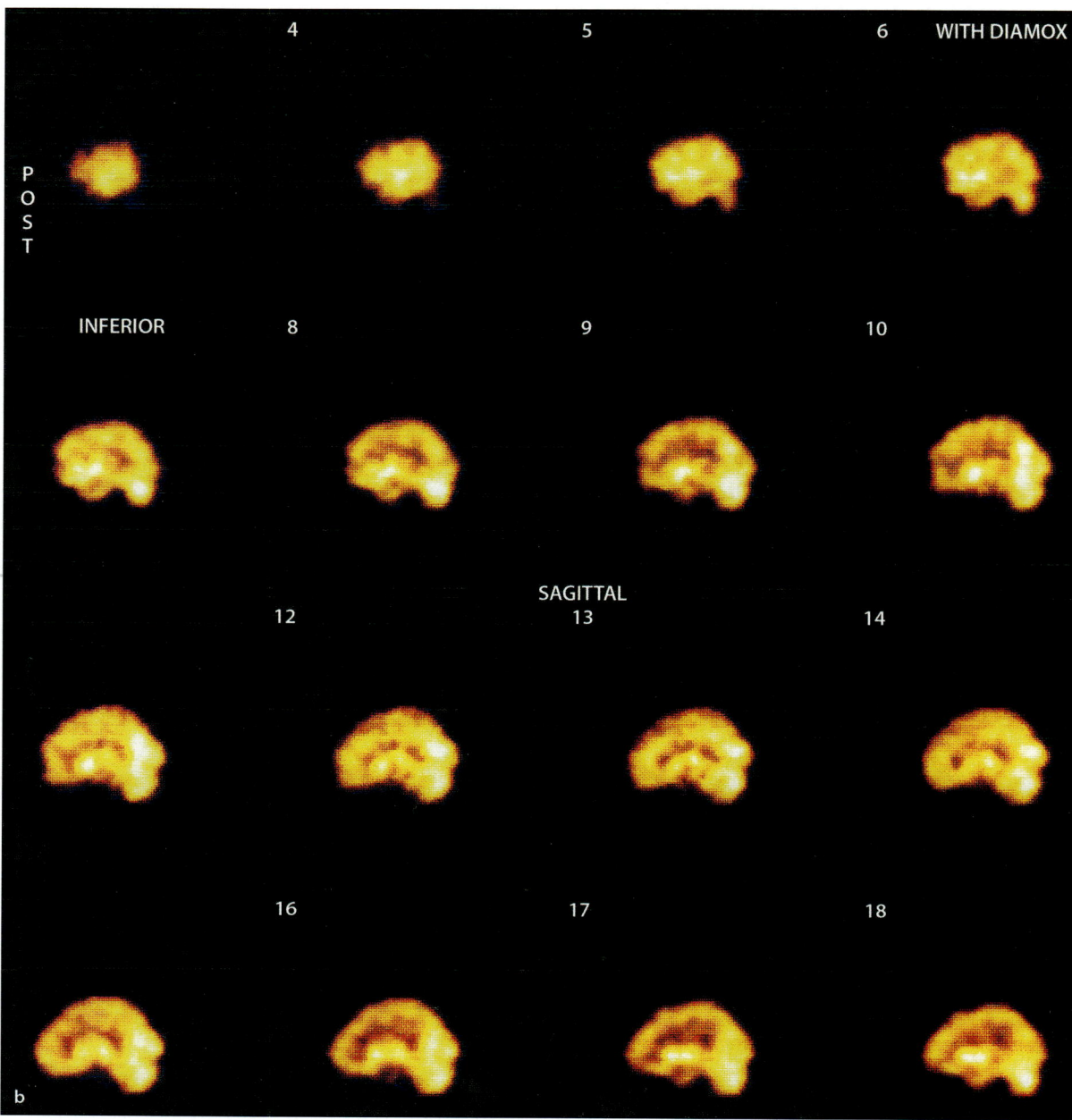

Fig. 1.6 a–d. Brain scan before (**a**) and after diamox (**b**) in a 39-year-old man complaining of headache shows a perfusion defect in the right frontal area with relatively high tracer uptake at the lesion periphery. This pattern suggests an avascular mass compressing the surrounding tissue. The lesion was identified by MRI (**c, d**) and postoperatively as an arachnoid cyst causing indentation and secondary hypertrophy of the adjacent brain parenchyma

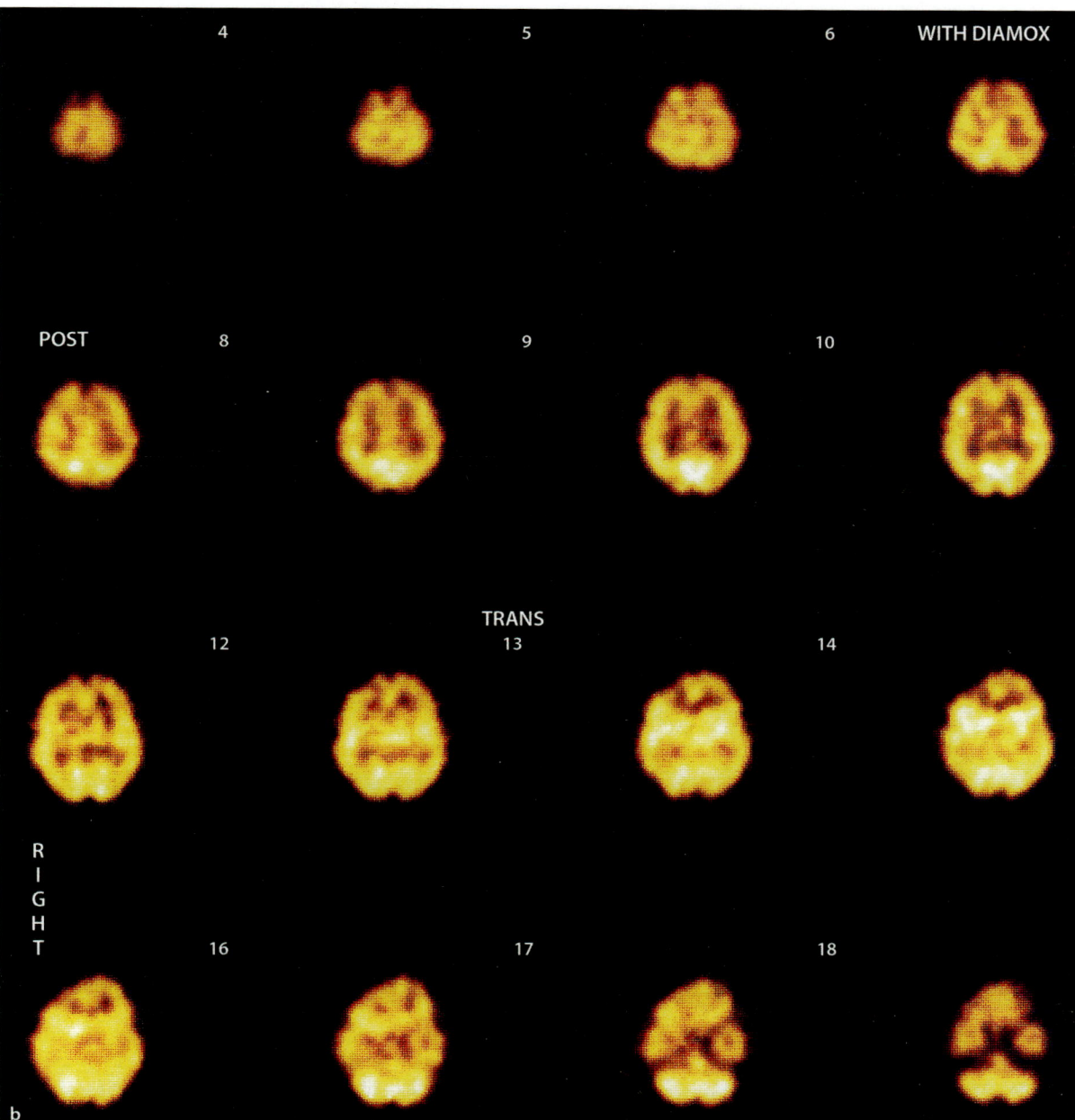

Fig. 1.6 b. *Continued*

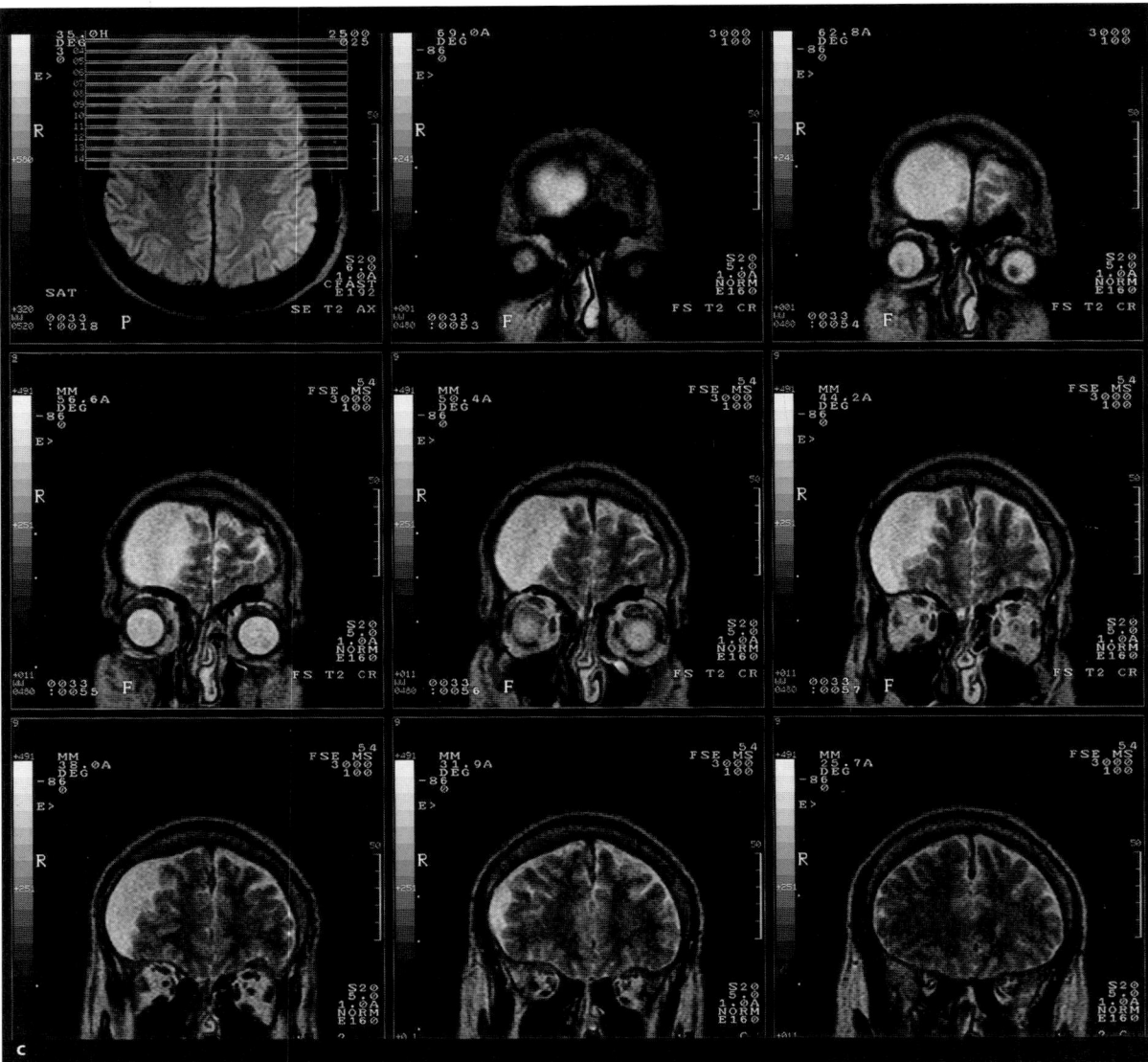

Fig. 1.6 a–d. Brain scan before (**a**) and after diamox (**b**) in a 39-year-old man complaining of headache shows a perfusion defect in the right frontal area with relatively high tracer uptake at the lesion periphery. This pattern suggests an avascular mass compressing the surrounding tissue. The lesion was identified by MRI (**c, d**) and postoperatively as an arachnoid cyst causing indentation and secondary hypertrophy of the adjacent brain parenchyma

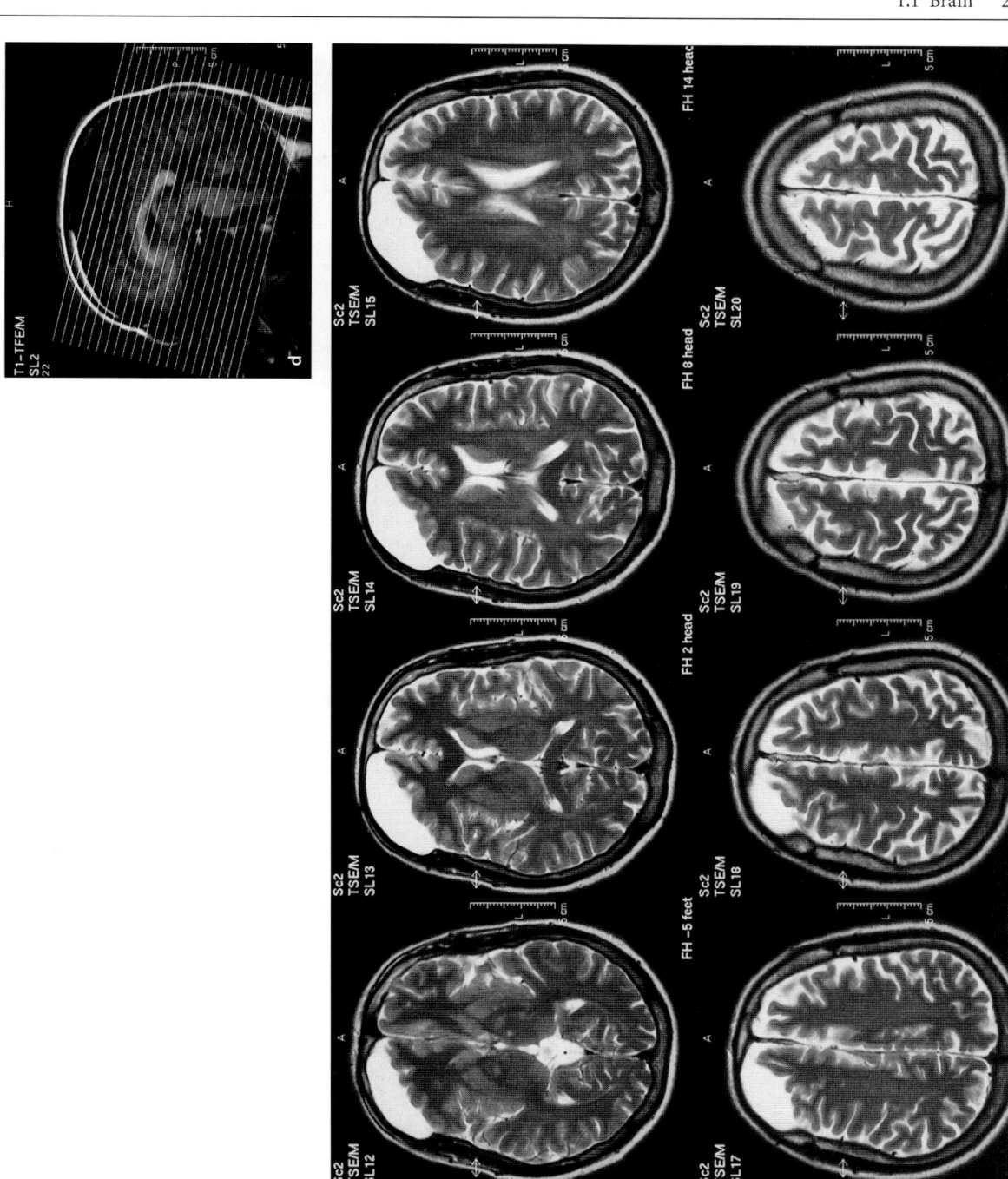

Fig. 1.6 d

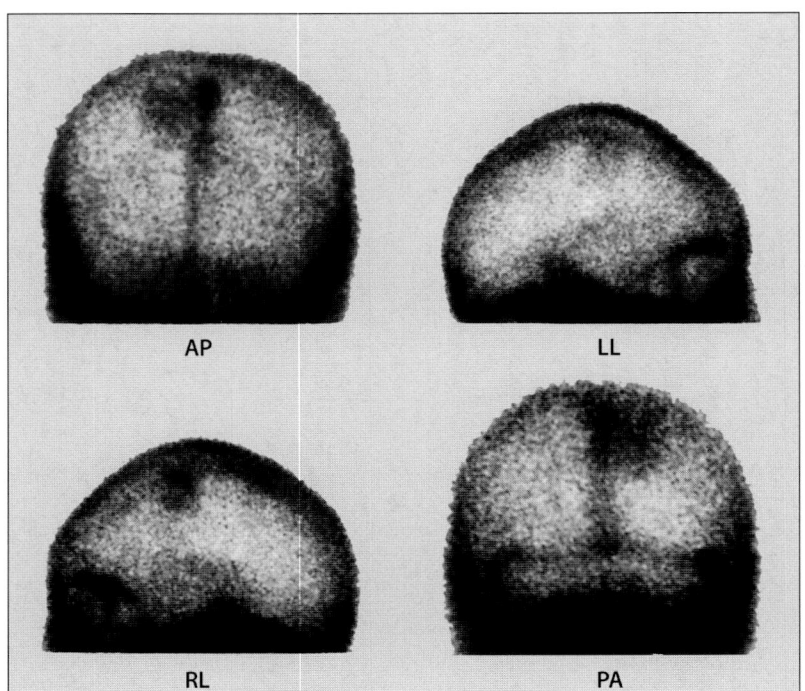

Fig. 1.7. Brain scan in a 43-year-old woman with unexplained headache shows a well-defined focus of increased uptake in the right parasagittal area with otherwise normal findings. This pattern is strongly suspicious for a metastatic tumor. Later the patient was found to have a microcarcinoma of the breast, establishing the diagnosis of metastatic breast cancer

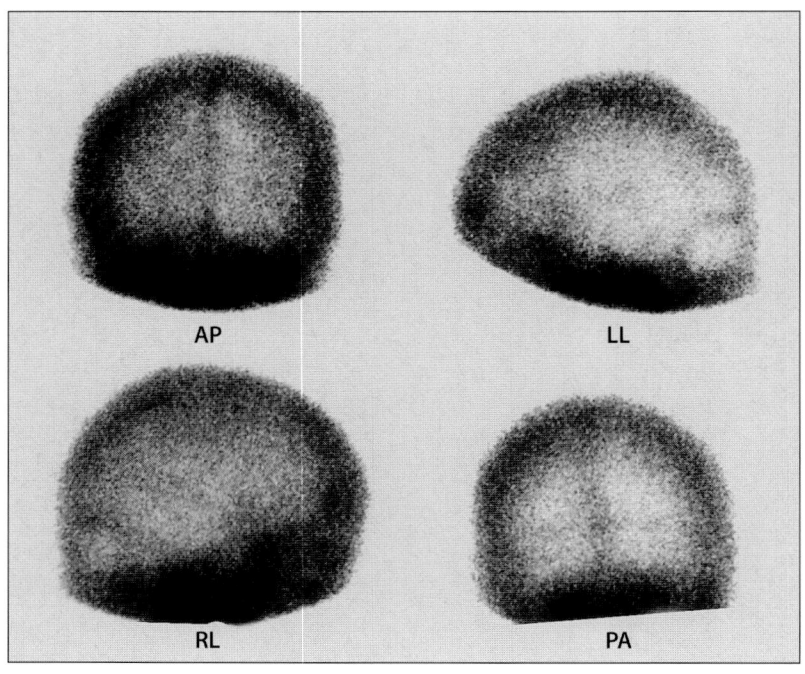

Fig. 1.8. Follow-up examination in a patient with breast carcinoma and vertigo. Brain scan shows a nonhomogeneous area of increased activity on the left side, localized mainly to the temporoparietal area and including ill-defined nodular foci. This pattern is strongly suspicious for incipient metastasis with perifocal edema, which was confirmed by CT

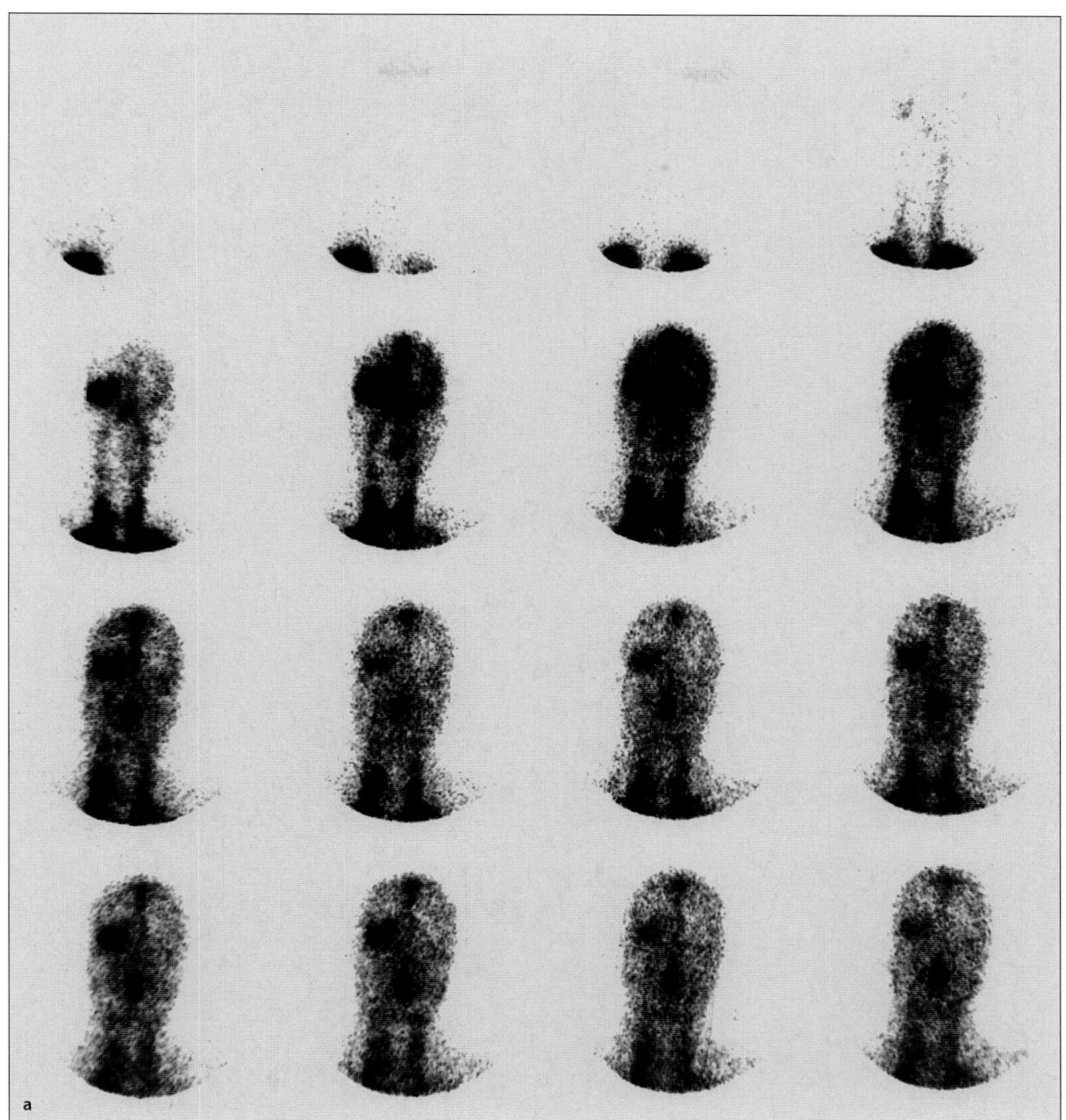

Fig. 1.9 a,b. This 15-year-old boy had epileptiform seizures since childhood and a 2-week history of left-sided arm weakness. Sequential images show focally increased uptake in the territory of the middle cerebral artery. Peak uptake occurs 17 seconds after radiotracer instillation and is accompanied by ipsilateral hypoperfusion (steal effect). The early static images show scalloped figures in the right temporal and occipital region along with multiple diffuse, less well-defined natural foci of slightly enhanced activity. This pattern signifies a hypervascular lesion consistent with AV angioma, and concomitant hemorrhages indicate a watershed infarction. The diagnosis was confirmed by CT and angiography

Fig. 1.9 b

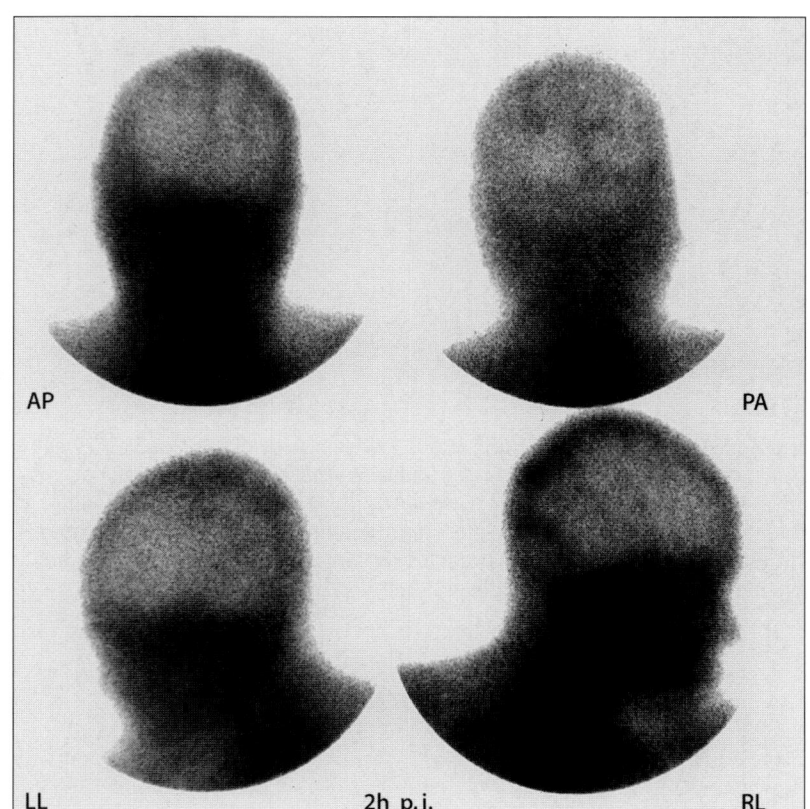

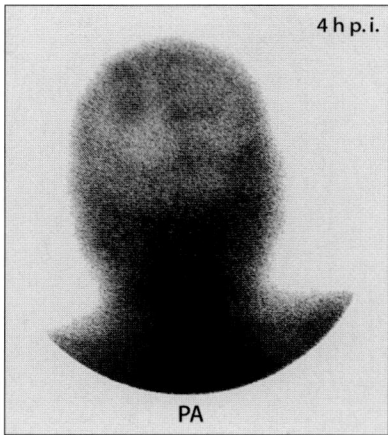

Fig. 1.10. Tl-201 chloride scan in a woman with impaired consciousness. The patient underwent previous surgery and postoperative irradiation for cervical carcinoma. The multiple foci of increased uptake in both hemispheres represent diffuse metastases

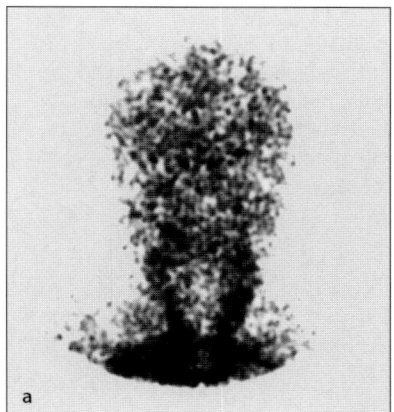

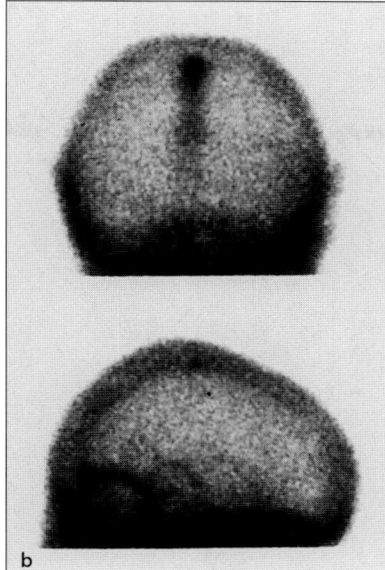

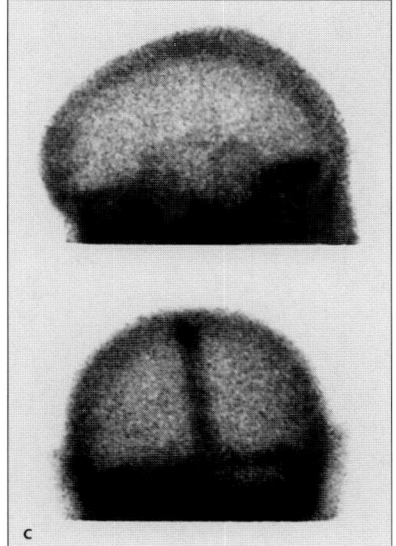

Fig. 1.11 a–c. Radionuclide study in a 60-year-old diabetic woman with dysphagic complaints. Side-to-side comparison of sequential images shows a faint increase in parasagittal and occipital uptake. A diffuse activity increase is seen in the delayed static views. Six weeks later, the clinical complaints and imaging changes were no longer present. The patient sustained a cerebral infarction due to hemorrhage in the territory of the posterior cerebral artery

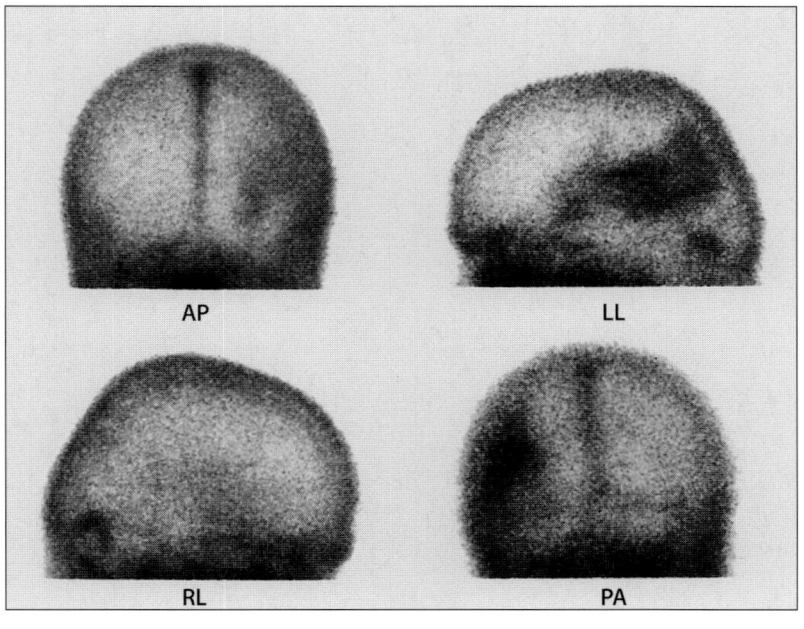

Fig. 1.12. Brain scan in a 71-year-old diabetic with gait and speech disturbance shows increased uptake in the left temporal area due to a cerebrovascular insult in the territory of the posterior temporal artery

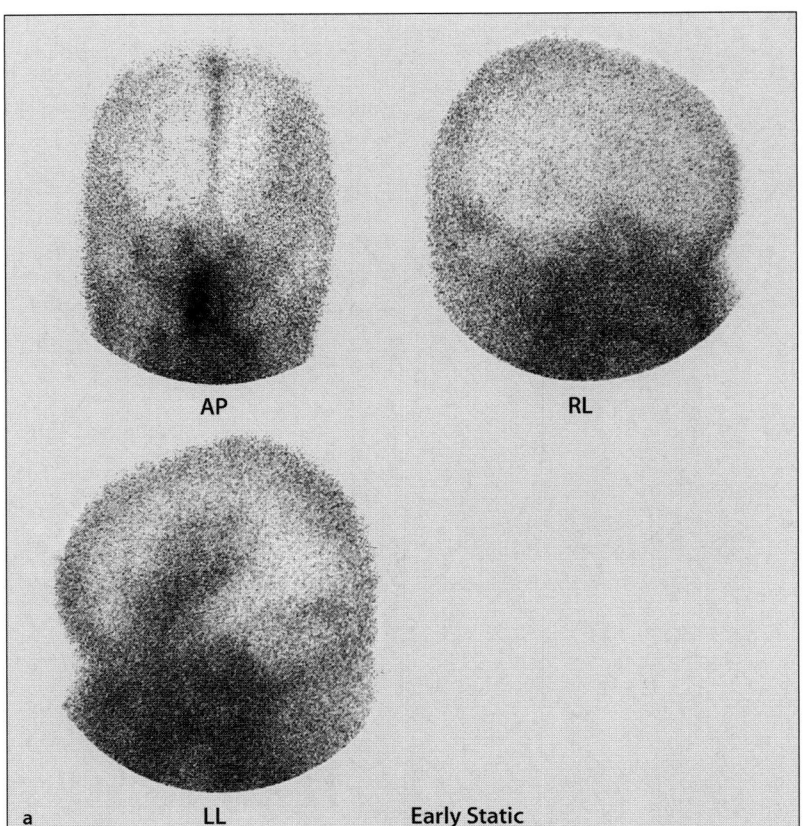

AP

RL

a   LL   Early Static

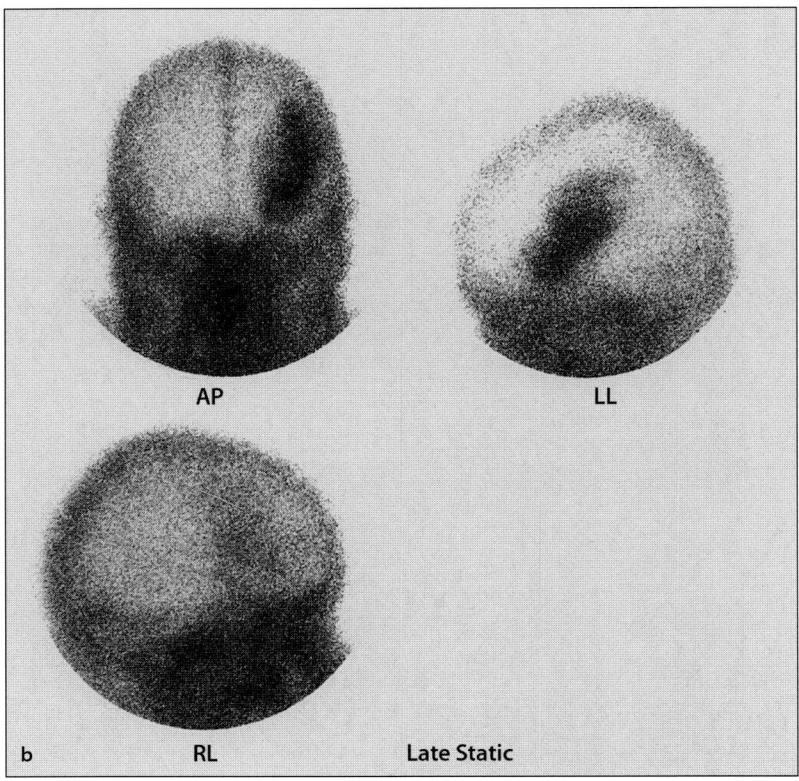

AP

LL

b   RL   Late Static

Fig. 1.13 a,b. A 50-year-old man was evaluated for dementia and gait disturbances. Early (**a**) and delayed (**b**) static radionuclide images show increased uptake in the territory of the middle cerebral artery due to a cerebrovascular insult

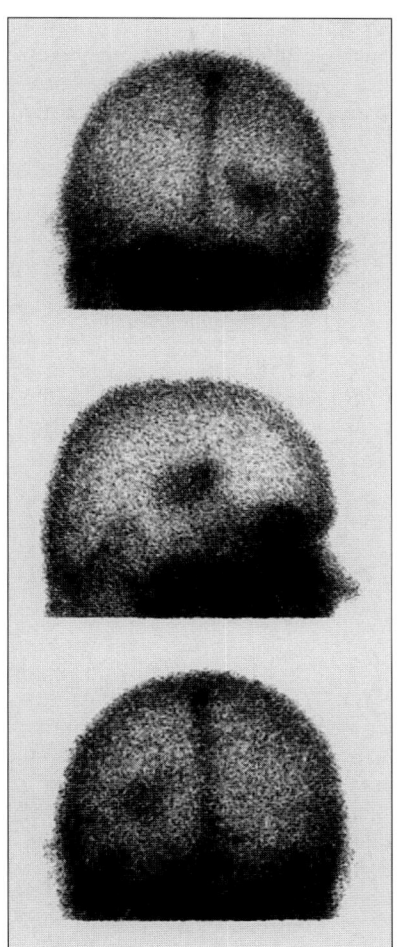

Fig. 1.14. Delayed static images in a 60-year-old woman with disorientation show areas of increased tracer uptake, some of which are sharply defined. The foci represent multiple metastases from an unknown primary tumor. The patient was later diagnosed with colon carcinoma

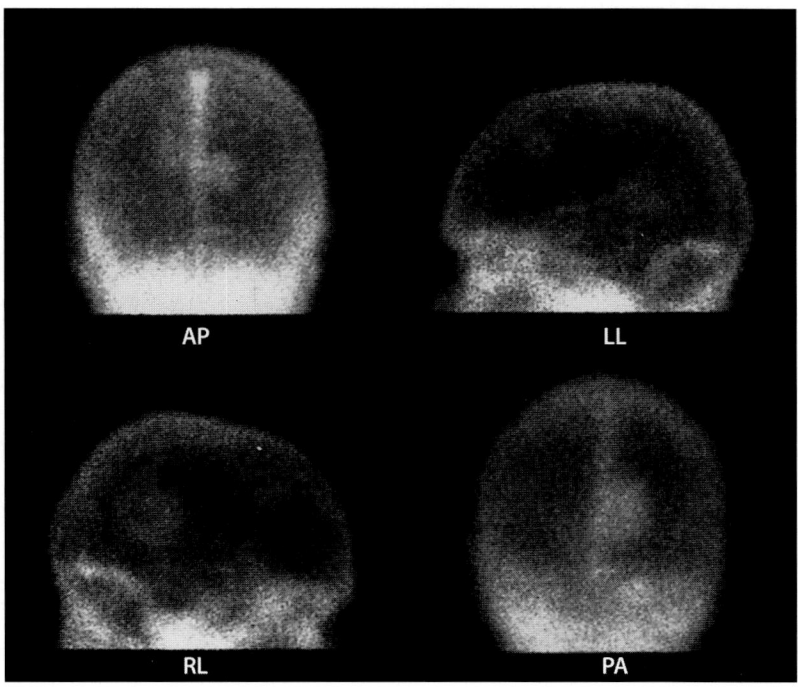

Fig. 1.15. Follow-up scan in a 35-year-old patient previously operated for breast carcinoma demonstrates multiple metastases, some with central necrosis

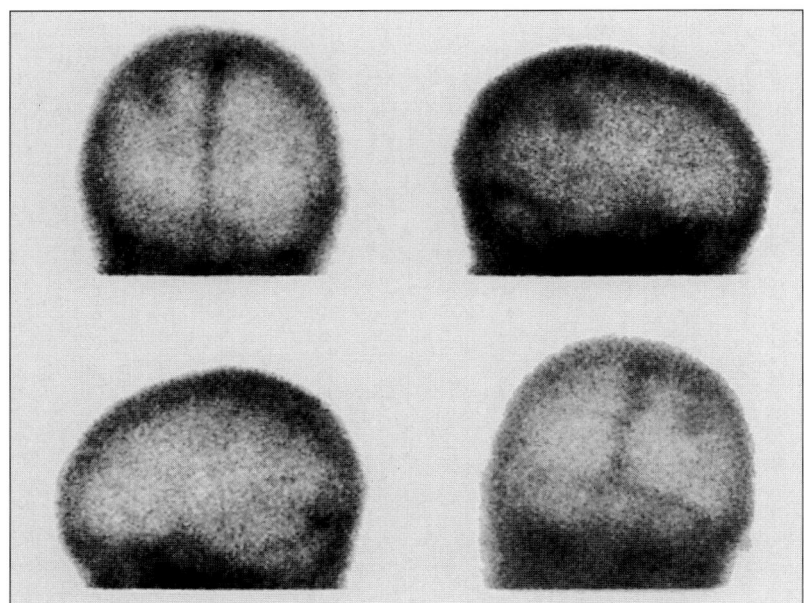

Fig. 1.16. Brain scan in a young leukemic patient with multiple neurologic symptoms shows multiple areas of increased uptake as a manifestation of leukemic involvement of the CNS

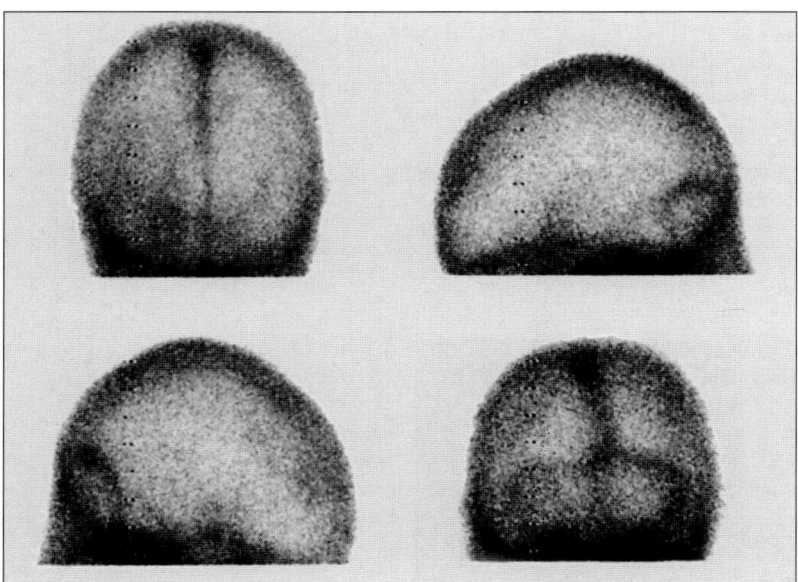

Fig. 1.17. This patient was evaluated for recurring headaches after trauma. Brain scan shows increased frontal uptake as a result of cerebral tissue injury. Follow-up examination several weeks later showed regression of the changes

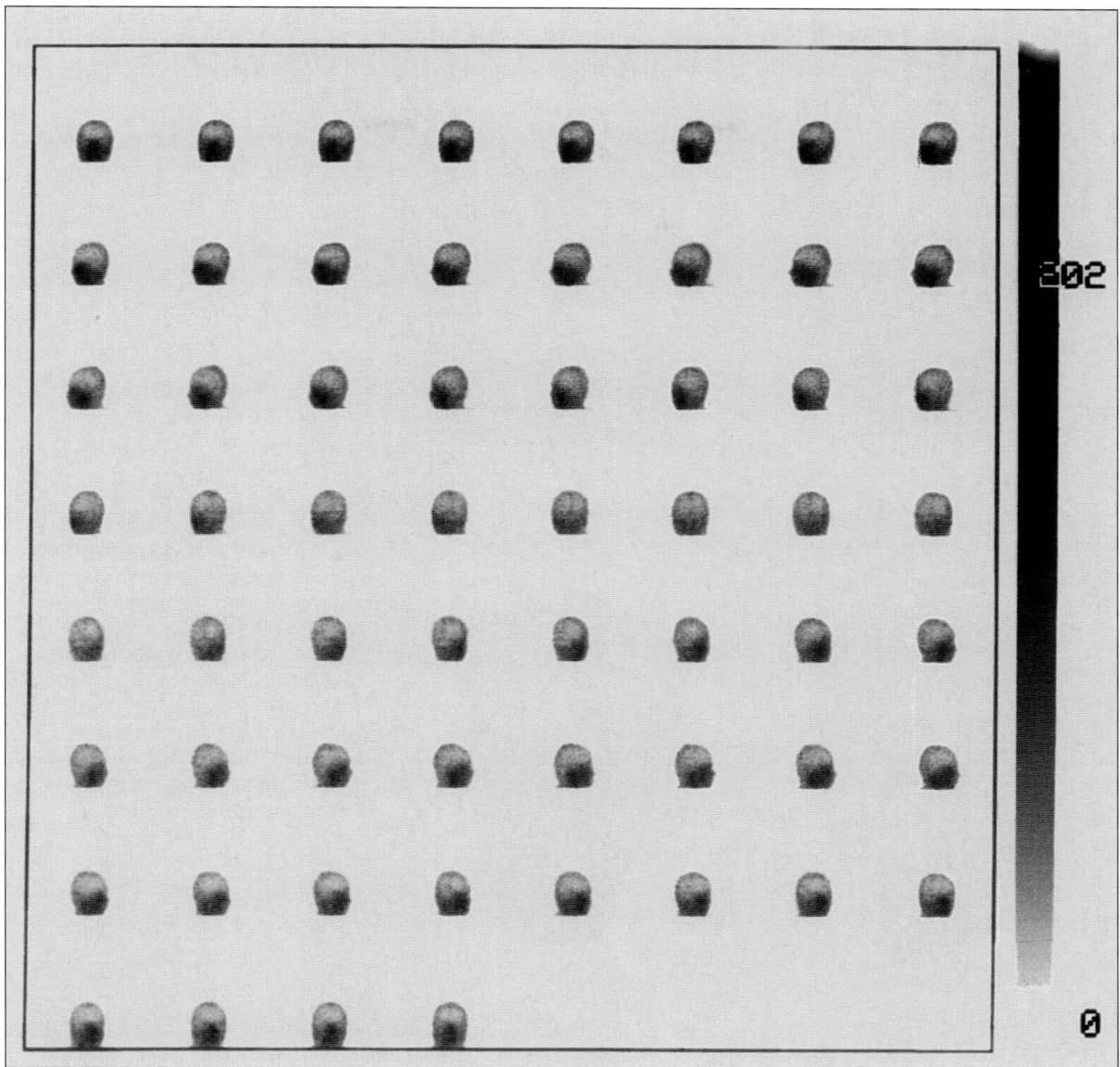

Fig. 1.18. SPECT brain scan. Unreconstructed image acquired by the step-and-shoot technique

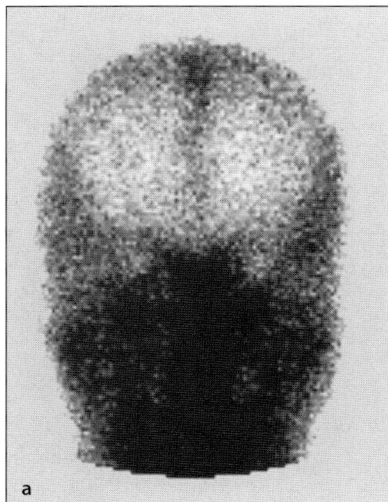

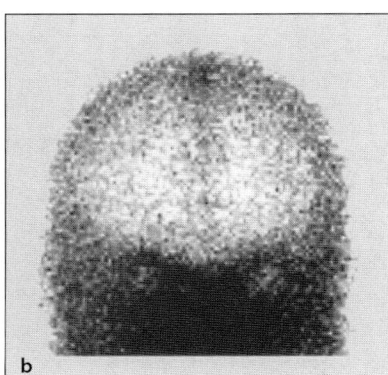

Fig. 1.19 a,b. This young woman was examined for headaches of three days' duration. **a** Slightly increased radiotracer uptake in the right frontoparietal area is due to thromboembolism resulting from oral contraceptive use ("pill embolism")

b The lesion resolved completely at follow-up

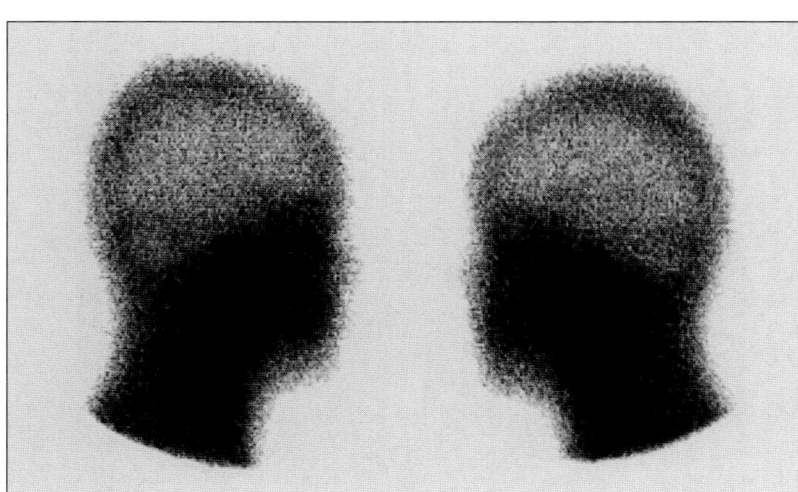

Fig. 1.20. A 19-year-old woman experienced a severe headache while swimming outdoors. The pain persisted for four days and was accompanied by slight nausea. Brain scan shows a diffuse activity increase in both hemispheres, which was no longer present when the scan was repeated one week later. The findings are consistent with transient meningeal irritation due to intense sun exposure

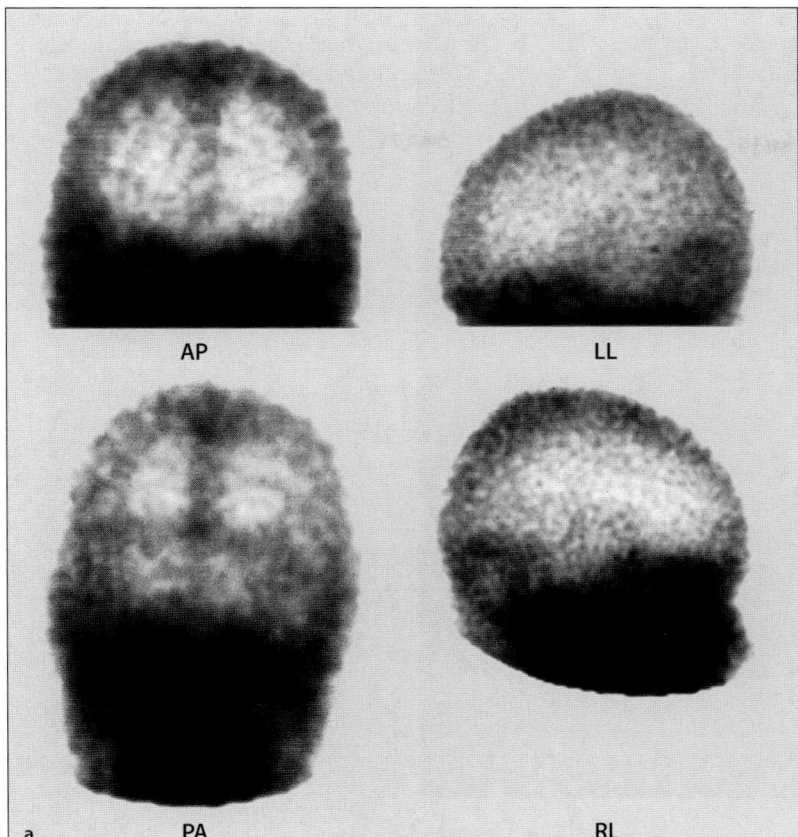

AP   LL

PA   RL

a

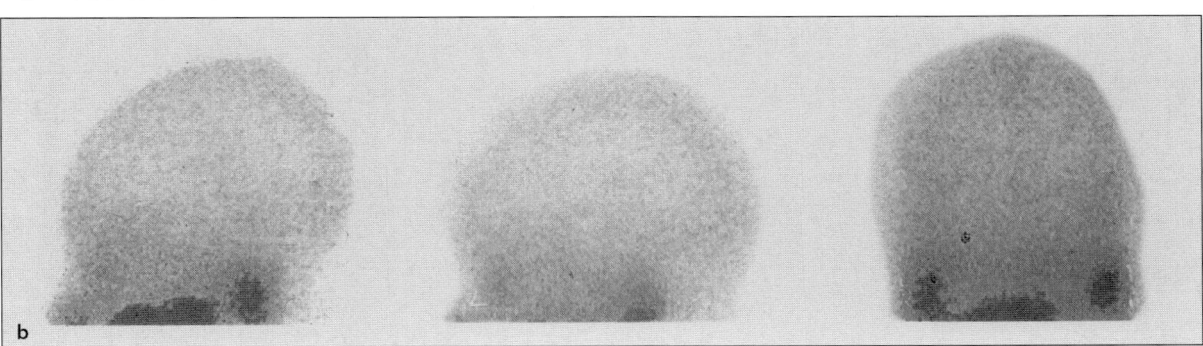

b

Fig. 1.21 a,b. A 40-year-old woman presented with diffuse headache and intermittent nuchal stiffness after visiting a tanning salon. **a** Brain scan shows a diffuse activity increase, which is most conspicuous on the static images. **b** Follow-up scan several weeks later shows complete resolution. The change was caused by transient, UV-induced meningeal irritation resulting in meningitis-like clinical symptoms

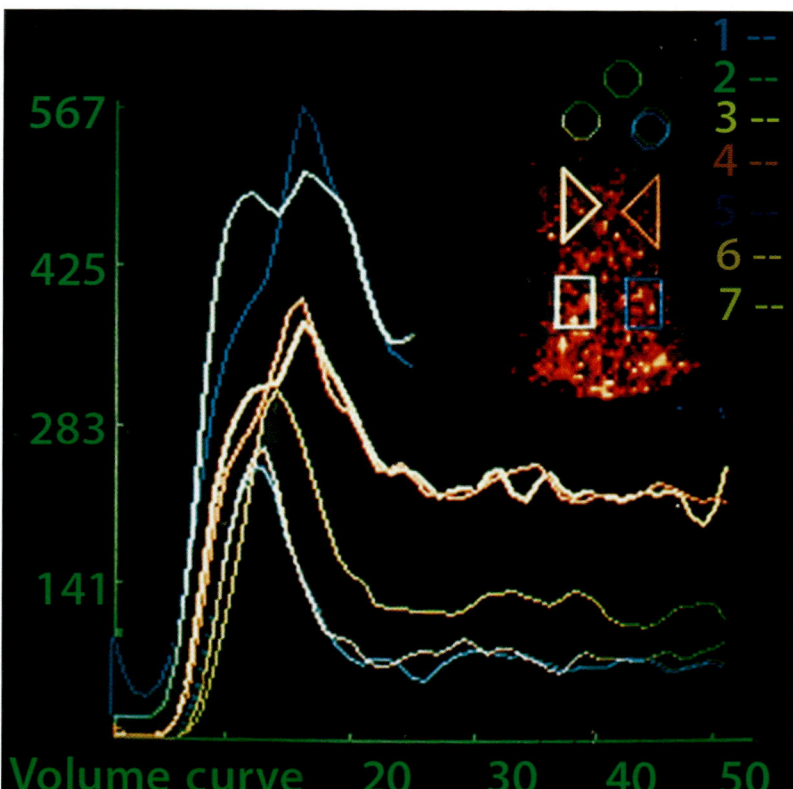

Fig. 1.22. Sequential functional brain scan with multiparameter analysis. Time-activity curves were recorded over the carotid arteries, middle cerebral arteries, and cerebral hemispheres

Brain/Early

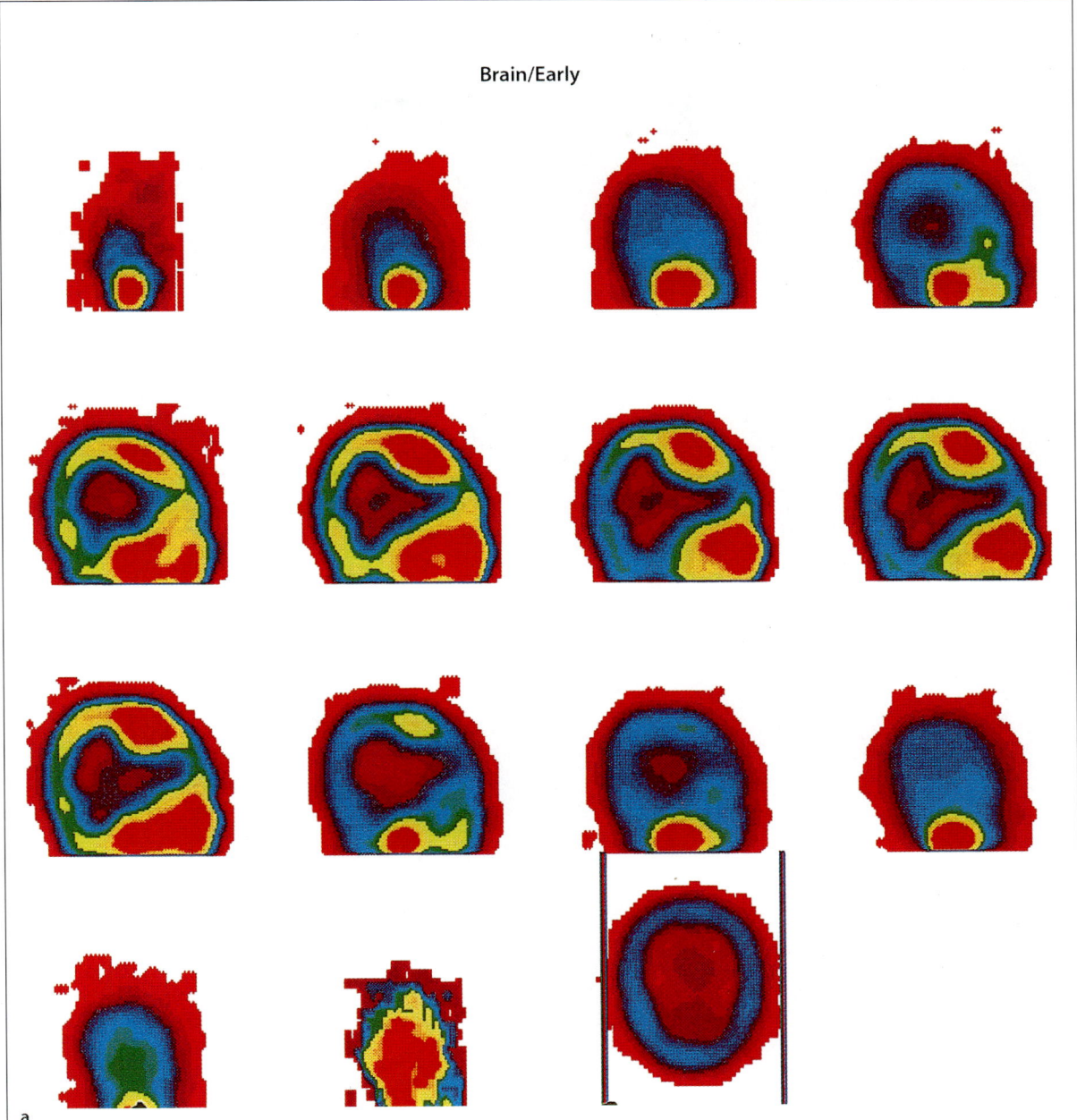

Fig. 1.23 a–c. Incidental finding in a 41-year-old man who told his brother that he felt as if his eye "bulged out" when he leaned forward. He had no other complaints. His brother, a patient, mentioned the complaint during an examination. Radionuclide scan shows a massive, hypervascular frontal tumor extending to the retrobulbar level. Immediate neurosurgical intervention was required to prevent impending blindness. The tumor was identified as a WHO grade-II bifrontal falx meningioma that was infiltrating the sinuses and both carotids

Brain/Early

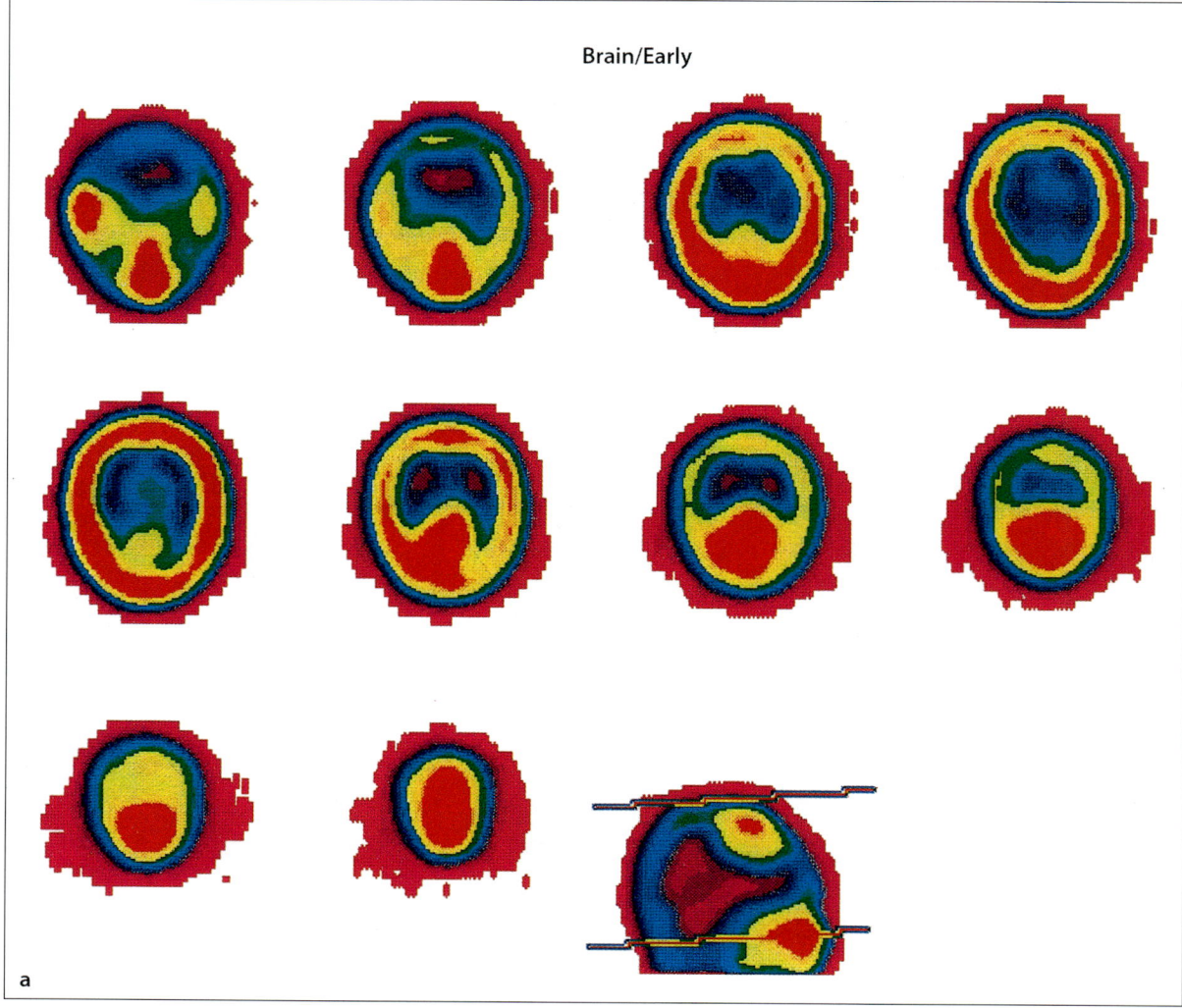

a

Fig. 1.23 a–c. Incidental finding in a 41-year-old man who told his brother that he felt as if his eye "bulged out" when he leaned forward. He had no other complaints. His brother, a patient, mentioned the complaint during an examination. Radionuclide scan shows a massive, hypervascular frontal tumor extending to the retrobulbar level. Immediate neuro-surgical intervention was required to prevent impending blindness. The tumor was identified as a WHO grade-II bifrontal falx meningioma that was infiltrating the sinuses and both carotids

Fig. 1.23 b

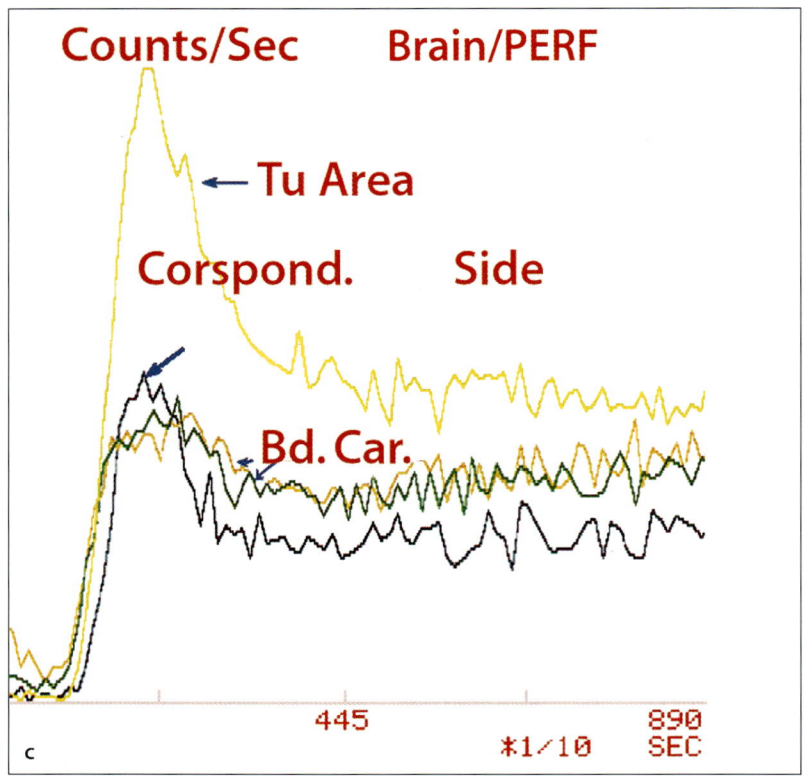

Fig. 1.23 a–c. Incidental finding in a 41-year-old man who told his brother that he felt as if his eye "bulged out" when he leaned forward. He had no other complaints. His brother, a patient, mentioned the complaint during an examination. Radionuclide scan shows a massive, hypervascular frontal tumor extending to the retrobulbar level. Immediate neurosurgical intervention was required to prevent impending blindness. The tumor was identified as a WHO grade-II bifrontal falx meningioma that was infiltrating the sinuses and both carotids

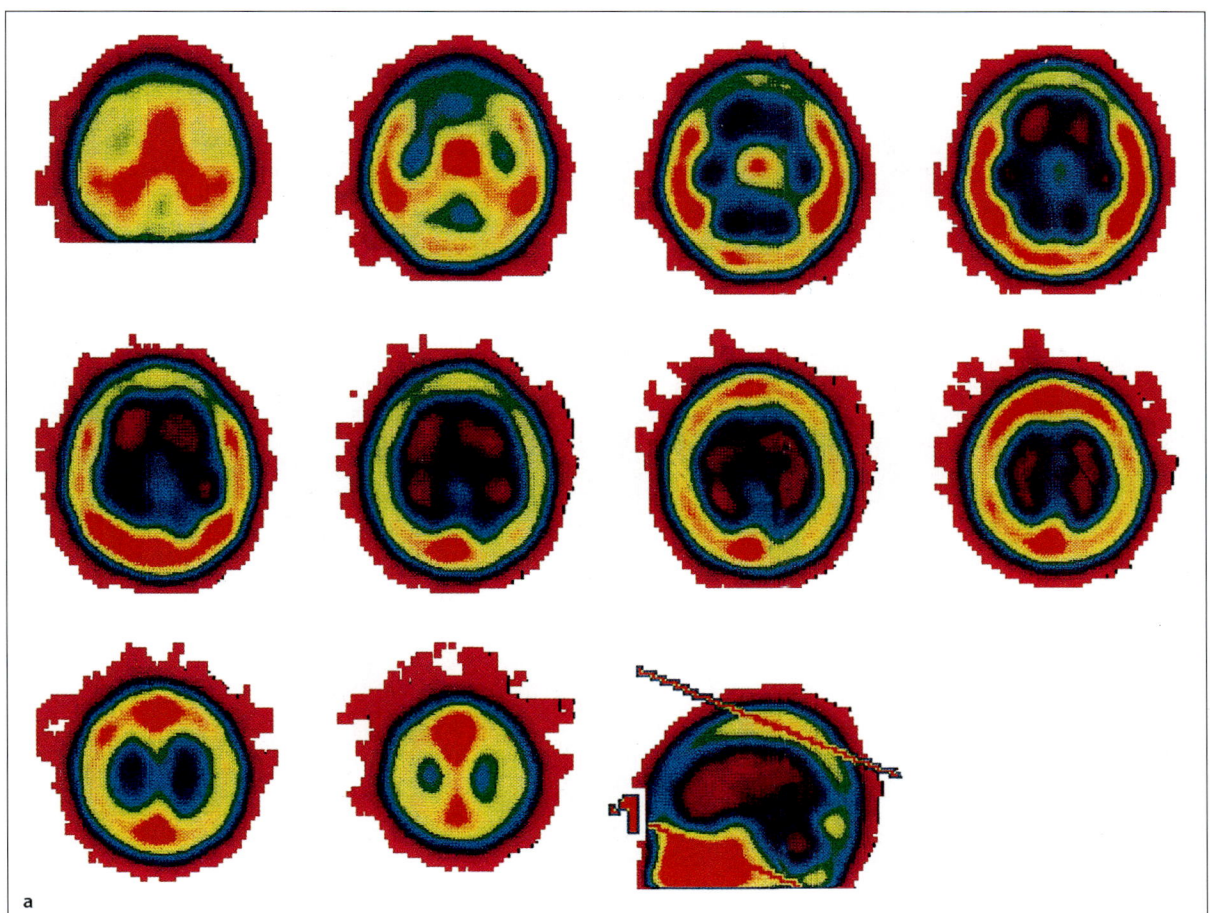

Fig. 1.24 a,b. A 31-year-old woman wanted to conceive but had been amenorrheic for years. She had a normal gyneco-logic examination and no other complaints. **a** Radionuclide imaging was performed to exclude a brain tumor. The scan shows slightly increased activity in the paramedian and basal area, raising suspicion of a hormone-producing neoplasm. This was confirmed by a prolactin assay of 1250 μg/L (<15 μg/L is normal). The patient was treated and achieved preg-nancy (bearing a healthy child). **b** Follow-up scan after treatment shows complete regression of the tumor

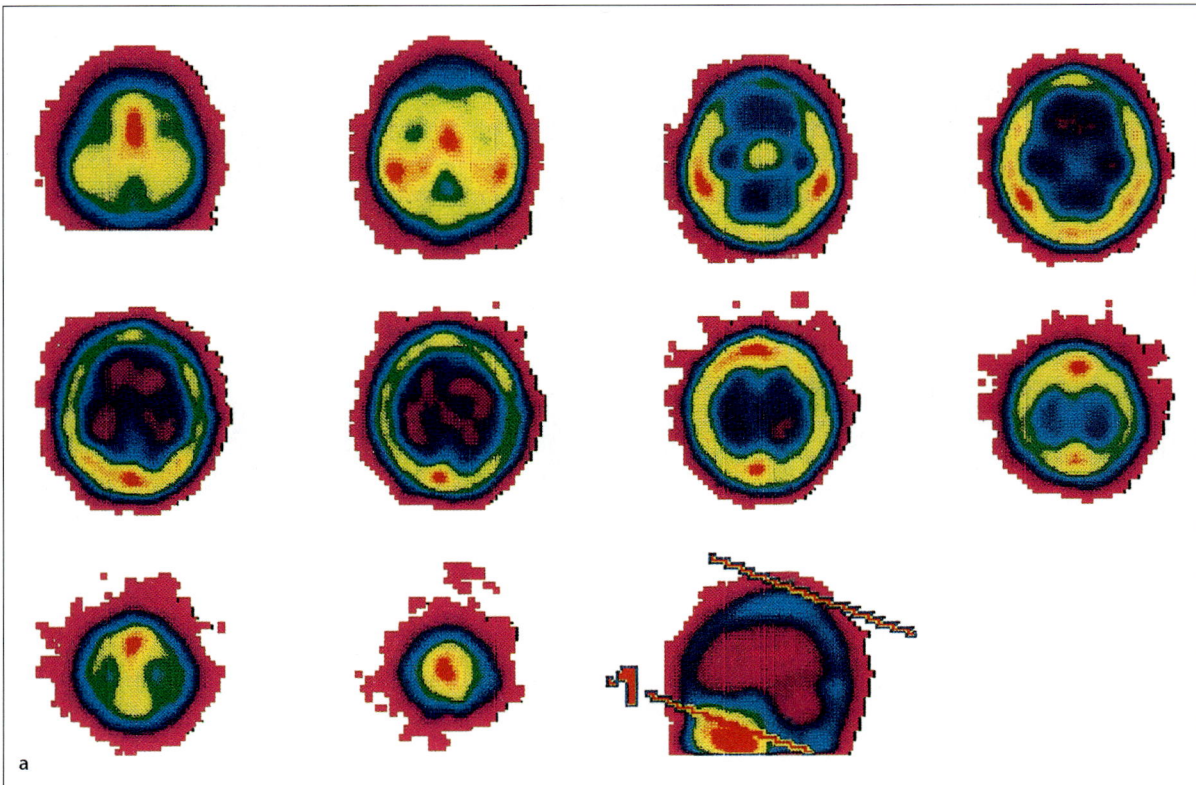

Fig. 1.24 a,b. A 31-year-old woman wanted to conceive but had been amenorrheic for years. She had a normal gyneco-logic examination and no other complaints. **a** Radionuclide imaging was performed to exclude a brain tumor. The scan shows slightly increased activity in the paramedian and basal area, raising suspicion of a hormone-producing neoplasm. This was confirmed by a prolactin assay of 1250 µg/L (<15 µg/L is normal). The patient was treated and achieved preg-nancy (bearing a healthy child). **b** Follow-up scan after treatment shows complete regression of the tumor

a

Fig. 1.24 a. *Continued*

b

Fig. 1.24 b

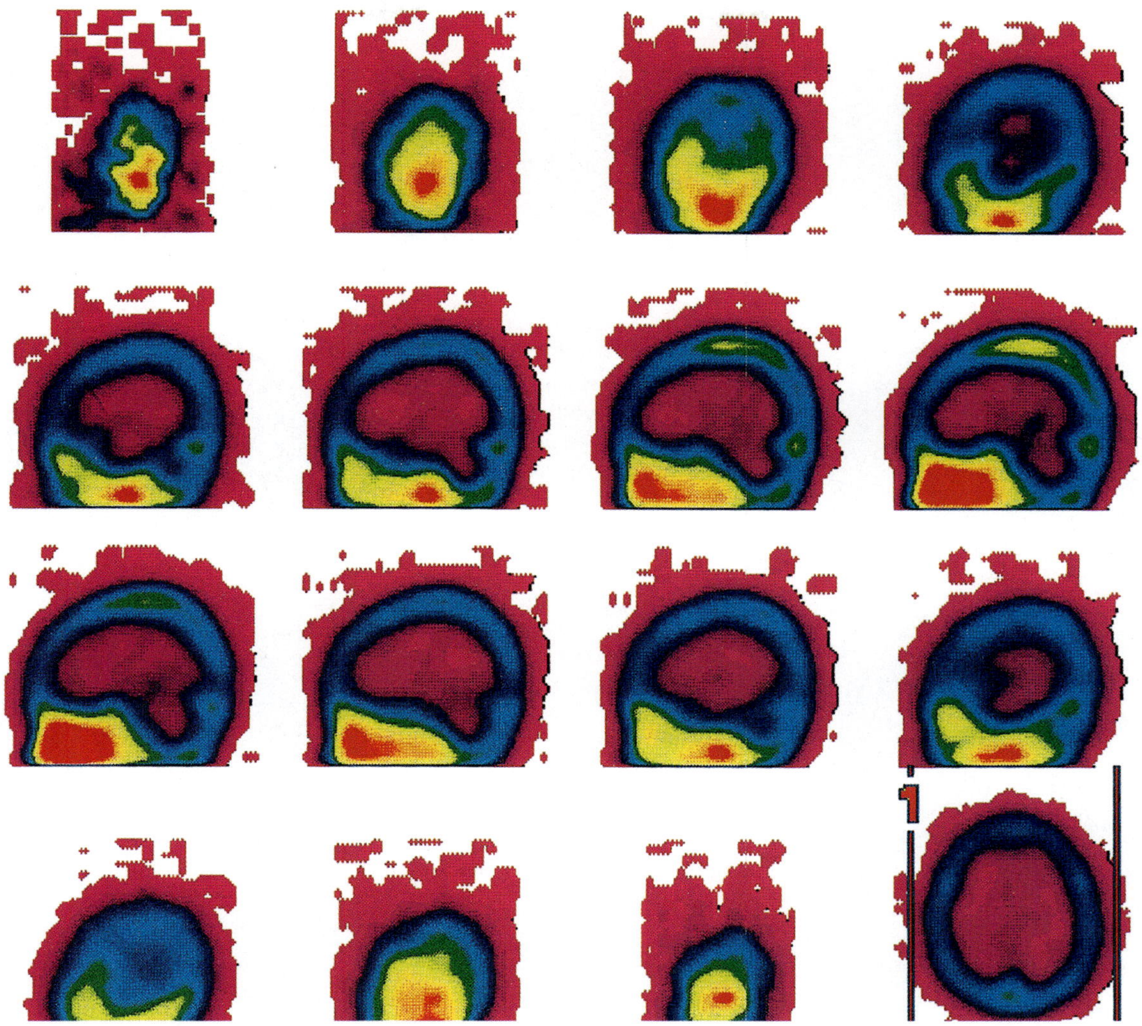

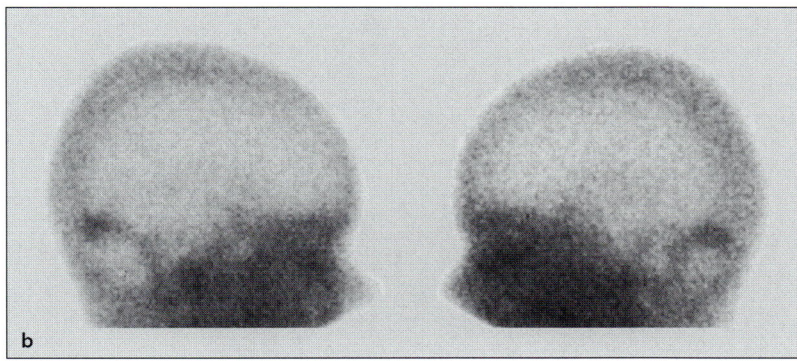

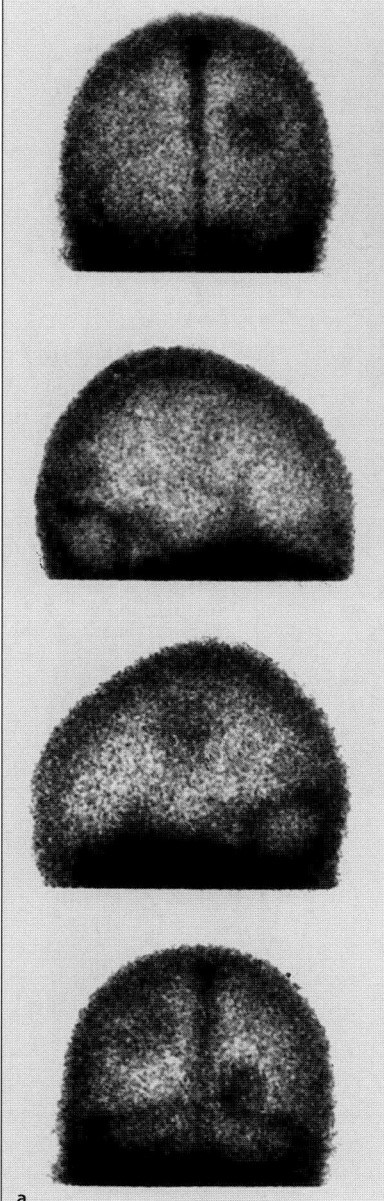

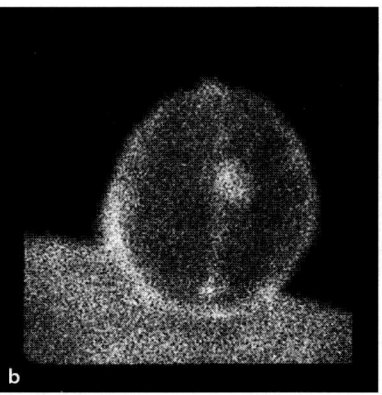

Fig. 1.25 a,b. Brain scan in a 35-year-old woman with vertigo shows multiple foci of increased uptake, some of which are poorly demarcated from surrounding tissue. This pattern is suggestive of multiple metastases, with perifocal edema accounting for the poorly demarcated foci. The patient was found to have cervical carcinoma

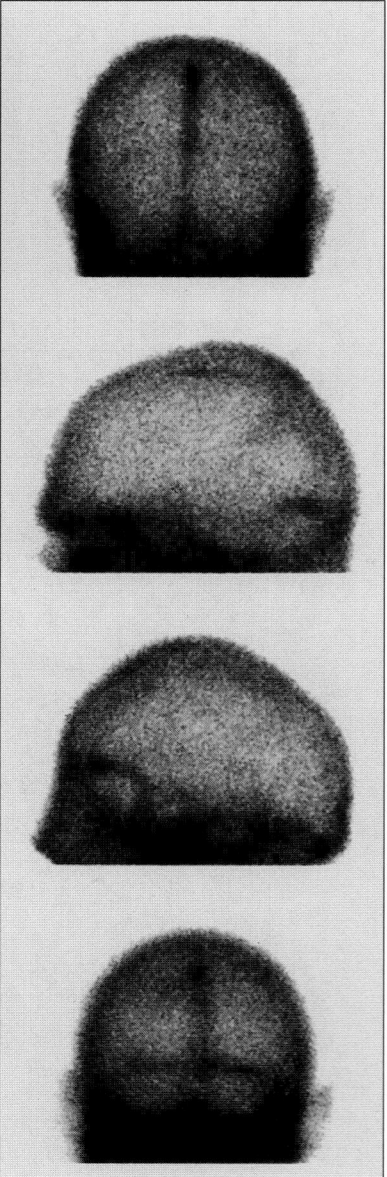

Fig. 1.26. Brain scan in a patient with intermittent headaches shows a wedge-shaped area of increased uptake in the left parieto-occipital region. The hot spot is visible only in one view. The initial impression of hemorrhage was incorrect, and the lesion proved to be a glioblastoma

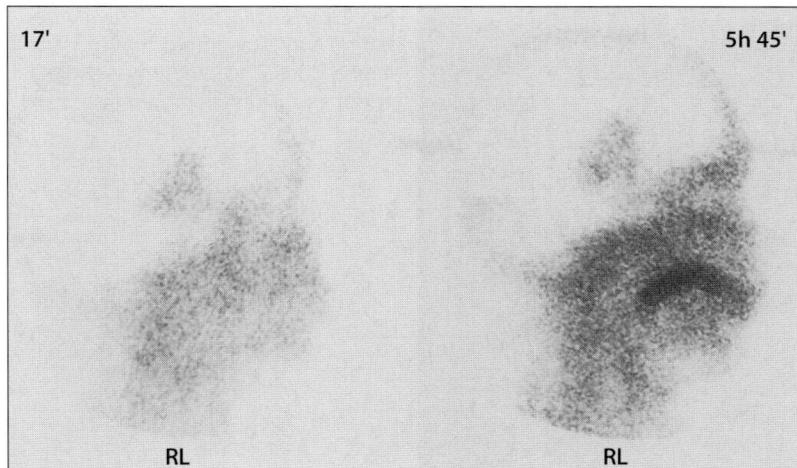

17'   5h 45'

RL   RL

Fig. 1.27. Brain abscess in a patient with a febrile infection and severe headache

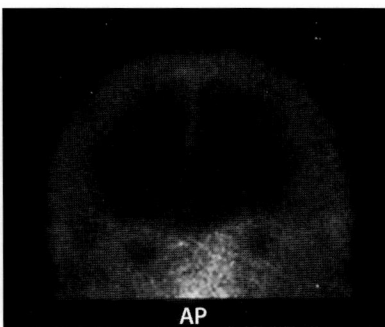

AP

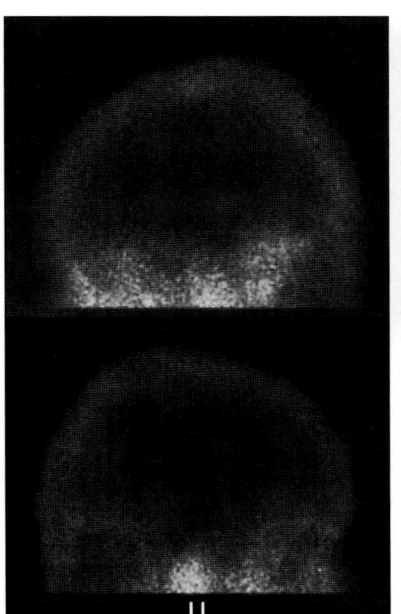

LL

Fig. 1.28. Increased uptake in the posterior fossa, diagnosed as acoustic neuroma

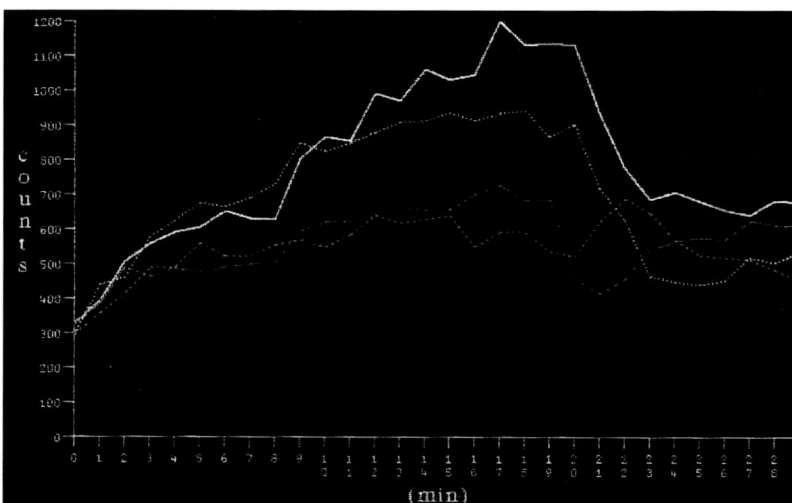

Fig. 1.29. Normal time-activity curve before and after administration of a lemon drink. The patient was evaluated for exclusion of Sjögren disease

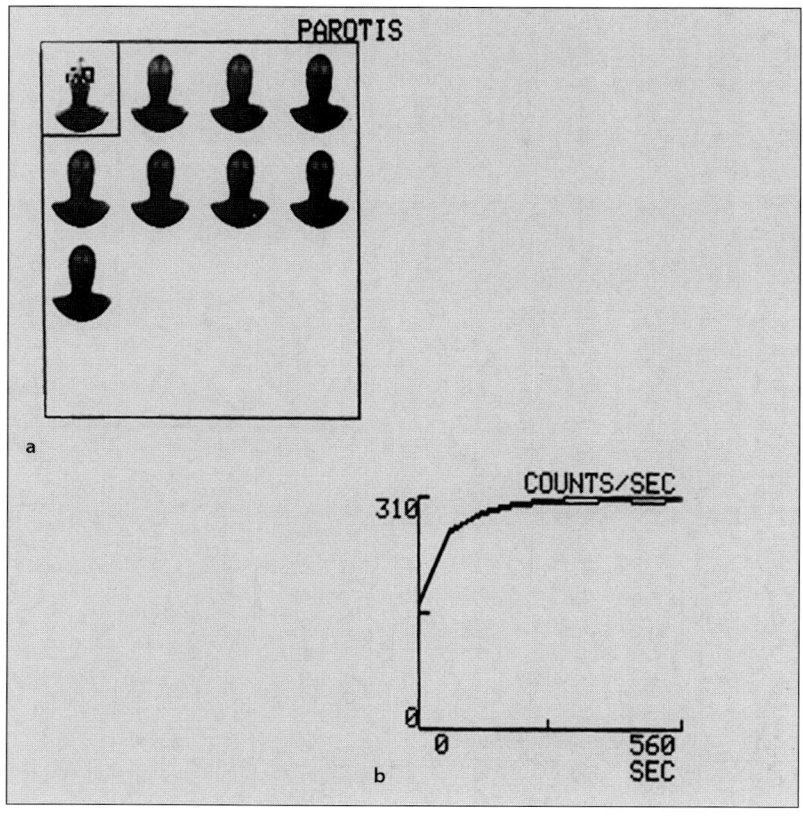

Fig. 1.30 a,b. This patient complained of dry mouth and fissuring of the oral mucosa following a strumectomy for thyroid carcinoma, multiple radioiodine treatments, and postoperative irradiation. The sequential images (**a**) and time-activity curve (**b**) demonstrate a complete loss of parotid function

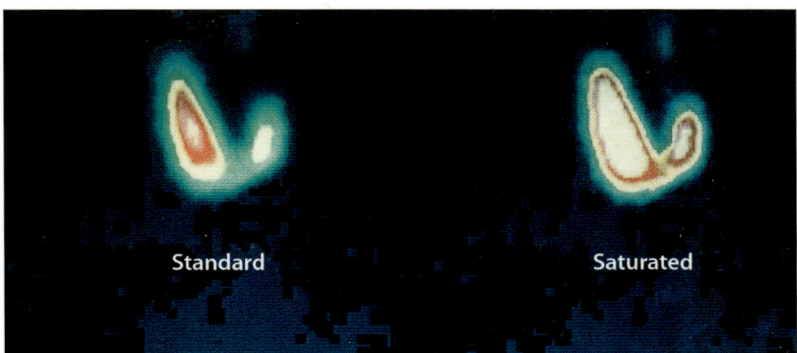

Fig. 1.31. Thyroid gland in a typical location. The right lobe is larger than the left

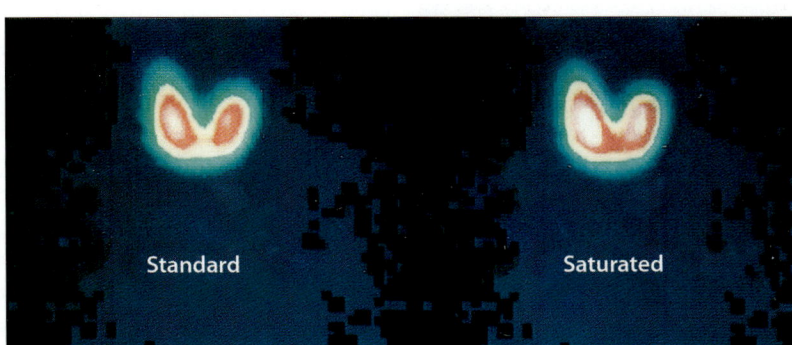

Fig. 1.32. U-shaped thyroid gland

Fig. 1.33. Right-sided thyroid gland with congenital absence of the left lobe

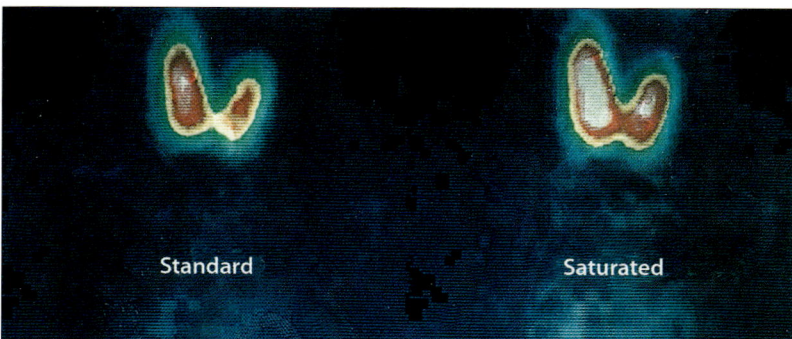

Fig. 1.34. V-shaped thyroid gland with right lobe larger than the left

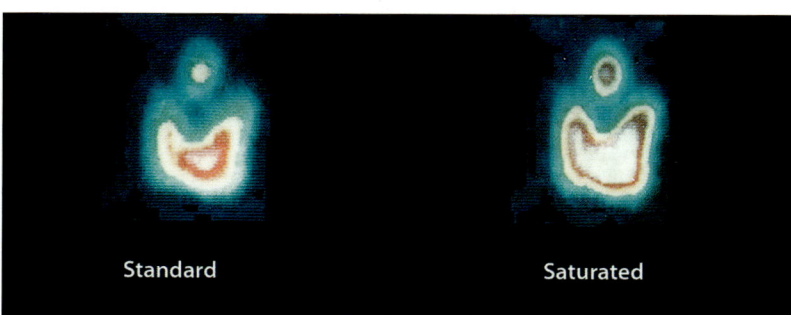

Fig. 1.35. Key-shaped thyroid gland with a pyramidal lobe

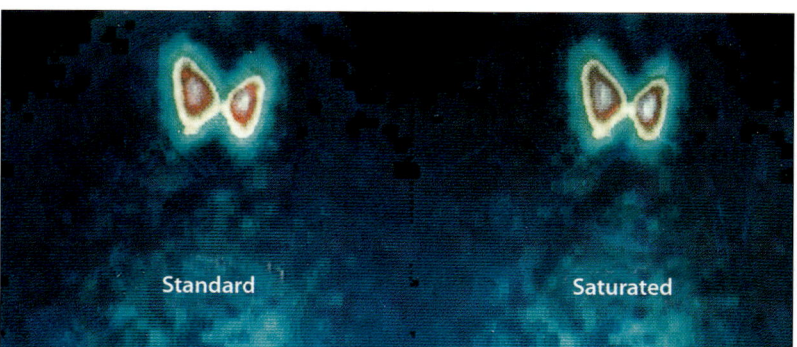

Fig. 1.36. Butterfly-shaped thyroid gland

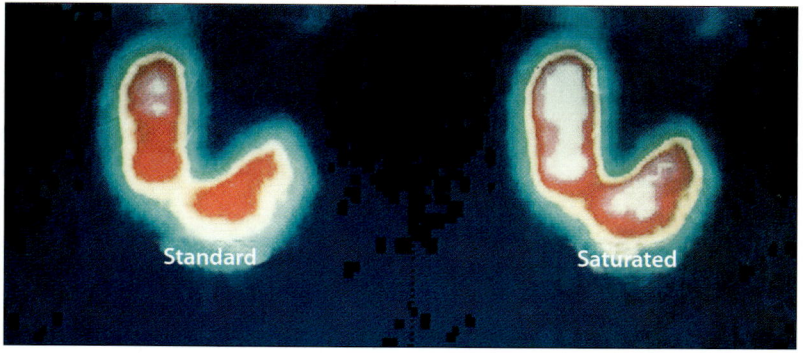

Fig. 1.37. Thyroid gland with an extended right lobe. The left lobe appears to blend with the widened isthmus

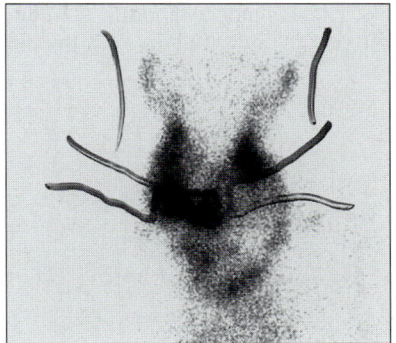

Fig. 1.38. The left lobe of this thyroid gland is larger than the right lobe and shows considerable substernal extension

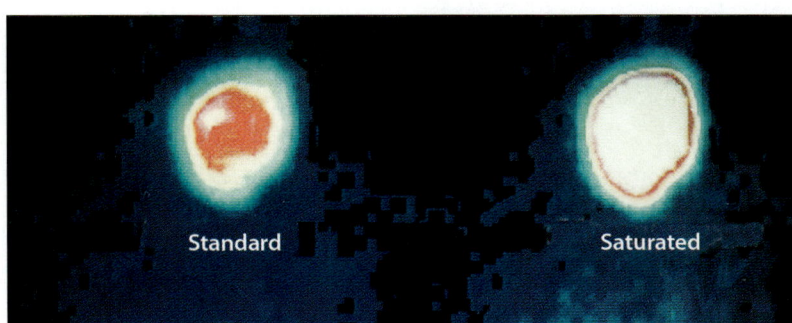

Fig. 1.39. Spherical thyroid gland (congenital variant)

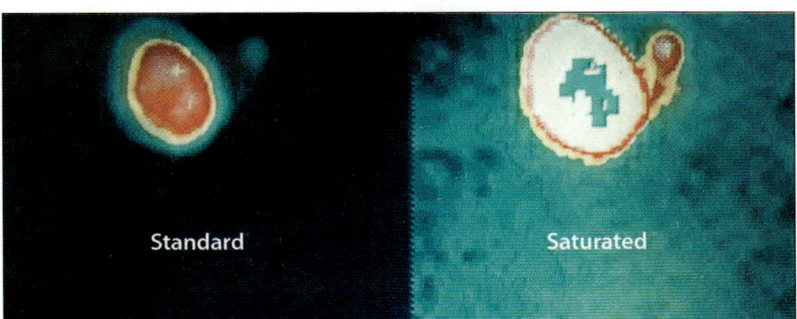

Fig. 1.40. Decompensated autonomous adenoma

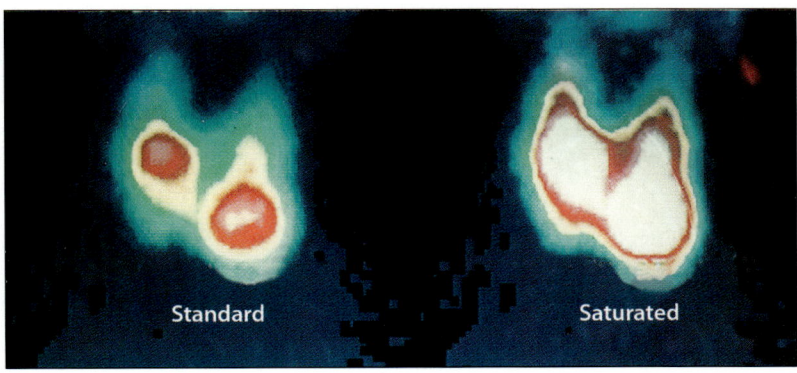

Fig. 1.41. Double decompensated autonomous adenoma

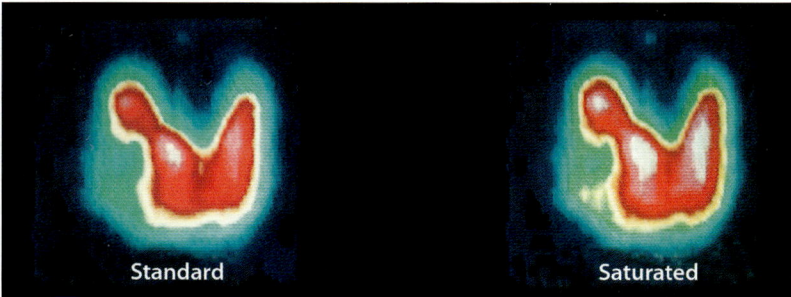

Fig. 1.42. Solitary cold nodule (cyst) in the central portion of the right thyroid lobe

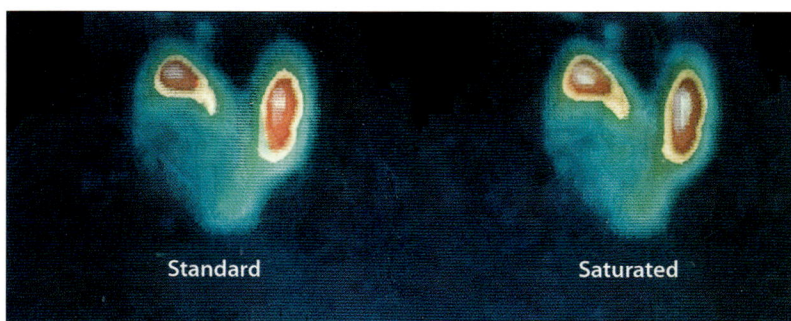

Fig. 1.43. Predominantly right-sided goiter. The central and lower portions of the lobe show only trace radionuclide uptake and substernal extension. With clinical correlation, the lesion is identified as a large right-sided cyst with extension to the isthmus

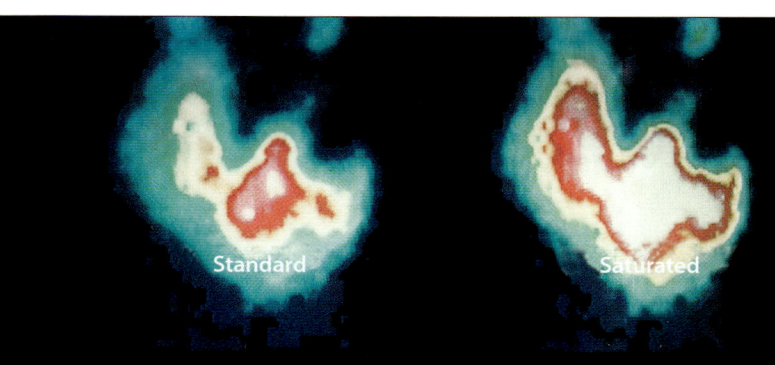

Fig. 1.44. Autonomous adenoma in the thyroid isthmus, accompanied by a large cyst in the central and lower portion of the left lobe. The inferior margin of the isthmus projects into the suprasternal notch

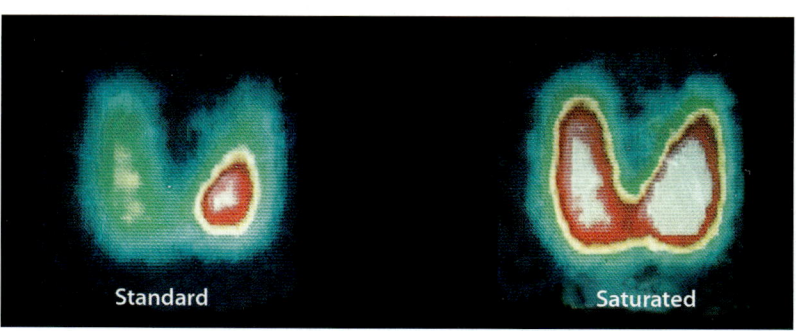

Fig. 1.45. Compensated autonomous adenoma in the lower pole of the left thyroid lobe

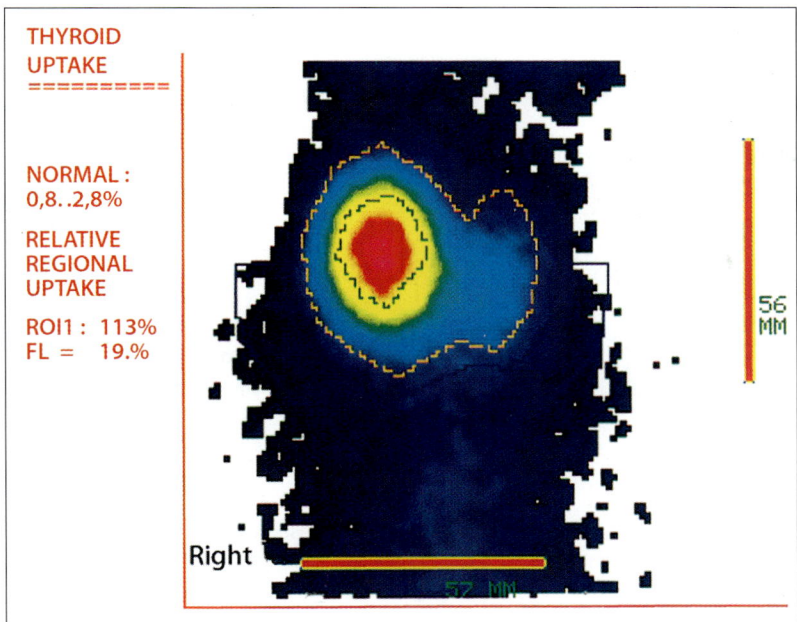

THYROID
UPTAKE
=========

NORMAL :
0,8..2,8%

RELATIVE
REGIONAL
UPTAKE

ROI1 : 113%
FL =   19.%

Right

56
MM

52 MM

Fig. 1.46. Compensated autonomous adenoma in the right lobe of a thyroid gland measuring 5.6×5.7 cm

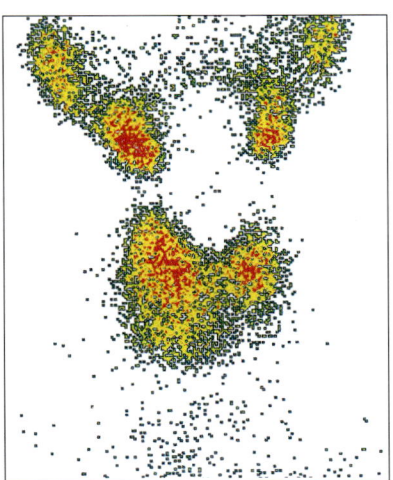

Fig. 1.47. Thyroid gland in which the lower pole of the larger right lobe shows decreased tracer uptake. Histology confirmed thyroid carcinoma. The right and left submandibular glands are visualized and show no abnormalities

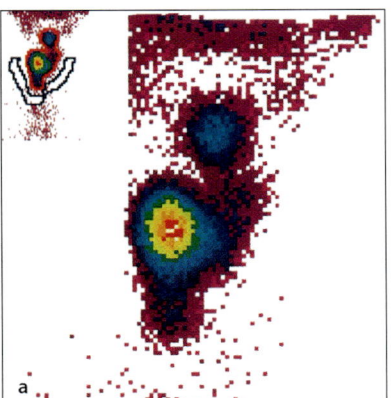

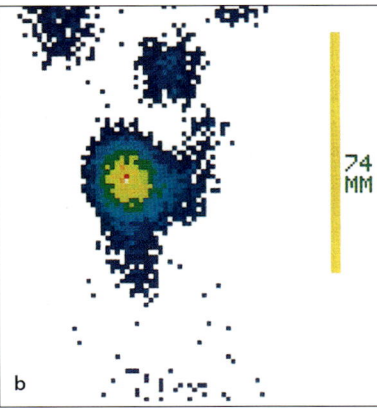

74
MM

Fig. 1.48. a Thyroid scan after subtotal strumectomy shows the round thyroid remnant on the right side along with a pyramidal lobe. **b** A suppression test was performed to exclude autonomy of the thyroid remnant. Uptake was reduced by more than half, confirming absence of autonomous function

a

b

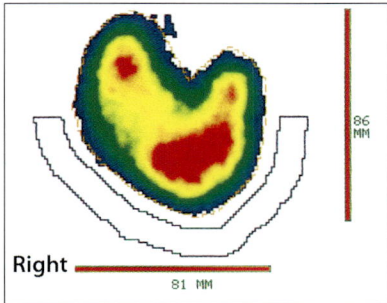

Right

86 MM

81 MM

Fig. 1.49

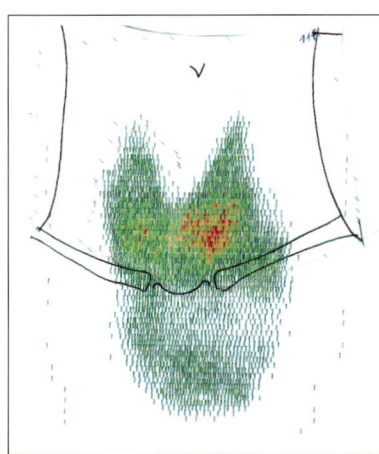

Fig. 1.49. Enlarged, asymmetric thyroid gland with decreased uptake in the central and lower portions of the left lobe. Histology established papillary carcinoma

Fig. 1.50. V-shaped thyroid gland whose isthmus shows 7 cm of substernal extension. The substernal tissue and upper left pole show significantly decreased uptake. Large goiter with a large substernal component. Histology established thyroid carcinoma

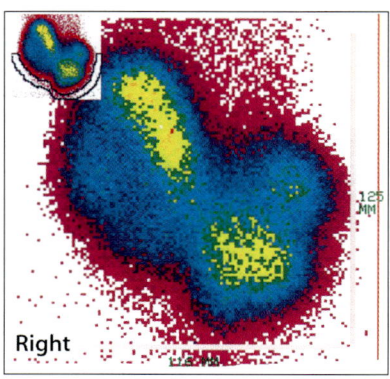

Right

125 MM

Fig. 1.51. Large cervical goiter with areas of decreased uptake. Histology showed regressive changes with no evidence of malignancy

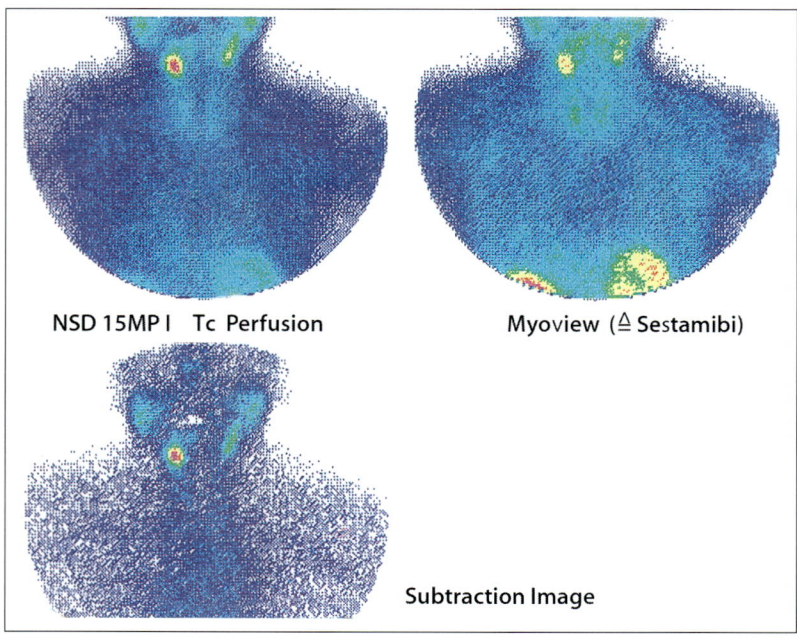

NSD 15MP I   Tc Perfusion   Myoview ($\triangleq$ Sestamibi)

Subtraction Image

Fig. 1.52. This patient with elevated hormone levels had equivocal findings at ultrasound. Double-tracer subtraction scanning with ^{99m}Tc pertechnetate and Myoview (sestamibi) clearly localizes the adenoma to the upper pole of the right thyroid lobe. The tumor was surgically removed

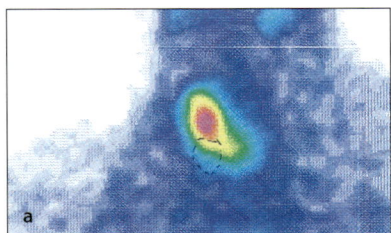 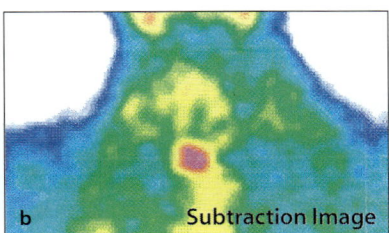

Fig. 1.53 a,b. This patient with elevated hormone levels underwent surgical resection of the left thyroid lobe. Subsequent double-tracer scanning (**a**) and image subtraction (**b**) localizes the adenoma to the inferolateral portion of the right lobe

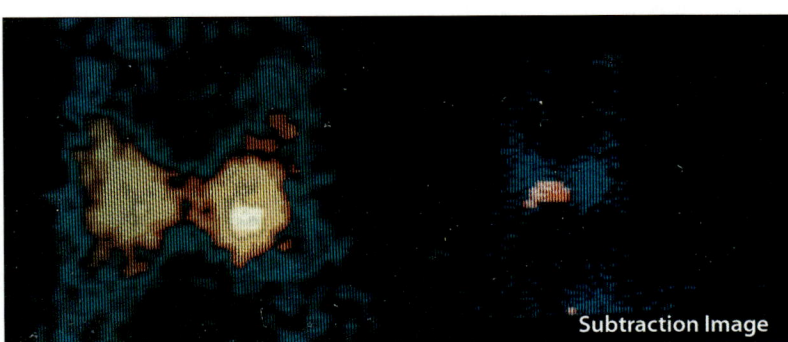

Fig. 1.54. Double-tracer subtraction imaging with ^{75}Se-labeled methionine and ^{99m}Tc pertechnetate demonstrates a subglandular adenoma in the right thyroid lobe of a patient with an elevated parathyroid hormone (PTH) level of 11.9 ng/mL (normal range = 0–1.3 ng/mL) and a midregion PTH (fragment 44–68) of 3.3 ng/mL (normal = 0.1–0.2 ng/mL)

2 Chest

2.1 Lungs

Perfusion lung scanning involves the intravenous injection of a suspension of radioactive particles, which are carried through the right heart and are trapped by the capillary filter in the lungs. Because this filter consists of terminal arterial branches that form a network surrounding the alveoli, the radiolabeled particles form microemboli that map the distribution of pulmonary blood flow and indicate the momentary status of lung perfusion.

Ventilation scanning is based on the precipitation of inhaled aerosol particles in the alveoli. This process involves the sedimentation or impaction of the particles on bronchial walls at sites of curvature or turbulence. Turbulence is caused by high flow velocities (hyperventilation) and also occurs at sites where airflow is impeded due to wall curvature or luminal obstruction. Because of its relatively complex protocols and diagnostic limitations, ventilation scanning has not achieved the same importance as perfusion scanning in pulmonary diagnosis.

The lung scan is currently recognized as the most sensitive method for the detection of pulmonary embolism. Its value has increased substantially as specific treatment measures for pulmonary embolism have improved. The decision whether to proceed with pulmonary angiography in patients with clinically suspected pulmonary embolism depends on the result of the perfusion lung scan. The presence of severe chronic obstructive lung disease complicates the differential diagnosis of pulmonary embolism, but the situation can be clarified by performing a ventilation scan and determining the ventilation-perfusion (V/Q) ratio. Areas affected by the embolism are characterized by a V/Q mismatch with an increase in the V/Q ratio.

The main clinical criteria for the diagnosis of pulmonary embolism, as described by Hornbostel et al. (1984), are dyspnea (46–100%), chest pain (55–73%), and hemoptysis (17–25%). These criteria were confirmed by a retrospective analysis of 71 confirmed pulmonary embolism cases (37 female, 34 male, 19–81 years of age) in which two subgroups (over or under age 40) were defined.

▌ Hemoptysis was present in 12.6% of the patients (57% female, half over age 40; 43% male, all over age 40).
▌ Chest pain was present in 100% of the patients (52% female, 34% under age 40; 48% male, 13% under age 40).
▌ Dyspnea was present in 84%.

In patients with frank chronic obstructive lung disease, both the perfusion scan and ventilation scan invariably show changes, such as a redistribution of radiotracer activity from the basal to the apical lung zones. Several causal mechanisms have been proposed for this phenomenon:

▌ Increased arteriolar resistance
▌ Functional constriction of the arterioles
▌ Increased alveolar pressure due to increased transbronchial flow resistance in the lower lung zones
▌ Increased vascular calibers in the upper lung zones due to pressure elevation in the pulmonary artery

Dynamic imaging at 0.24-second intervals for 25 seconds after bolus tracer injection is useful for investigating pulmonary hypertension, which by ROI definition is measured over the right ventricle (Fig. 2.1).

The uptake pattern in the lung scan is useful for the differentiation of pulmonary edema, as the defects associated with pulmonary embolism are more sharply defined in their shape, size, and contrast than the defects seen in interstitial lung edema. Perfusion defects due to chronic lung disease tend to be focal and show very little change on follow-up. With central mass lesions of the lung, the perfusion defects that appear on lung scans are larger than the corresponding radiographic lesions. This suggests that radionuclide imaging detects perihilar bronchial tumors more sensitively and at an earlier stage than chest radiographs.

The outstanding feature of pulmonary sarcoidosis is an abnormality of lung diffusion. Perfusion appears essentially normal in stage I cases, and stage II a is associated with little or no change in the scan pattern. Stages II b, II c, and II d present a mottled or patchy pattern of tracer uptake. Stage III is associated with conspicuous perfusion defects, which appear as large, poorly marginated areas of decreased activity.

Pleural effusions can lead to a local perfusion defect by compressing the surrounding lung tissue.

2.2
Breast

Breast carcinoma is the most common cancer that affects women in western industrialized countries. Its incidence has been steadily rising while the average age of onset has declined. It is incumbent upon medical professionals to use all available imaging techniques to advance the early detection of this disease.

2.3
Mediastinum

2.3.1
Major Vessels

While nuclear medicine usually employs organ-specific protocols, it is usually nonspecific in the diagnosis of mediastinal diseases, where it serves as a primary study for detecting circumscribed mediastinal masses or recognizing the diffuse widening of a structure such as the aorta.

**2.3.2
Heart**

A number of radionuclides and their labeled compounds have been tested in recent years for the nuclear medicine imaging of cardiovascular disease, but thallium-201 (^{201}Tl) has proven the most effective agent for clinical myocardial imaging. The following radiopharmaceuticals have been employed for cardiac imaging:

- ^{203}Hg chlormerodrin
- ^{203}Hg mercurifluorescein
- ^{99m}Tc tetracycline
- ^{67}Ga
- ^{99m}Tc glucoheptonate
- ^{99m}Tc phosphonate
- ^{201}Tl chloride
- $^{17-123}$I heptadecanic acid (HDA)
- ^{99m}Tc methoxyisobutylisonitrile (MIBI)

The introduction of Fourier analysis for the evaluation of radionuclide ventriculography has further advanced the use of thallium myocardial imaging. As a result, nuclear medicine imaging has become an indispensable tool in diagnostic cardiology.

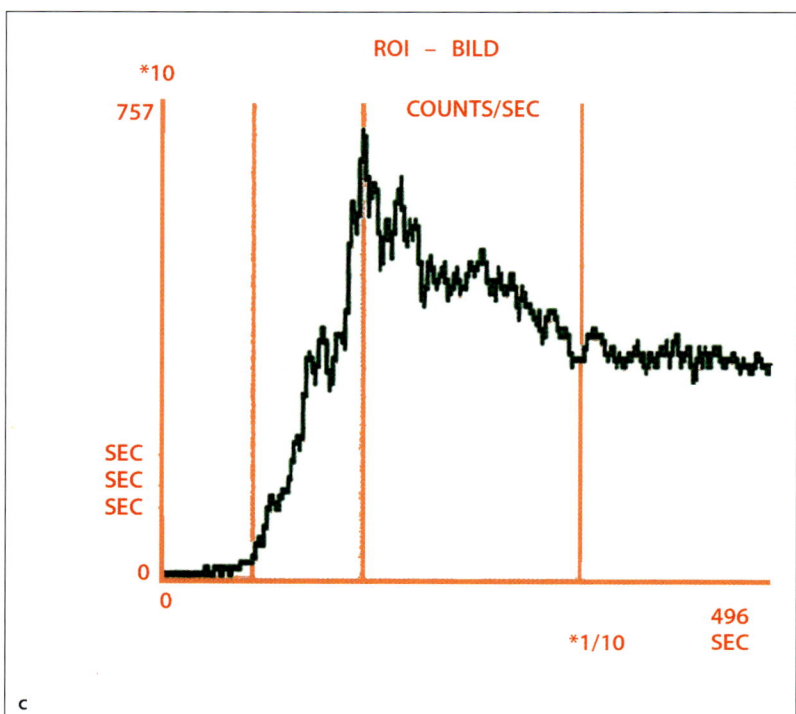

Fig. 2.1 a–c. Pulmonary hypertension is measured over the right ventricle by ROI definition. Q is defined as integral I/integral II, where integral I is the area under the time-activity curve to maximum counts and integral II is the area from maximum counts to minimum counts. **a** Sequential images. **b** Summation image. **c** Time-activity curve

ROI – BILD

*10

757

COUNTS/SEC

SEC
SEC
SEC

0

0

*1/10

496
SEC

c

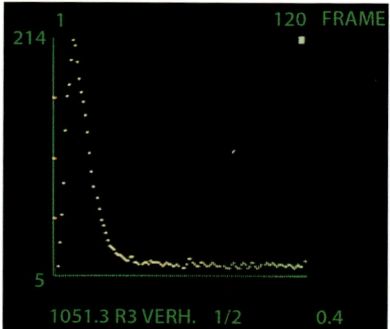

Fig. 2.2. Lung scan in a patient with normal chest radiographs, normal pulmonary function tests, and no pulmonary complaints. Q = 0.4 (<5.5 is normal)

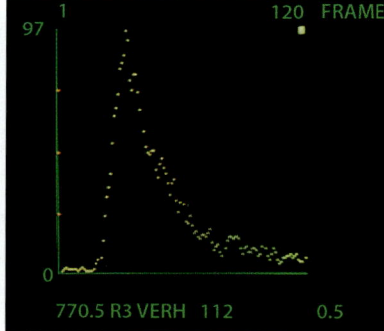

Fig. 2.3. Lung scan a 35-year-old man with incipient pulmonary emphysema. Q is within normal limits

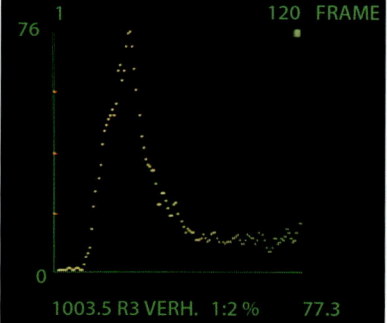

Fig. 2.4. Lung scan in a 22-year-old woman with obstructive lung disease and pulmonary embolism. Q = 77.3

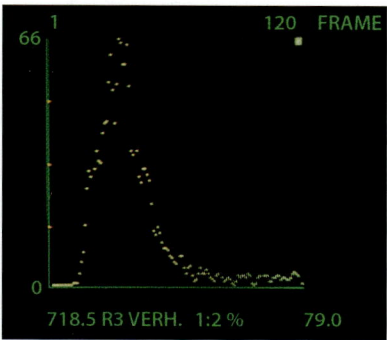

Fig. 2.5. Lung scan in a 60-year-old man with pulmonary fibrosis. Q = 79

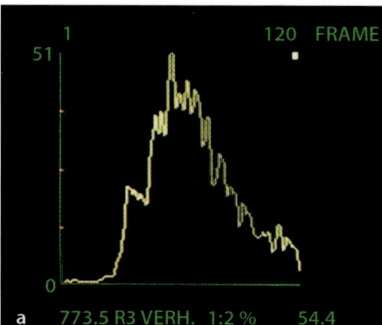

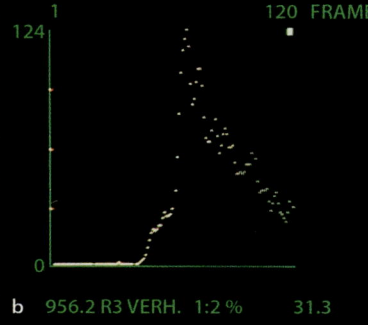

Fig. 2.6 a,b. This patient, a 69-year-old pacemaker wearer with heart failure, experienced immediate respiratory distress after the initiation of lower-extremity venography. Lung scan shows a pulmonary embolism originating from varicosity in the lower leg. Q1=54.4, Q2=31.3

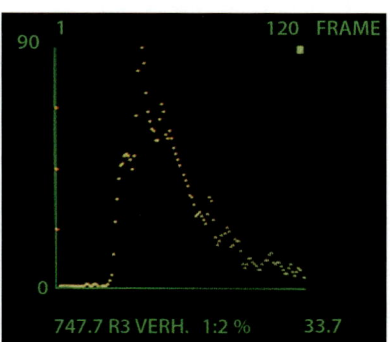

Fig. 2.7. Man 70 years of age with a history of pulmonary tuberculosis. Ventilation scan and chest films indicate chronic obstructive bronchitis with pulmonary emphysema. Q = 33.7

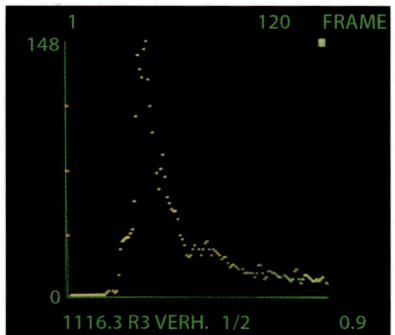

Fig. 2.8. Pleuropneumonia in a 70-year-old man. Q = 0.9

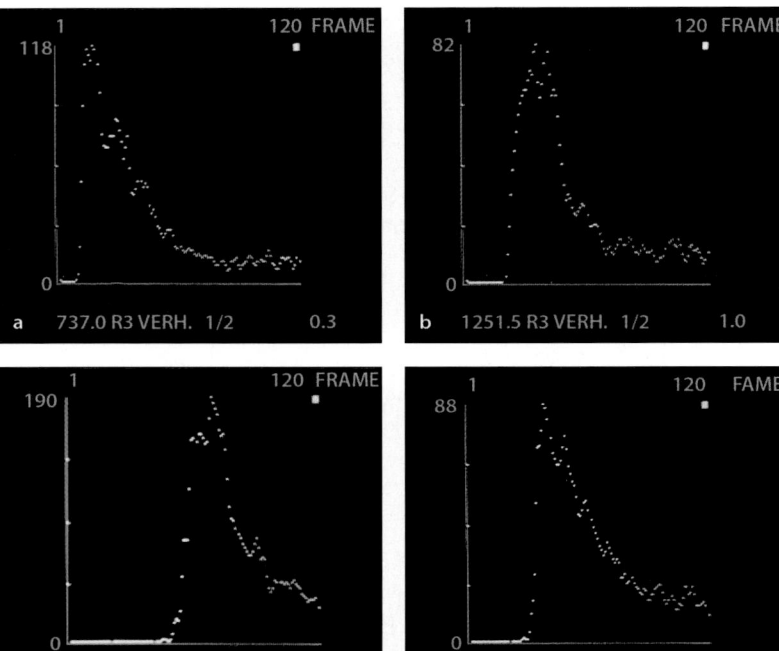

Fig. 2.9 a–d. This 51-year-old man with thrombophlebitis underwent several lung scans to exclude a pulmonary embolism. Lower-left-quadrant chest pain occurred on 30 March, and pulmonary embolism was diagnosed on 14 April. Q1=0.3, Q2=1.0, Q3=0.5, Q4=55.5

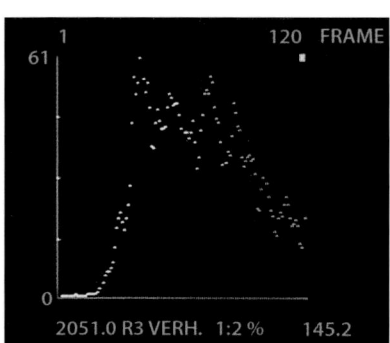

Fig. 2.10. Multiple pulmonary emboli in a 50-year-old man. Q = 145.2

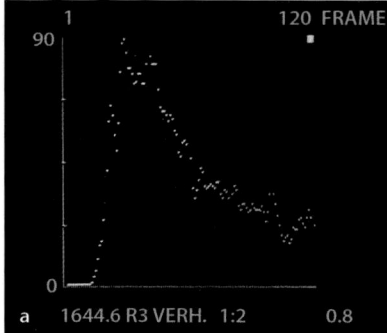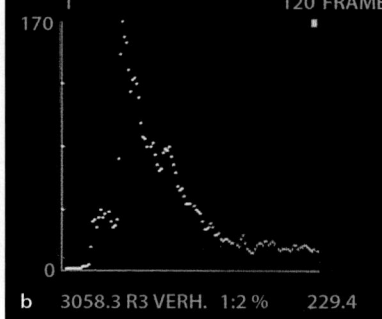

Fig. 2.11 a,b. A 76-year-old man with a history of CHD developed chest pain and respiratory distress while hospitalized. Chest radiographs showed no change compared with admission films. Lung scan shows a conspicuous pulmonary embolism. Q increased from 0.6 to 229.4

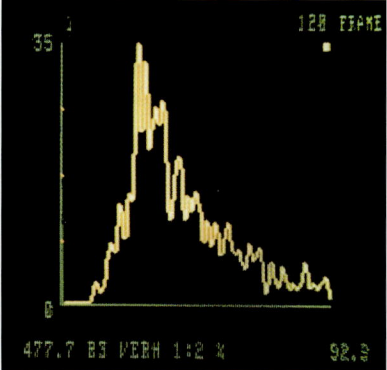

Fig. 2.12. Lung scan in a 76-year-old man with pulmonary fibrosis and bullous emphysema. Q = 92.9

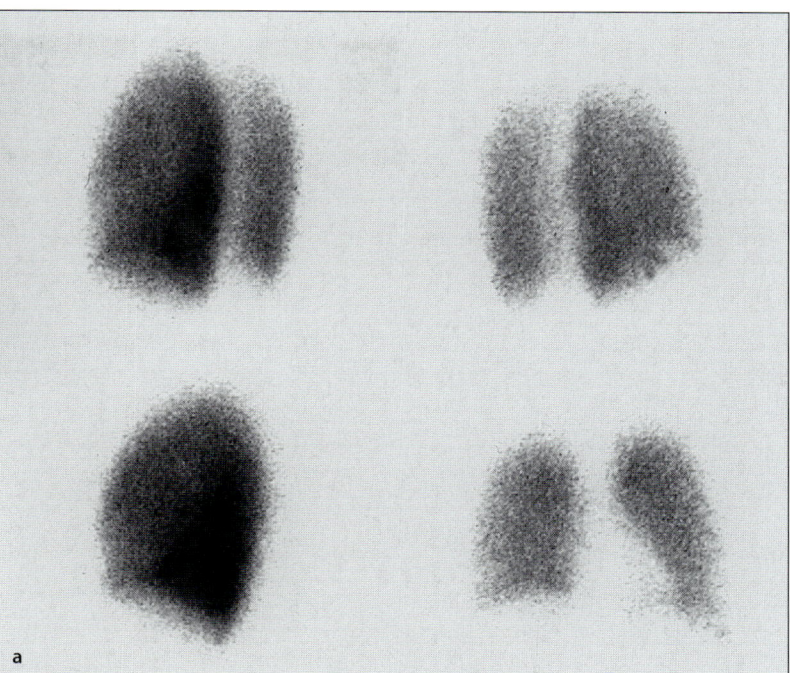

a

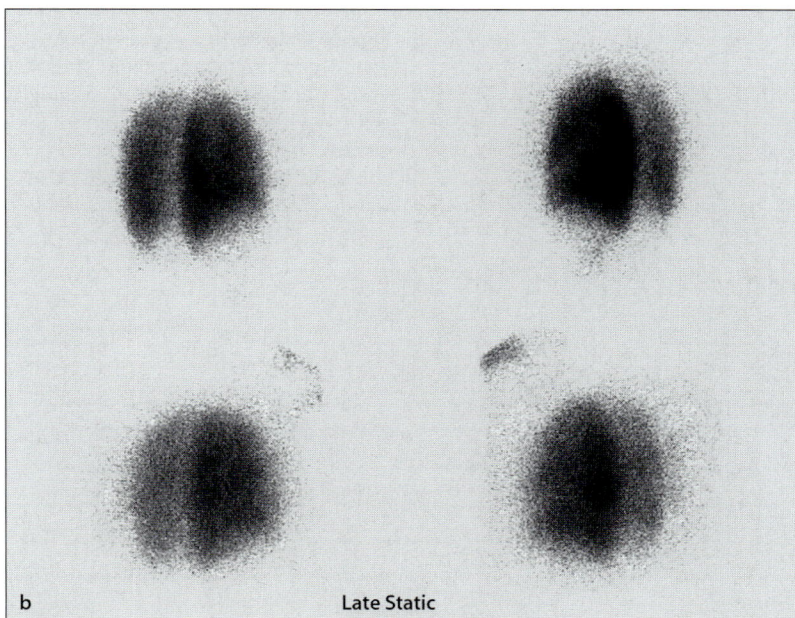

b   Late Static

Fig. 2.13 a,b. Normal ventilation-perfusion lung scan

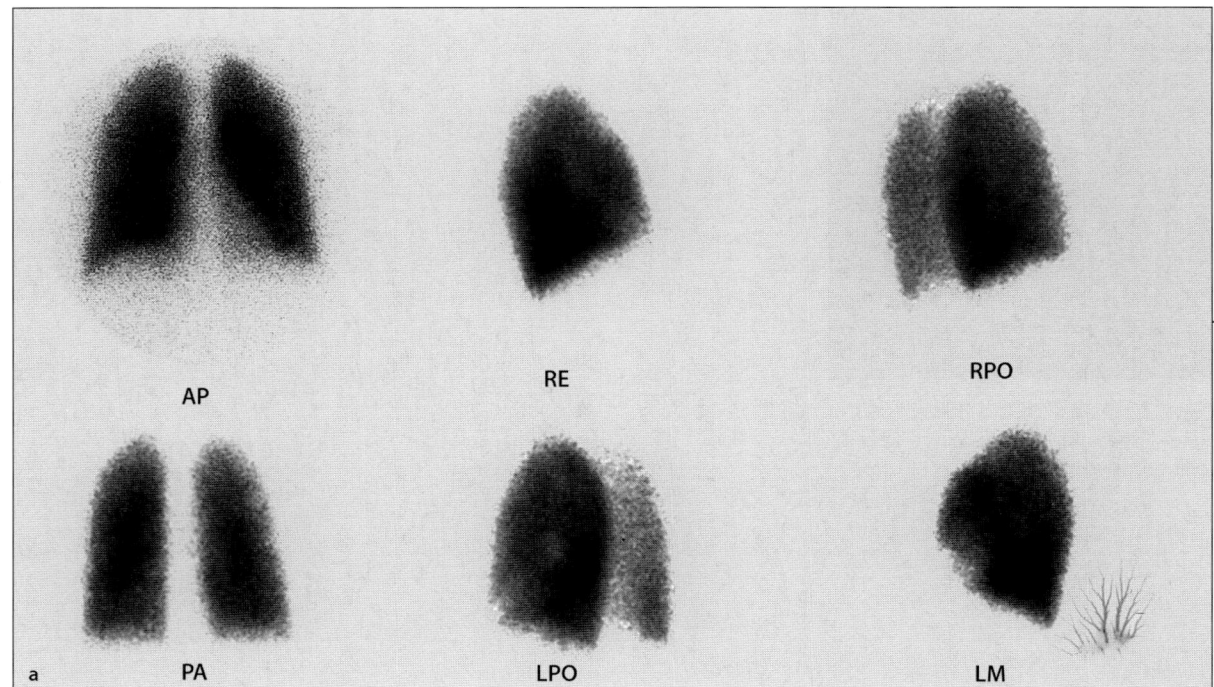

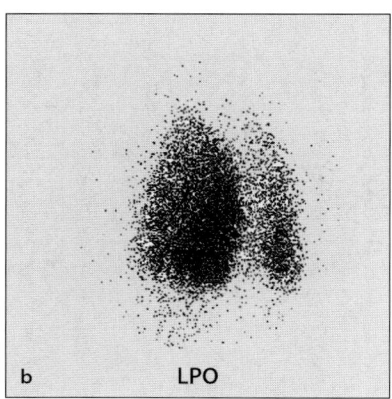

Fig. 2.14 a,b. Perfusion scan in a 41-year-old woman shows slight straightening of the lower lung border with normal width of the mediastinum and cardiac shadow. Ventilation scan shows a slight nonhomogeneity consistent with mild or incipient emphysema

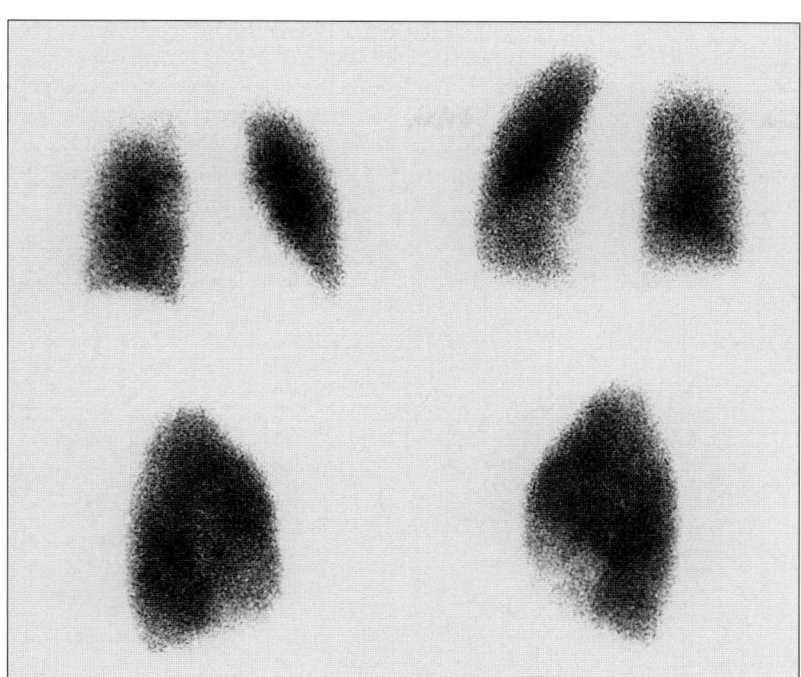

Fig. 2.15. Perfusion scan in a 50-year-old obese woman shows slight mediastinal widening with marked elevation of the lower lung border and an absence of apical perfusion in the right lung. The diaphragmatic elevation is obesity-related and has caused upward displacement of the heart. The apparent mediastinal widening is an artifact caused by the camera head or equipment settings. Apical induration is responsible for the perfusion defect in the right lung

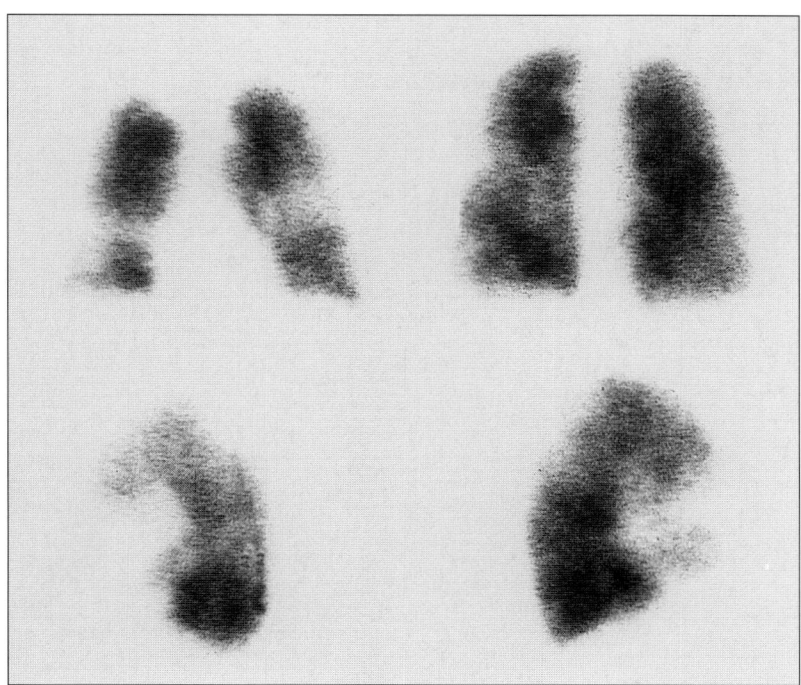

Fig. 2.16. Lung scan in a patient with stage II Boeck disease shows midzone perfusion defects in both lungs accompanied by widening of the mediastinum

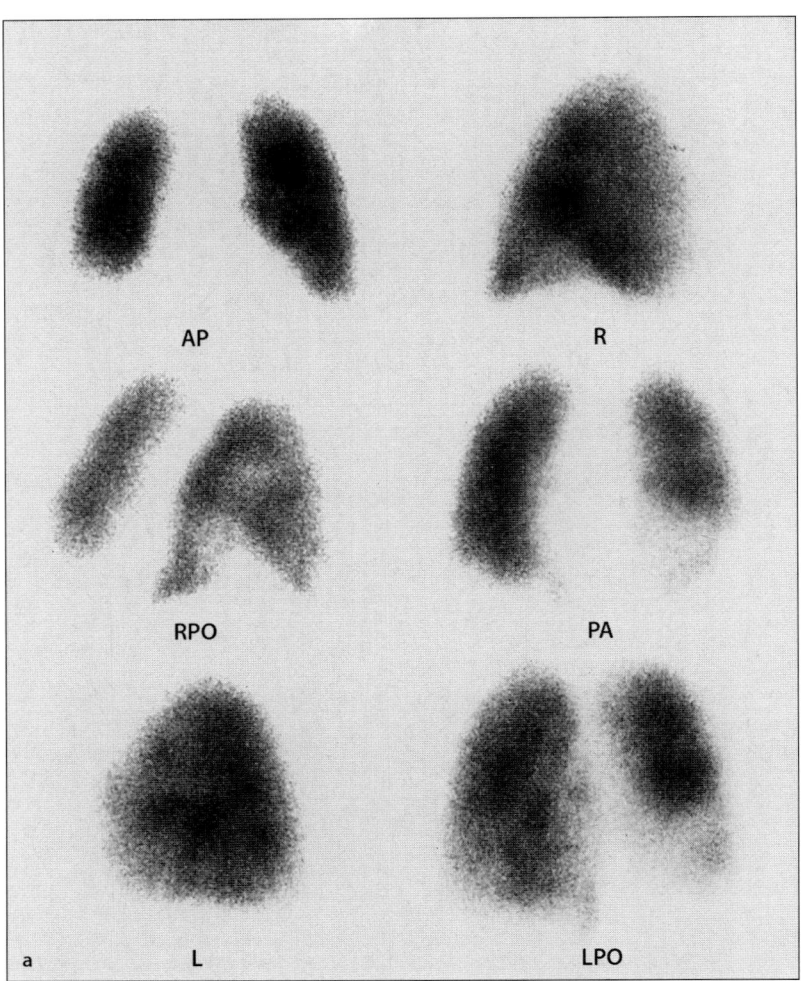

a

AP

R

RPO

PA

L

LPO

Fig. 2.17 a. Perfusion scan in a 40-year-old woman with sudden right-sided chest pain and dyspnea shows an absence of perfusion in segment 9 and a portion of segment 10, indicating fresh emboli in both segments.

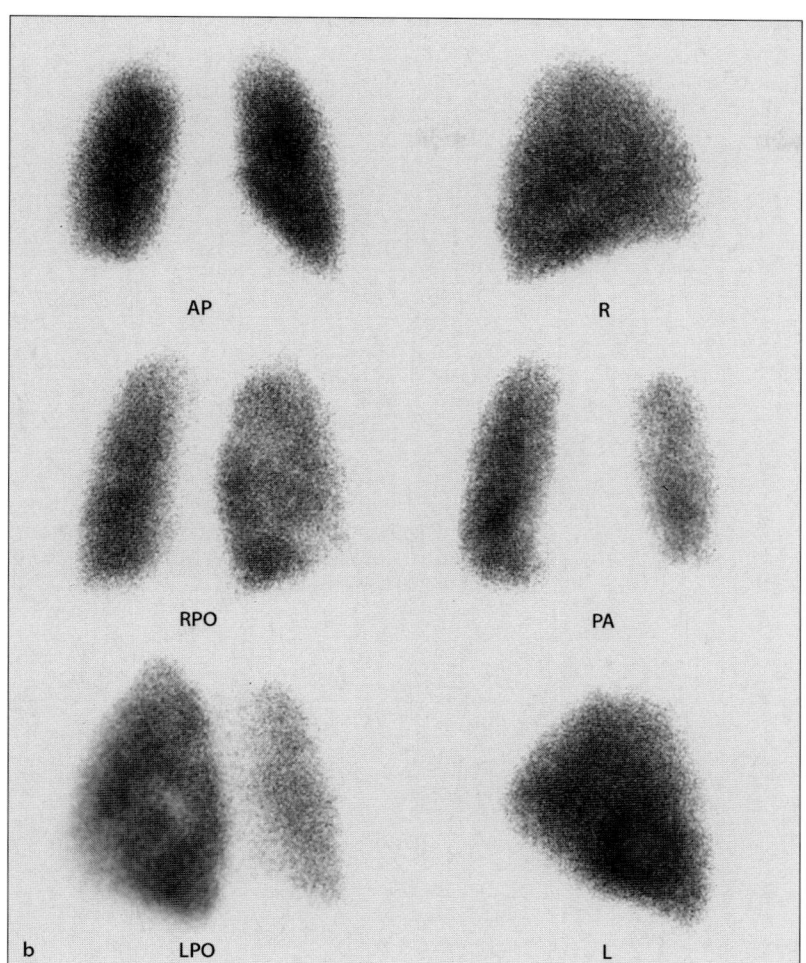

Fig. 2.17 b. Post-treatment follow-up scan 2 weeks later shows complete reperfusion. The uneven radionuclide distribution is a result of postural guarding due to chest pain

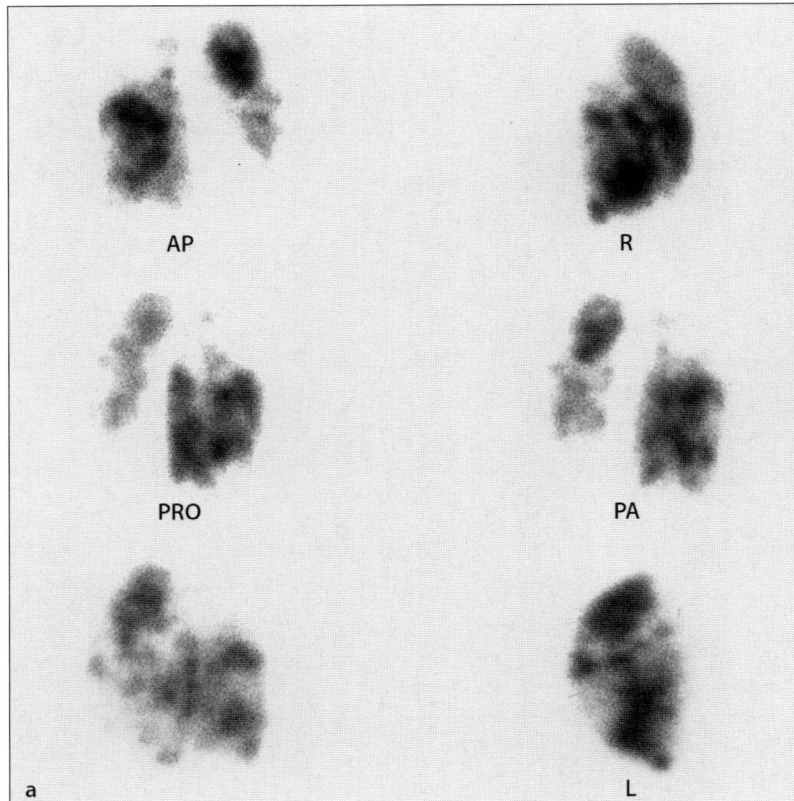

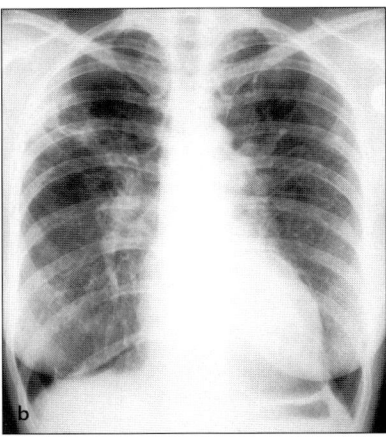

Fig. 2.18 a,b. Lung scan in a patient with pulmonary cysts shows multiple hypoperfused areas in both lungs with an absence of marked clinical symptoms

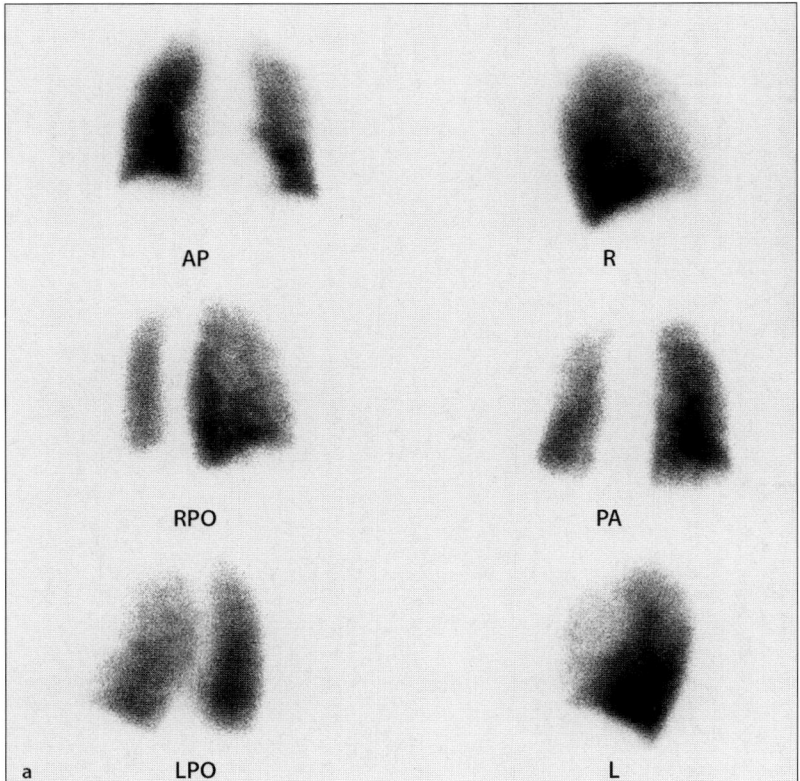

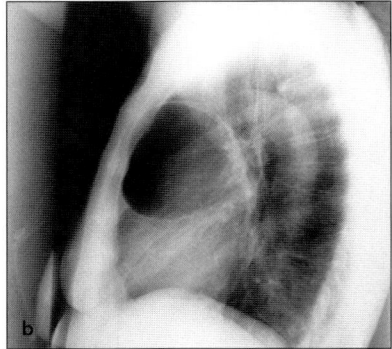

Fig. 2.19 a,b. Anterolateral scan view shows a perfusion deficit involving all of the middle and upper zones of the left lung and a nonhomogeneous perfusion pattern in the right lung with a straightened lower lung border. The patient has a left-sided lung cyst displacing the surrounding healthy tissue, accompanied by compensatory emphysema in the right lung

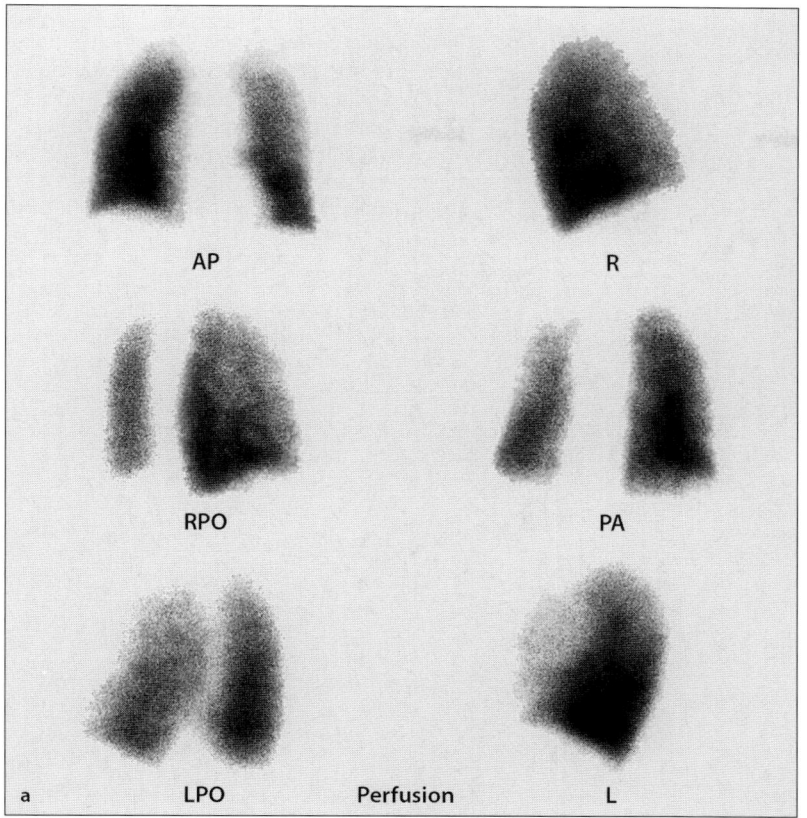

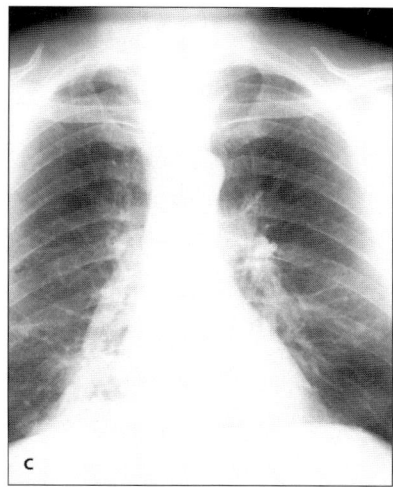

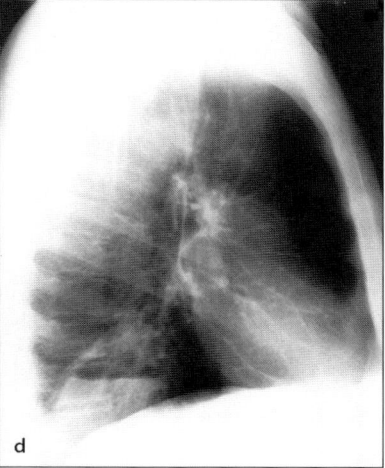

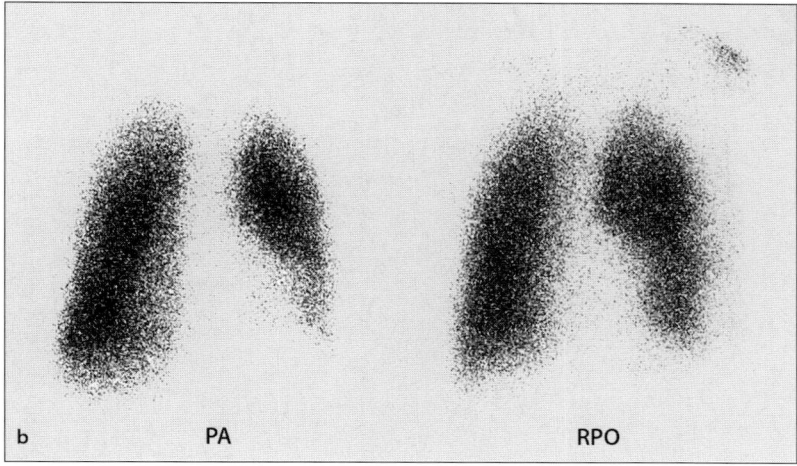

Fig. 2.20 a–d. Absent perfusion and ventilation in the right lower lung, caused by areas of bronchiectasis displacing the healthy tissue

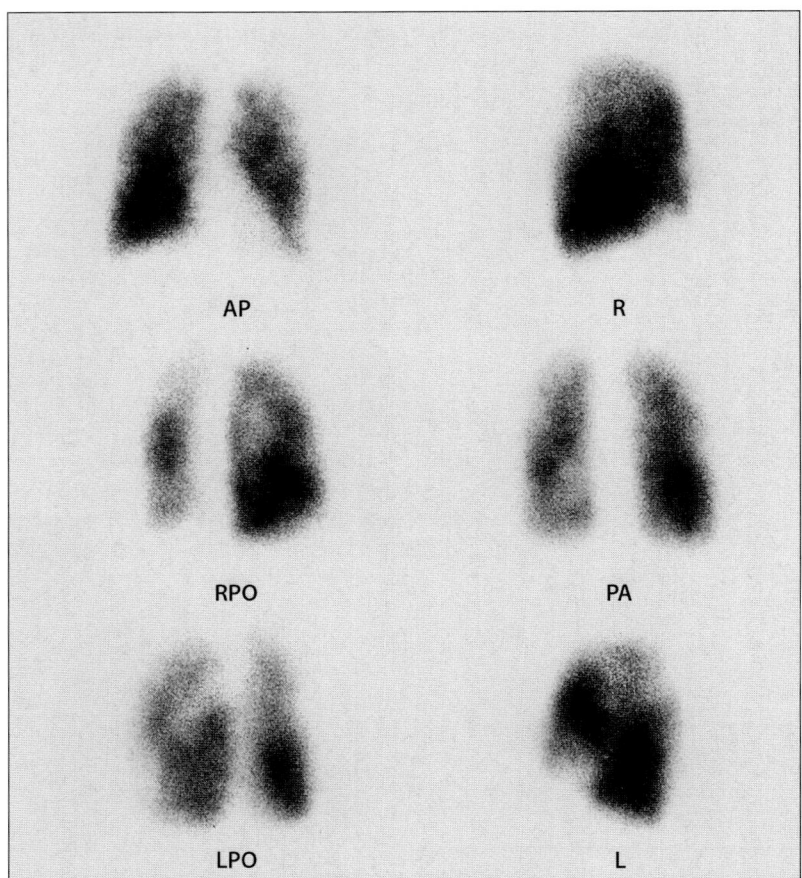

Fig. 2.21. Bilateral nonhomogeneous lung perfusion in a 30-year-old smoker with shallow respiratory excursions and a whistling sound audible over both lungs. The perfusion deficits are a result of spastic bronchitis

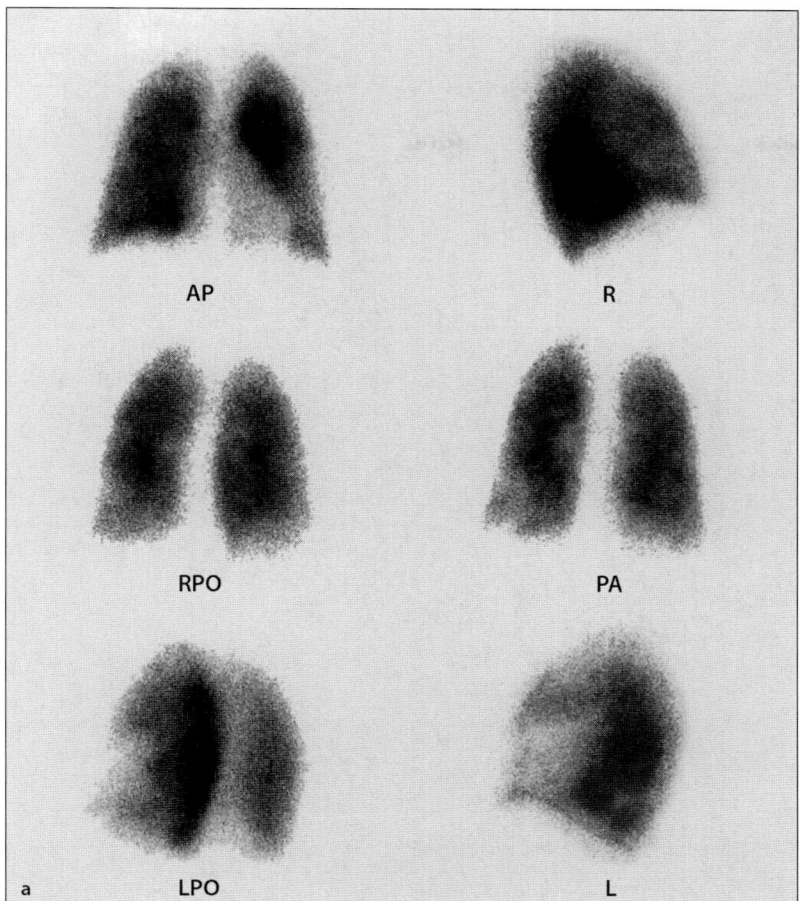

AP

R

RPO

PA

LPO

L

a

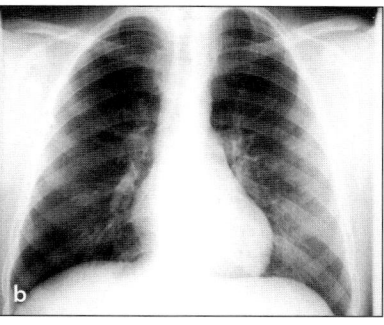

b

Fig. 2.22 a,b. Lung scan in an adolescent male with cyanosis, dyspnea, tachycardia, and vomiting shows widespread hypoperfusion chiefly involving the lower portion of each lung. The patient was diagnosed with Ceelen-Gellerstedt syndrome (hemosiderosis due to pulmonary hemorrhage)

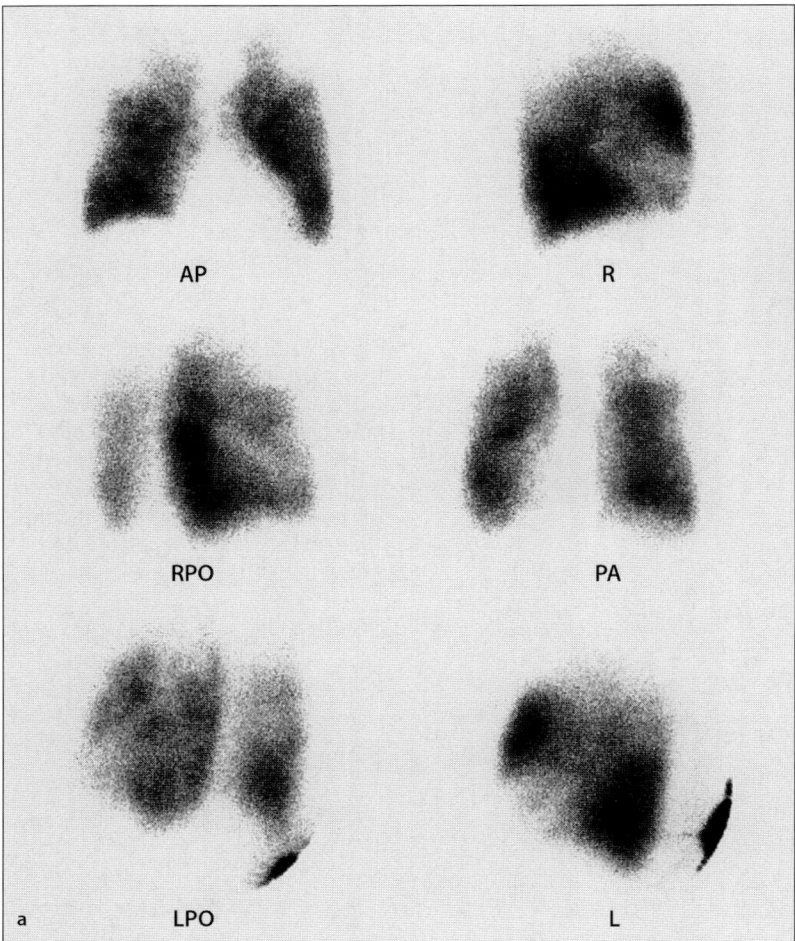

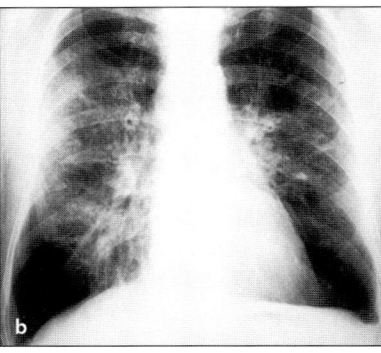

Fig. 2.23 a,b. A 45-year-old mineworker was admitted with cough, dyspnea, and cyanosis. The lung scan shows a disseminated pattern of coarse and fine perfusion defects chiefly involving the middle and upper lung zones. Pneumoconiosis with emphysema

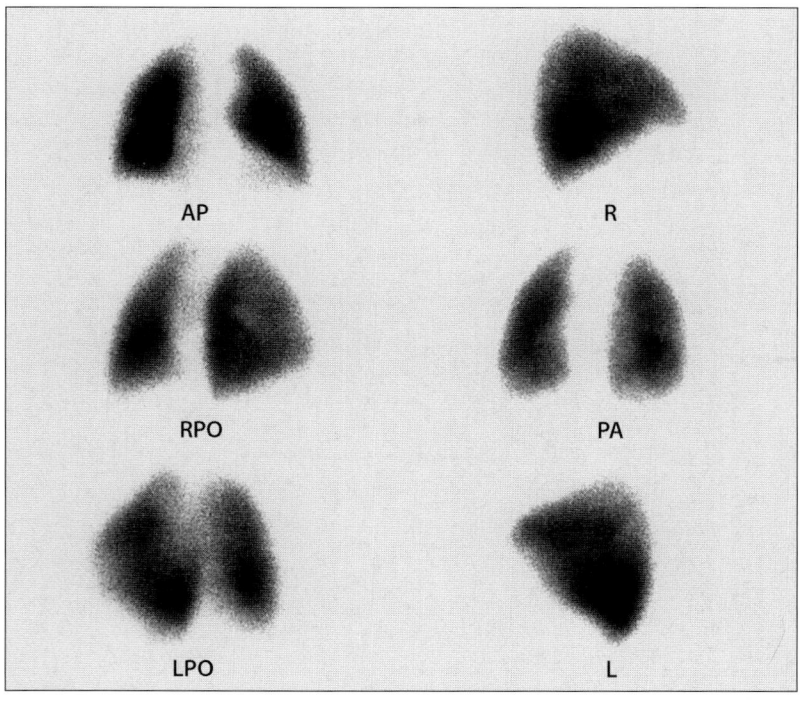

Fig. 2.24. Lung scan in a patient with hemoptysis and rhinitis shows a mild perfusion deficit in the posterosuperior left lung and anterosuperior right lung. Pulmonary vasculitis in Wegener syndrome

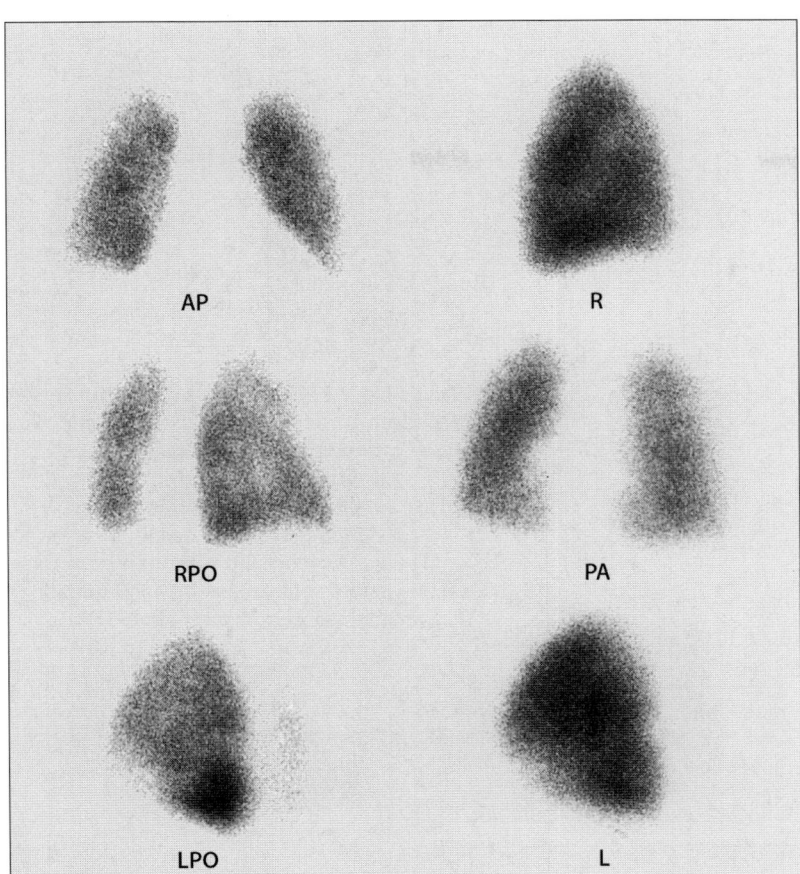

Fig. 2.25. Patient admitted with high fever shows widespread perfusion defects involving most of the lung tissue. Some of the defects appear as coarse patches. Goodpasture syndrome with extensive areas of necrotic lung parenchyma

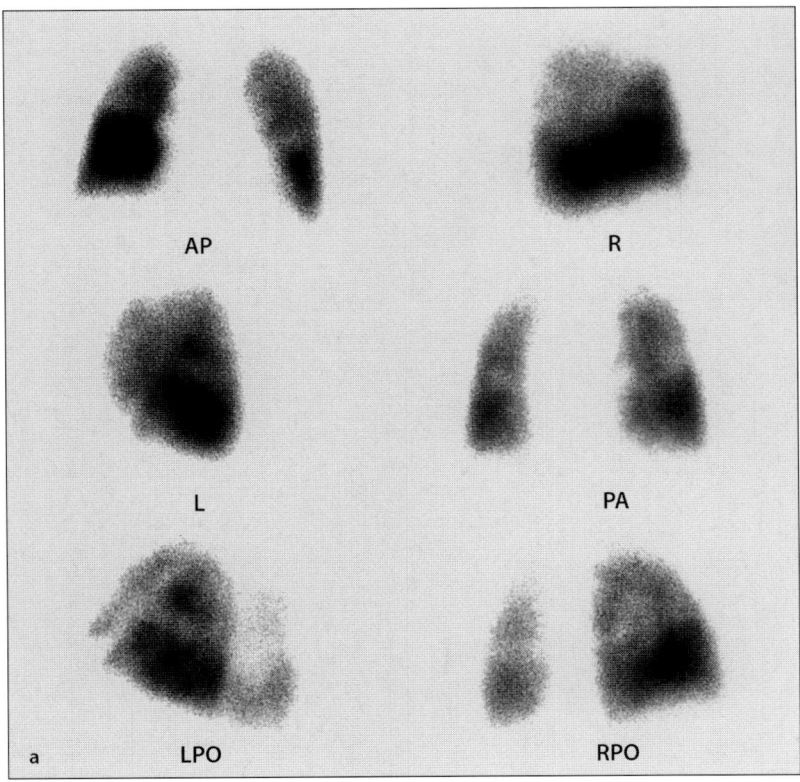

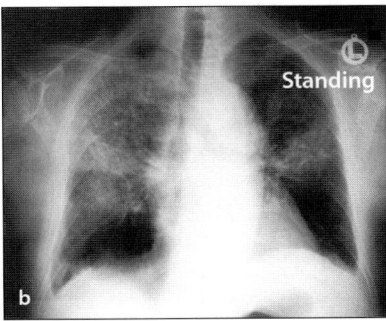

Fig. 2.26 a,b. Diffuse to patchy perfusion defects are found in the upper and midlung zones of an emaciated patient with cough and sputum production. Miliary tuberculosis

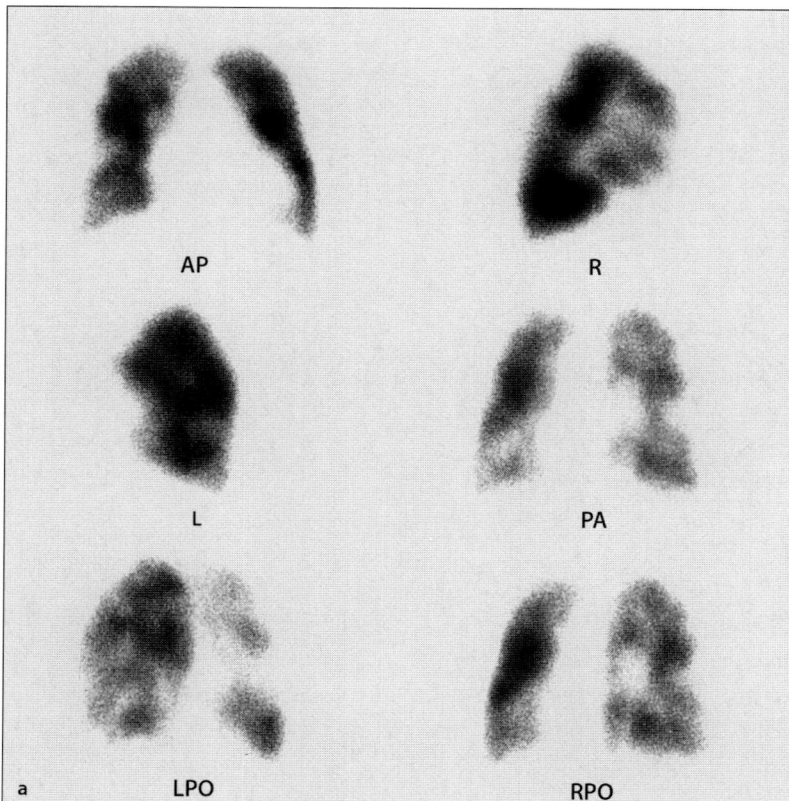

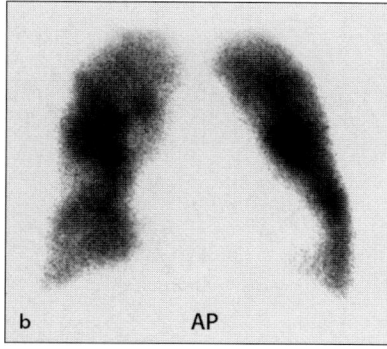

Fig. 2.27 a–d. Patient with a history of an aortic-mitral valve defect was admitted in a moribund state with dyspnea, tachyarrhythmia, and cold sweats. Lung scan shows general widening of the mediastinum and cardiac shadow and a nonhomogeneous pattern of tracer uptake. Pulmonary edema due to heart failure

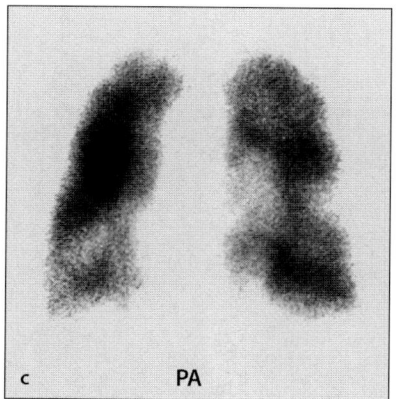

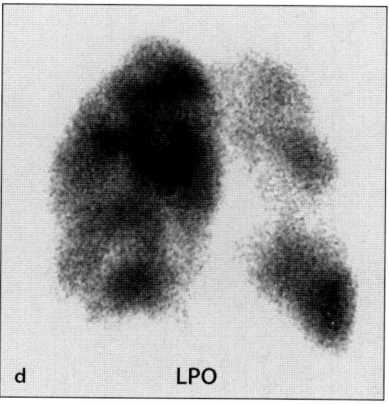

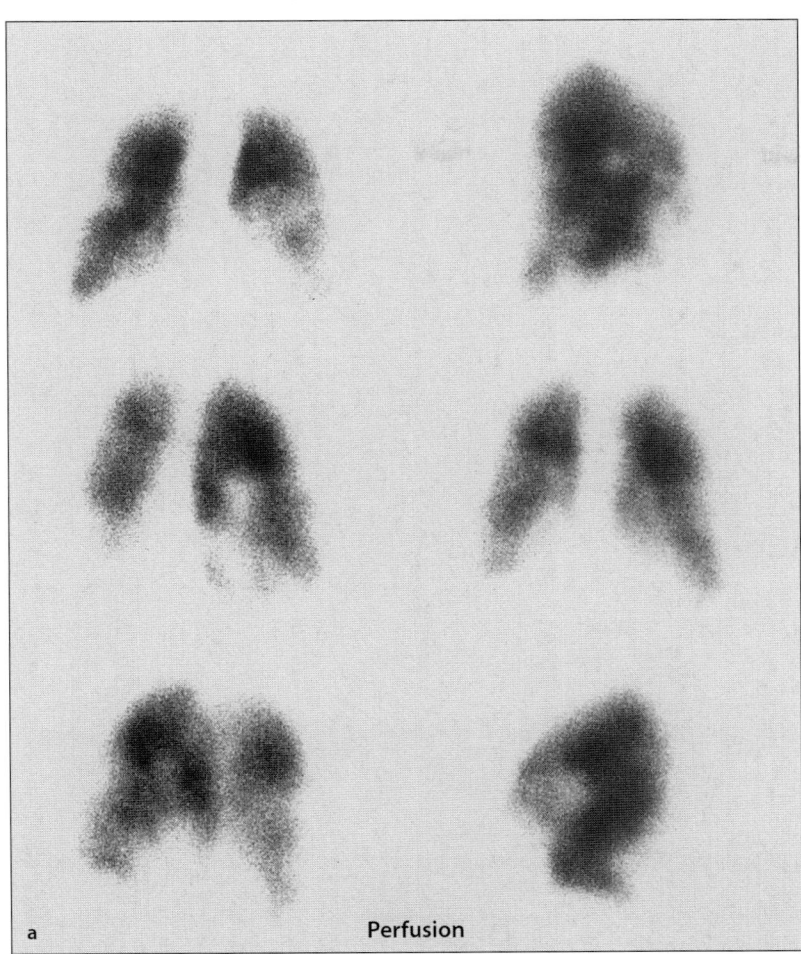

a   Perfusion

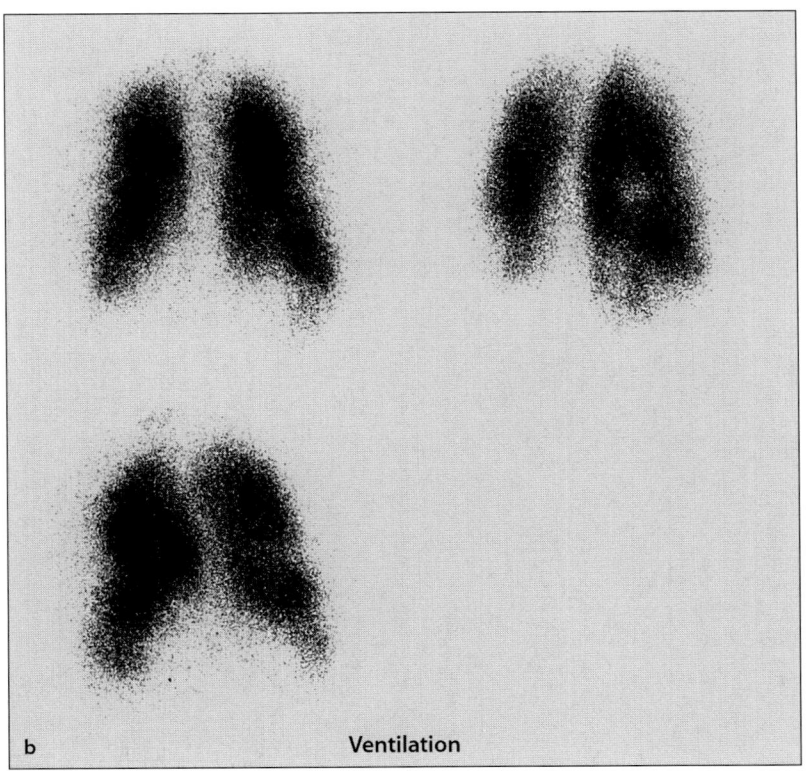

b   Ventilation

Fig. 2.28 a,b. Lung scan shows patchy areas of decreased activity in the middle and lower zones of both lungs, which are still well ventilated. The perfusion and ventilation scans also show a nodular defect projected over the major fissure of the right lung. Bilateral pneumonia with an encapsulated effusion in the right major fissure

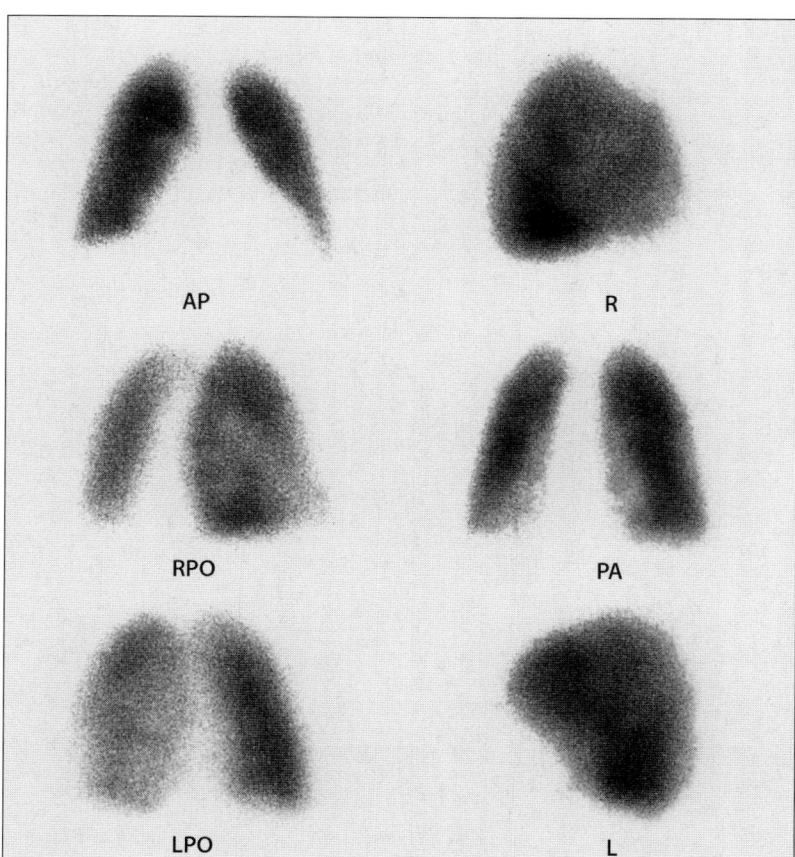

Fig. 2.29. Lung scan shows general widening of the cardiac shadow, decreased perihilar activity on both sides, straightened lower lung borders, and a relative accentuation of tracer uptake in the apical zones. Heart failure with central pulmonary congestion and upper-zone predominance of lung perfusion

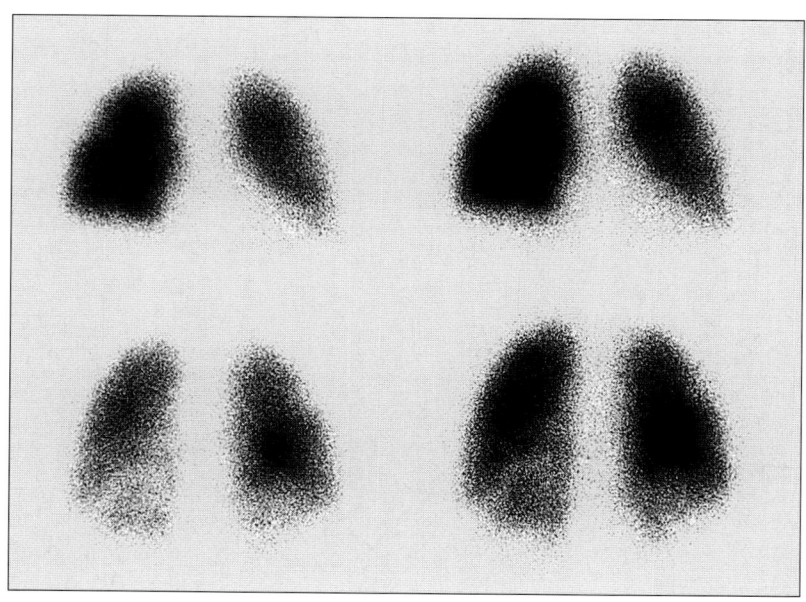

Fig. 2.30. Hypoperfusion in the posterobasal portion of the right lung with bilateral blunting of the costophrenic angles. Posterobasal pneumonia of the right lung with bilateral angle effusions

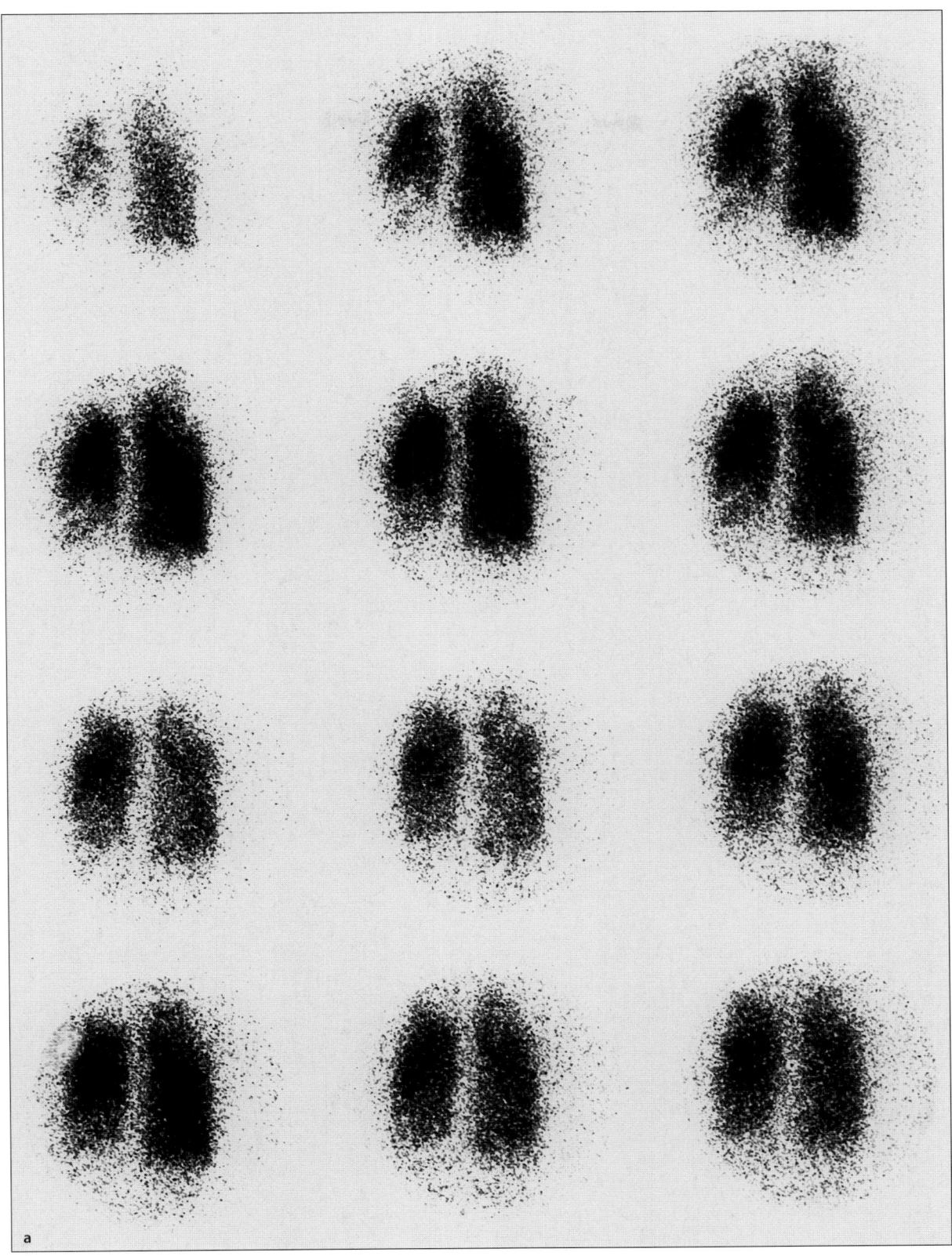

Fig. 2.31 a,b. A 38-year-old oral contraceptive user was admitted to the emergency room with painful tachypnea, cyanosis, and tachycardia. Perfusion lung scan shows multiple peripheral perfusion defects, some wedge-shaped, in both lungs with poor visualization of the left lung. Ventilation study shows good ventilation of both lungs but different exhalation times. The patient was diagnosed with multiple thromboemboli secondary to oral contraceptive use. Some of the emboli are peripheral and some are in the reperfusion stage

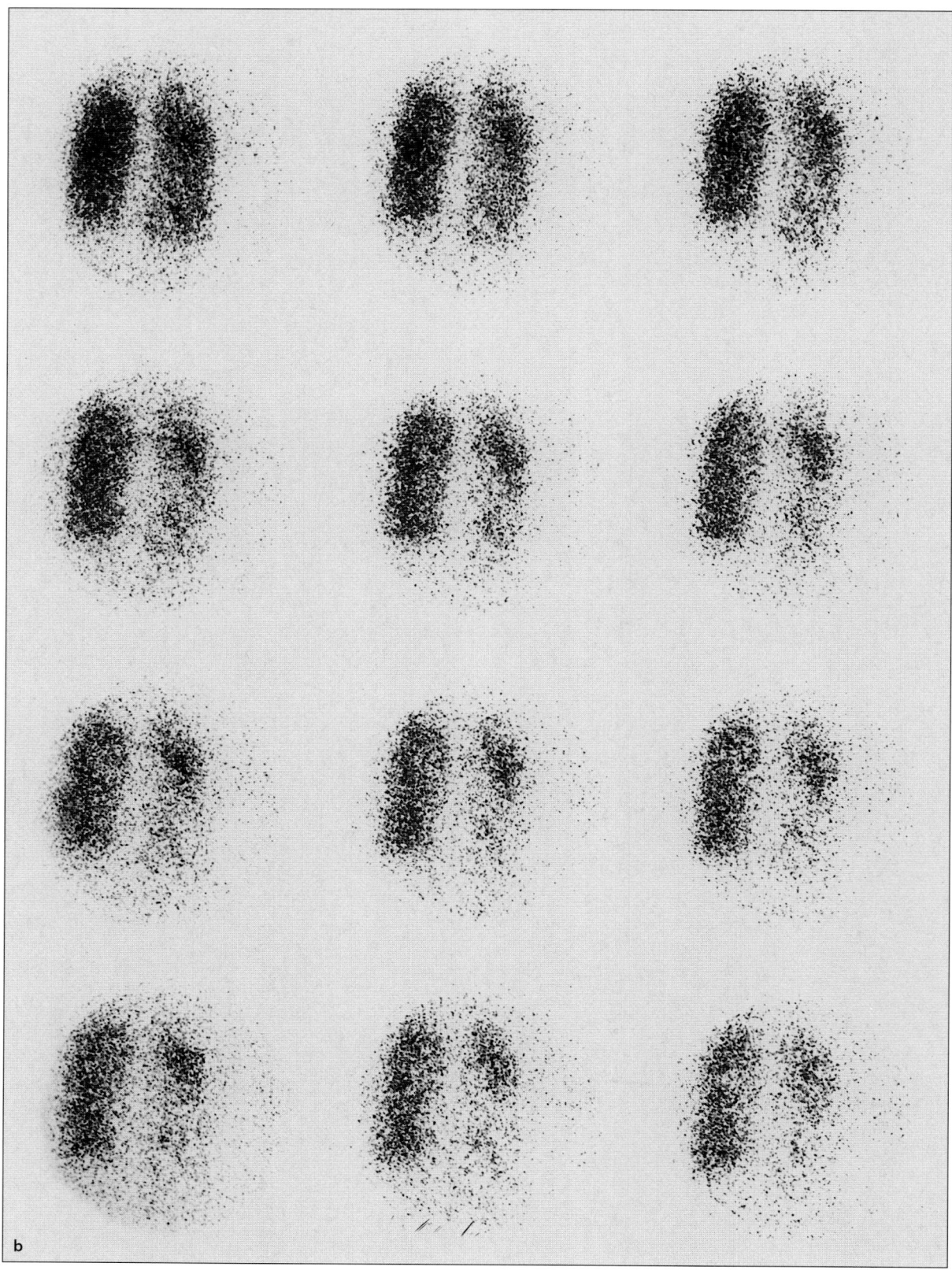

Fig. 2.31 a,b. A 38-year-old oral contraceptive user was admitted to the emergency room with painful tachypnea, cyanosis, and tachycardia. Perfusion lung scan shows multiple peripheral perfusion defects, some wedge-shaped, in both lungs with poor visualization of the left lung. Ventilation study shows good ventilation of both lungs but different exhalation times. The patient was diagnosed with multiple thromboemboli secondary to oral contraceptive use. Some of the emboli are peripheral and some are in the reperfusion stage

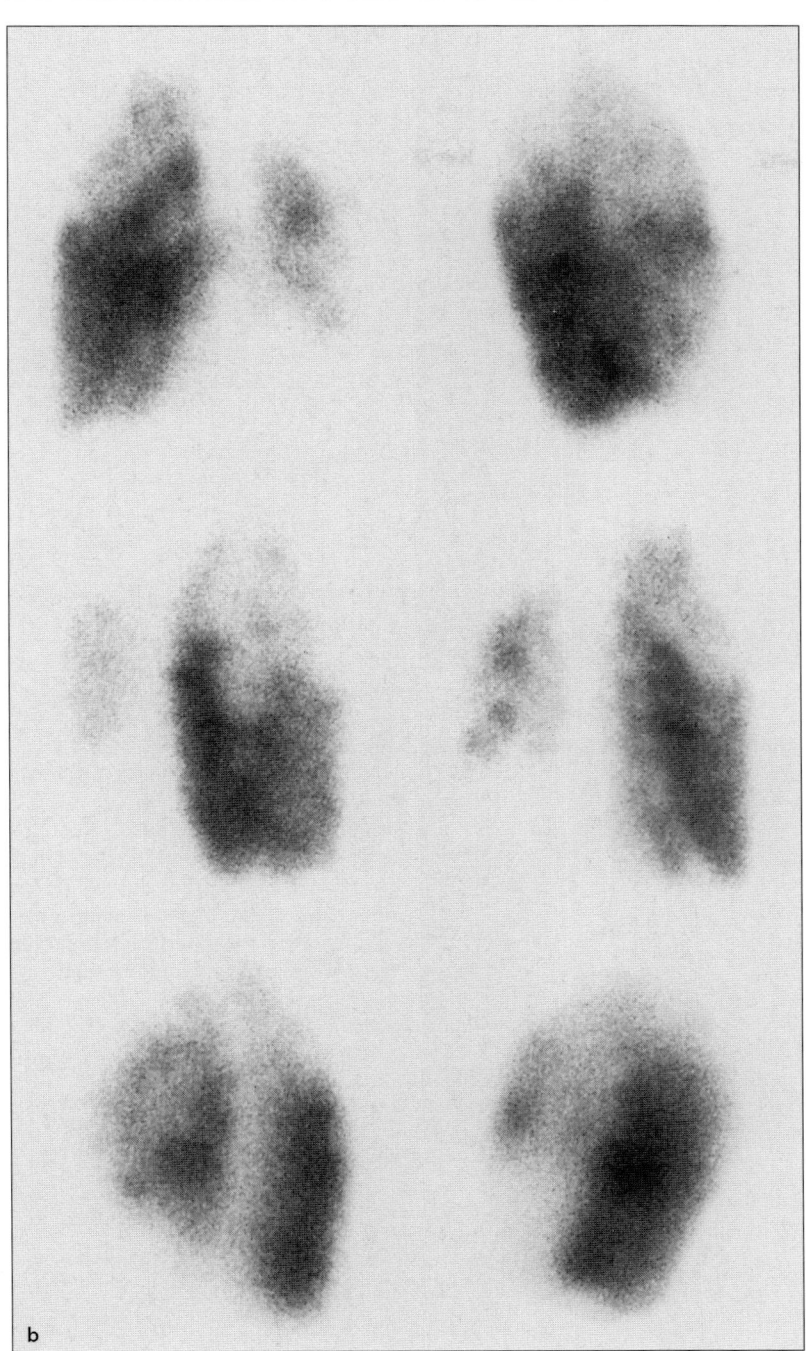

Fig. 2.31 b. *Continued*

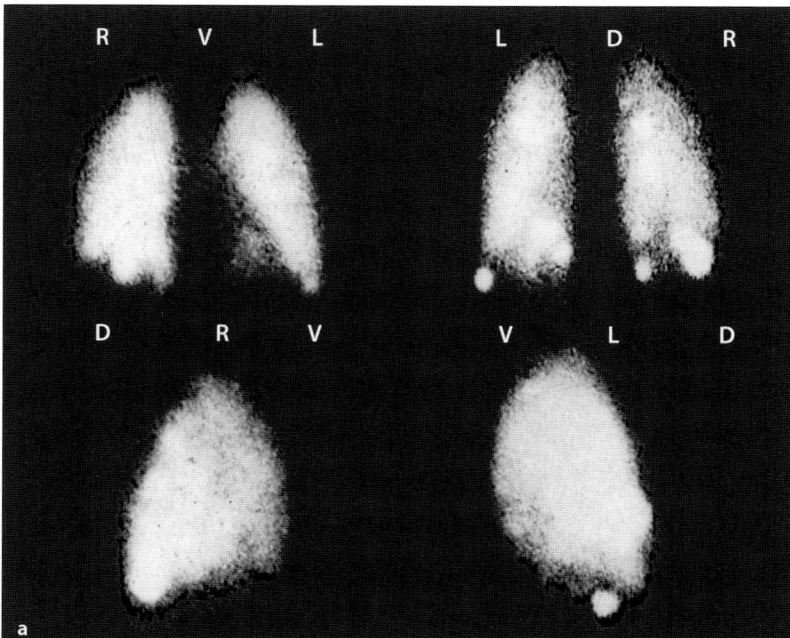

Fig. 2.32. Lung scan demonstrates hot spots in the posterobasal and lateral portions of the left lung and the mediobasal right lung. These areas represent technical artifacts without pathologic significance

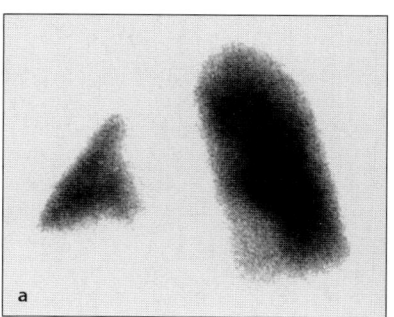

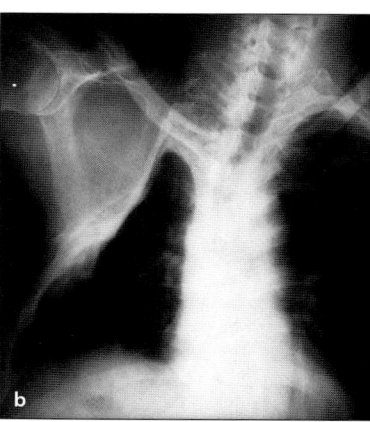

Fig. 2.33. a Perfusion scan shows a perfusion defect involving almost the entire right lung. Only a small mediobasal portion of the lung is visualized. **b** Chest radiograph shows plombage material that was inserted during World War II for the treatment of tuberculosis. The perfusion defect was caused by pressure from the plombage mass

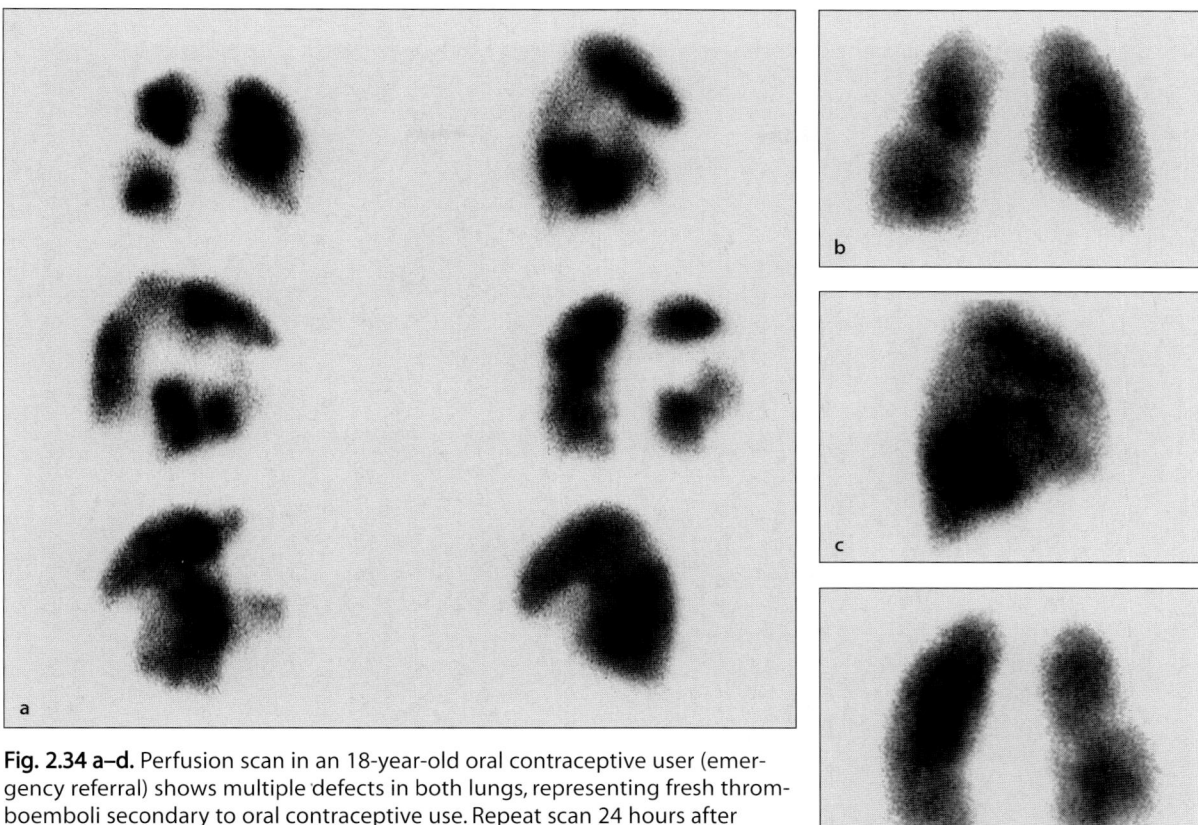

Fig. 2.34 a–d. Perfusion scan in an 18-year-old oral contraceptive user (emergency referral) shows multiple defects in both lungs, representing fresh thromboemboli secondary to oral contraceptive use. Repeat scan 24 hours after treatment shows almost complete reperfusion

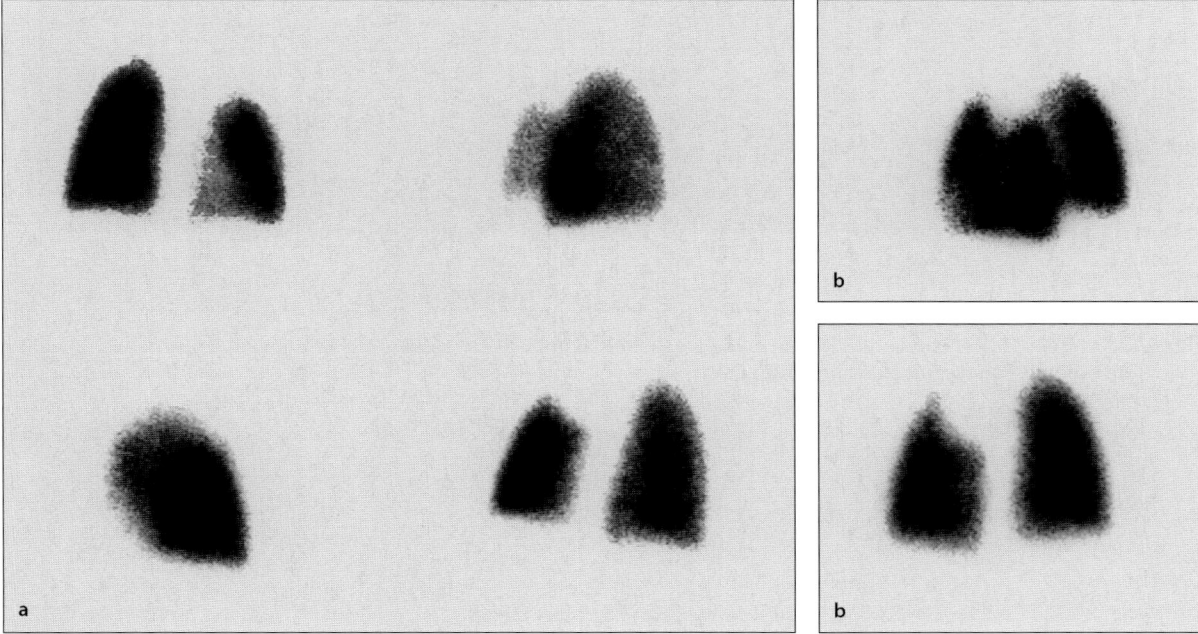

Fig. 2.35 a,b. Perfusion defect involving segments 1 and 2 and part of segment 3 in the left lung. Embolism of the left upper lobe

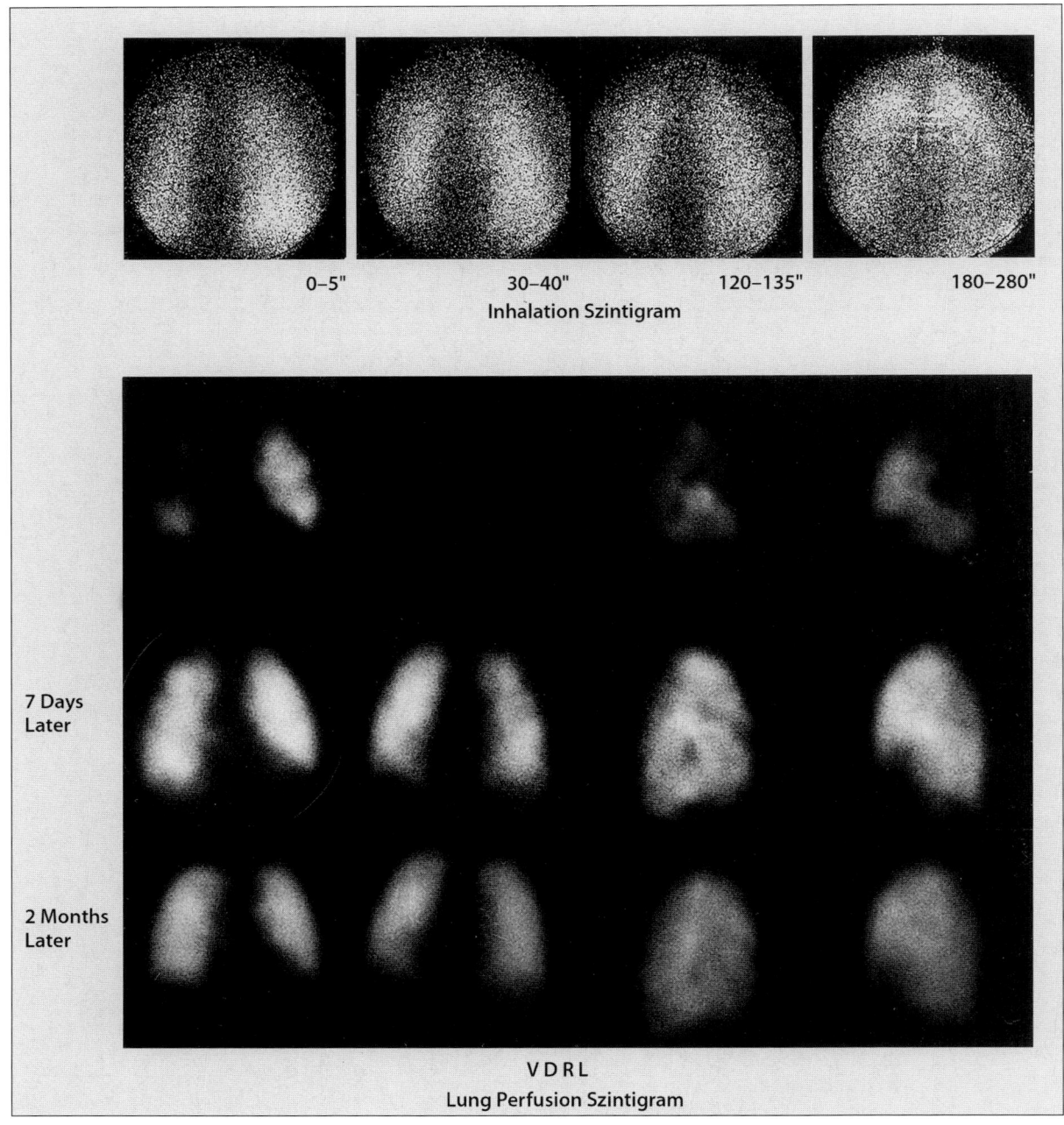

0–5"   30–40"   120–135"   180–280"
Inhalation Szintigram

7 Days
Later

2 Months
Later

VDRL
Lung Perfusion Szintigram

Fig. 2.36. Ventilation-perfusion scan demonstrates fresh emboli in both lungs secondary to thrombosis in the lower leg. Follow-ups showed good reperfusion in both lungs

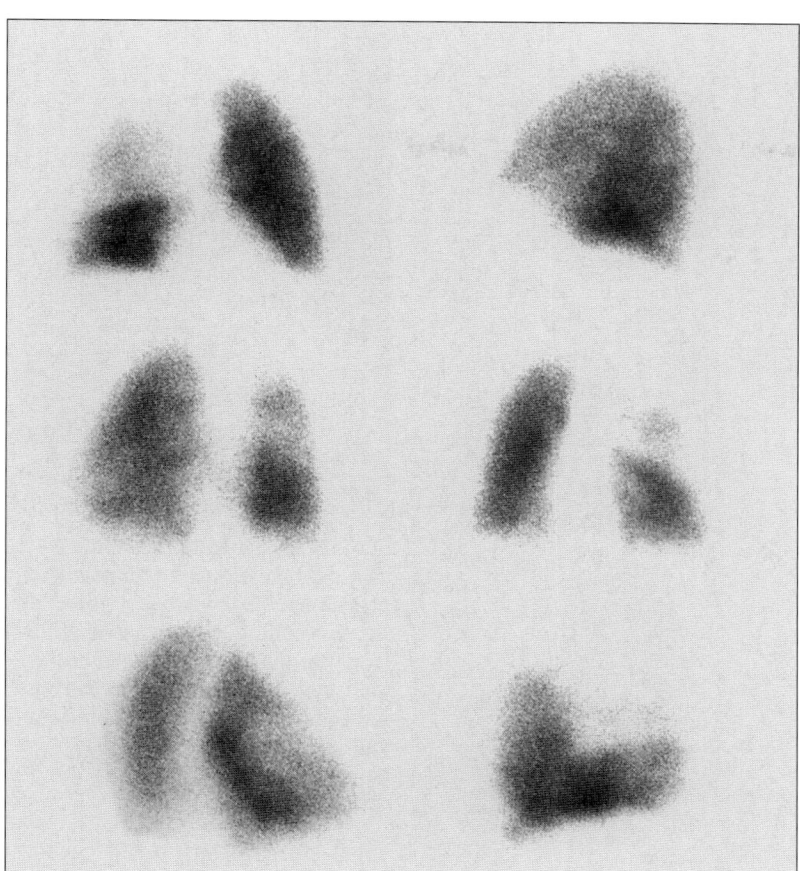

Fig. 2.37. Perfusion scan in a patient who previously underwent a partial upper lobectomy of the right lung shows a perfusion defect involving segments 1 and 3 of the right upper lobe with marked hypoperfusion of segments 4 and 5. The scan also shows bilateral nonhomogeneous tracer distribution and flattened diaphragmatic leaflets. The changes are due to fresh emboli in segments 4 and 5 of the right lung and bilateral compensatory emphysema of the remaining lung tissue

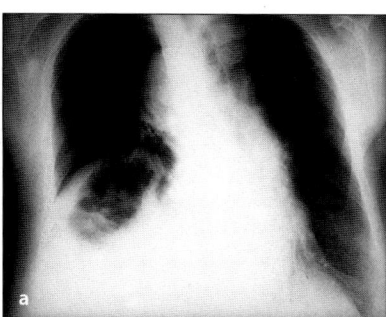

Fig. 2.38 a,b. Lung scan shows a perfusion defect involving all of the middle and lower zones of the right lung and a nonhomogeneous, somewhat patchy activity pattern in the left lung. The perfusion defect is caused by compression of the right lung by a diaphragmatic hernia (herniating colon), leading to compensatory emphysema in the left lung

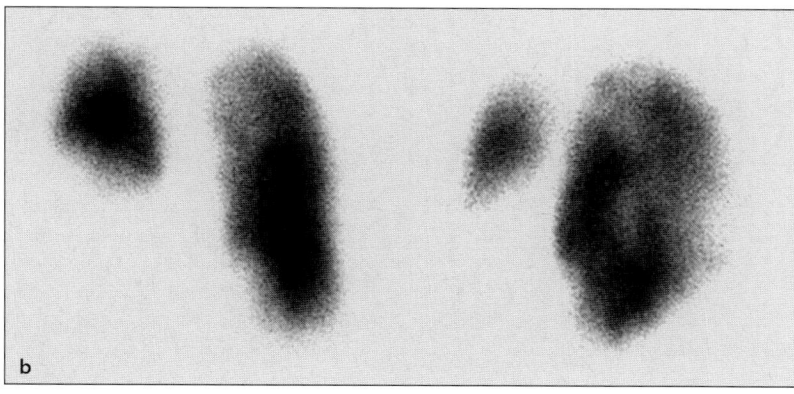

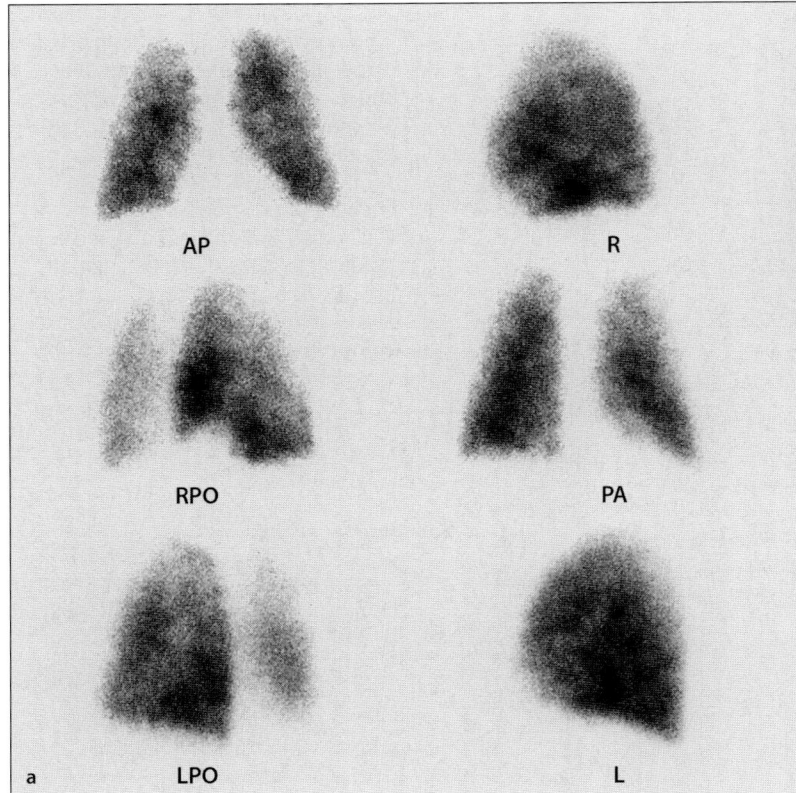

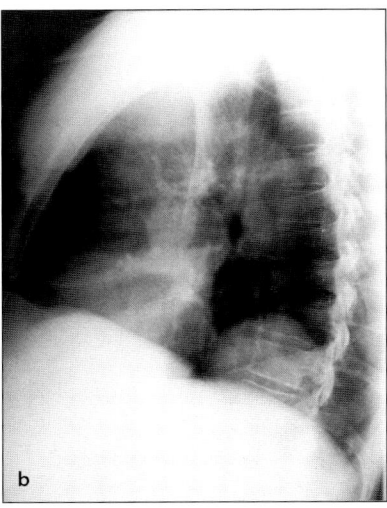

Fig. 2.39 a,b. Perfusion scan in a 71-year-old man evaluated for pain and pressure in the lower half of the chest shows a combined patchy and nodular pattern of tracer uptake in both lungs and a curved defect in the posterobasal portion of the left lung. Bullous emphysema. The perfusion defect in the left lung is caused by a supraphrenic mass

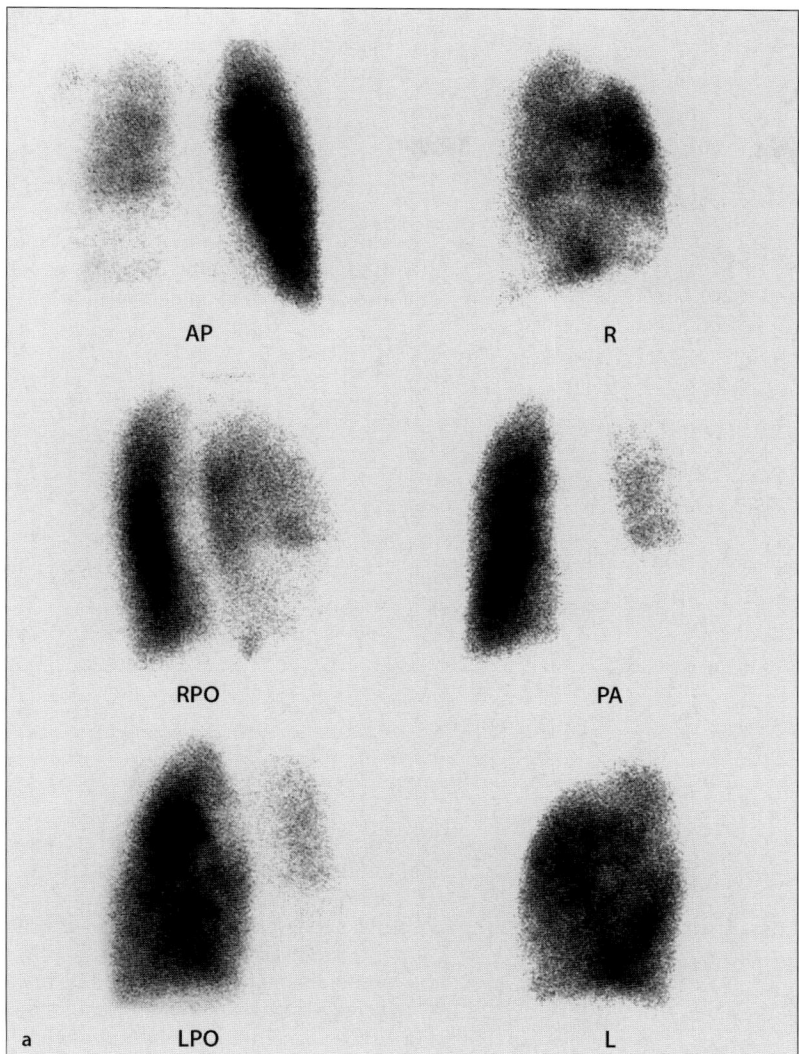

AP

R

RPO

PA

a   LPO

L

Fig. 2.40 a,b. Ventilation and perfusion scans show an almost complete absence of function in the right lung. There is minimal uptake in the upper zone, and the faint area of basal uptake shows a straight linear boundary with the lung above it. These findings are caused by a peripheral effusion ("mantle effusion") over the right lung, compressing the lung tissue and also causing radiation absorption

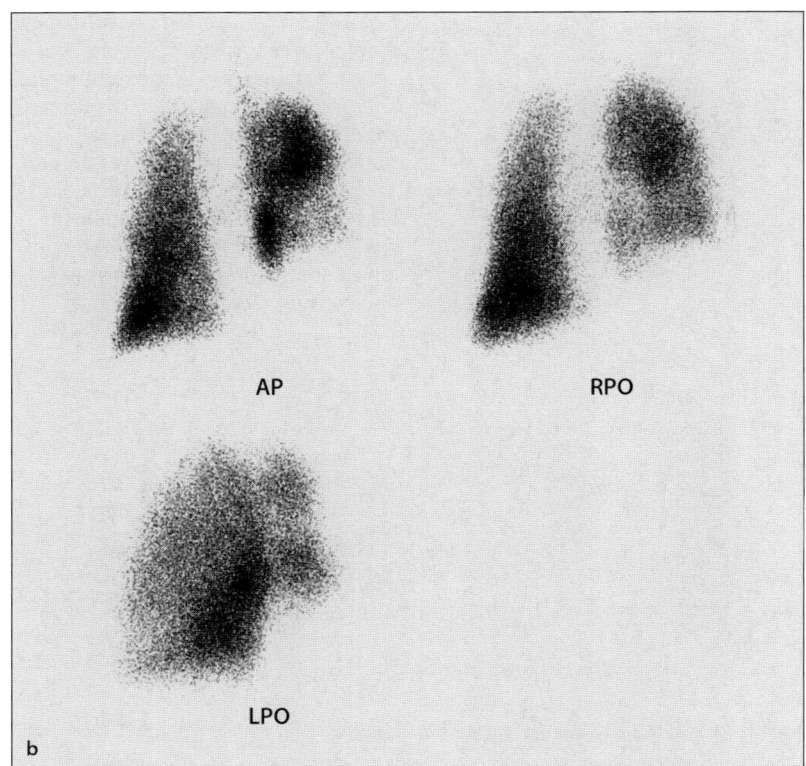

Fig. 2.40 a,b. Ventilation and perfusion scans show an almost complete absence of function in the right lung. There is minimal uptake in the upper zone, and the faint area of basal uptake shows a straight linear boundary with the lung above it. These findings are caused by a peripheral effusion ("mantle effusion") over the right lung, compressing the lung tissue and also causing radiation absorption

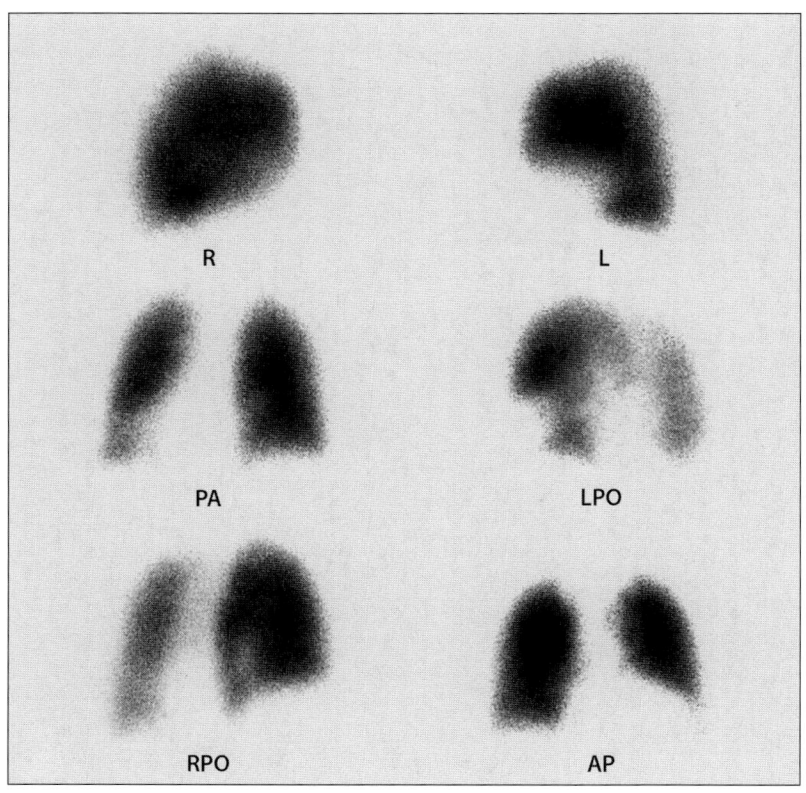

Fig. 2.41. Perfusion scan in an emaciated, dyspneic elderly man had to be performed in the supine position. The LPO and left lateral views show absent and diminished perfusion posteriorly and in the major fissure with a relative increase of activity in the apical zones (upper-zone predominance of perfusion). Posterobasal hypoperfusion is noted in the right lung. Cytology indicated a tuberculous pleural effusion. The right-sided angle effusion is nonspecific and is probably due to heart failure

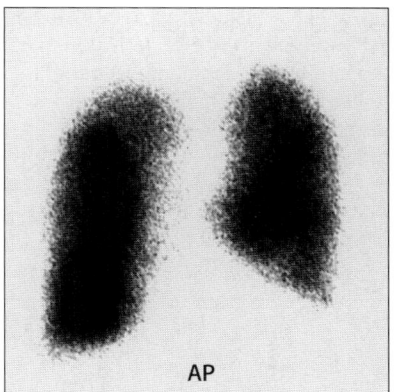 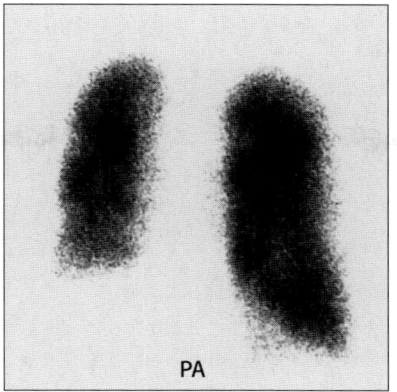 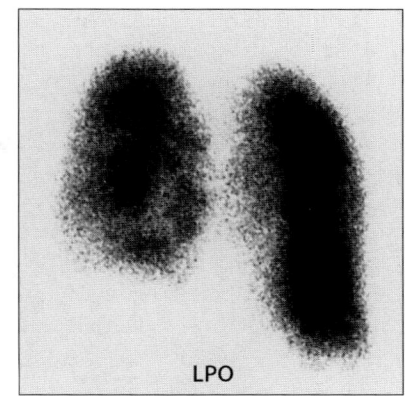

Fig. 2.42. Position-related discrepancy in the heights of the pulmonary apices. There is apparent widening of the cardiac shadow, and the lower part of the left lung is not visualized. These changes are caused by elevation of the diaphragm. The right lung is well perfused

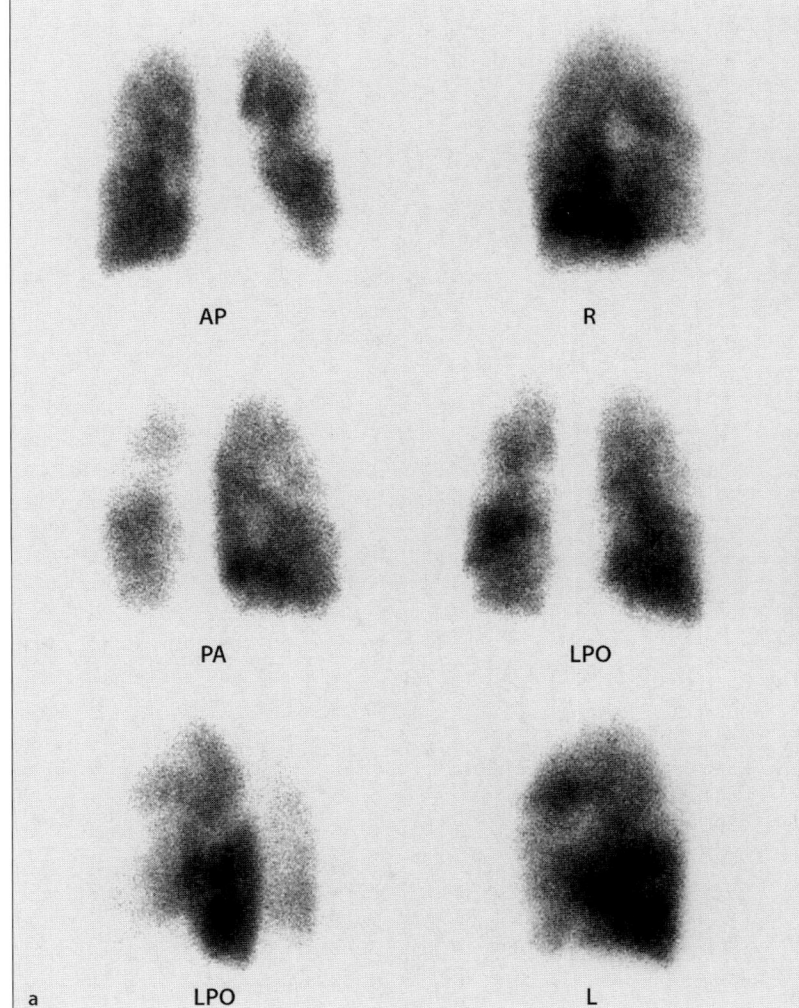

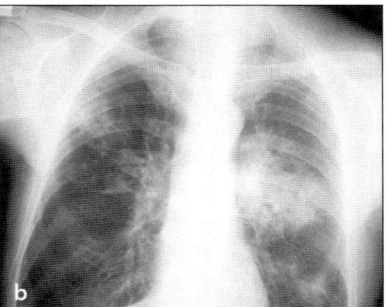
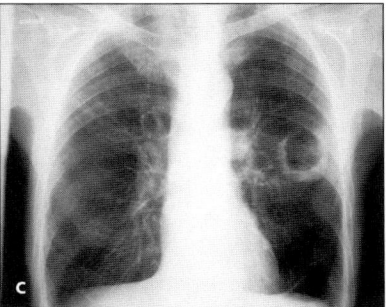

Fig. 2.43 a–c. Follow-ups in a patient with a four-year history of tuberculosis and intermittent sputum production. **a** Perfusion scan shows multiple areas of decreased activity mainly affecting the upper and middle zones of both lungs and including several nodular defects. The decreased activity results from scarring and emphysema formation associated with the remission of miliary tuberculosis. The nodular perfusion defects are due to cavitation

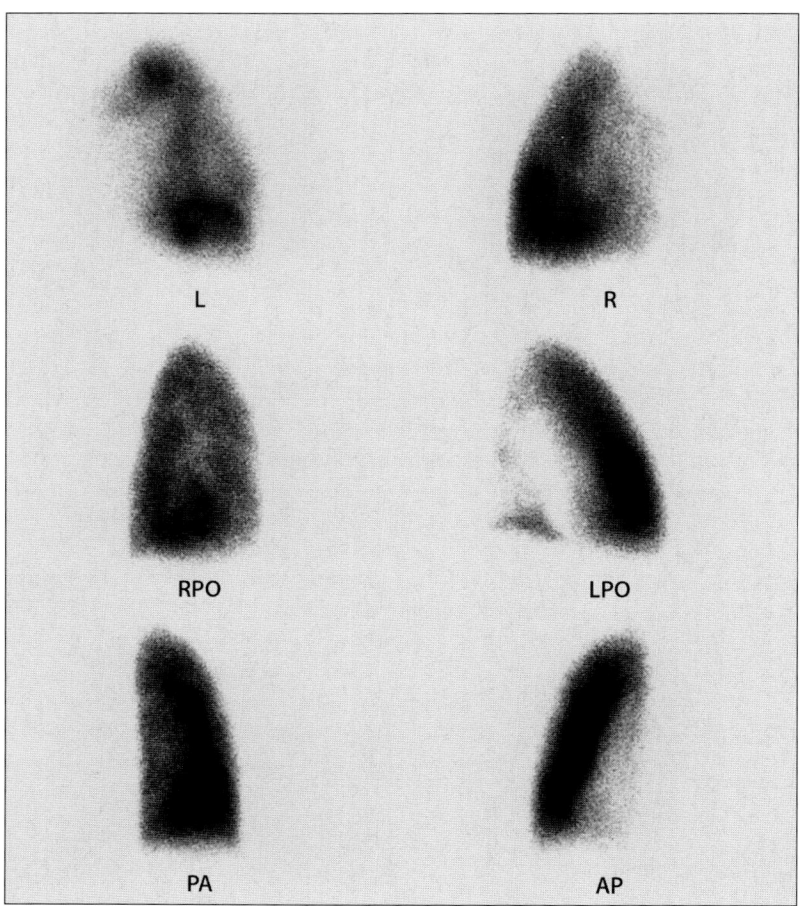

Fig. 2.44. Perfusion scan demonstrates a complete absence of perfusion in the left lung in a patient evaluated for severe dyspnea. The mediastinum is displaced to the right. Left-sided pneumothorax

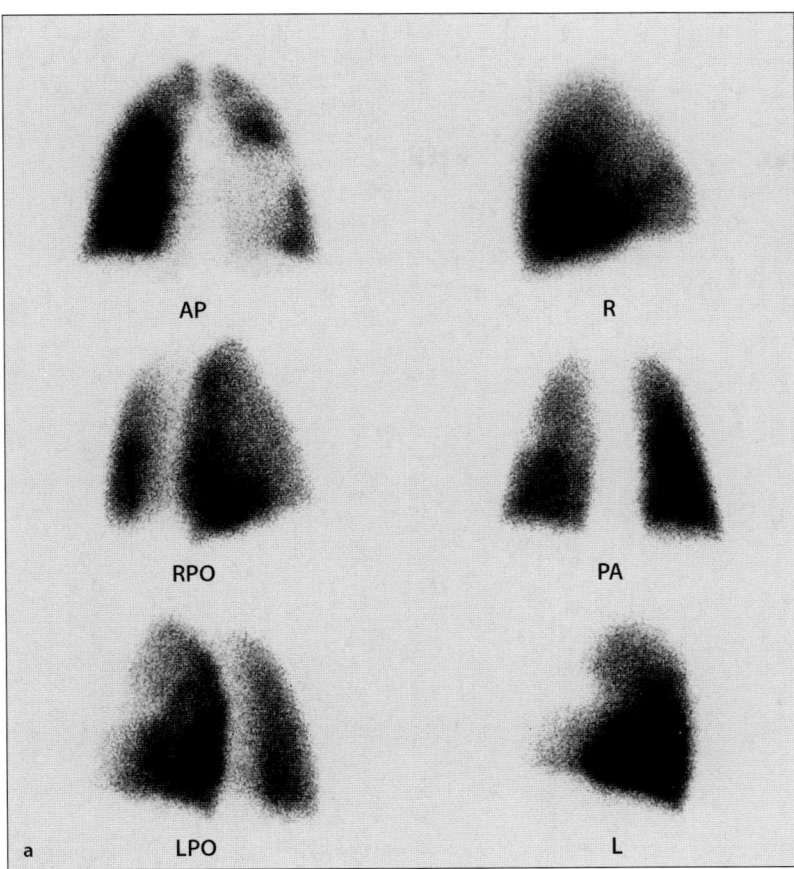

AP

R

RPO

PA

LPO

L

a

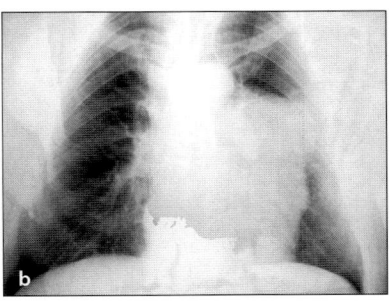

b

Fig. 2.45 a,b. Most of the upper lobe of the left lung is devoid of perfusion, and only a portion of segment 1 is visualized in the perfusion scan. The right lung and the lower lobe of the left lung are homogeneously perfused, but the diaphragmatic leaflets are obscured. These findings suggest a mass lesion in the upper lobar region of the left lung, with no evidence of metastasis or extension to the contralateral side. Bronchial carcinoma with compensatory emphysema

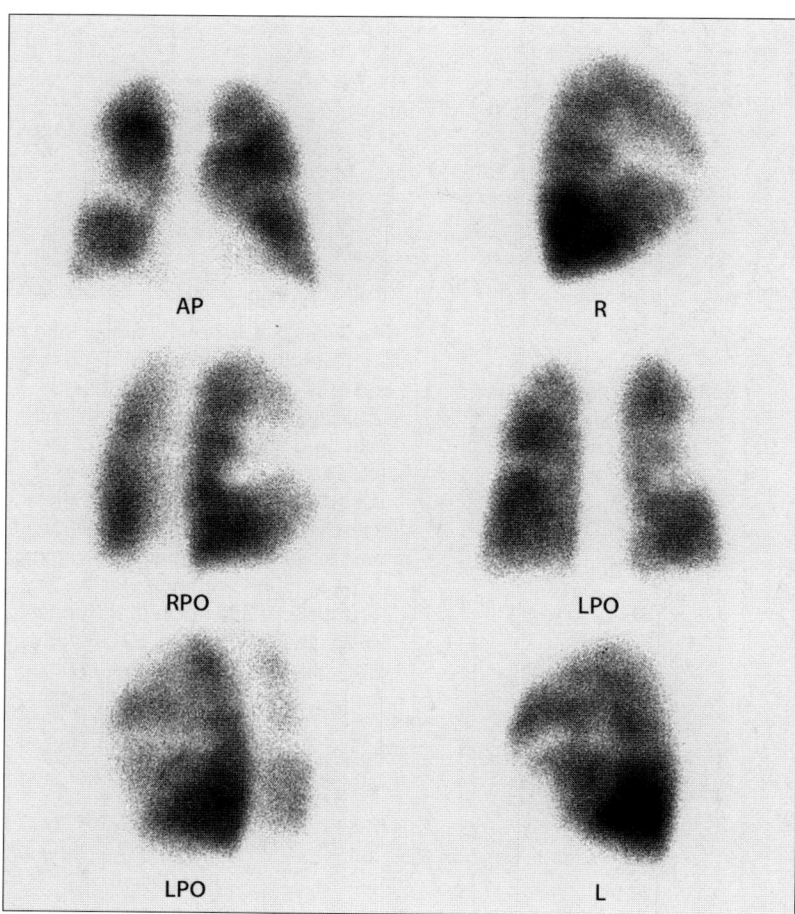

AP

R

RPO

LPO

LPO

L

Fig. 2.46. This scan shows a substantial perfusion defect involving the upper and middle zones of both lungs, particularly the right. The cause is a central bronchial carcinoma that originated in the right lung and has metastasized to the opposite side. Lymph node metastases are also present

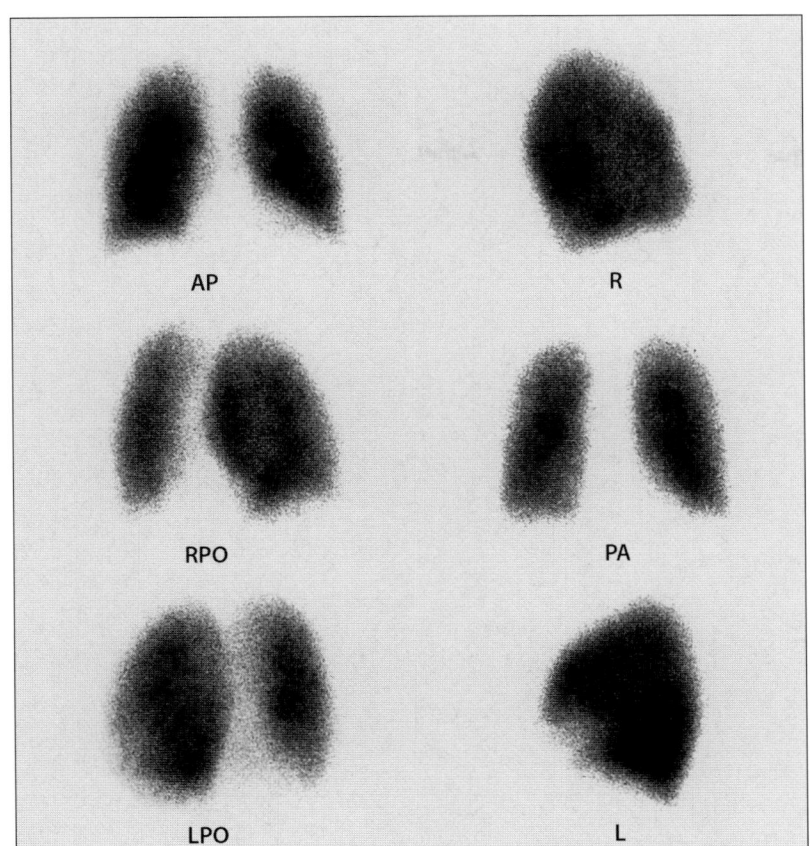

Fig. 2.47. Local neoplastic thickening has caused a perfusion defect in the posterobasal portion of the right lung. The rest of the parenchyma is unaffected

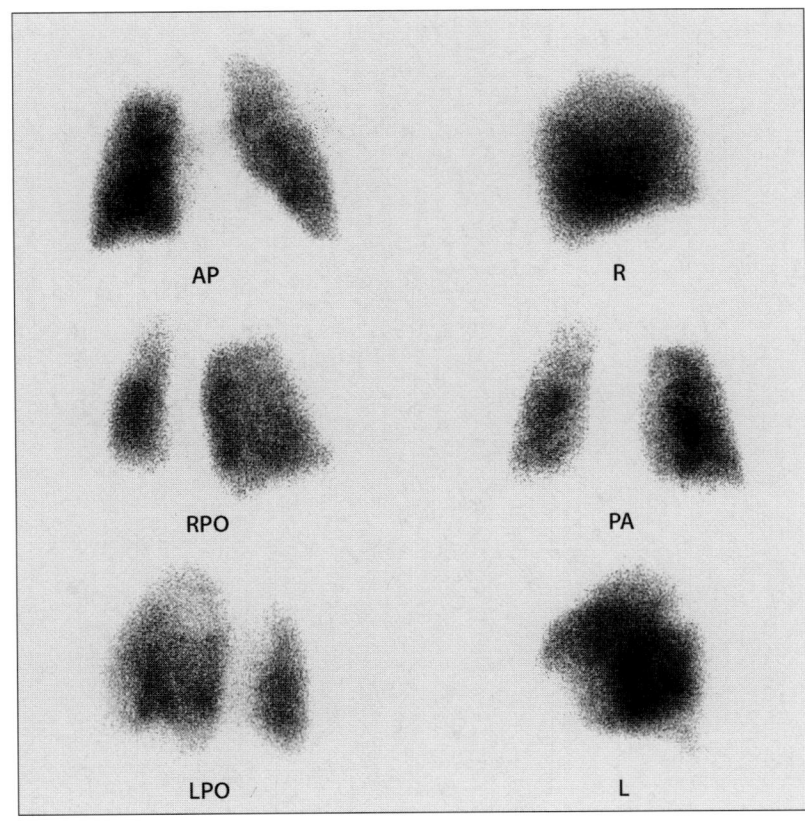

Fig. 2.48. Lung scan shows a perfusion defect in the apical portion of the right lung and a nonhomogeneous pattern of uptake in the left lung. Right-sided Pancoast tumor and emphysema

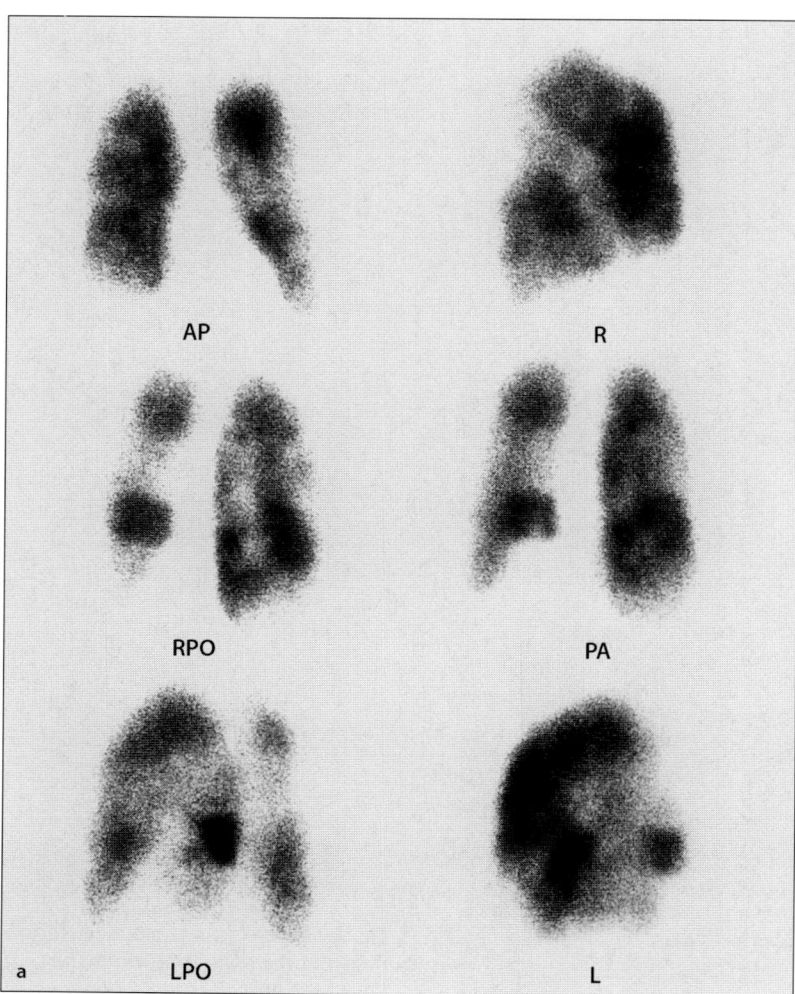

a   AP   R

RPO   PA

LPO   L

Fig. 2.49 a,b. Scattered islands of lung tissue are still perfused and can just be visualized on ventilation and perfusion scans. The defects are caused by a central mass lesion, identified as anaplastic carcinoma

Fig. 2.49 b

PA

PRO

b   LPO

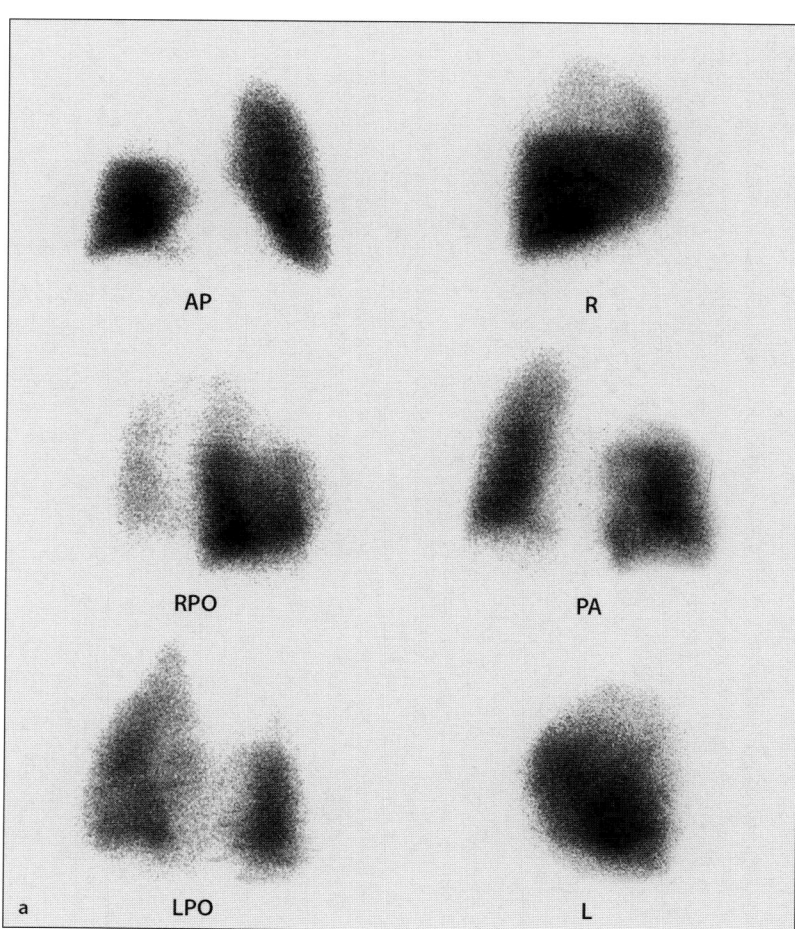

AP

R

RPO

PA

a   LPO

L

Fig. 2.50 a,b. Perfusion defect in the right lung caused by upper lobar carcinoma. Follow-up at one year (postirradiation) shows slight regression

Fig. 2.50 b

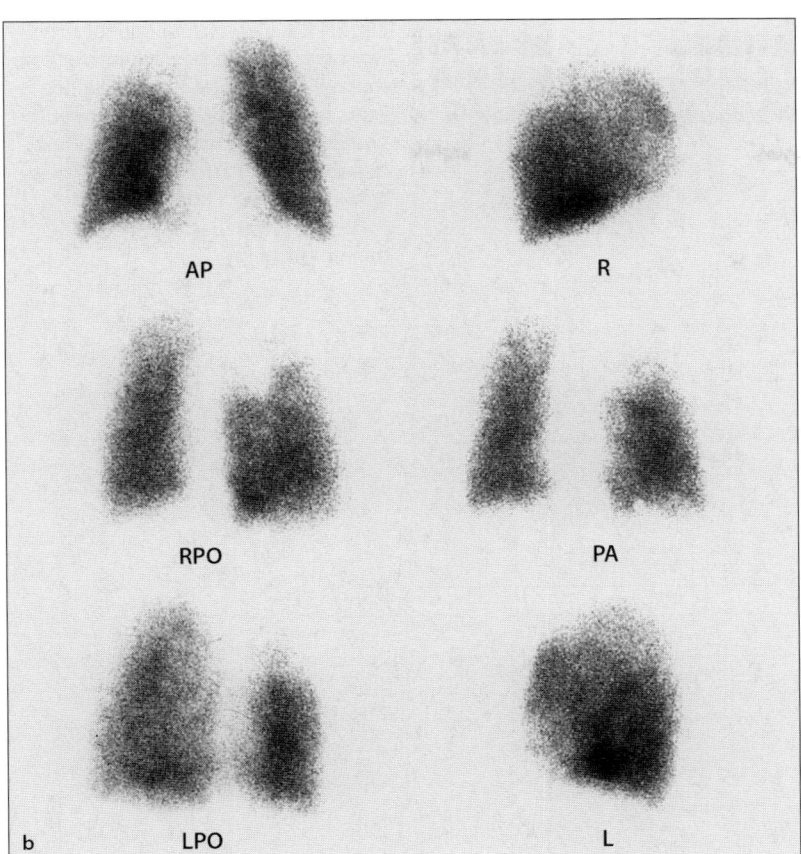

AP   R

RPO   PA

b   LPO   L

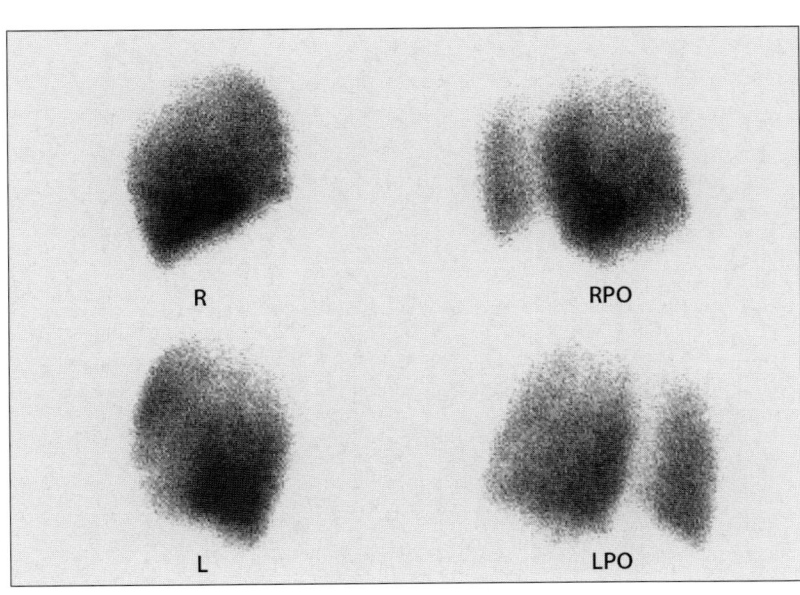

R   RPO

L   LPO

Fig. 2.51. A 59-year-old patient underwent surgery and postoperative radiotherapy for tonsillar carcinoma two years before. He presented now with swallowing difficulties and poor exercise tolerance. Perfusion scan shows hypoperfusion in both upper lung zones, interpreted as late sequelae of the radiotherapy

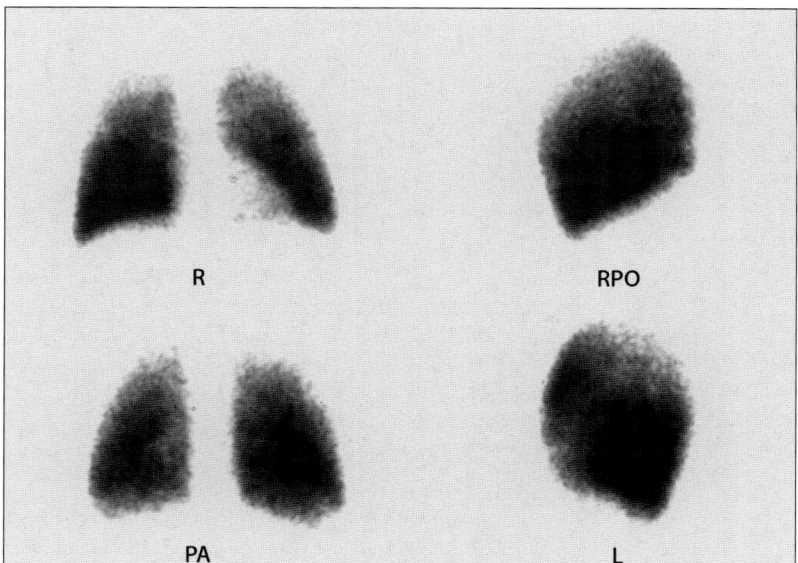

Fig. 2.51. A 59-year-old patient underwent surgery and postoperative radiotherapy for tonsillar carcinoma two years before. He presented now with swallowing difficulties and poor exercise tolerance. Perfusion scan shows hypoperfusion in both upper lung zones, interpreted as late sequelae of the radiotherapy

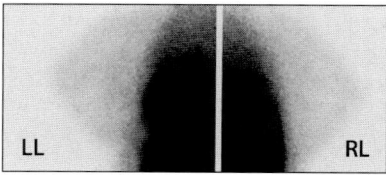

Fig. 2.52. During a routine examination, this patient complained of tenderness in both breasts. Radionuclide scan shows homogeneous breast uptake with no abnormal findings

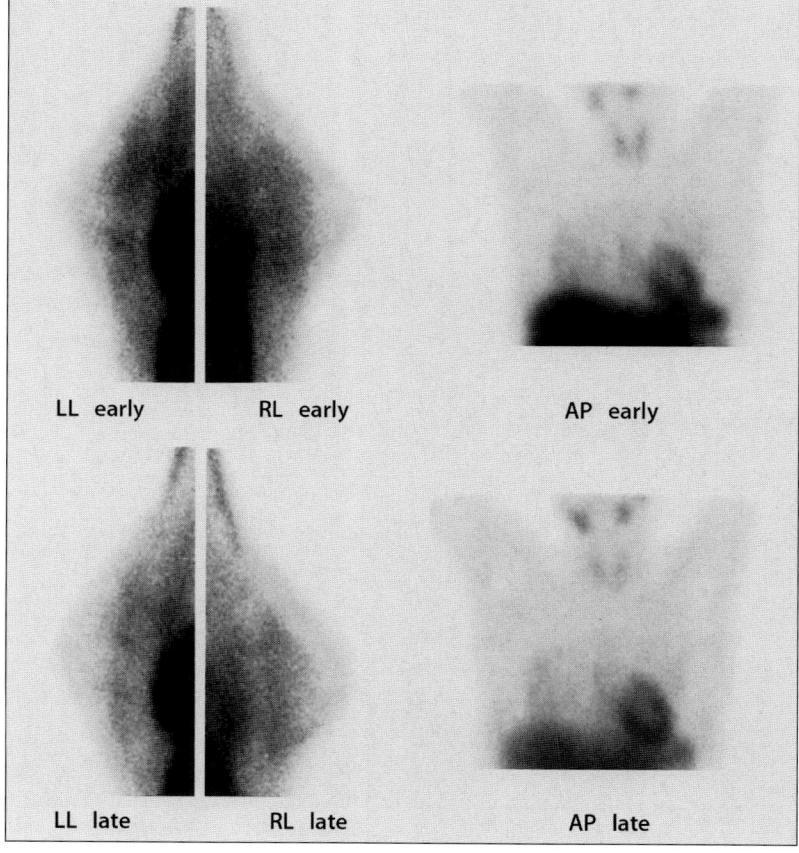

Fig. 2.53. This patient presented with bilateral breast tenderness with slight palpable firmness but no focal abnormalities. Radionuclide breast scan shows a striate to diffuse pattern of moderately increased radionuclide uptake in the relatively small breasts, consistent with fibrocystic change

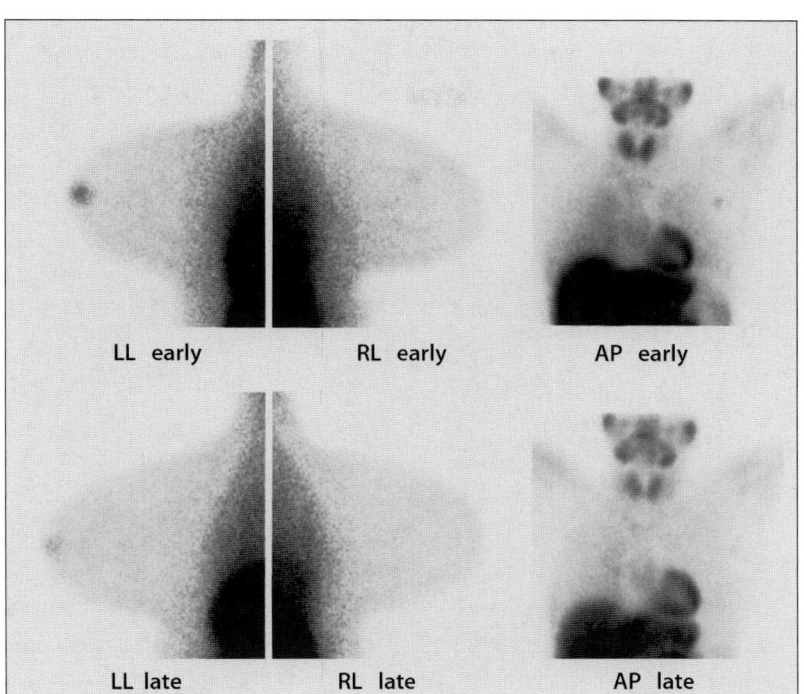

Fig. 2.54. This patient noticed an area of firmness deep to her left nipple. Breast scan demonstrates a well-defined retroareolar focal lesion. The suspicion of carcinoma was confirmed histologically

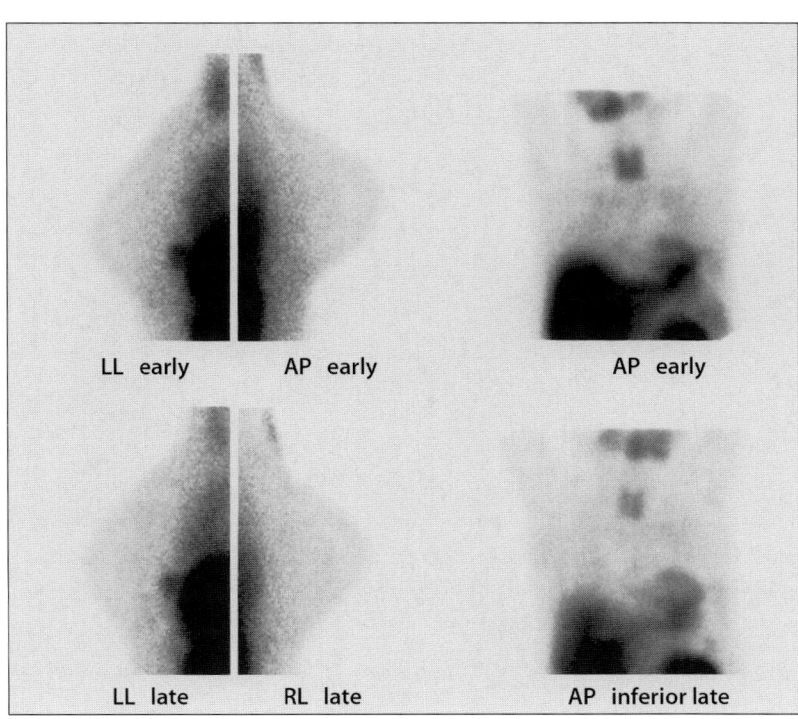

Fig. 2.55. This patient, who had previously undergone a left partial mastectomy for carcinoma, noticed sudden tension in the residual breast. Mammograms were negative. Breast scan shows a well-defined focus of increased uptake at the level of the chest wall, which proved to be recurrent tumor. It is noteworthy that focal lesions at this location are frequently missed on mammograms

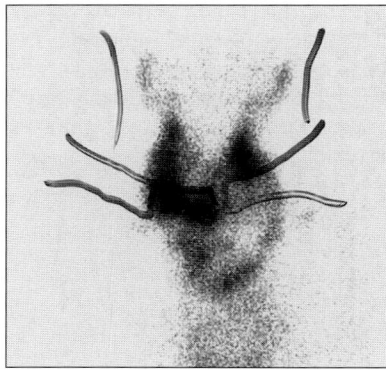

Fig. 2.56. Radionuclide scan shows mediastinal widening in a 42-year-old man complaining of a globus sensation in the neck. The thyroid gland is retrosternal, and the central and lower portions of the left lobe are hypoperfused. Thyroid carcinoma

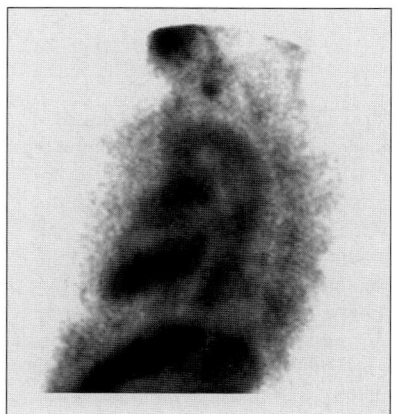

Fig. 2.57. Radionuclide aortography in a patient with mediastinal widening demonstrates a clotted aortic aneurysm

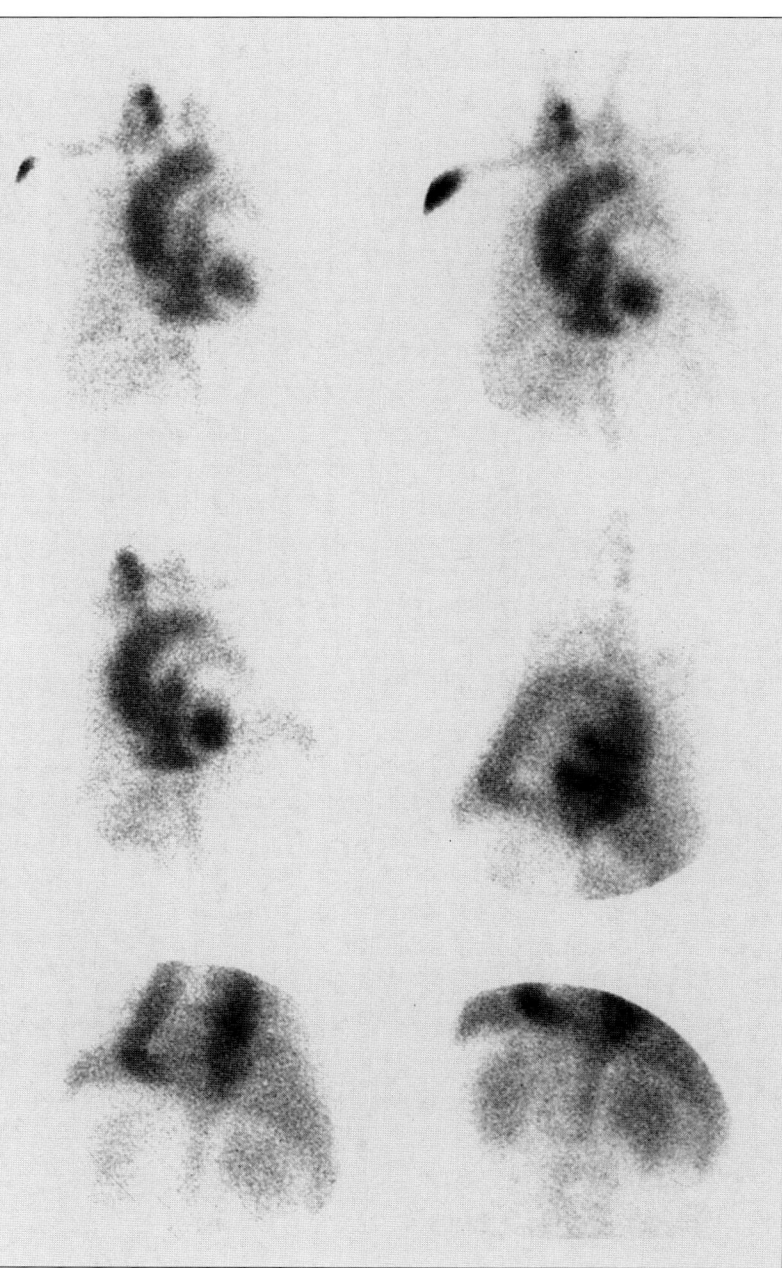

Fig. 2.58. Irregular mediastinal contour secondary to kyphoscoliosis. Radionuclide aortography shows a tortuous, ectatic thoracic aorta

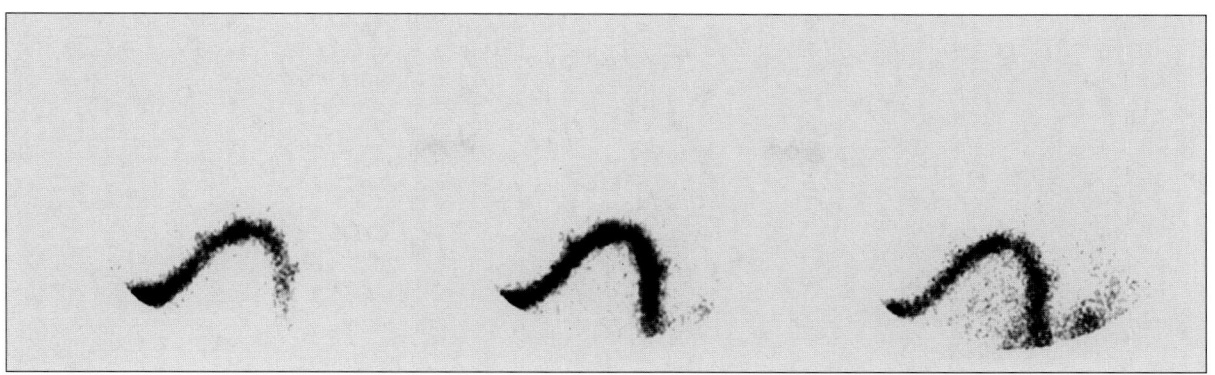

Fig. 2.59. Swelling in the right upper arm of a patient with suspected extrinsic compression of the superior vena cava. Radionuclide scan of the superior vena cava shows a completely normal pattern

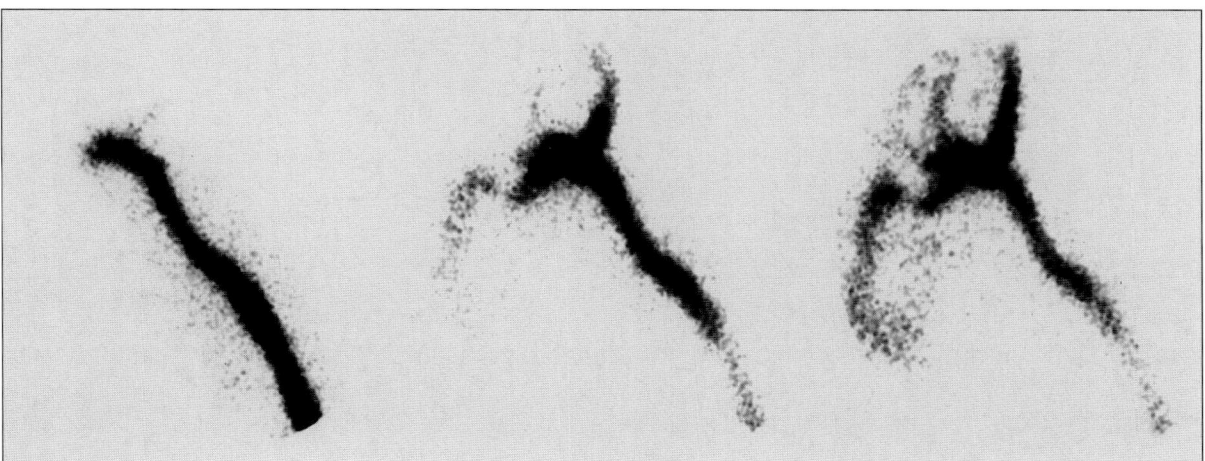

Fig. 2.60. Radionuclide angiogram in a 63-year-old woman with vertigo and exertional dyspnea shows an outflow obstruction in the brachiocephalic trunk and right common carotid artery. It is likely that a vascular anomaly is also present

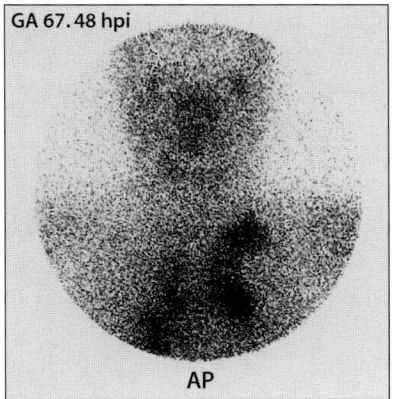

Fig. 2.61. Mediastinal widening in a patient with Hodgkin's disease. Respiratory distress recurred while the patient was in remission. Radionuclide scan shows multiple mediastinal lymphomas

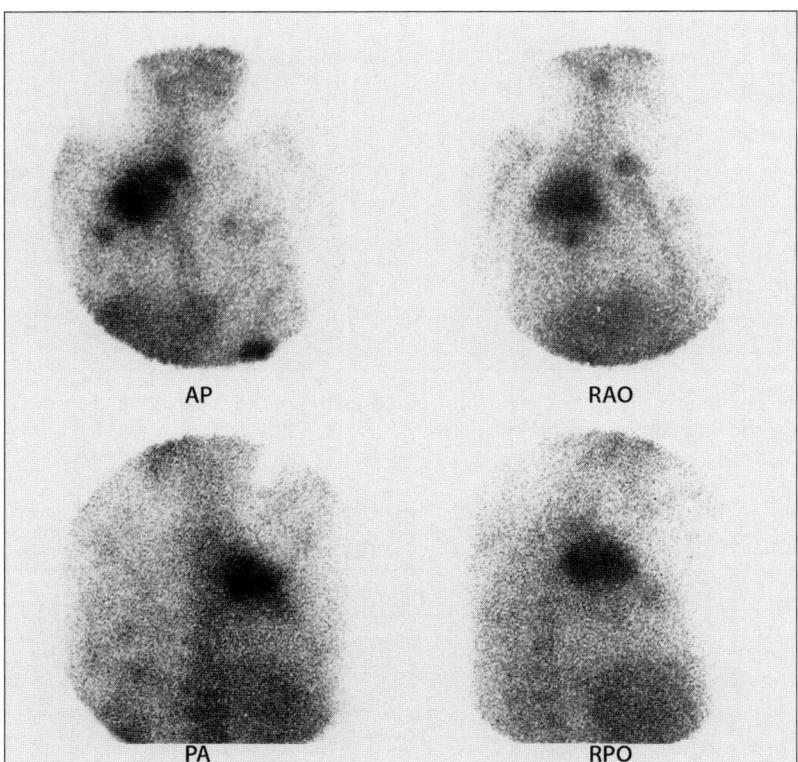

AP

RAO

PA

RPO

Fig. 2.62. Dyspnea and cough in a smoker. Radionuclide scan shows bronchial carcinoma with bilateral hilar lymph node metastases

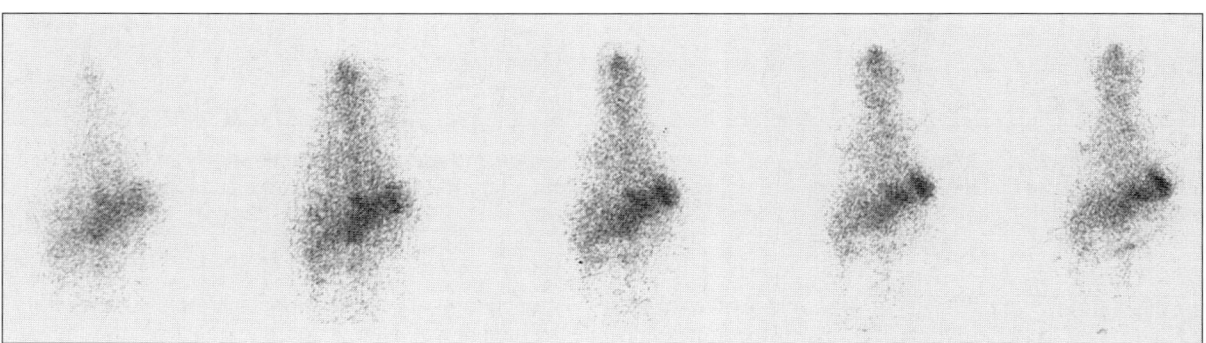

Fig. 2.63. Ga-67 imaging in a patient with burning retrosternal pain and a widened cardiac shadow shows relative thickening of the myocardium due to syphilitic myocarditis (phoconte Technik)

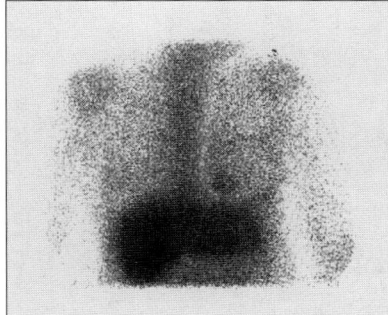

Fig. 2.64. This patient, who had a history of bilateral mastectomy (for carcinoma) and silicone implant reconstruction, complained of a burning sensation in the lower half of the chest, most pronounced in the left parasternal area. Radionuclide scanning was performed to exclude mediastinal neoplasia. The scan shows a ringlike, predominantly parasternal area of increased uptake on the left side caused by an allergic inflammatory reaction to the breast implant. The implant was immediately removed

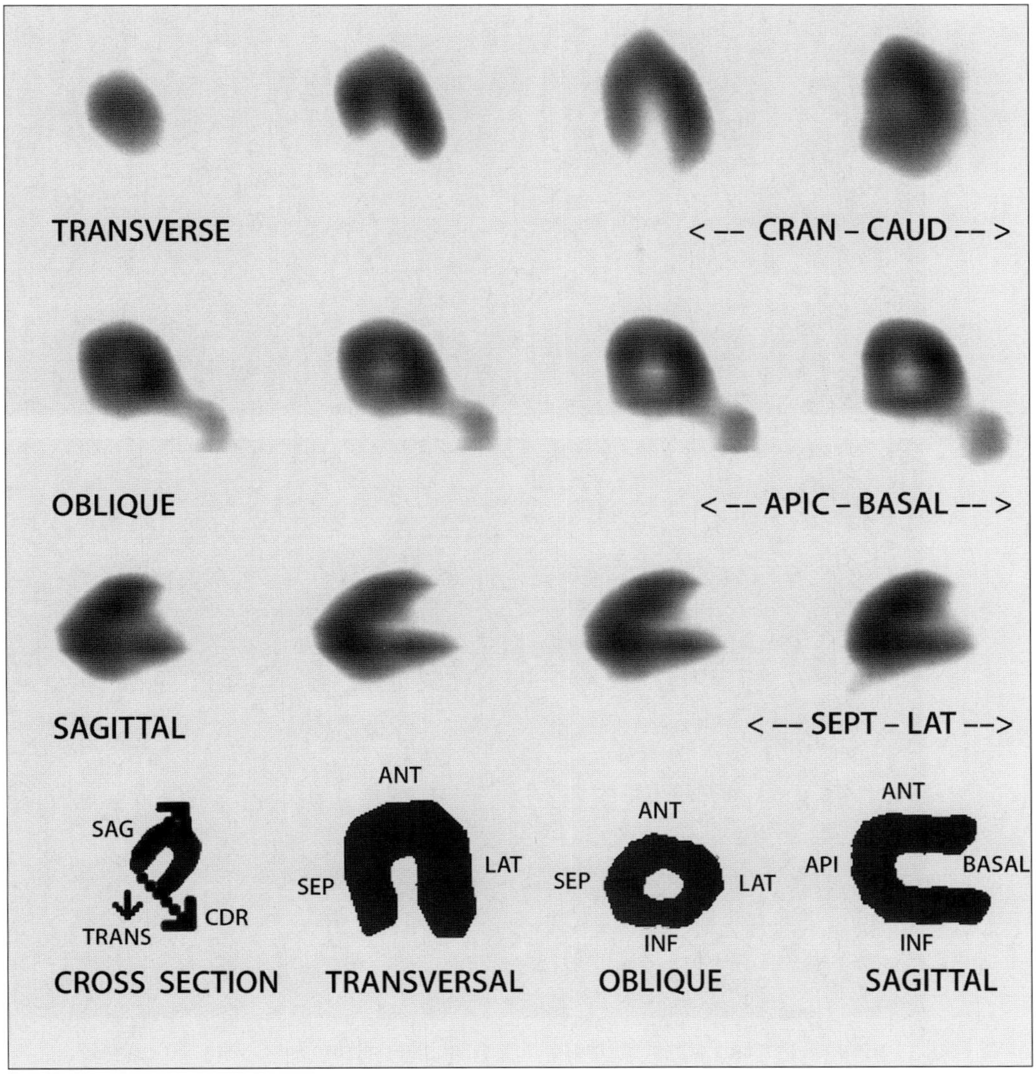

TRANSVERSE
<-- CRAN - CAUD -->
OBLIQUE
<-- APIC - BASAL -->
SAGITTAL
<-- SEPT - LAT -->
SAG
TRANS
CDR
CROSS SECTION
ANT
SEP
LAT
TRANSVERSAL
ANT
SEP
LAT
INF
OBLIQUE
ANT
API
BASAL
INF
SAGITTAL

Fig. 2.65

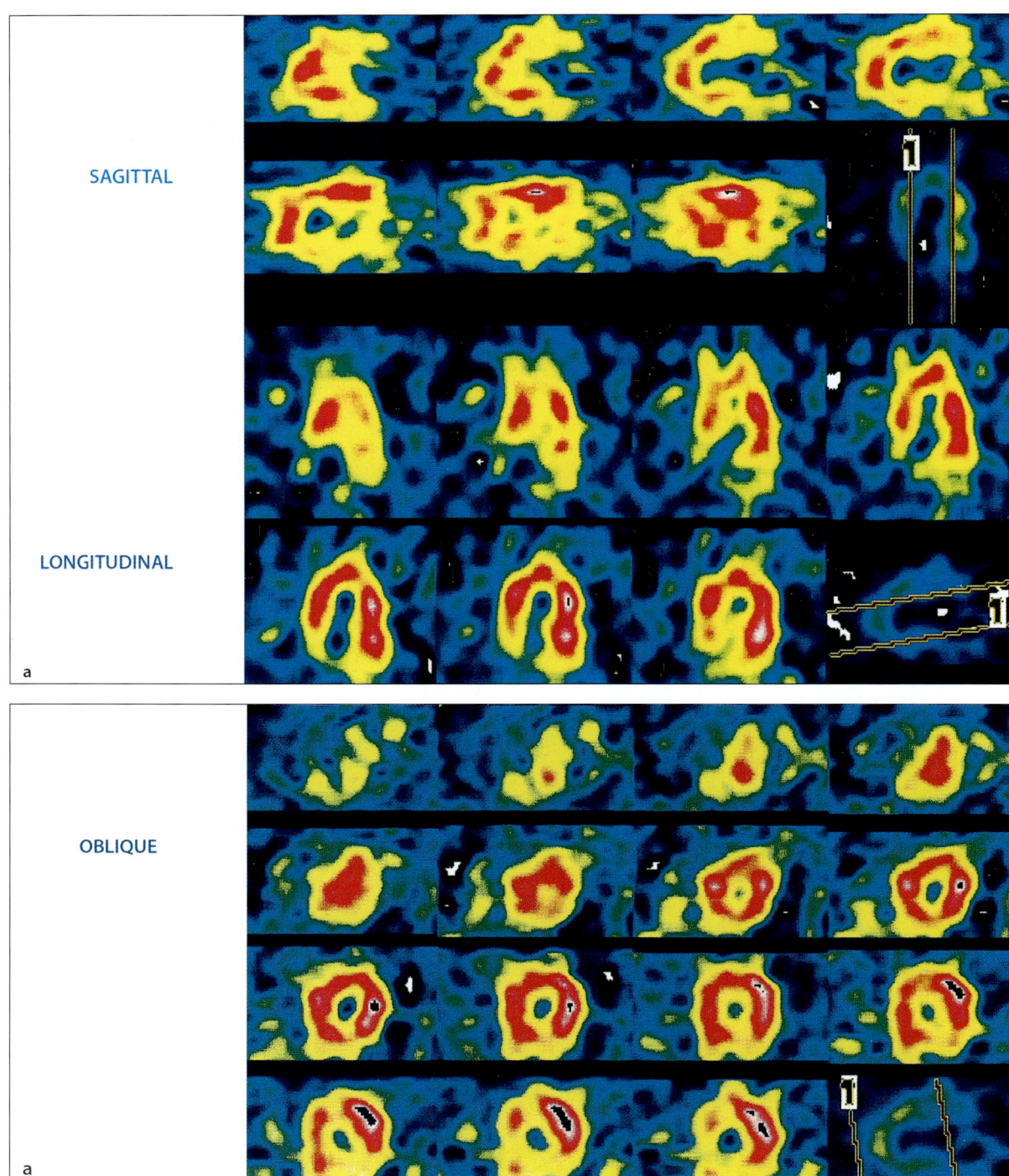

SAGITTAL

LONGITUDINAL

OBLIQUE

Fig. 2.66 a,b. Patient 72 years of age with dyspnea at rest and suspicion of multivessel disease. Due to difficulties in scheduling coronary angiography, the patient was initially referred to a health spa. [201]Tl myocardial scanning before (**a**) and after (**b**) spa treatment shows significant improvement in myocardial perfusion and tone. The patient's exercise tolerance after the spa treatment was normal for age

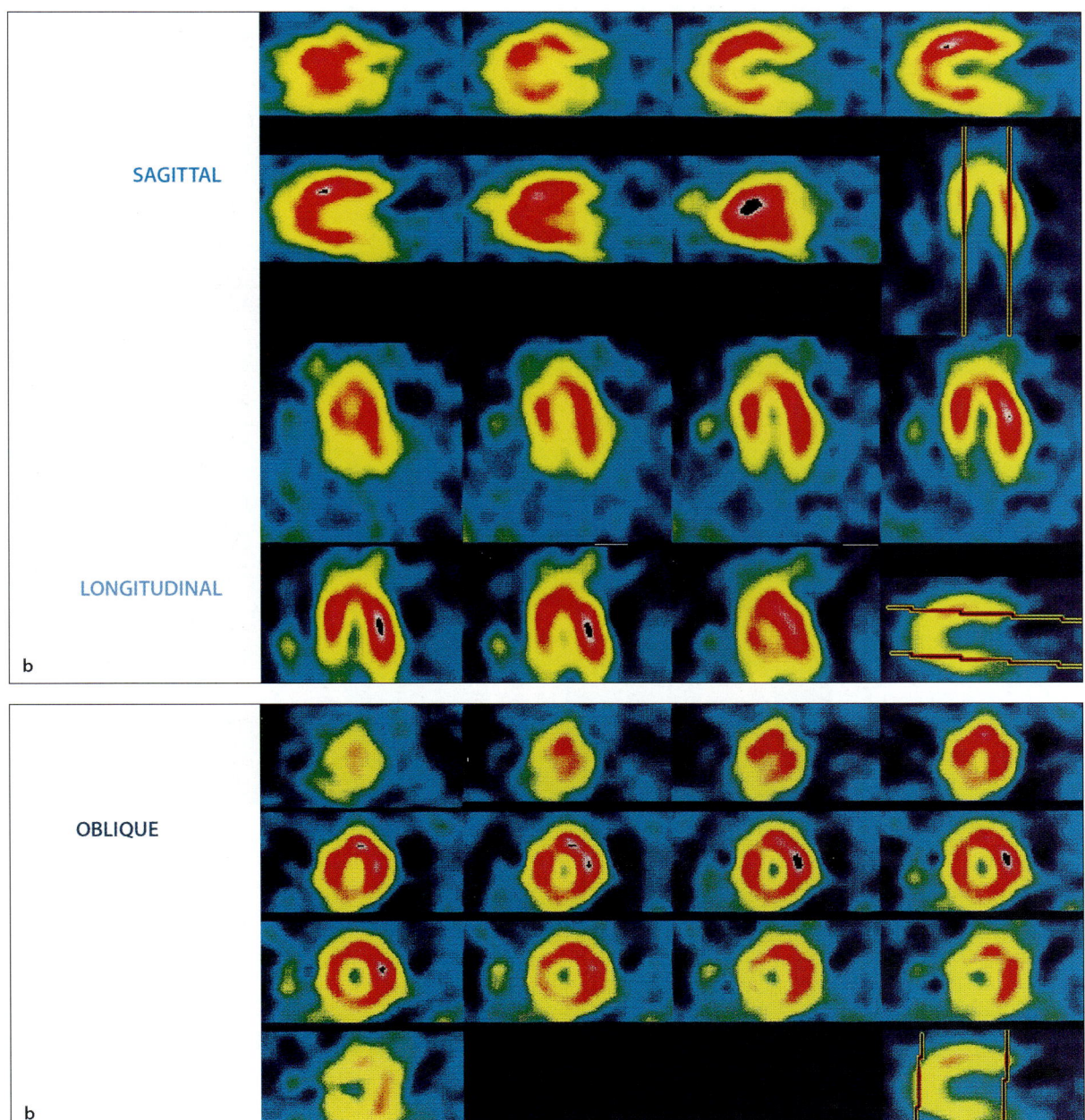

SAGITTAL

LONGITUDINAL

OBLIQUE

Fig. 2.66 b

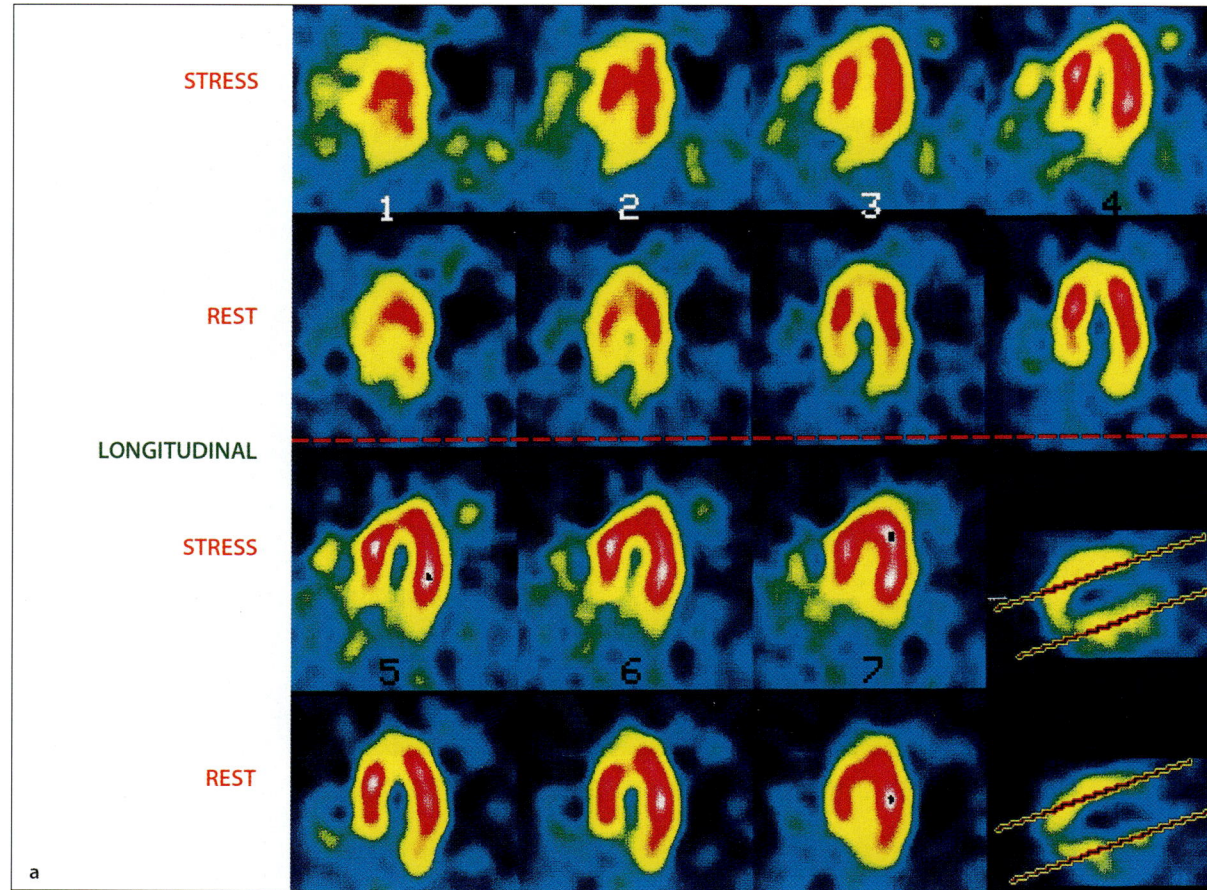

STRESS

REST

LONGITUDINAL

STRESS

REST

a

Fig. 2.67 a–d. A 59-year-old man had taken various analgesic tablets for several years since suffering a stroke, increasing his consumption to 18 tablets daily during the past three months. His presenting complaint was exertional dyspnea.
a Stress myocardial perfusion scanning was performed to 50 W of exercise, at which point exercise was stopped because of dyspnea. Both the resting and exercise study show multiple focal defects that are difficult to assign to a particular vessel. Abnormal amplitude and phase analysis with a global decrease in ejection fraction (global EF). **b** Follow-ups at 4 months and 1 year after discontinuance of analgesics show significant improvement of thallium fixation in the left myocardium. The patient's general state of health is also improved

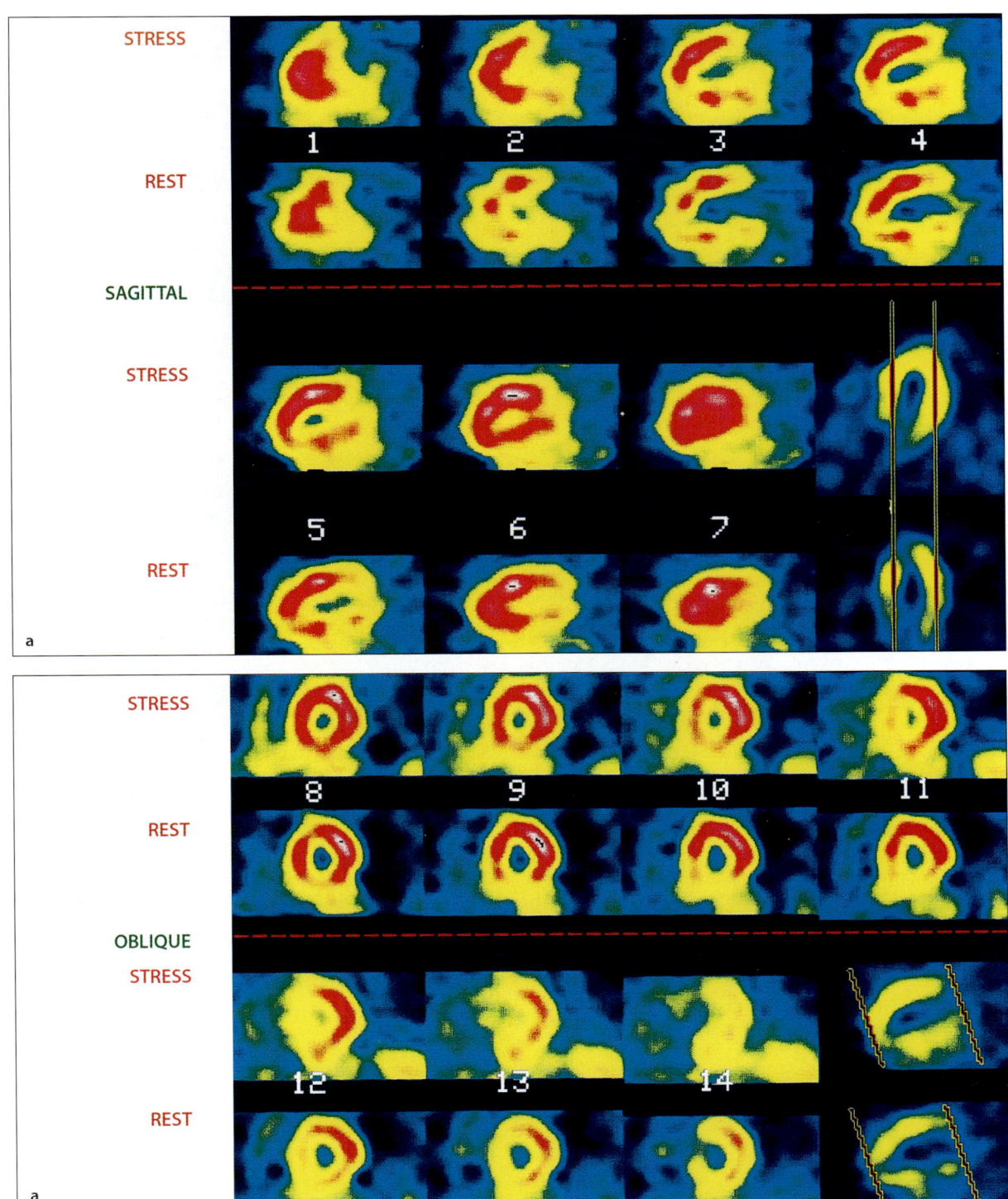

Fig. 2.67 a. *Continued*

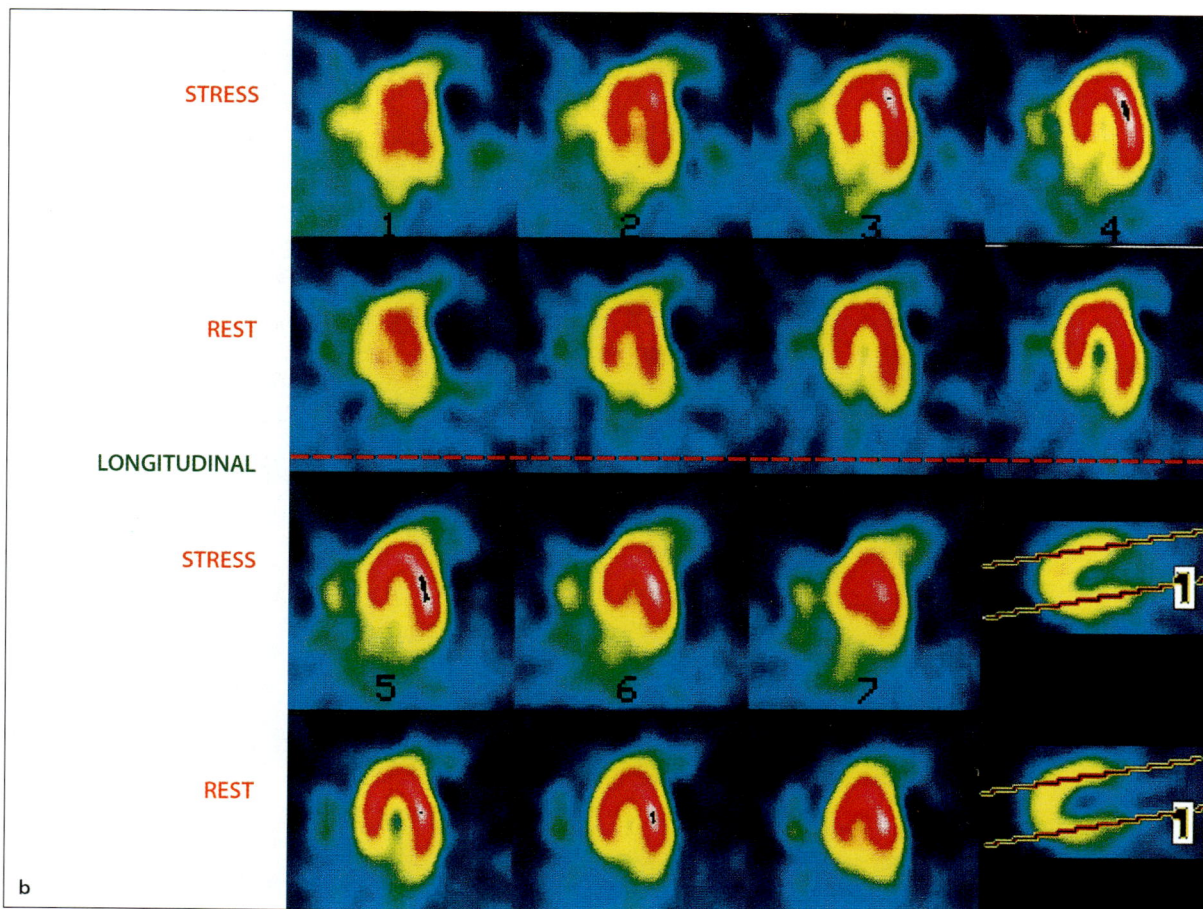

b

Fig. 2.67 a–d. A 59-year-old man had taken various analgesic tablets for several years since suffering a stroke, increasing his consumption to 18 tablets daily during the past three months. His presenting complaint was exertional dyspnea. **a** Stress myocardial perfusion scanning was performed to 50 W of exercise, at which point exercise was stopped because of dyspnea. Both the resting and exercise study show multiple focal defects that are difficult to assign to a particular vessel. Abnormal amplitude and phase analysis with a global decrease in ejection fraction (global EF). **b** Follow-ups at 4 months and 1 year after discontinuance of analgesics show significant improvement of thallium fixation in the left myocardium. The patient's general state of health is also improved

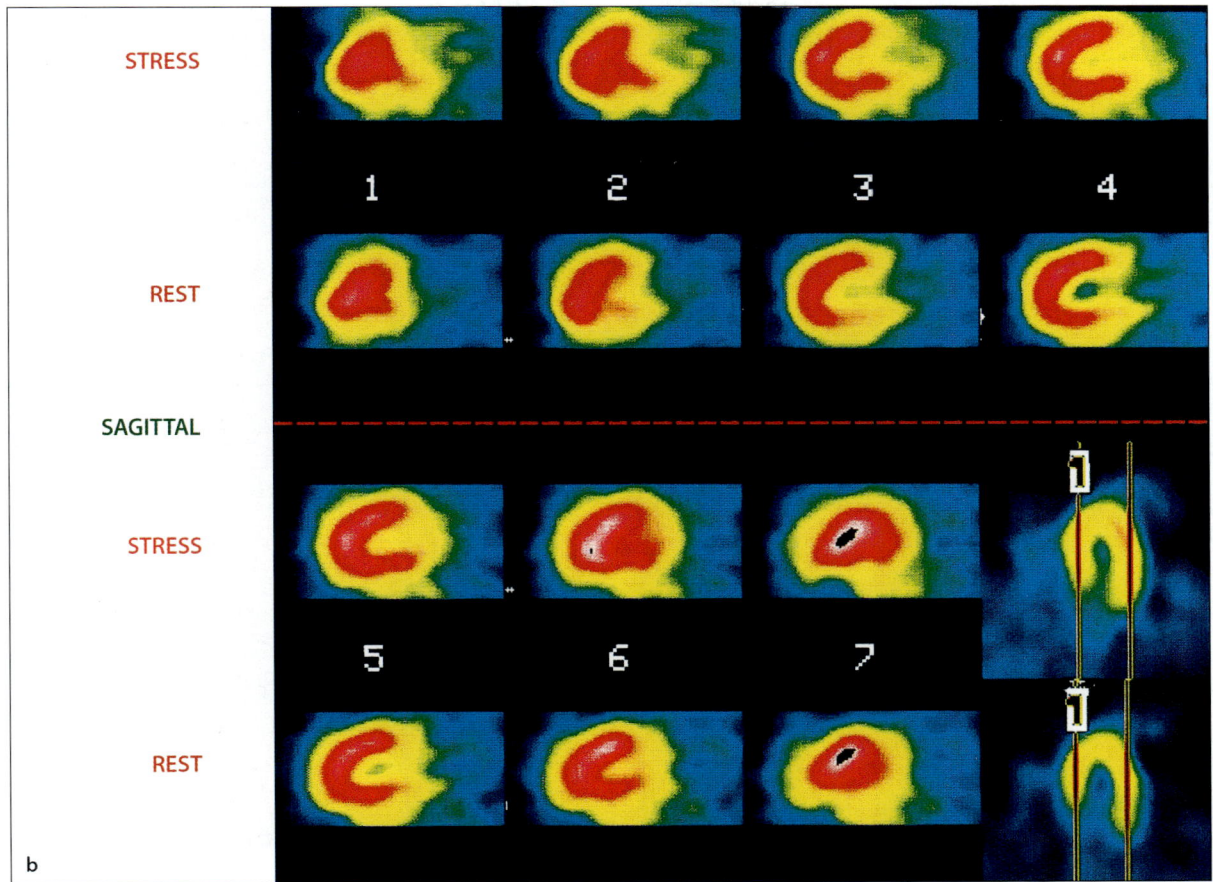

Fig. 2.67 b. *Continued*

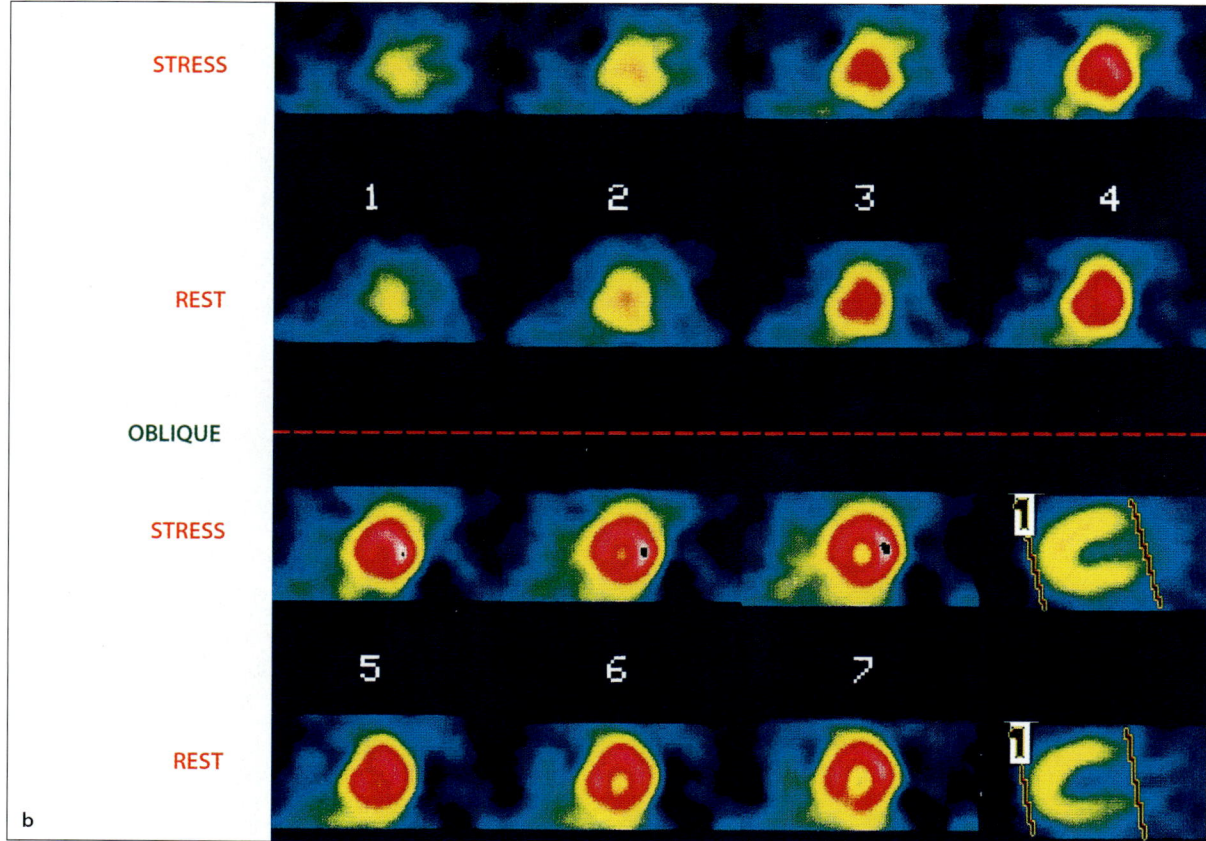

Fig. 2.67 a–d. A 59-year-old man had taken various analgesic tablets for several years since suffering a stroke, increasing his consumption to 18 tablets daily during the past three months. His presenting complaint was exertional dyspnea. **a** Stress myocardial perfusion scanning was performed to 50 W of exercise, at which point exercise was stopped because of dyspnea. Both the resting and exercise study show multiple focal defects that are difficult to assign to a particular vessel. Abnormal amplitude and phase analysis with a global decrease in ejection fraction (global EF). **b** Follow-ups at 4 months and 1 year after discontinuance of analgesics show significant improvement of thallium fixation in the left myocardium. The patient's general state of health is also improved

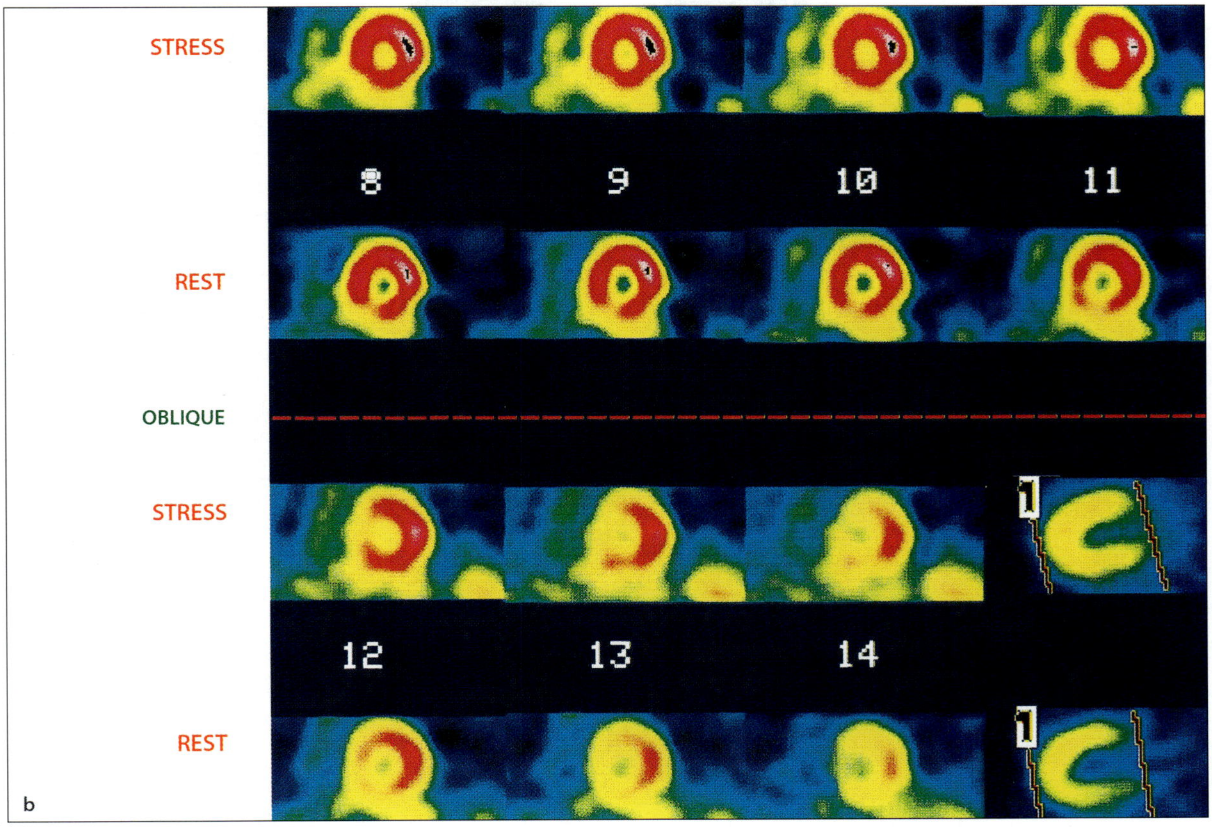

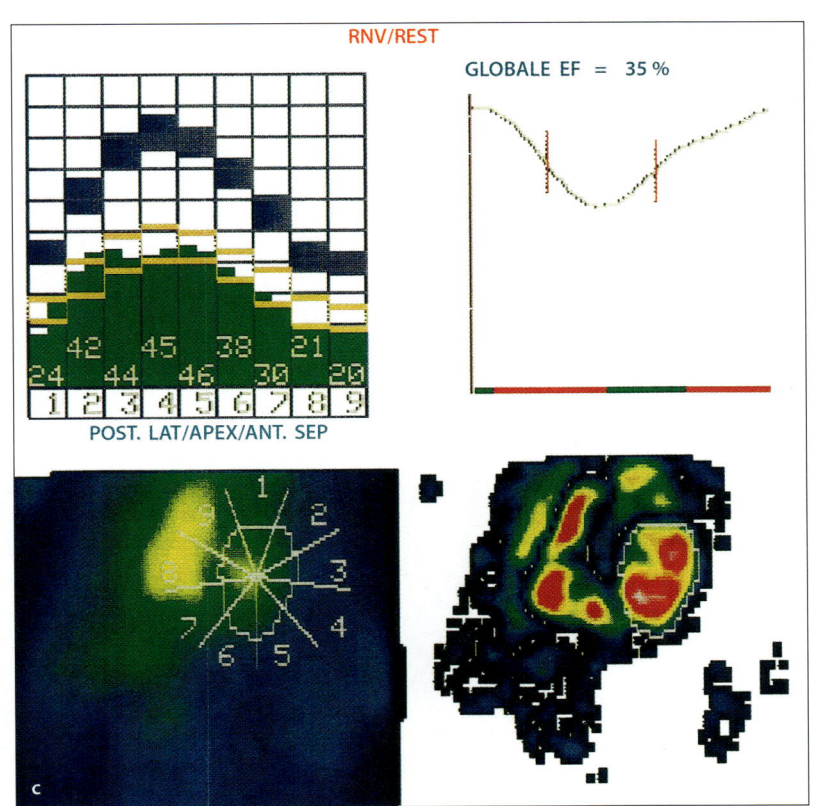

Fig. 2.67 b. *Continued*

Fig. 2.67 c

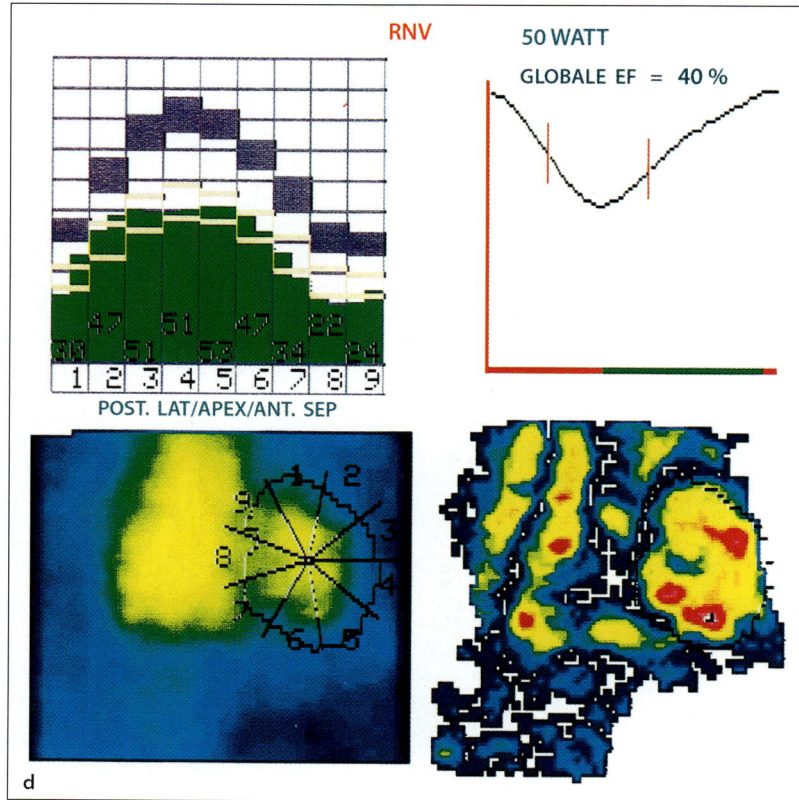

RNV

50 WATT

GLOBALE EF = 40 %

POST. LAT/APEX/ANT. SEP

d

Fig. 2.67 a–d. A 59-year-old man had taken various analgesic tablets for several years since suffering a stroke, increasing his consumption to 18 tablets daily during the past three months. His presenting complaint was exertional dyspnea. **a** Stress myocardial perfusion scanning was performed to 50 W of exercise, at which point exercise was stopped because of dyspnea. Both the resting and exercise study show multiple focal defects that are difficult to assign to a particular vessel. Abnormal amplitude and phase analysis with a global decrease in ejection fraction (global EF). **b** Follow-ups at 4 months and 1 year after discontinuance of analgesics show significant improvement of thallium fixation in the left myocardium. The patient's general state of health is also improved

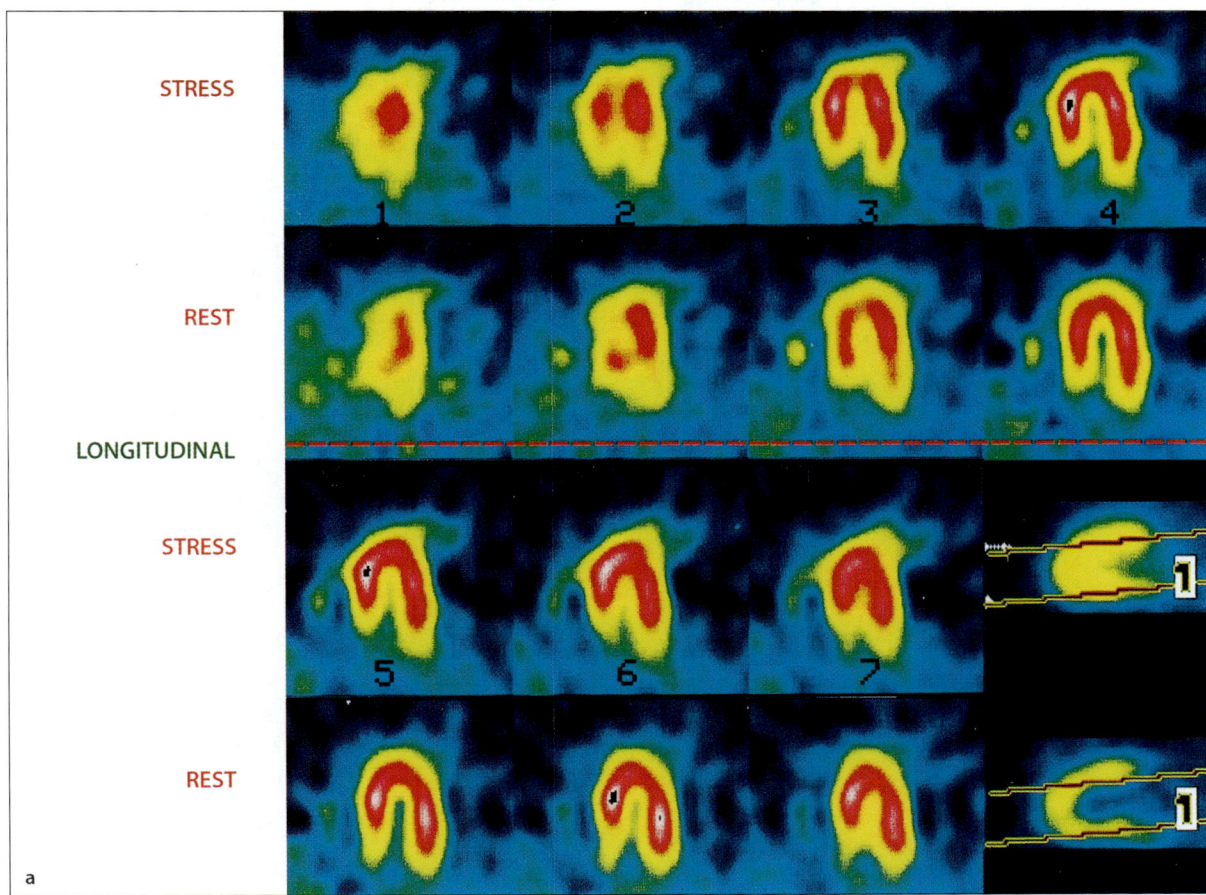

Fig. 2.68 a–c. This 56-year-old man had a long history of analgesic use for treatment of noncardiac chest pain. **a** Myocardial perfusion scan shows no change at rest, but exercise to 140 W shows hypoperfusion in the territory of the right coronary artery. **b** Radionuclide ventriculography shows a slight segmental EF decrease in the perfused region at rest, with involvement of the adjacent segments during exercise

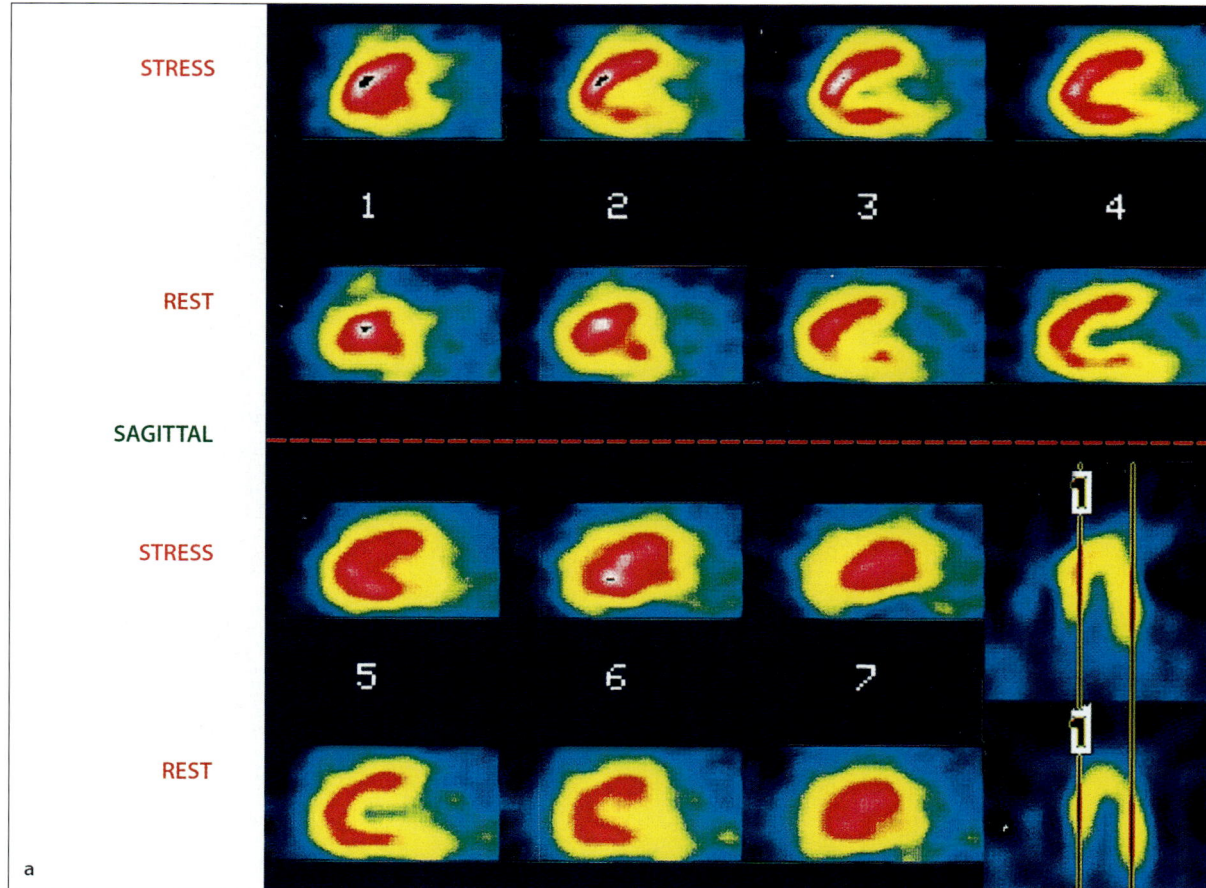

Fig. 2.68 a–c. This 56-year-old man had a long history of analgesic use for treatment of noncardiac chest pain. **a** Myocardial perfusion scan shows no change at rest, but exercise to 140 W shows hypoperfusion in the territory of the right coronary artery. **b** Radionuclide ventriculography shows a slight segmental EF decrease in the perfused region at rest, with involvement of the adjacent segments during exercise

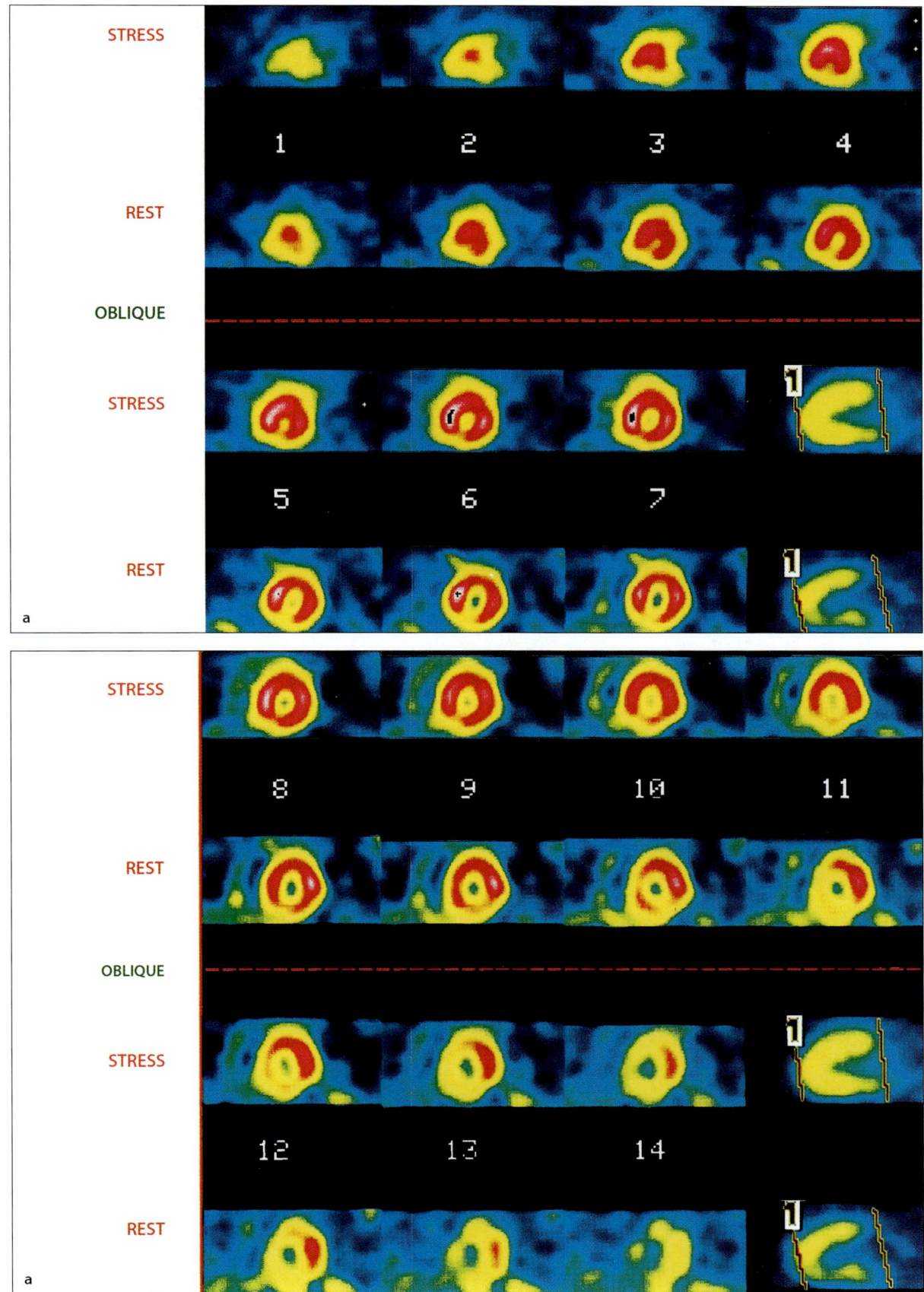

Fig. 2.68 a. *Continued*

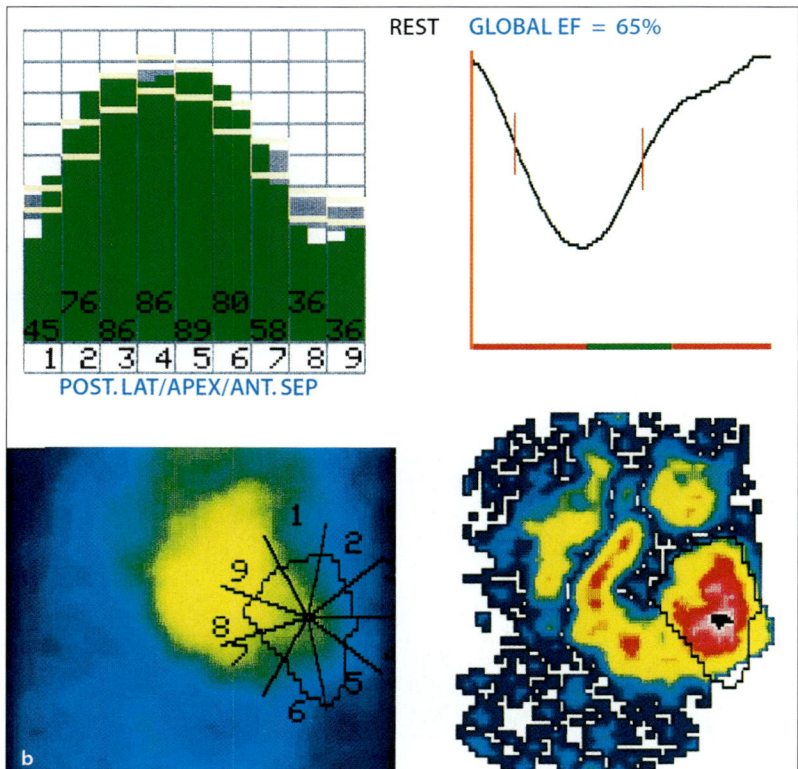

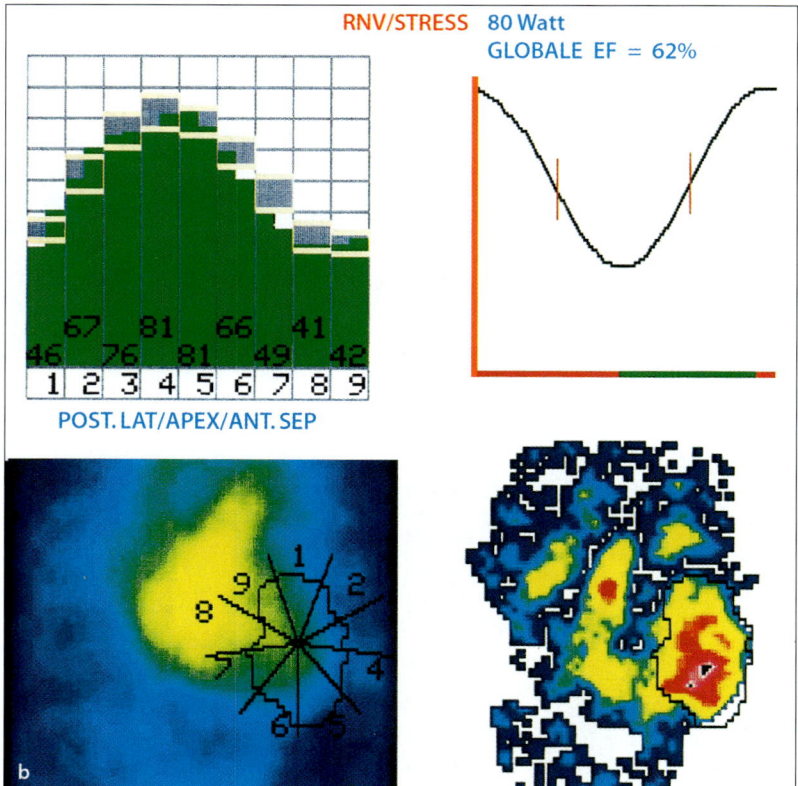

Fig. 2.68 a–c. This 56-year-old man had a long history of analgesic use for treatment of noncardiac chest pain. **a** Myocardial perfusion scan shows no change at rest, but exercise to 140 W shows hypoperfusion in the territory of the right coronary artery. **b** Radionuclide ventriculography shows a slight segmental EF decrease in the perfused region at rest, with involvement of the adjacent segments during exercise

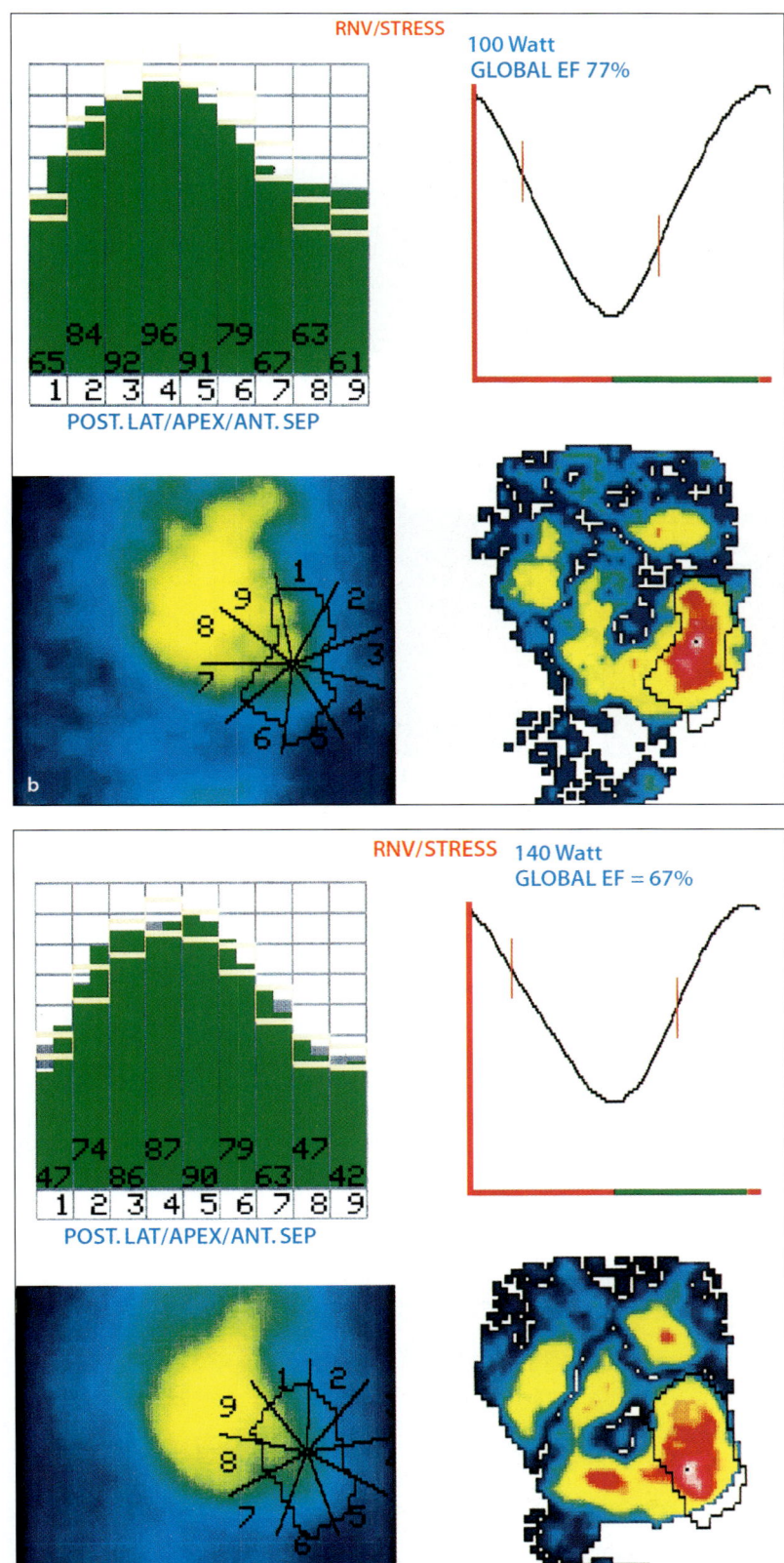

Fig. 2.68 b. *Continued*

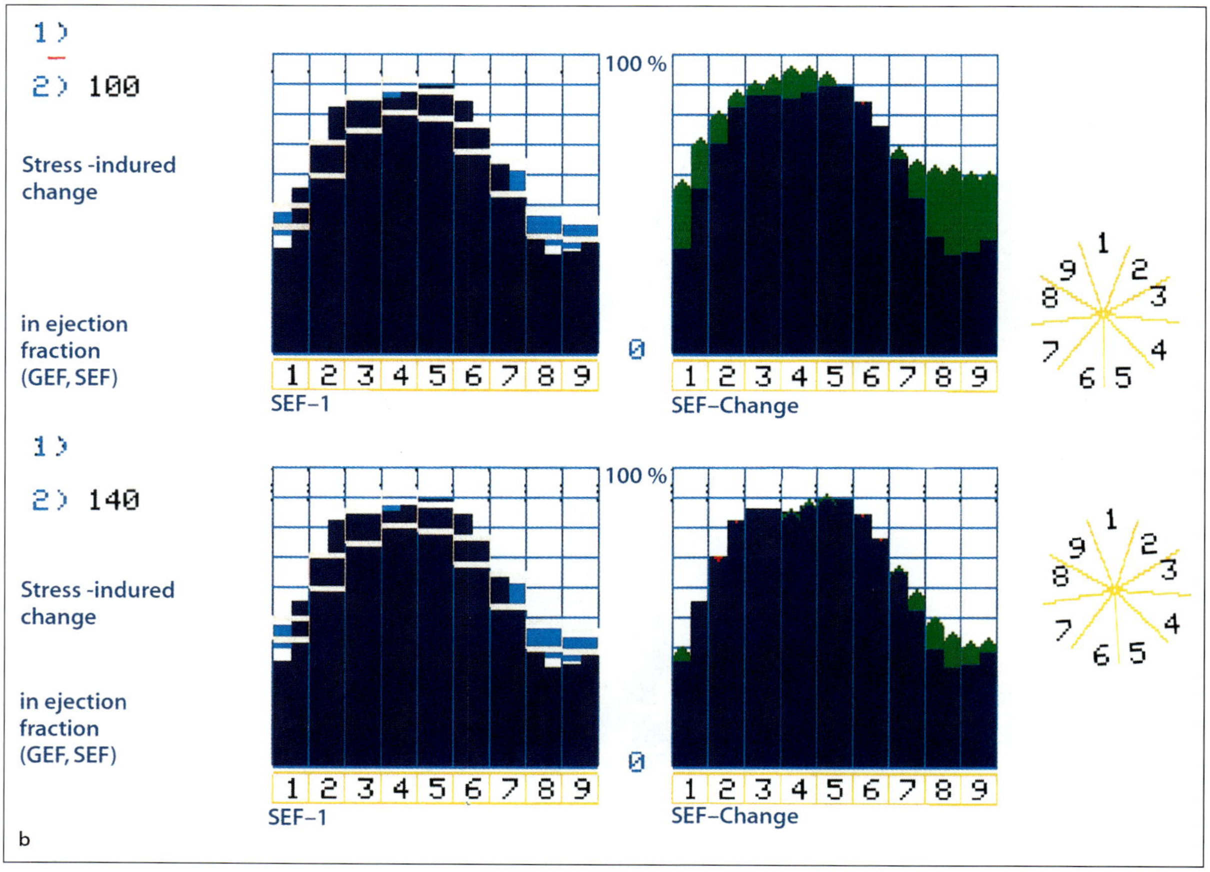

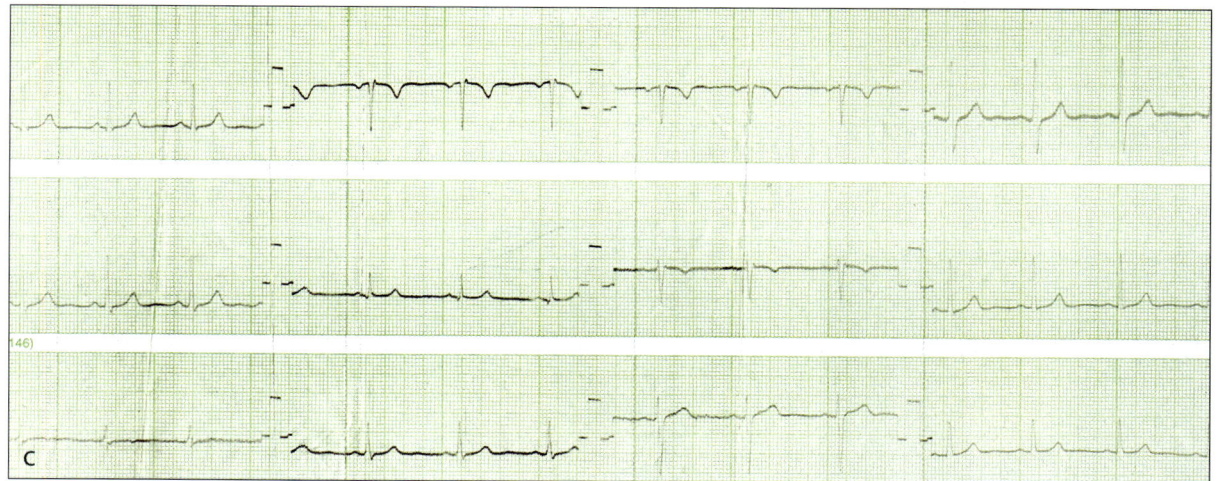

Fig. 2.68 a–c. This 56-year-old man had a long history of analgesic use for treatment of noncardiac chest pain. **a** Myocardial perfusion scan shows no change at rest, but exercise to 140 W shows hypoperfusion in the territory of the right coronary artery. **b** Radionuclide ventriculography shows a slight segmental EF decrease in the perfused region at rest, with involvement of the adjacent segments during exercise

Fig. 2.68 c

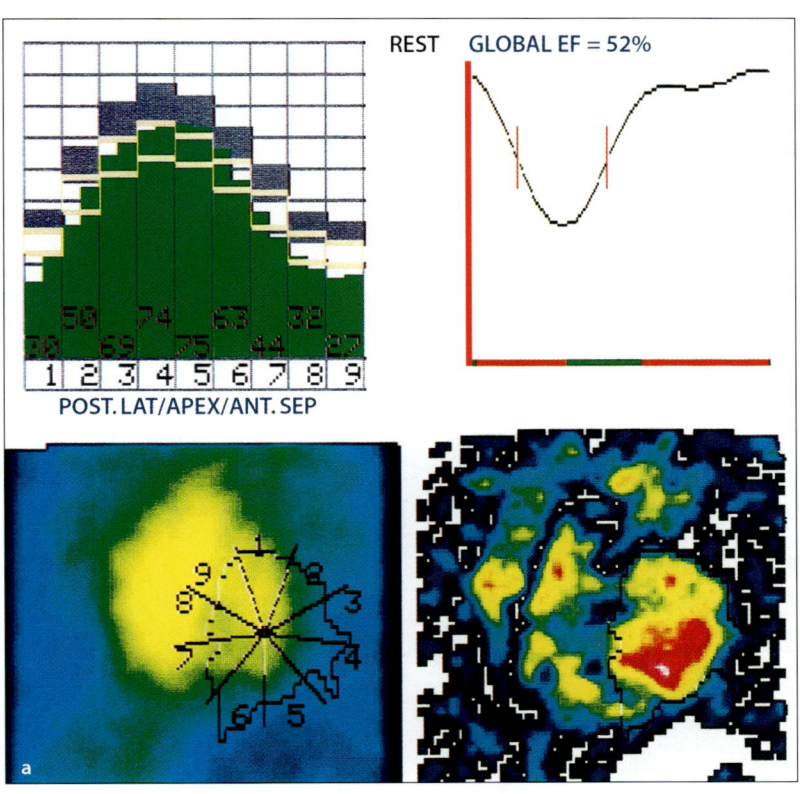

REST   GLOBAL EF = 52%

POST. LAT/APEX/ANT. SEP

Fig. 2.69 a,b. Radionuclide ventriculography was performed to evaluate myocardial stress tolerance during incremental graded exercise (**a**). Study at 90 W shows a decrease in segmental myocardial ejection volume (**b**). SEF segmental ejection fraction

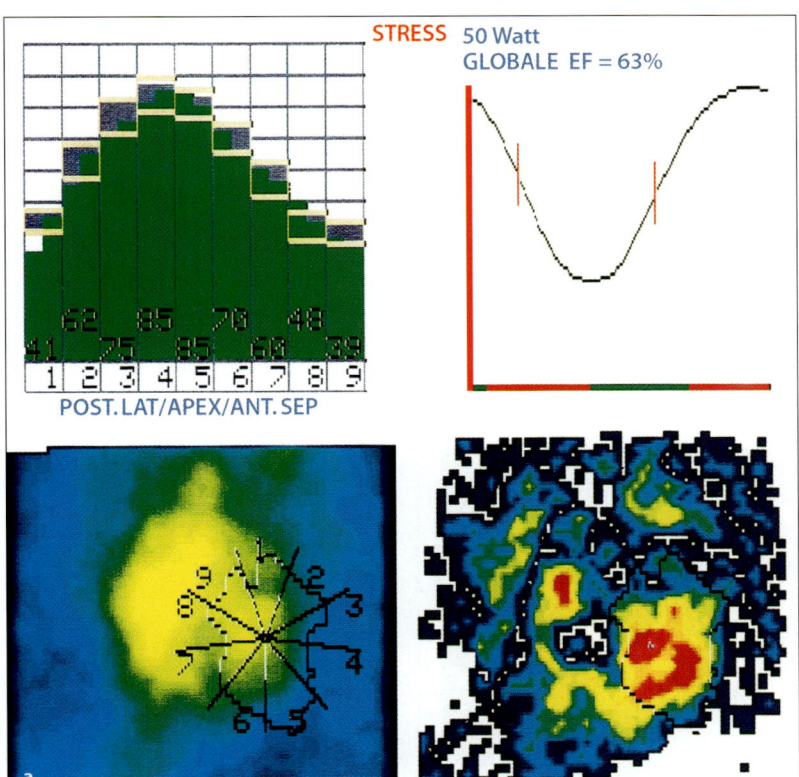

STRESS   50 Watt
GLOBALE EF = 63%

POST. LAT/APEX/ANT. SEP

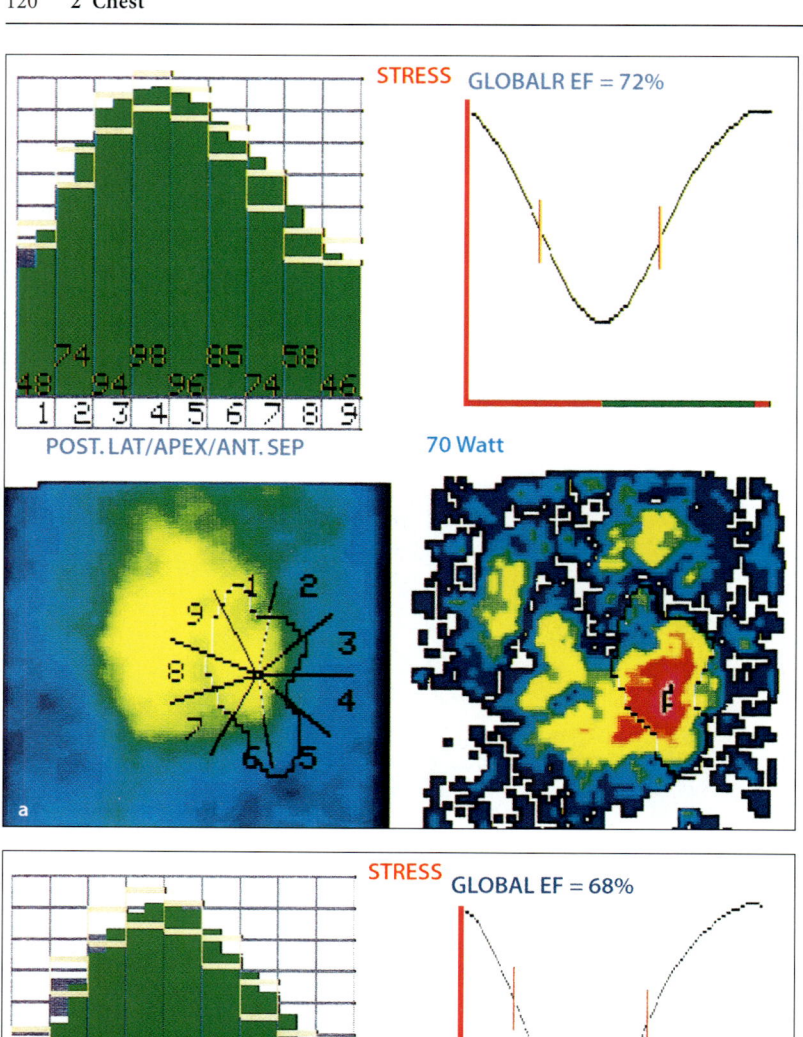

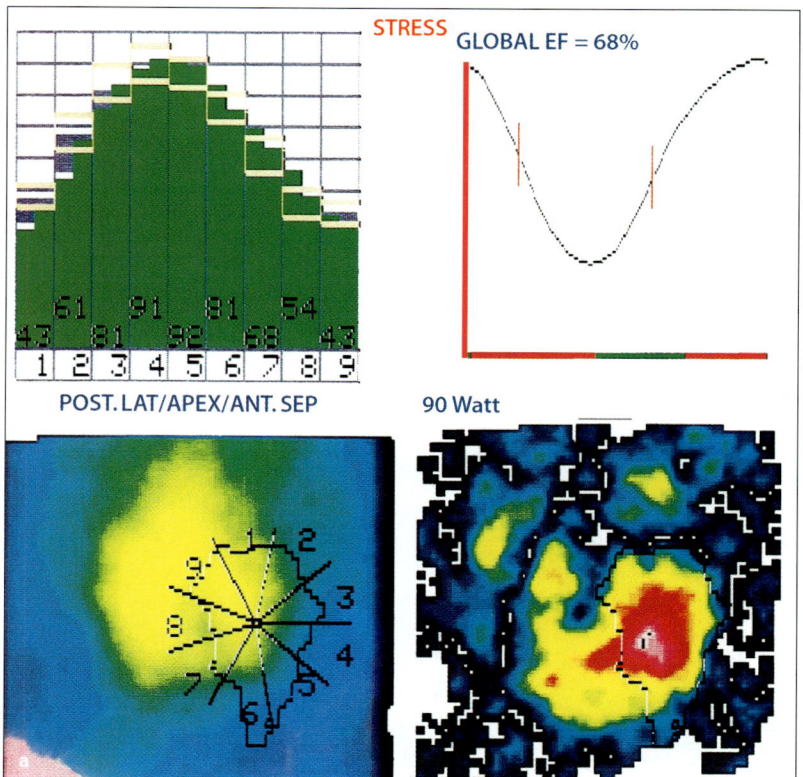

Fig. 2.69 a. *Continued*

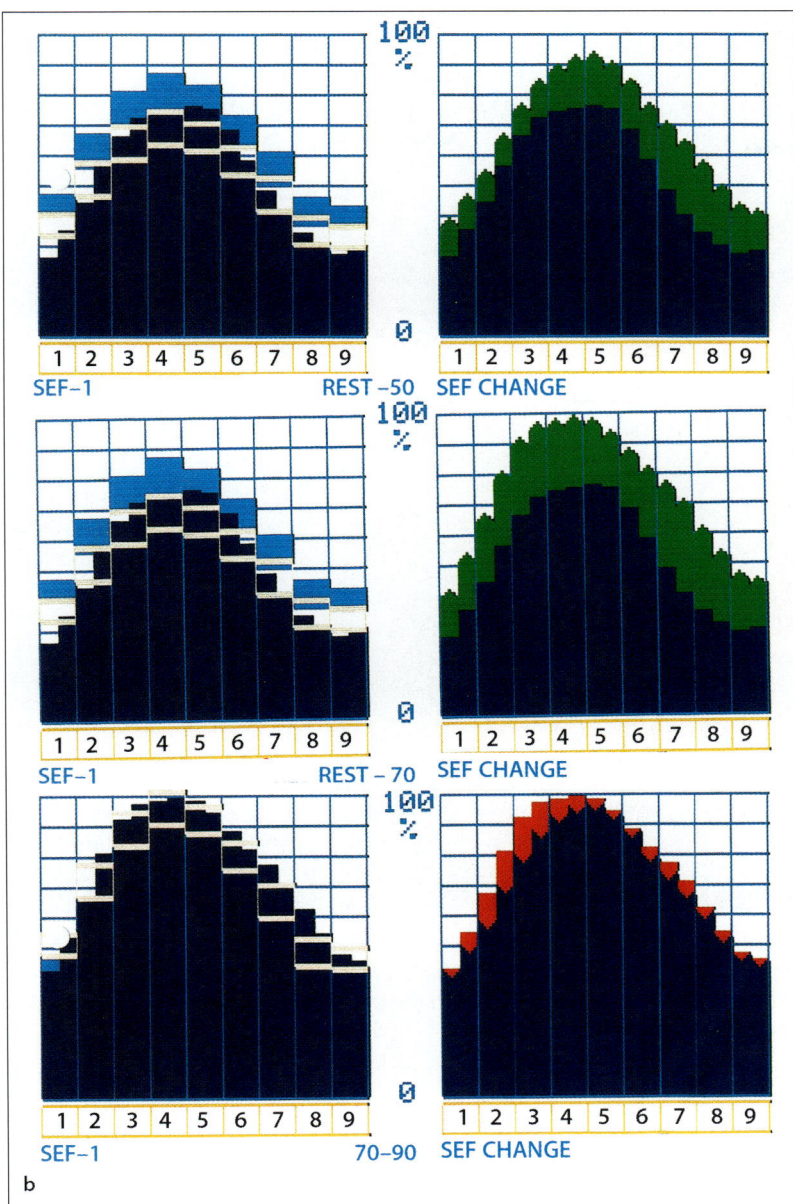

b

Fig. 2.69 a,b. Radionuclide ventriculography was performed to evaluate myocardial stress tolerance during incremental graded exercise (**a**). Study at 90 W shows a decrease in segmental myocardial ejection volume (**b**). SEF segmental ejection fraction

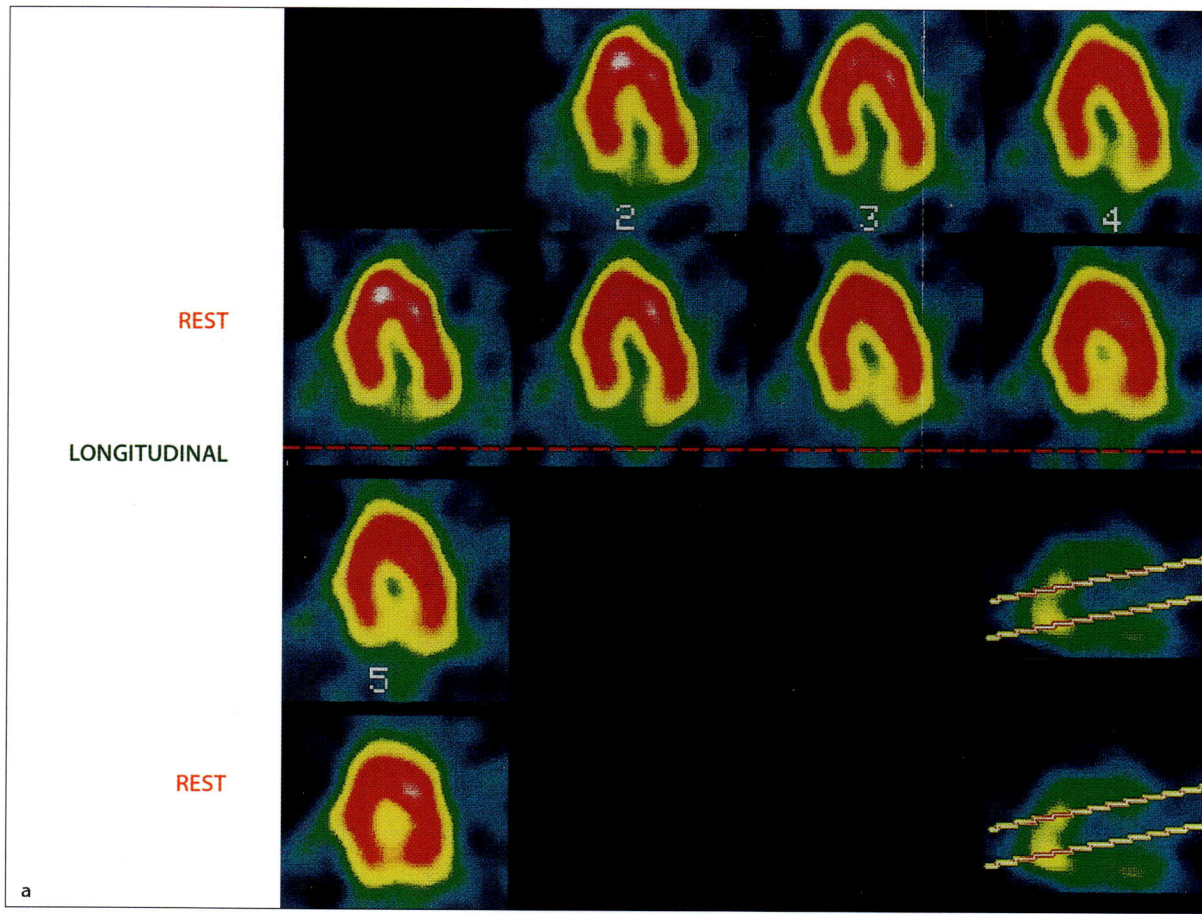

REST

LONGITUDINAL

REST

a

Fig. 2.70 a,b. Woman 59 years of age presented with sharp chest pains, anxiety, and varicose veins. **a** ^{201}Tl myocardial scan shows no evidence of CHD but does show intense uptake throughout the left myocardium, suggestive of a hyperfunctioning thyroid. **b** Thyroid scan demonstrates an autonomous adenoma in the thyroid gland. After 3 months' radioiodine therapy, the patient is free of complaints

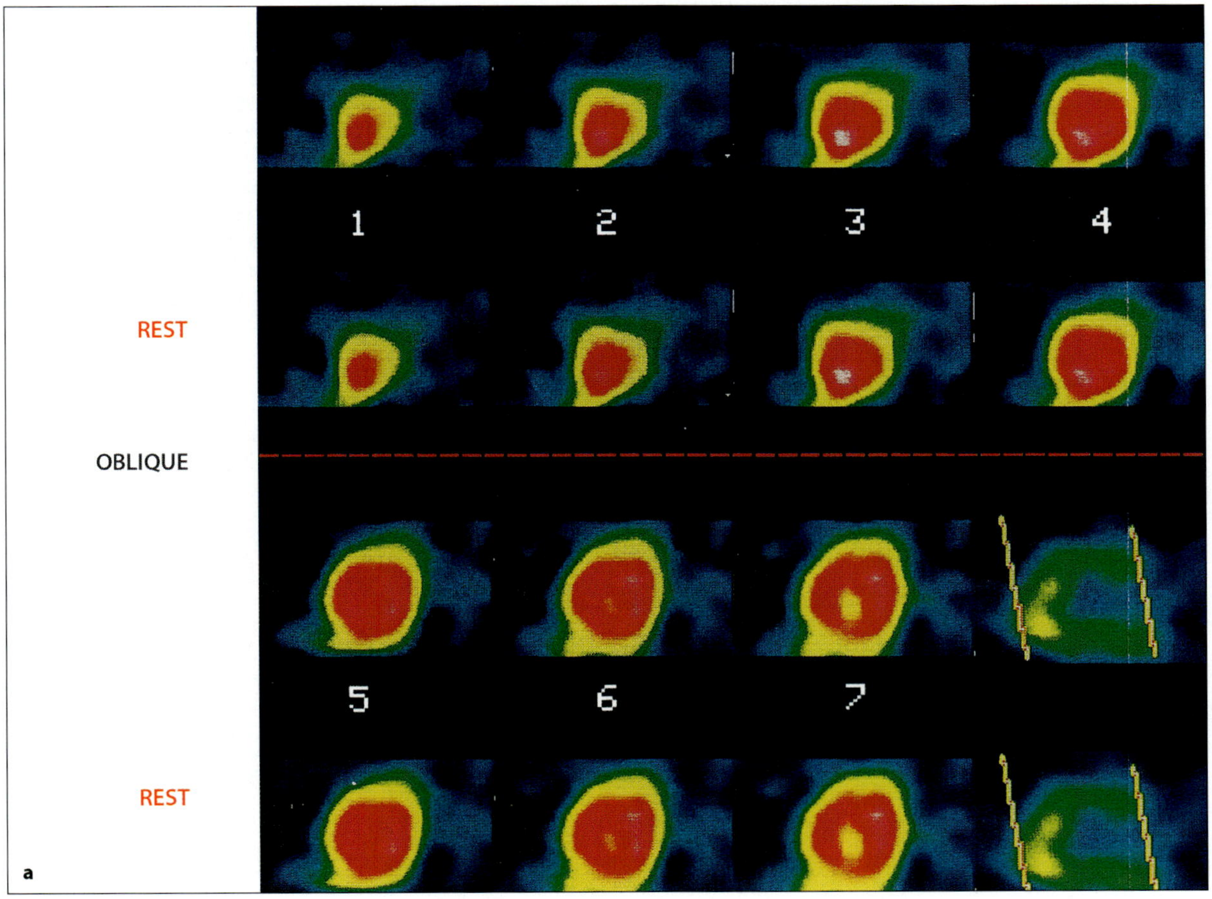

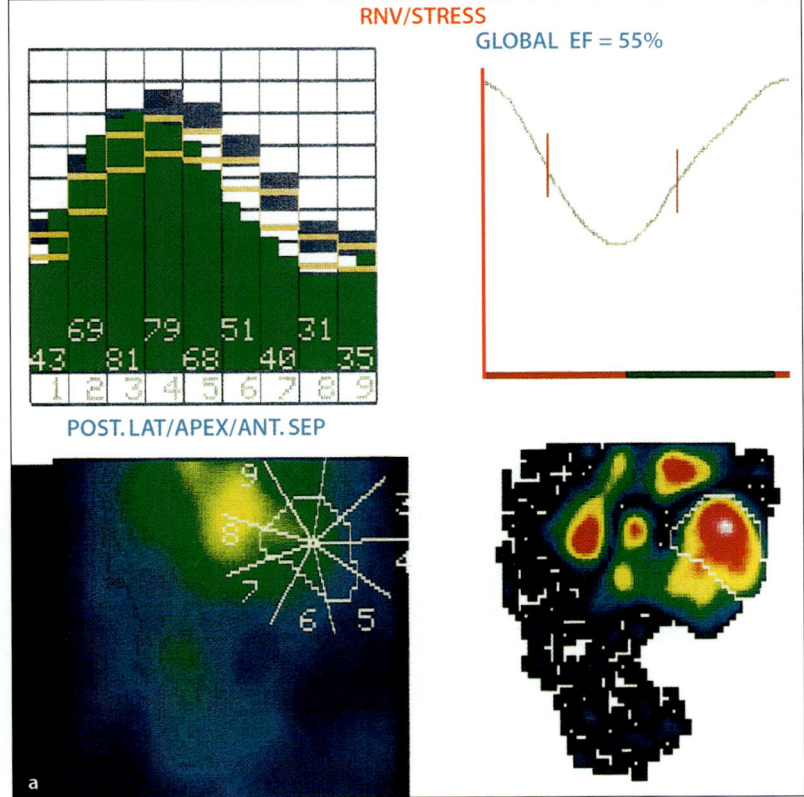

REST

OBLIQUE

REST

1 2 3 4

5 6 7

RNV/STRESS

GLOBAL EF = 55%

69 79 51 31
43 81 68 40 35
1 2 3 4 5 6 7 8 9

POST. LAT/APEX/ANT. SEP

Fig. 2.70 a. *Continued*

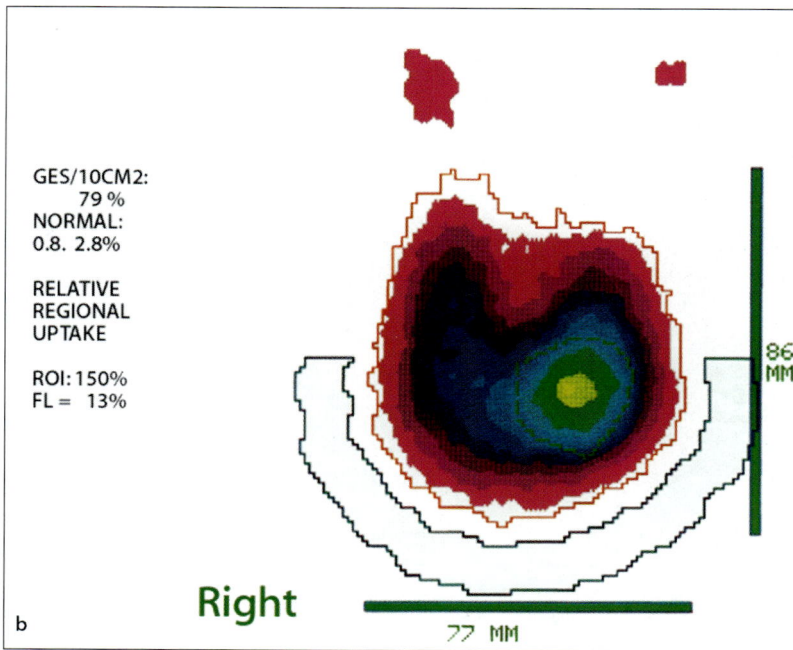

GES/10CM2:
    79 %
NORMAL:
0.8. 2.8%

RELATIVE
REGIONAL
UPTAKE

ROI: 150%
FL = 13%

86
MM

Right

77 MM

b

Fig. 2.70 a,b. Woman 59 years of age presented with sharp chest pains, anxiety, and varicose veins. **a** [201]Tl myocardial scan shows no evidence of CHD but does show intense uptake throughout the left myocardium, suggestive of a hyperfunctioning thyroid. **b** Thyroid scan demonstrates an autonomous adenoma in the thyroid gland. After 3 months' radioiodine therapy, the patient is free of complaints

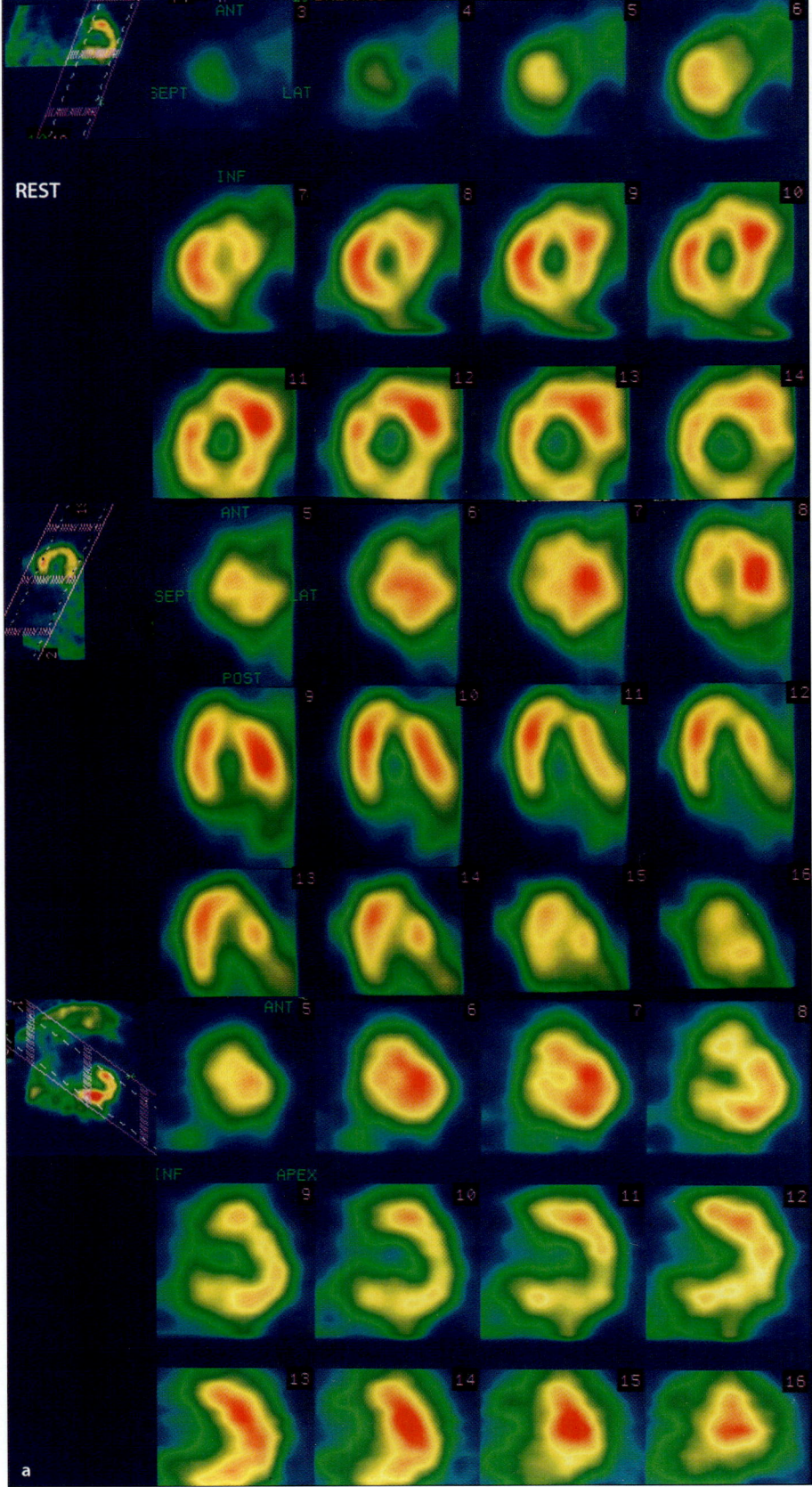

Fig. 2.71 a,b. Man 33 years of age sustained seafood poisoning abroad and complained of burning retrosternal pain. Myocardial perfusion scan at rest (**a**) and during exercise (**b**). The patient was exercised at 25 W for 2 min; this was the highest level tolerated due to severe pain and faintness. The study shows diffuse, nonhomogeneous uptake through the left myocardium during rest and exercise. Toxic cardiomyopathy

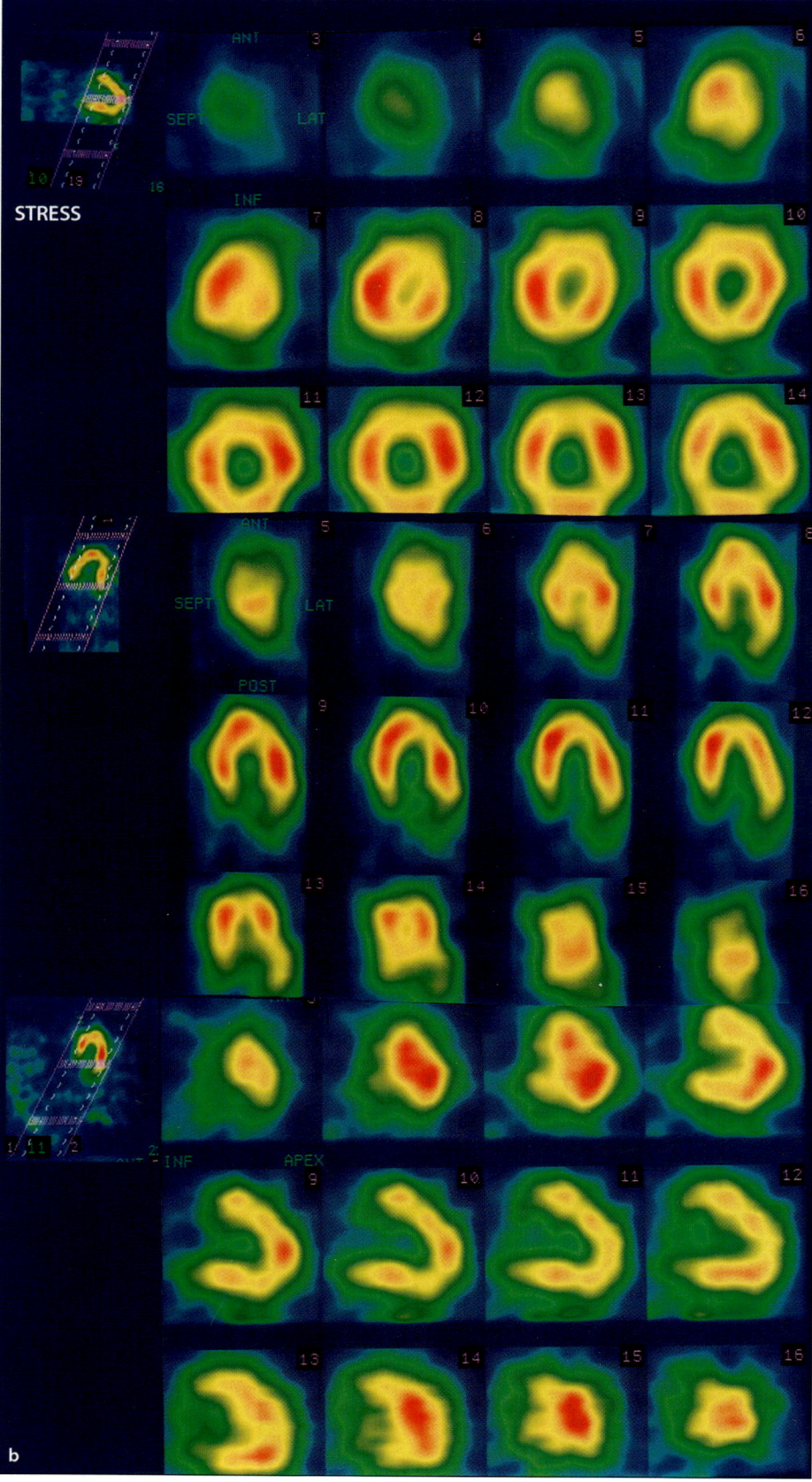

STRESS

b

Fig. 2.71 a,b. Man 33 years of age sustained seafood poisoning abroad and complained of burning retrosternal pain. Myocardial perfusion scan at rest (**a**) and during exercise (**b**). The patient was exercised at 25 W for 2 min; this was the highest level tolerated due to severe pain and faintness. The study shows diffuse, nonhomogeneous uptake through the left myocardium during rest and exercise. Toxic cardiomyopathy

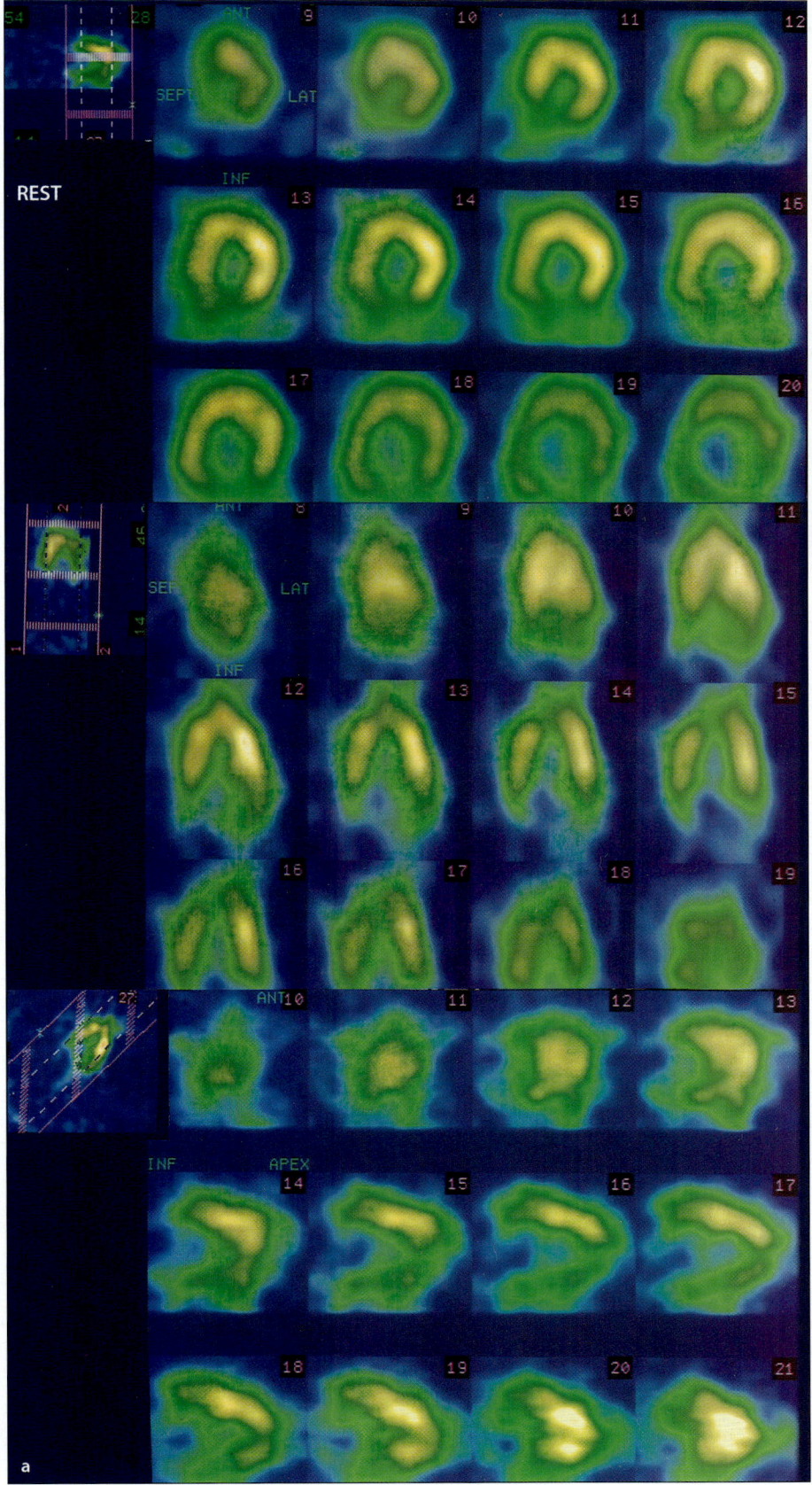

Fig. 2.72 a,b. Stress myocardial perfusion scan in an obese 56-year-old man (body weight 154 kg) with resting and exertional dyspnea. Exercise was terminated at 25 W due to retrosternal pain, shortness of breath, and cyanosis. Scans at rest (**a**) and during exercise (**b**) show diffusely decreased uptake throughout the left myocardium. The pronounced posterior wall defect may be a position-related artifact due to the patient's obesity or may result from absorption by the elevated diaphragm. The scan pattern is a result of fatty degeneration ("tiger heart")

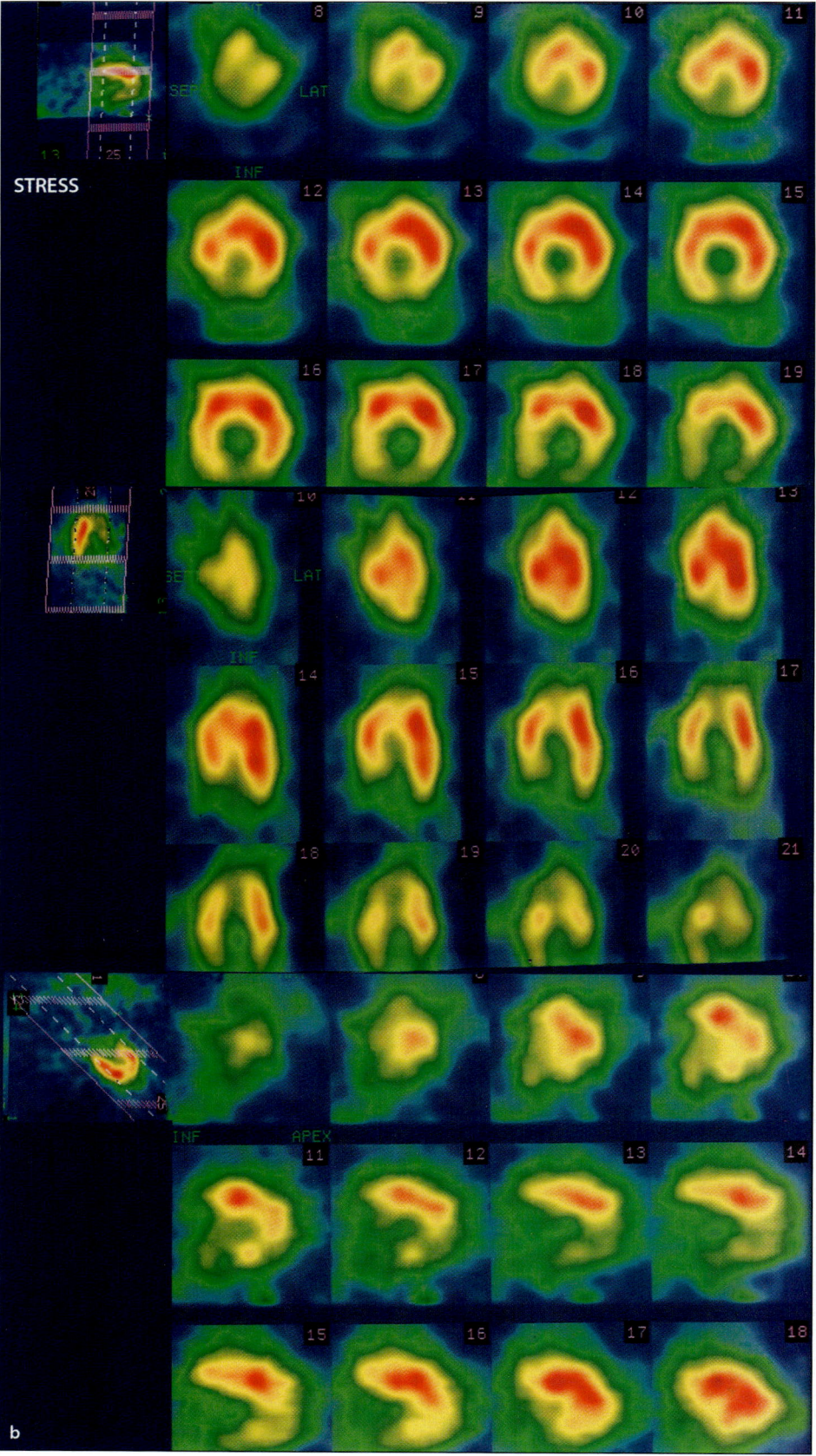

Fig. 2.72 a,b. Stress myocardial perfusion scan in an obese 56-year-old man (body weight 154 kg) with resting and exertional dyspnea. Exercise was terminated at 25 W due to retrosternal pain, shortness of breath, and cyanosis. Scans at rest (**a**) and during exercise (**b**) show diffusely decreased uptake throughout the left myocardium. The pronounced posterior wall defect may be a position-related artifact due to the patient's obesity or may result from absorption by the elevated diaphragm. The scan pattern is a result of fatty degeneration ("tiger heart")

Early 20 min.

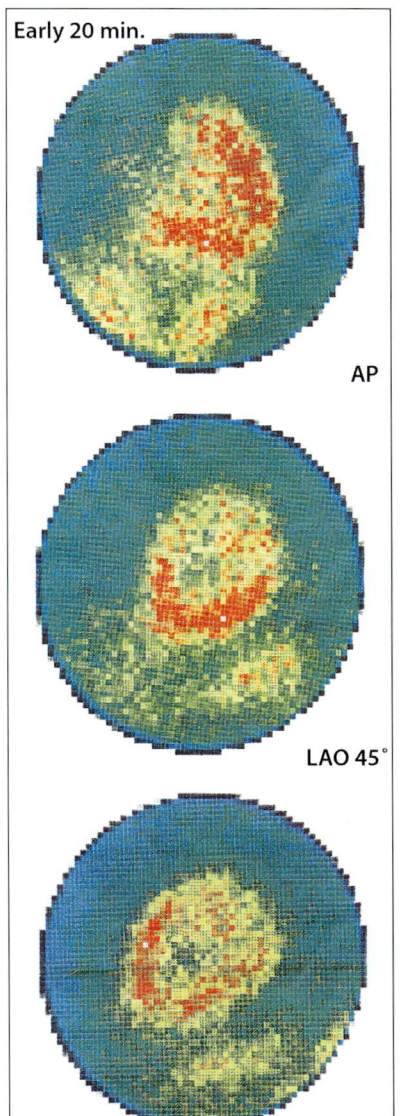

AP

LAO 45°

LAO 70°

a

Late 2 h pi

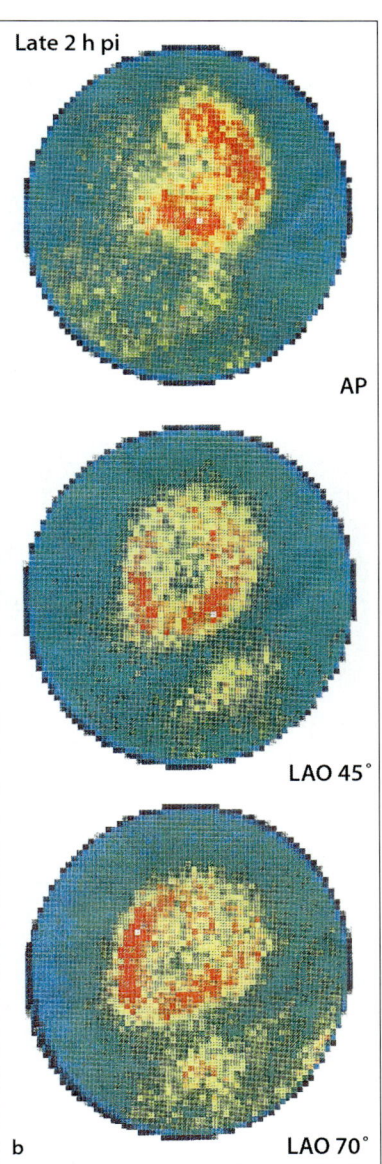

AP

LAO 45°

LAO 70°

b

Fig. 2.73 a,b. Myocardial perfusion scan in a 41-year-old man with dyspnea and a known history of sarcoidosis with multiorgan involvement. The early (**a**) and late (**b**) static images show nonhomogeneous, diffusely decreased uptake through the myocardium at rest. Biopsy confirmed cardiac involvement by sarcoidosis

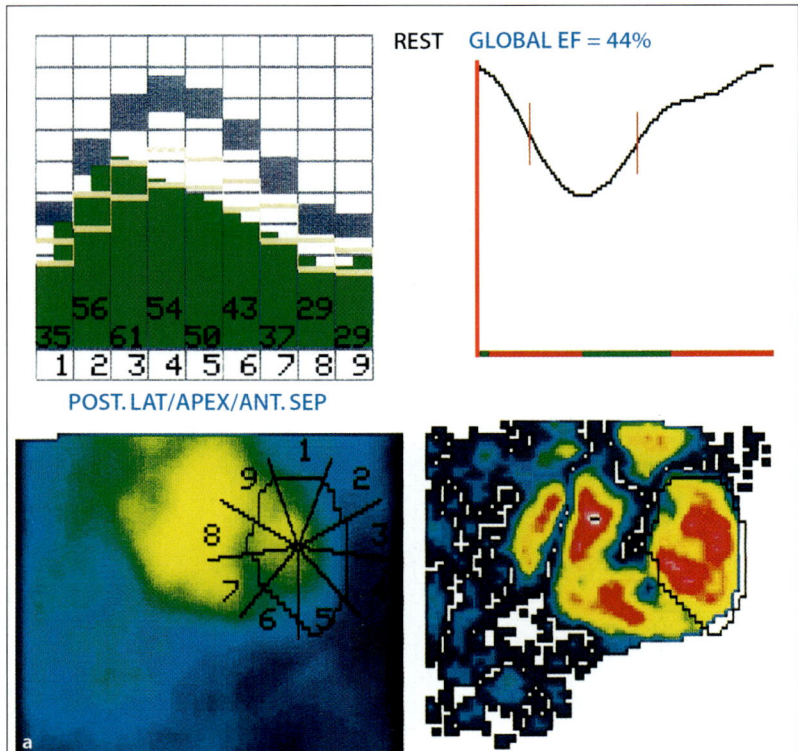

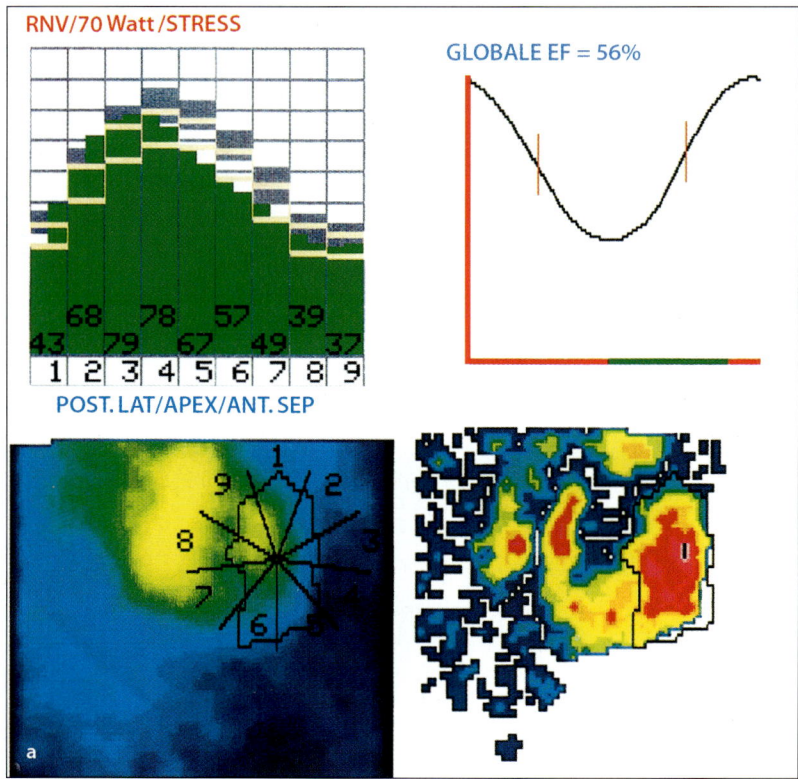

Fig. 2.74 a–c. Man 49 years of age with hyperthyroid-related cardiac complaints, treated with cardimazol. Stress ventriculography shows global restriction in the left myocardium as a result of hyperthyroidism and cardimazol therapy

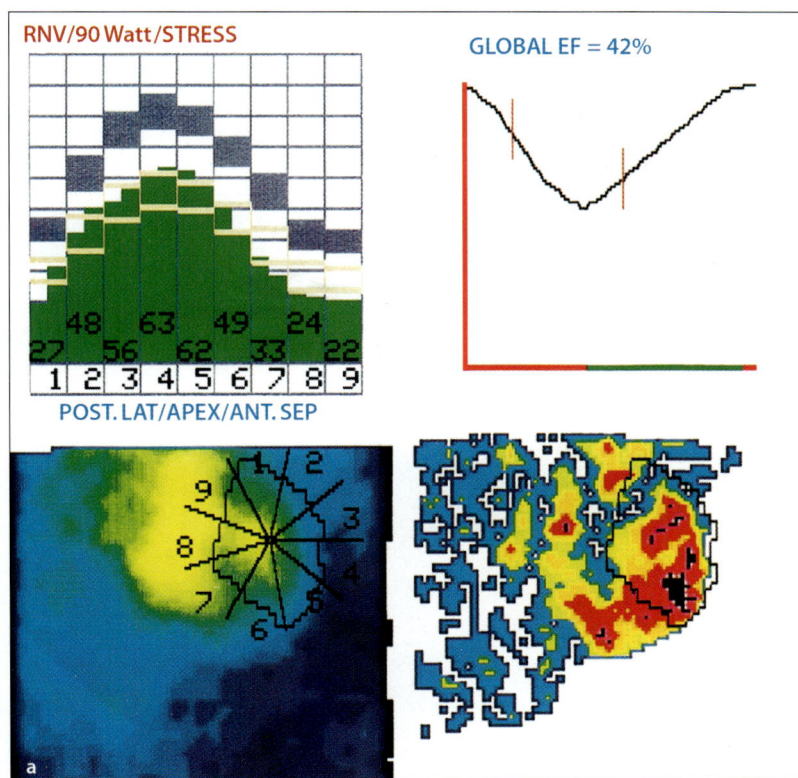

Fig. 2.74 a. *Continued*

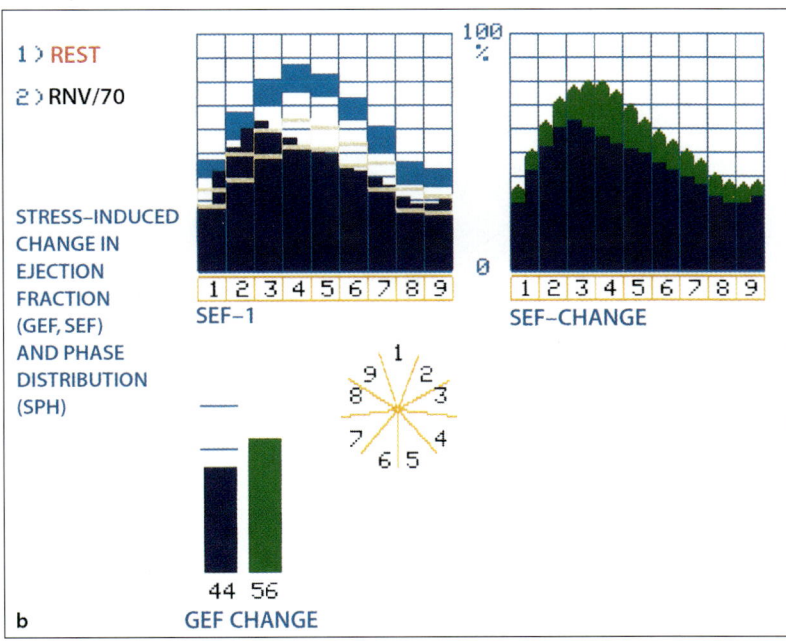

Fig. 2.74 b

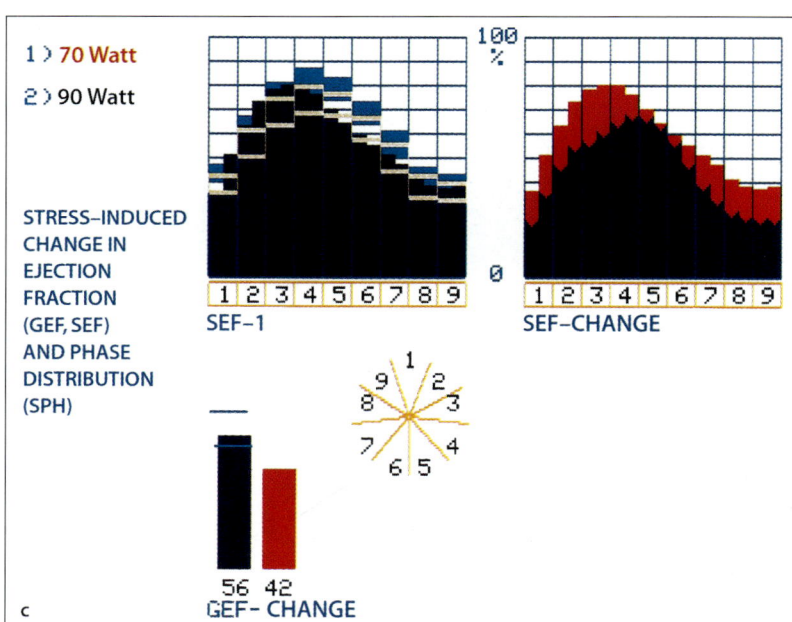

c

Fig. 2.74 a–c. Man 49 years of age with hyperthyroid-related cardiac complaints, treated with cardimazol. Stress ventriculography shows global restriction in the left myocardium as a result of hyperthyroidism and cardimazol therapy

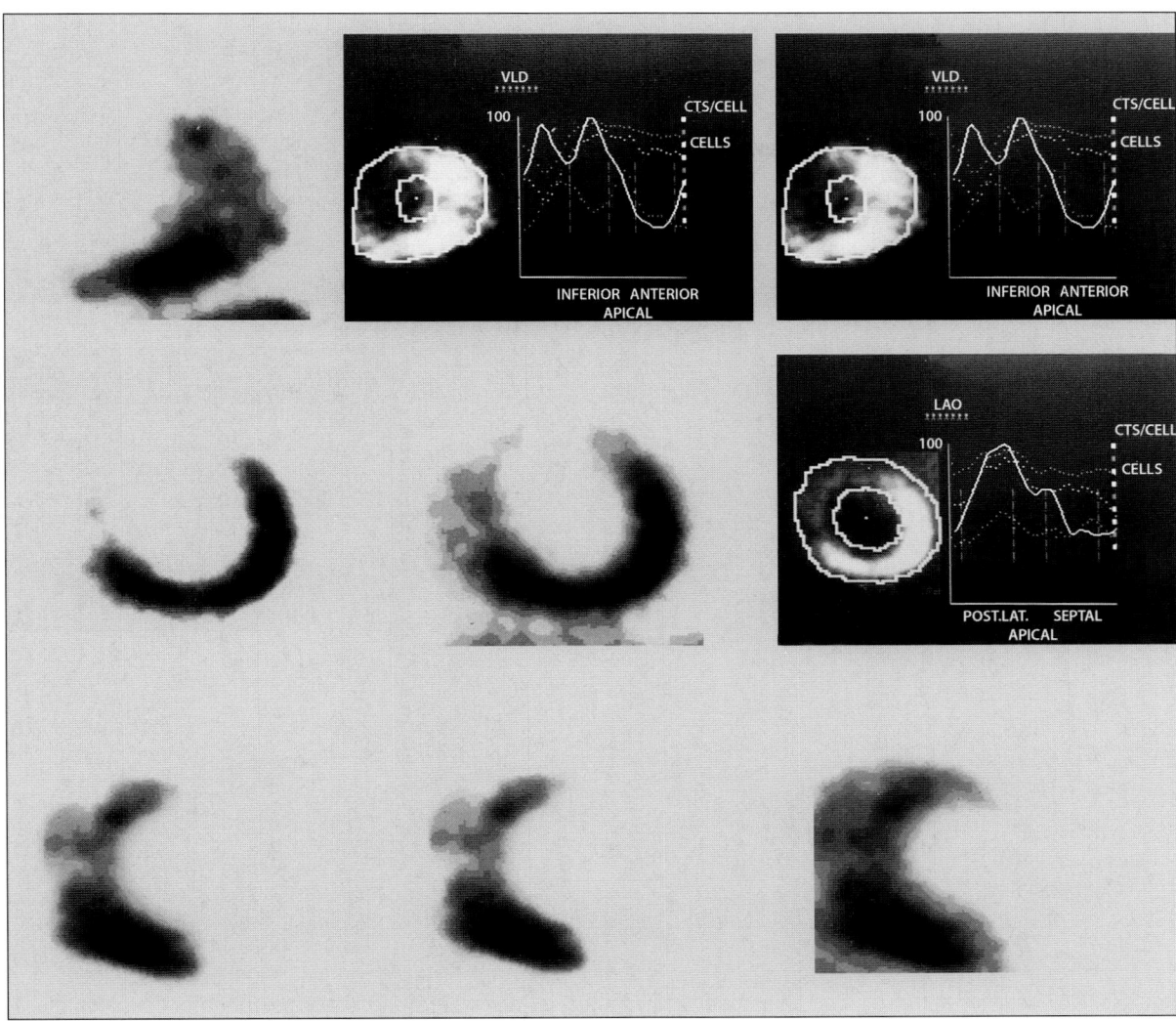

Fig. 2.75. A 61-year-old man sustained an anterior wall infarction two years ago and a recurrent anterior infarction one year later. Resting myocardial perfusion scan shows a defect in the anterior wall and apex of an axially rotated heart (cor bovinum). The activity profile is difficult to visualize in the apex and adjacent anterior wall, suggesting that an aneurysm has formed in that region

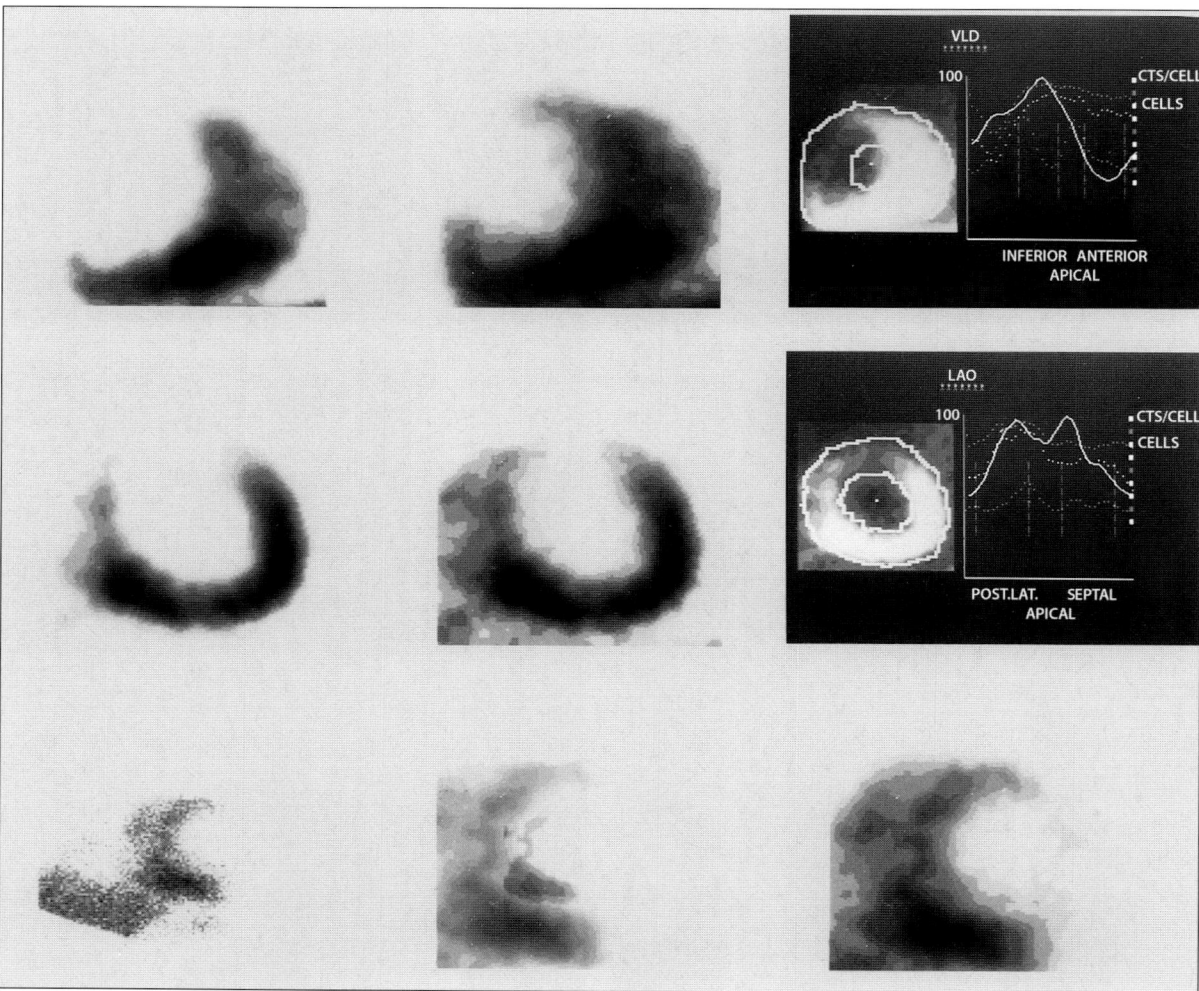

Fig. 2.75. A 61-year-old man sustained an anterior wall infarction two years ago and a recurrent anterior infarction one year later. Resting myocardial perfusion scan shows a defect in the anterior wall and apex of an axially rotated heart (cor bovinum). The activity profile is difficult to visualize in the apex and adjacent anterior wall, suggesting that an aneurysm has formed in that region

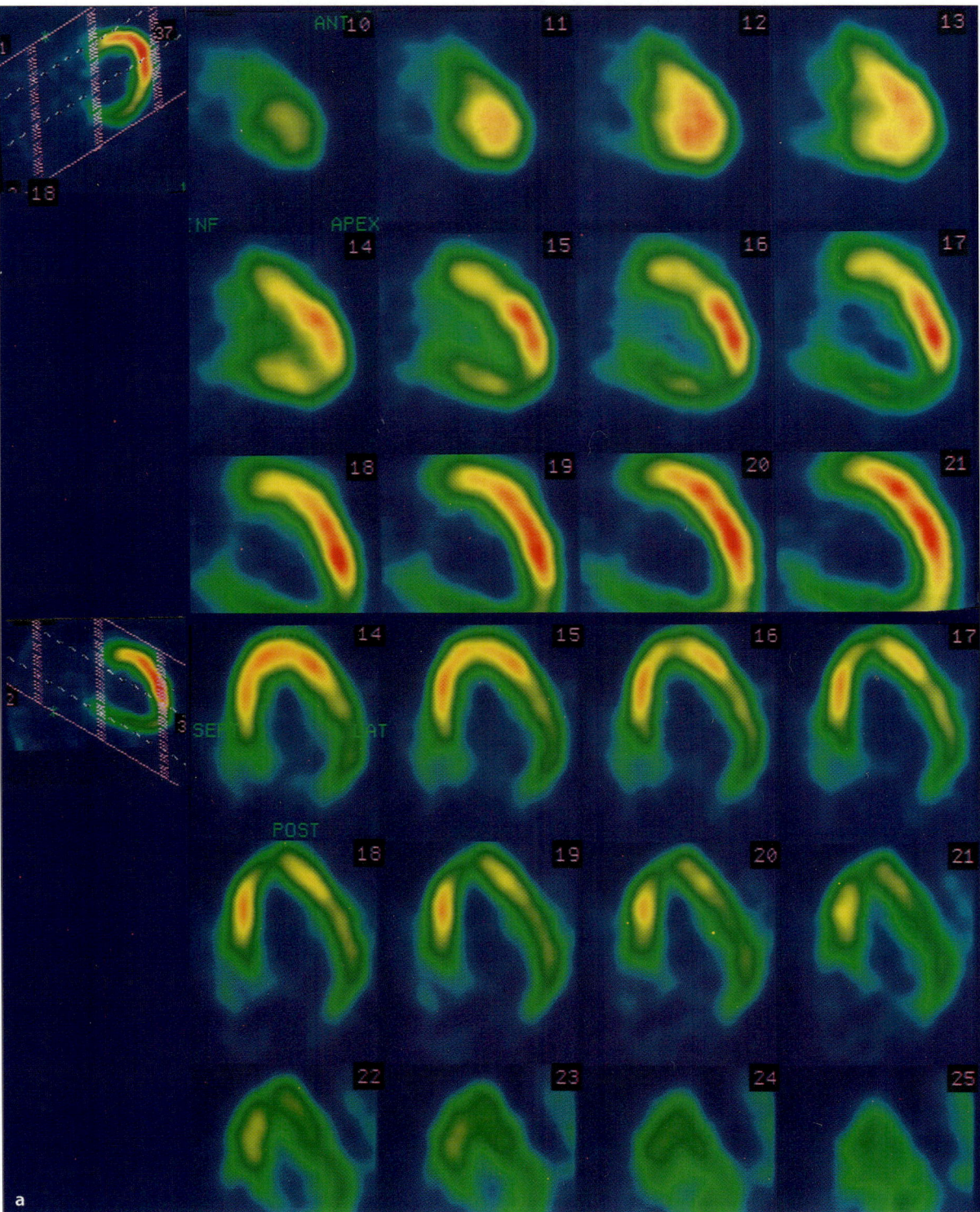

Fig. 2.76 a–c. A 79-year-old man experienced tachycardia during preparations for surgery. **a** Stress ^{201}Tl myocardial perfusion scan. Exercise was stopped at 30 W because of tachycardia to 114 bpm. Stress scan shows diffusely decreased uptake through the left myocardium with an enlarged ventricular cavity. **b** Resting scan shows no change except for better visualization of the anterior wall. Heart failure

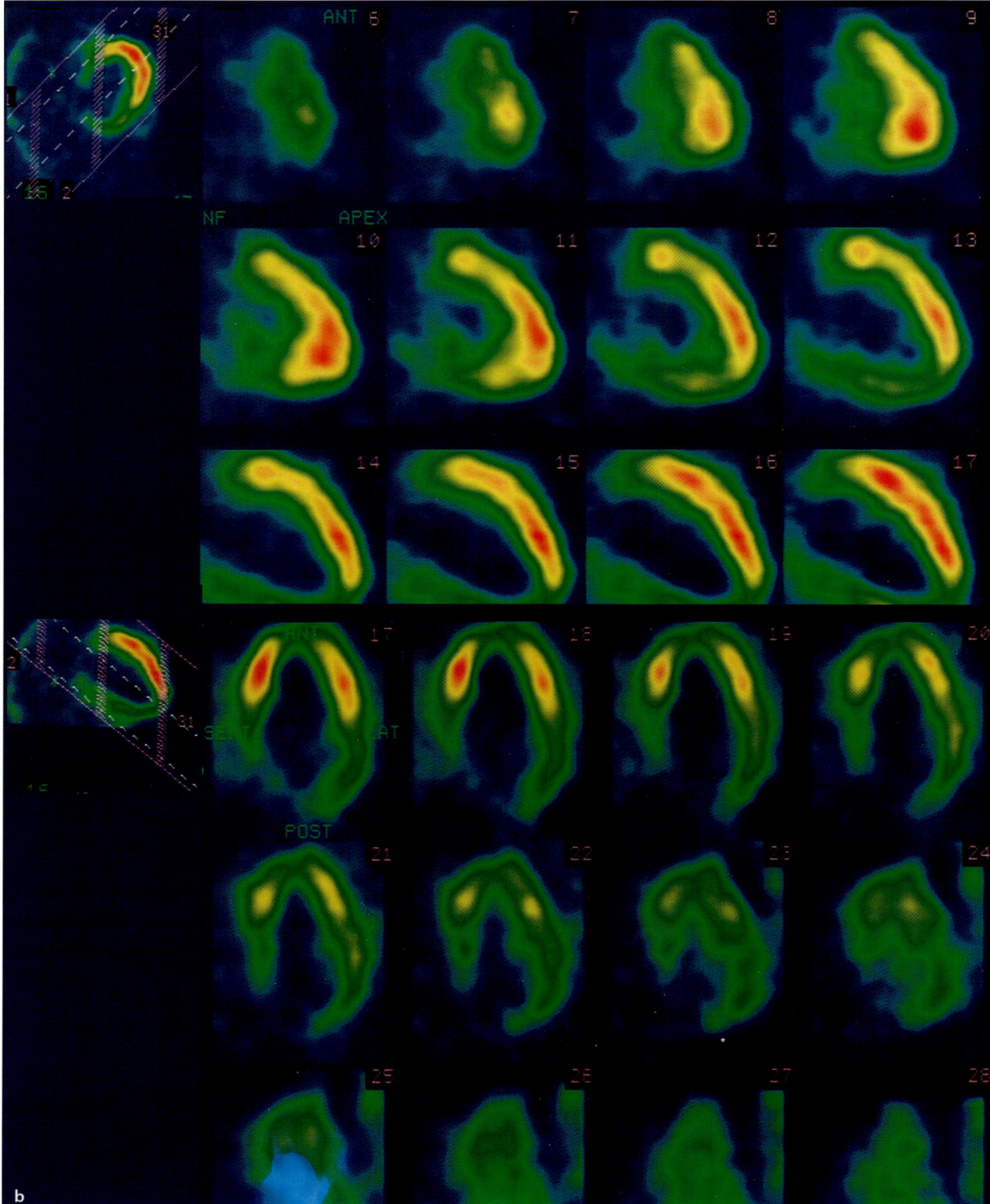

Fig. 2.76 a–c. A 79-year-old man experienced tachycardia during preparations for surgery. **a** Stress ^{201}Tl myocardial per-fusion scan. Exercise was stopped at 30 W because of tachycardia to 114 bpm. Stress scan shows diffusely decreased uptake through the left myocardium with an enlarged ventricular cavity. **b** Resting scan shows no change except for better visualization of the anterior wall. Heart failure

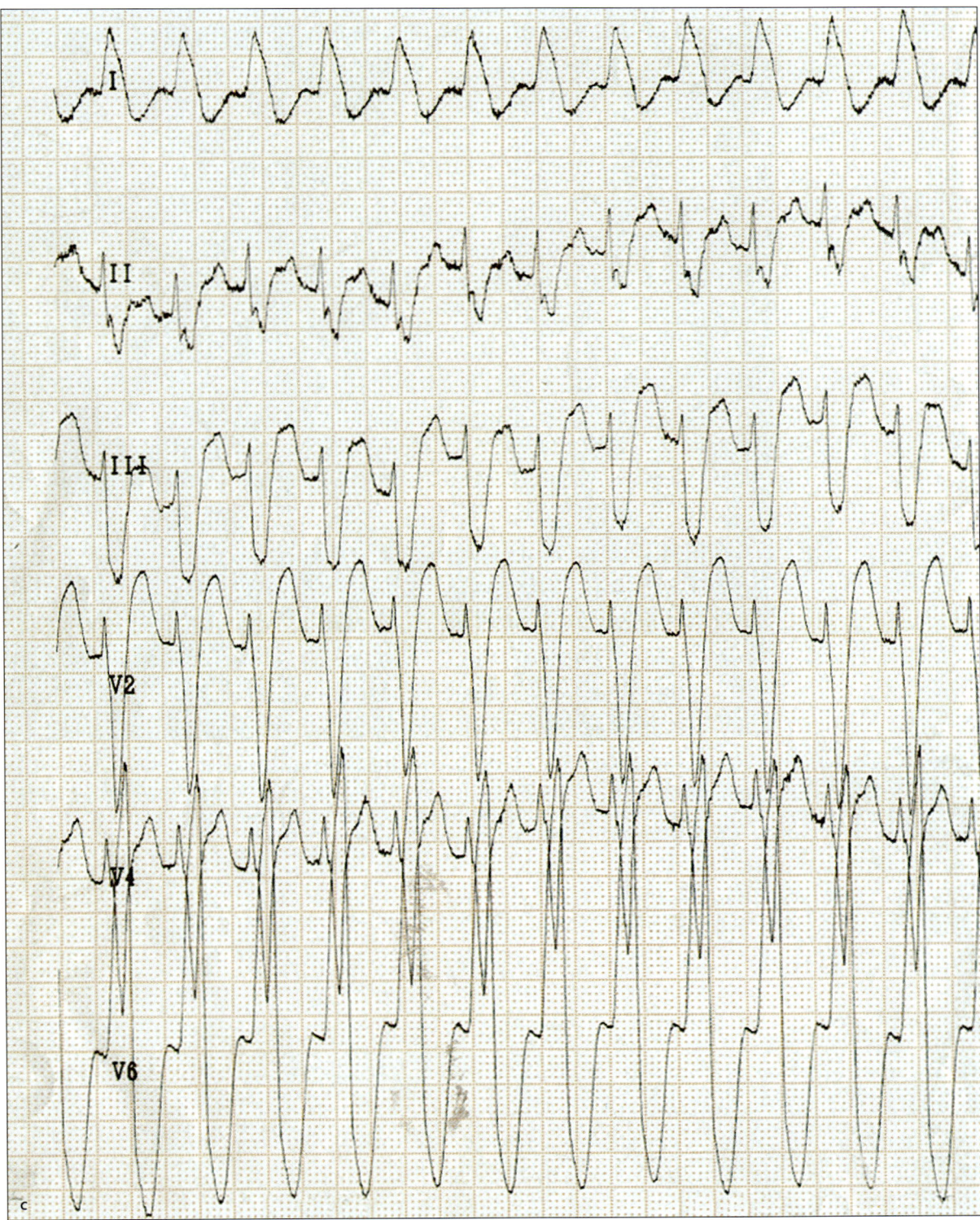

Fig. 2.76 c

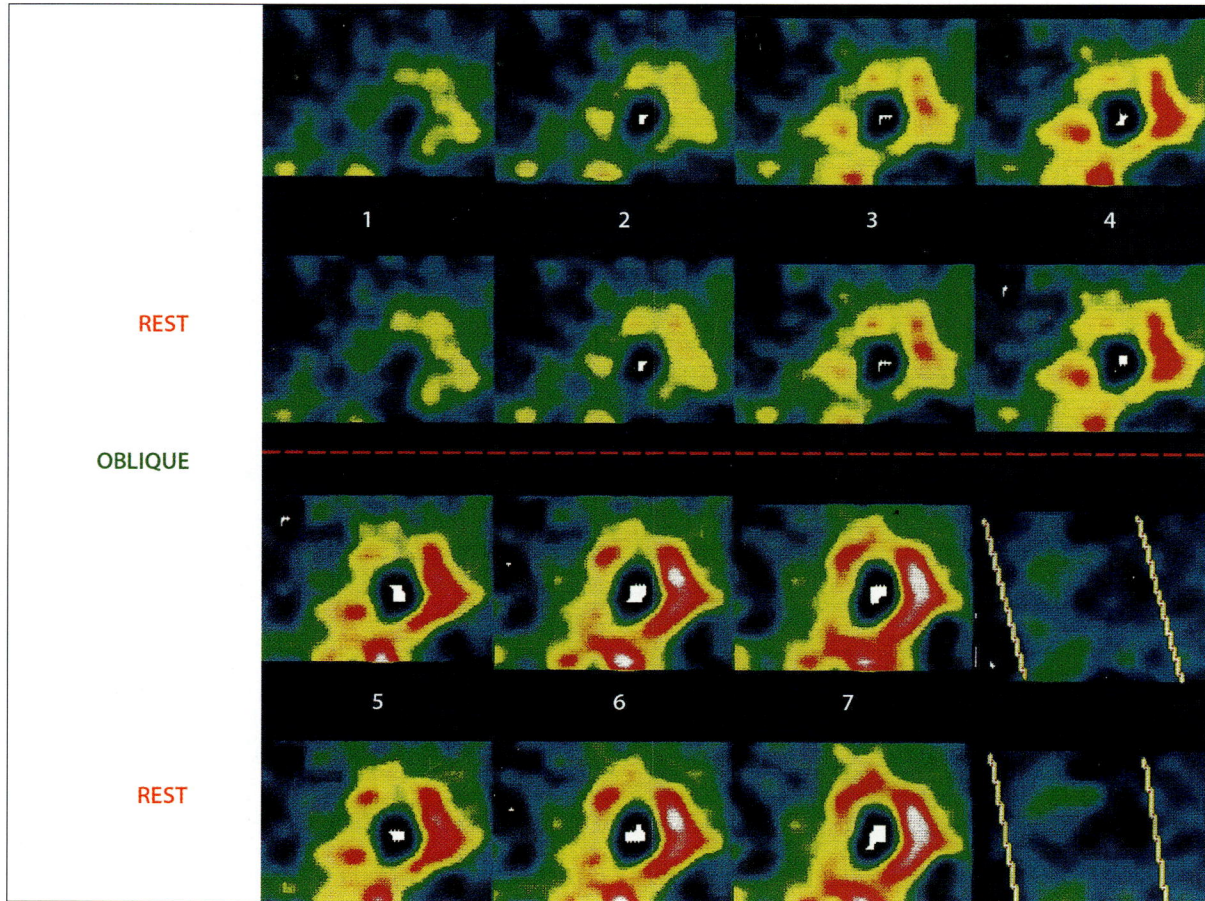

REST

OBLIQUE

REST

Fig. 2.77. A 49-year-old man was referred for workman's compensation assessment due to limitation of stress tolerance. The patient complained of exertional dyspnea. Resting perfusion scan shows scattered myocardial defects with nonperfusion of the anterior wall region and most of the posterior wall. EF is 23% (poorly reproducible). The perfusion defects are caused by scarring of the left myocardium with aneurysm formation in the anterior wall

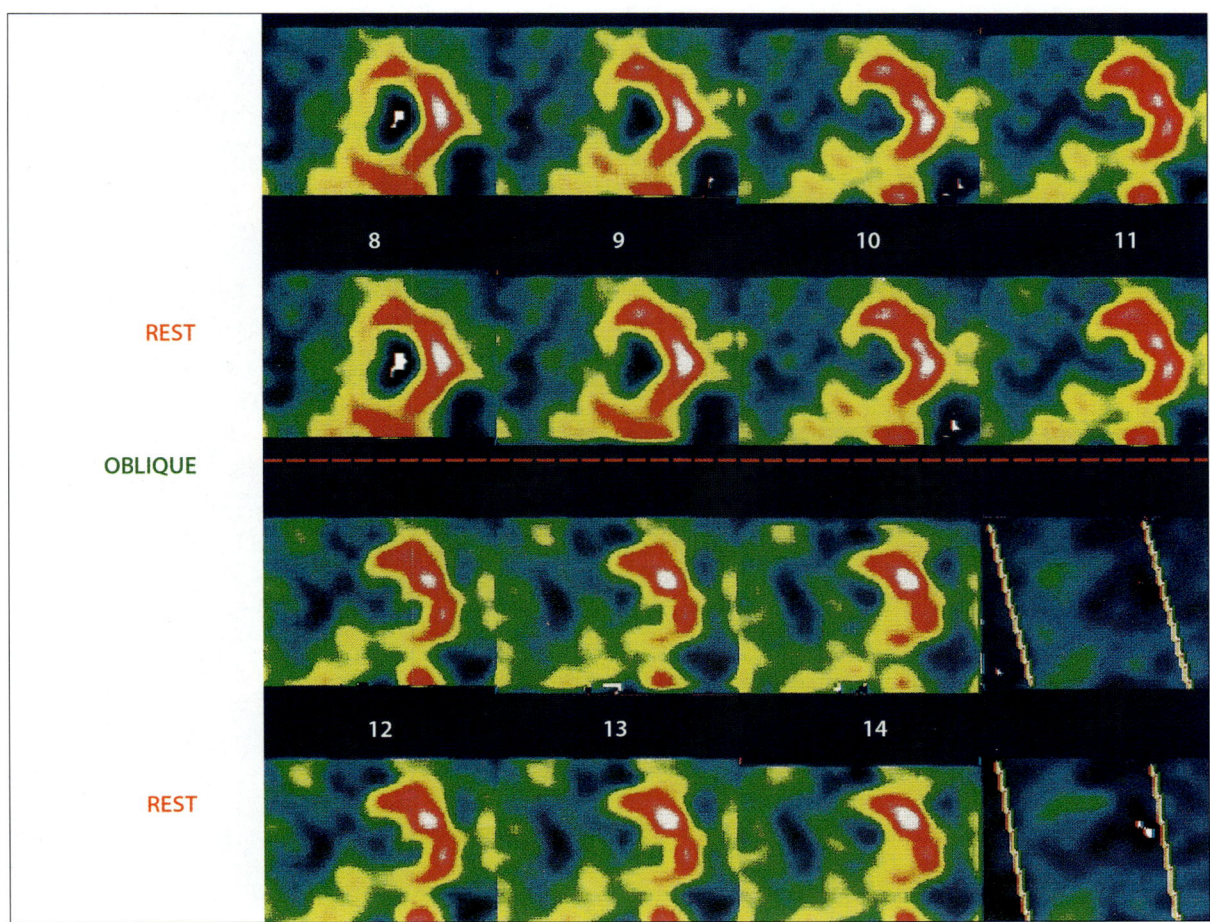

REST

OBLIQUE

REST

Fig. 2.77. *Continued*

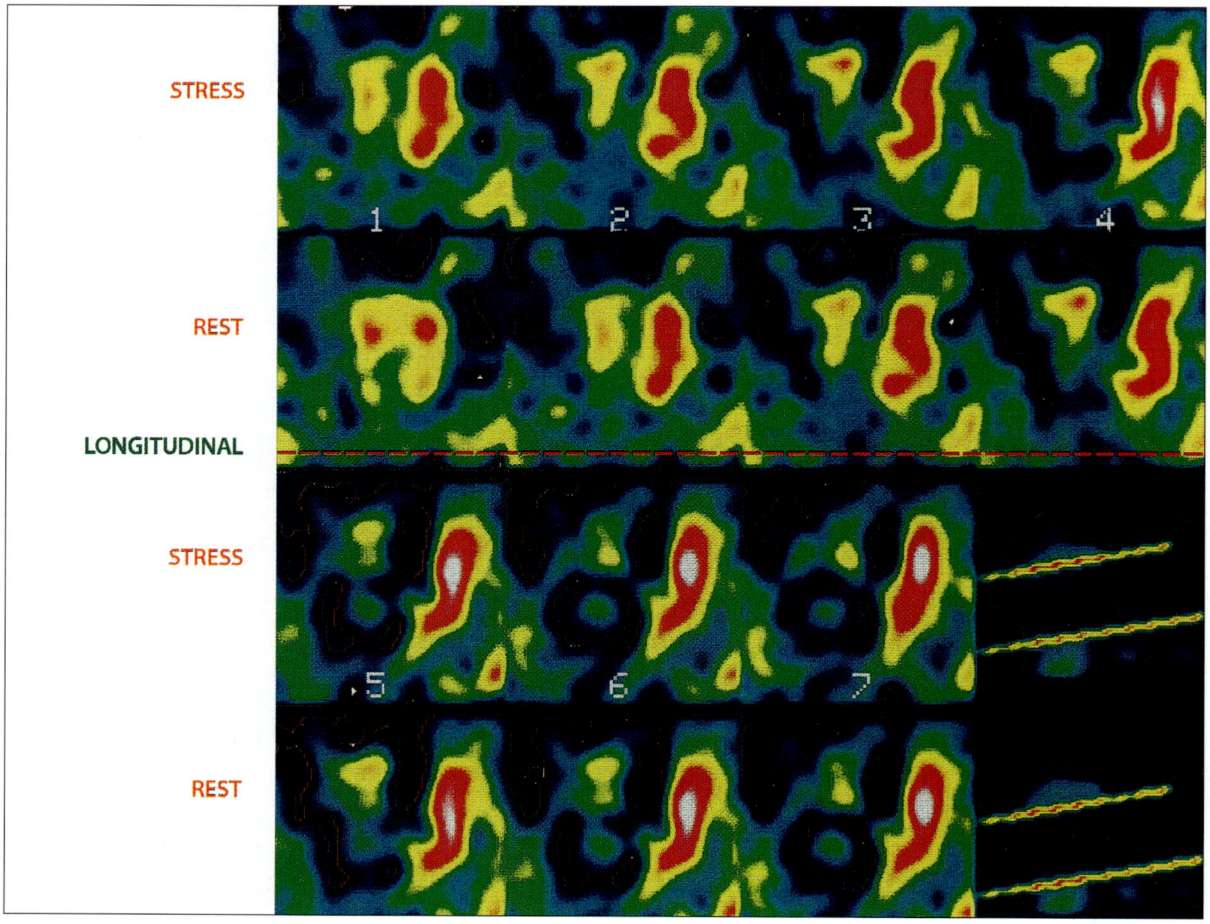

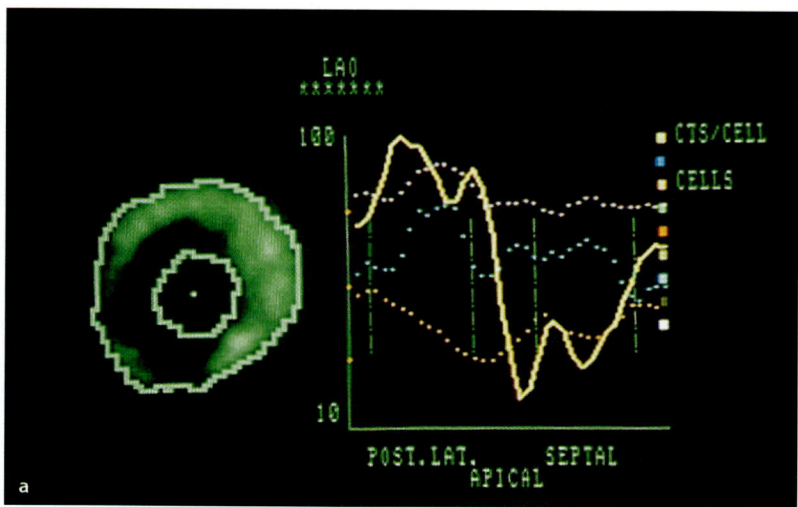

Fig. 2.77. A 49-year-old man was referred for workman's compensation assessment due to limitation of stress tolerance. The patient complained of exertional dyspnea. Resting perfusion scan shows scattered myocardial defects with nonperfusion of the anterior wall region and most of the posterior wall. EF is 23% (poorly reproducible). The perfusion defects are caused by scarring of the left myocardium with aneurysm formation in the anterior wall

Fig. 2.78 a–c. Resting ^{201}Tl myocardial scan in a 40-year-old woman with unexplained retrosternal burning shows a perfusion defect in the anterior wall and interventricular septum. Amplitude and phase analysis consistent with an anterior wall aneurysm

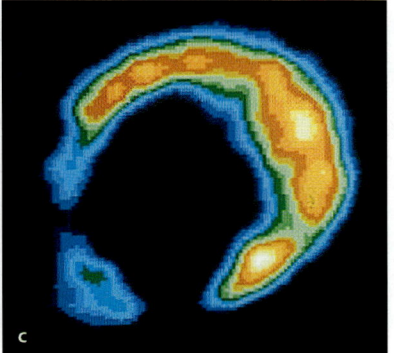

Fig. 2.78 b–c

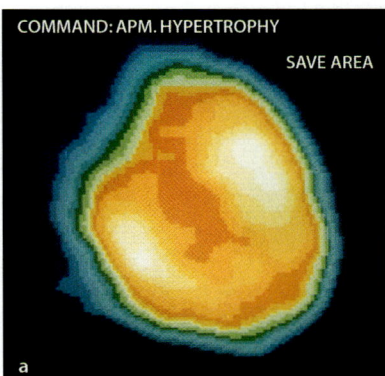

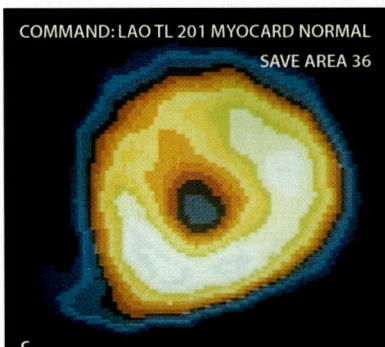

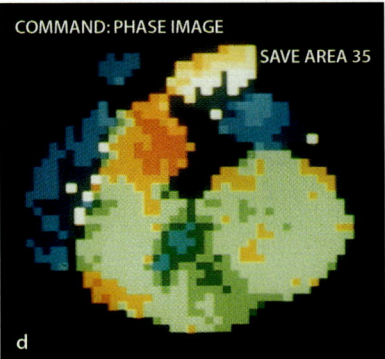

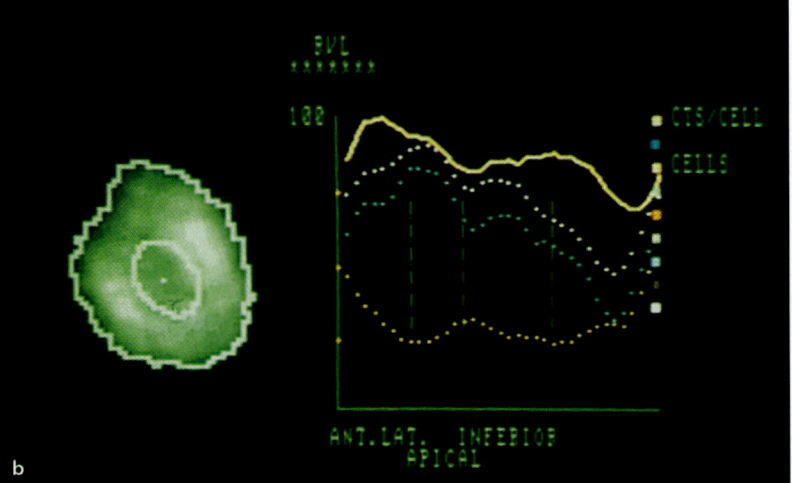

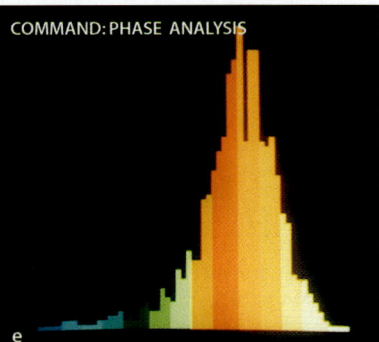

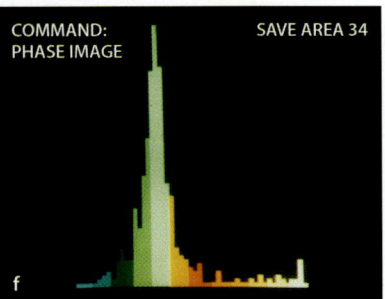

Fig. 2.79 a–f. A 35-year-old woman had a febrile infection for four weeks and a four-day history of exertional dyspnea and cyanotic lips. Resting ^{201}Tl perfusion study shows prolonged retention of the radionuclide in the myocardium with no defects. Amplitude and phase analysis (**e**) indicates significant dissociation. Post-treatment follow-up (**f**) shows regression of the changes

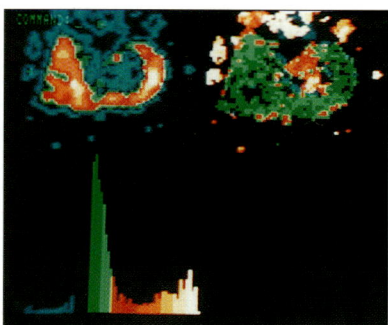

Fig. 2.80. Amplitude and phase analysis in a 44-year-old woman with burning retrosternal pain. Anterior wall aneurysm near the base of the heart

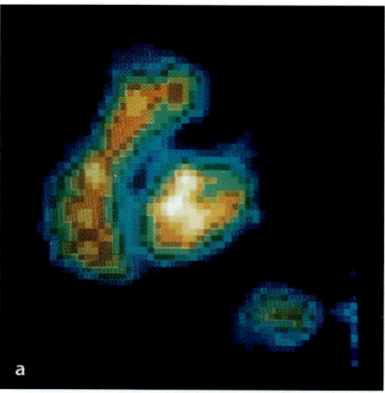
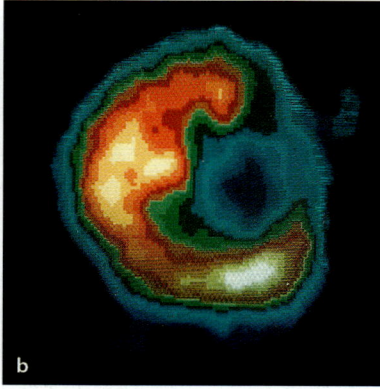

Fig. 2.81 a,b. Serial images document paradoxical wall motion associated with a ventricular aneurysm. **a** Radionuclide ventriculography. **b** ^{201}Tl myocardial perfusion scan

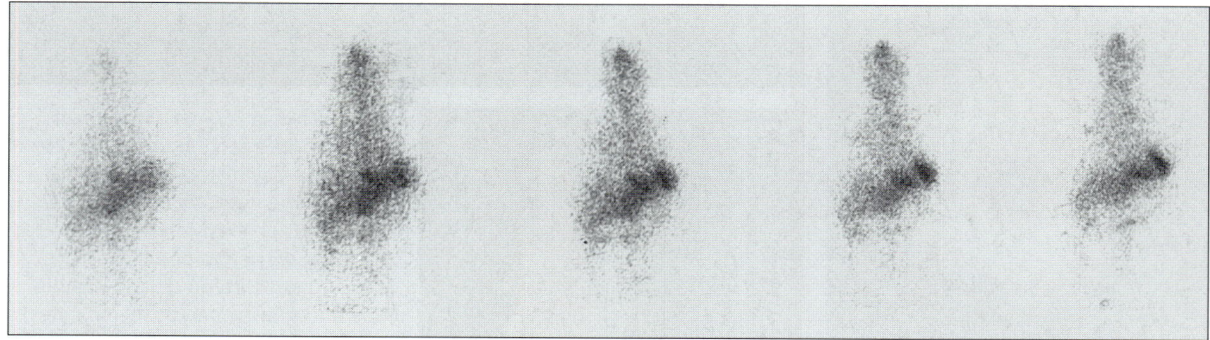

Fig. 2.82. ^{67}Ga myocardial scan in a 38-year-old woman with burning retrosternal pain, fever, and exertional dyspnea shows a diffuse increase in tracer uptake and relative thickening of the left ventricular wall (Phocon technique). Histology confirmed syphilitic myocarditis

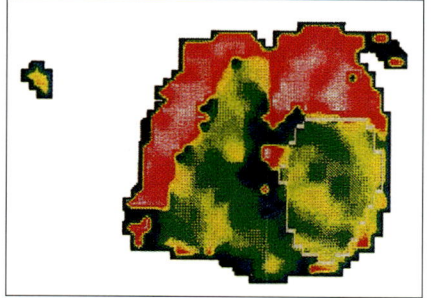

Fig. 2.83. Phase analysis shows irregular, ill-defined phase distribution in the presence of absolute arrhythmia

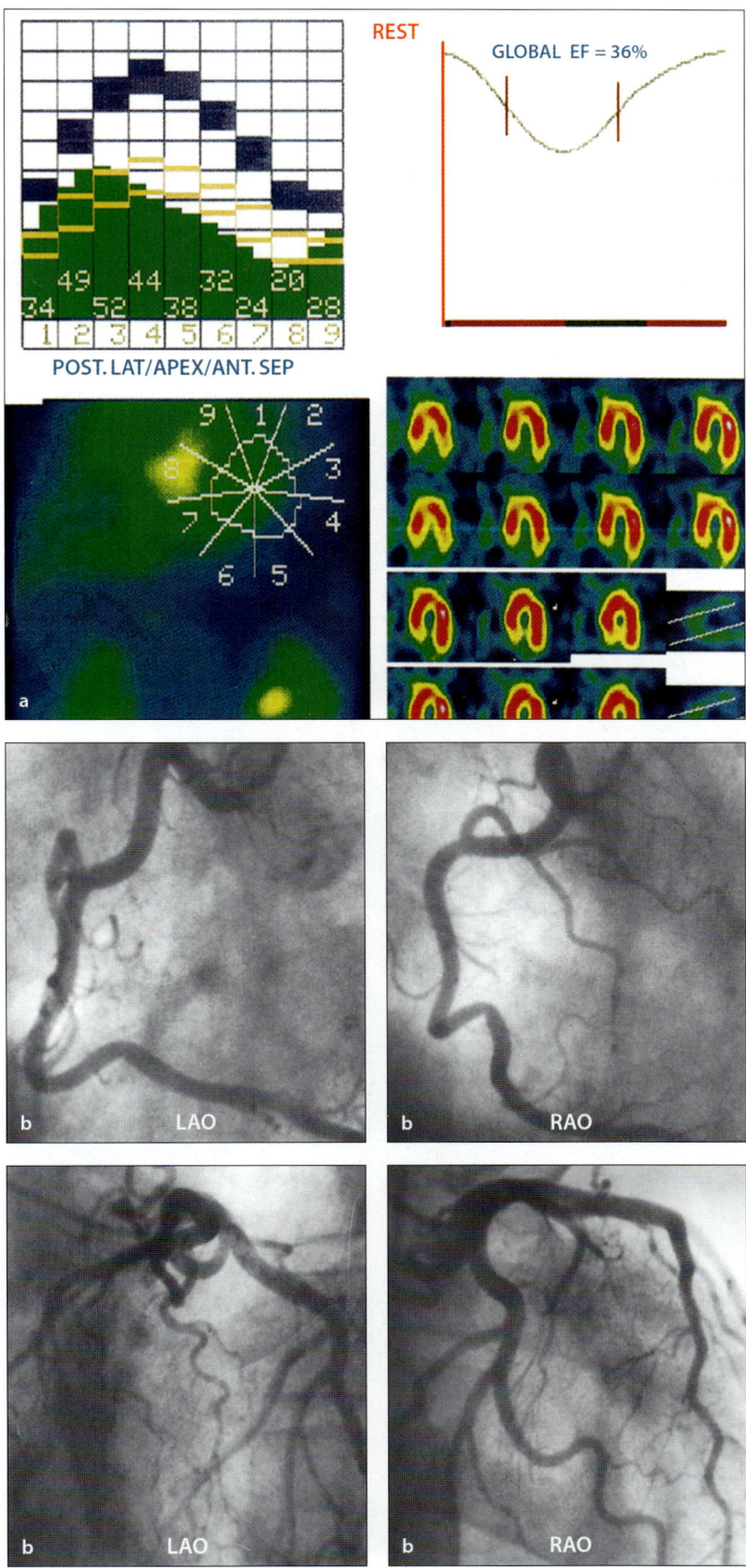

Fig. 2.84 a–c. Man 41 years of age presented with constant angina pectoris and low back pain. Myocardial perfusion scan and radionuclide ventriculography (**a**) show a hypoplastic myocardium with a diminished global and regional EF. Angiography (**b**) and ECG (**c**) show no evidence of CHD

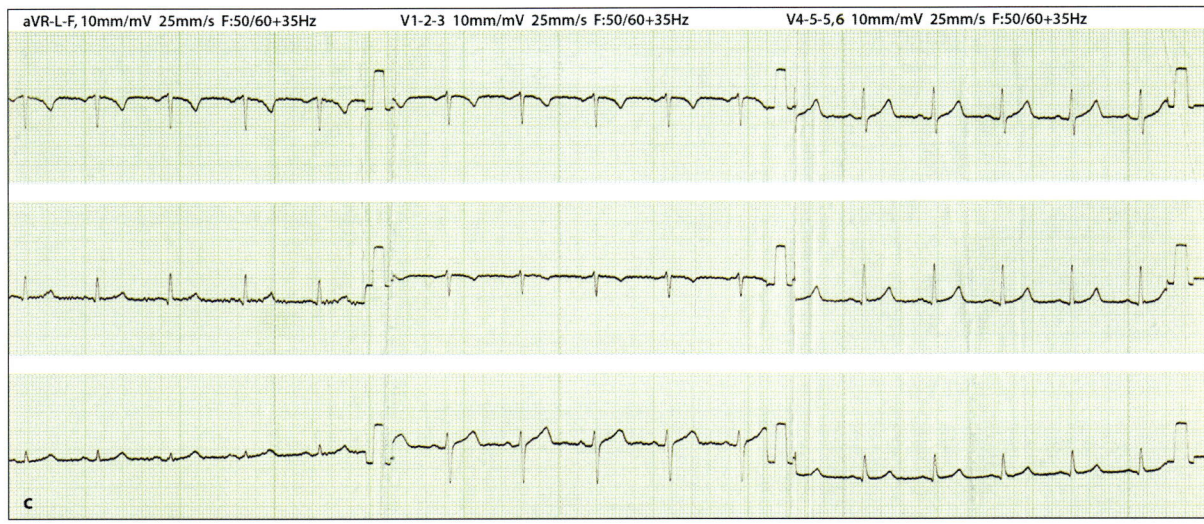

aVR-L-F, 10mm/mV 25mm/s F:50/60+35Hz   V1-2-3 10mm/mV 25mm/s F:50/60+35Hz   V4-5-5,6 10mm/mV 25mm/s F:50/60+35Hz

Fig. 2.84 a–c. Man 41 years of age presented with constant angina pectoris and low back pain. Myocardial perfusion scan and radionuclide ventriculography (**a**) show a hypoplastic myocardium with a diminished global and regional EF. Angiography (**b**) and ECG (**c**) show no evidence of CHD

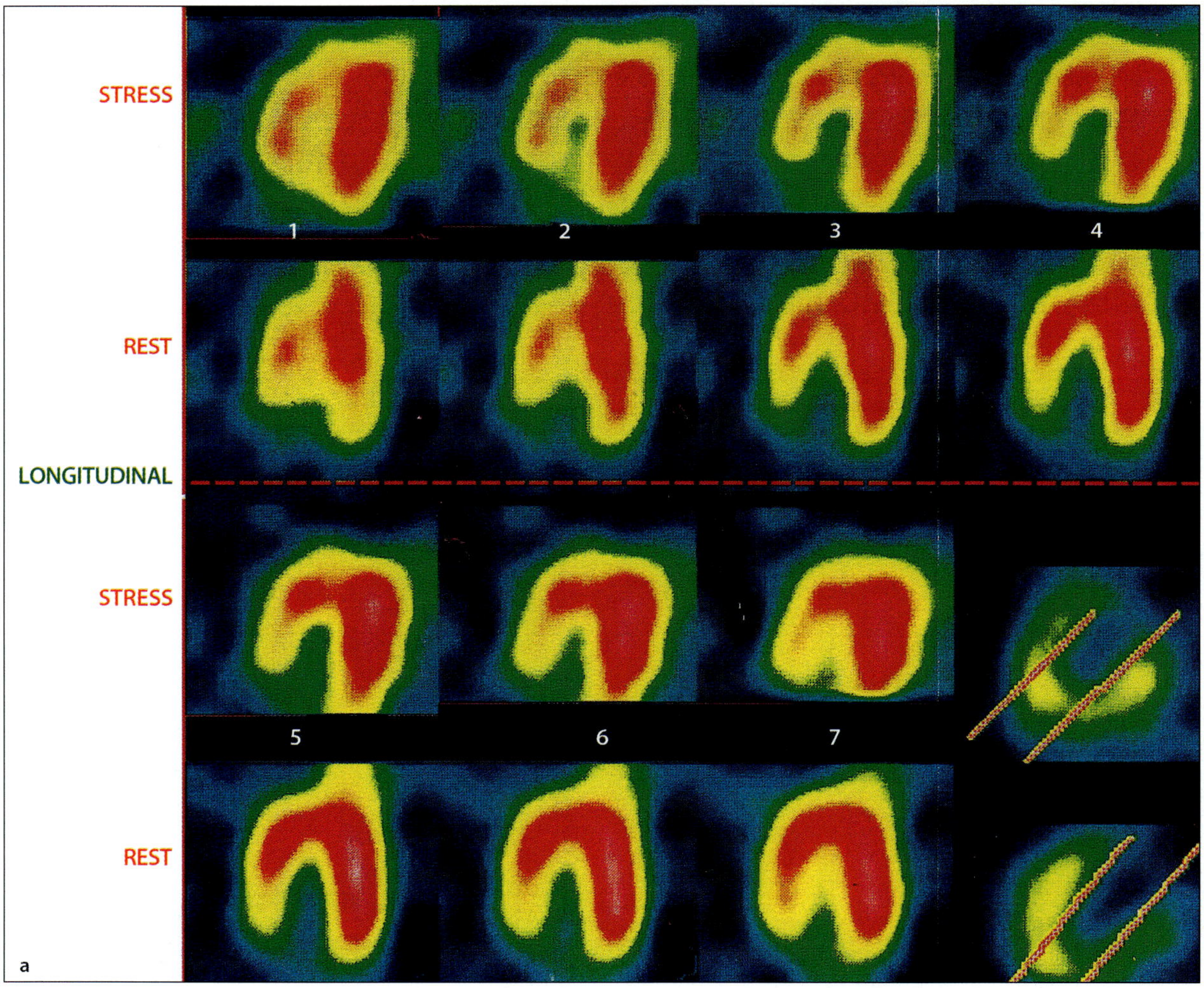

STRESS

REST

LONGITUDINAL

STRESS

REST

Fig. 2.85 a,b. Radionuclide findings in a 51-year-old male hypochondriac. **a** Stress myocardial perfusion scan in the anxious patient shows hypoperfusion of the anterior wall

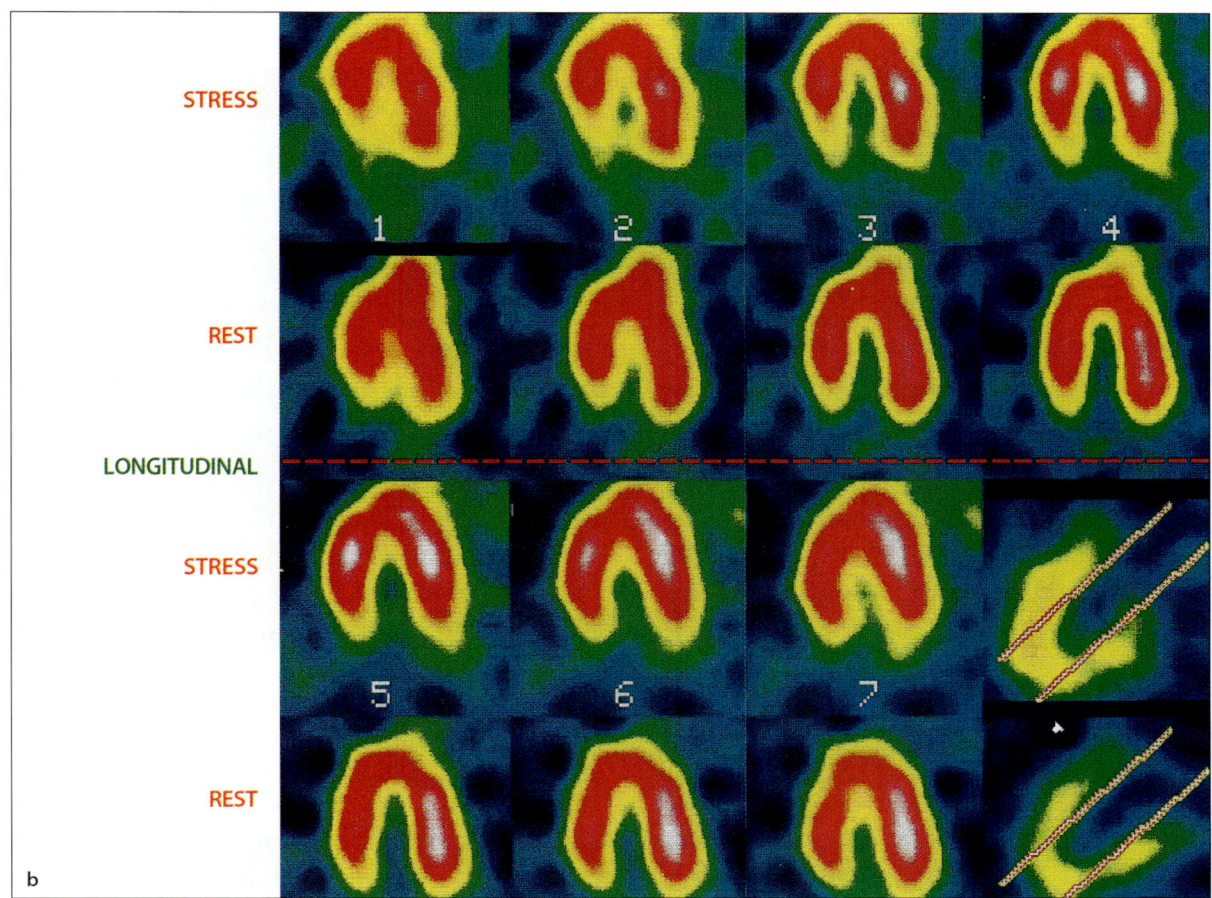

STRESS

REST

LONGITUDINAL

STRESS

REST

b

Fig. 2.85 b. Repeat scan after psychological counseling (no medication) shows excellent perfusion of the left myocardium at rest and during exercise

TL/REST

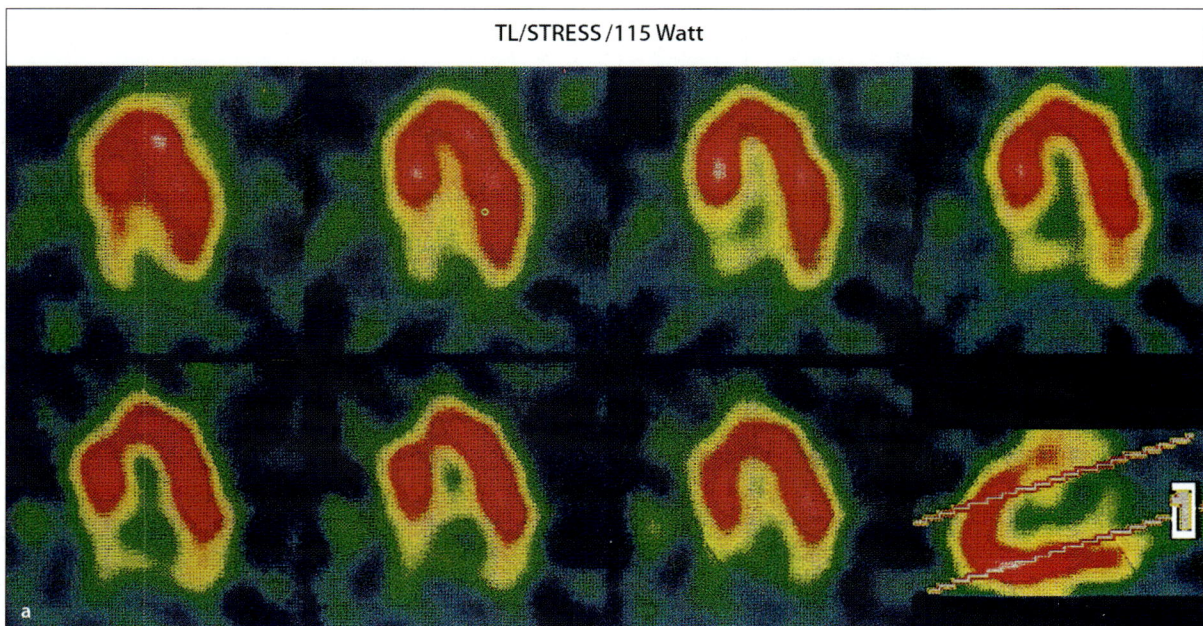

Fig. 2.86 a,b. A 42-year-old woman with unexplained tachycardia was referred for exclusion of CHD. Exercise ECG to 115 W showed no abnormalities. **a** ^{201}Tl myocardial perfusion study with graded exercise to 115 W shows good perfusion at rest and during exercise. **b** Ventriculography shows good global and segmental EF

TL/STRESS /115 Watt

Fig. 2.86 a. *Continued*

TL/STRESS /115 Watt

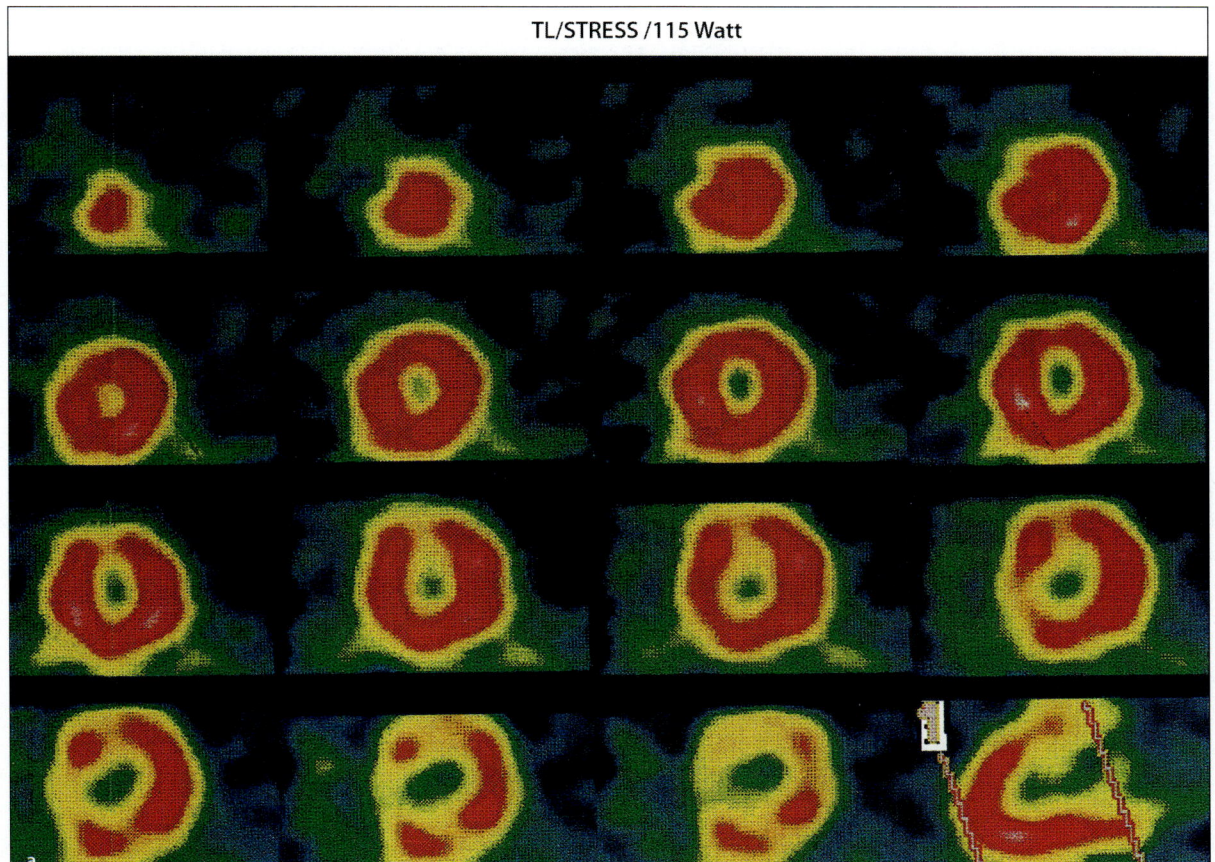

Fig. 2.86 a. *Continued*

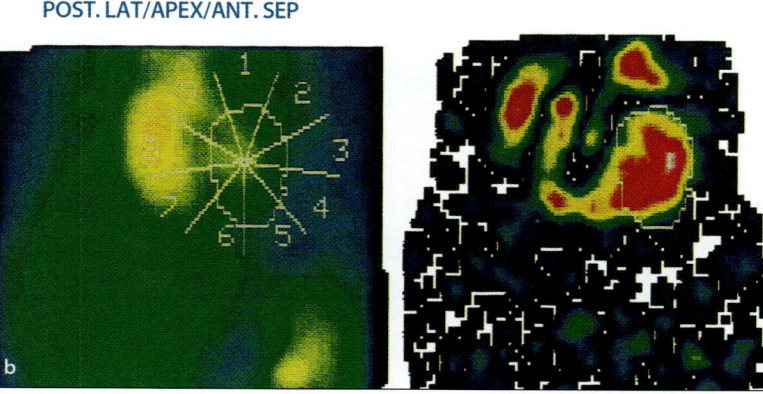

RNV/REST

GLOBAL   EF = 59%

67   78   59   39
43   78   68   49   38
1 / 2   3   4   5   6   7   8   9

POST. LAT/APEX/ANT. SEP

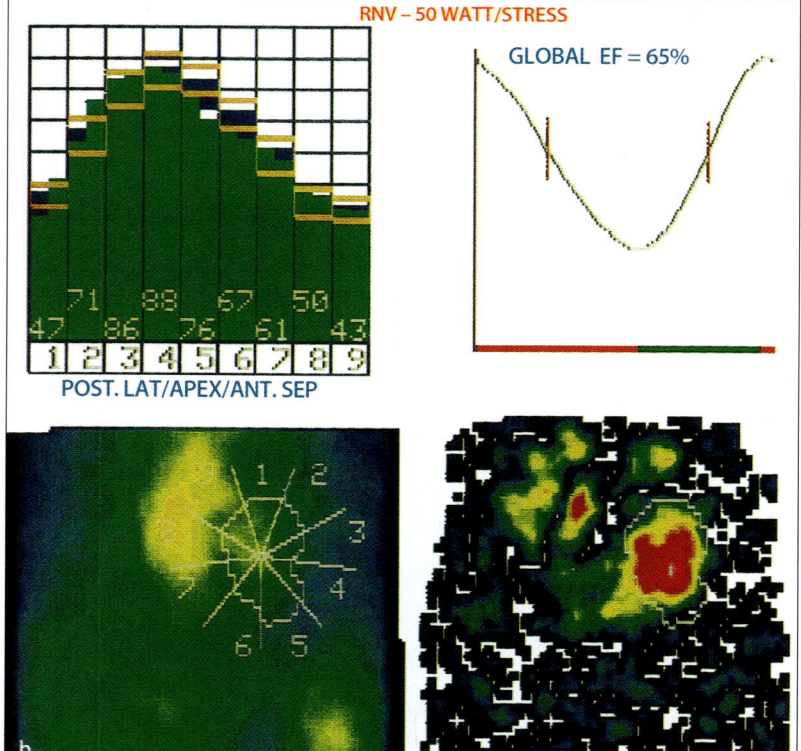

RNV – 50 WATT/STRESS

GLOBAL EF = 65%

71   88   67   50
47   86   76   61   43
1   2   3   4   5   6   7   8   9

POST. LAT/APEX/ANT. SEP

Fig. 2.86 a,b. A 42-year-old woman with unexplained tachycardia was referred for exclusion of CHD. Exercise ECG to 115 W showed no abnormalities. **a** ^{201}Tl myocardial perfusion study with graded exercise to 115 W shows good perfusion at rest and during exercise. **b** Ventriculography shows good global and segmental EF

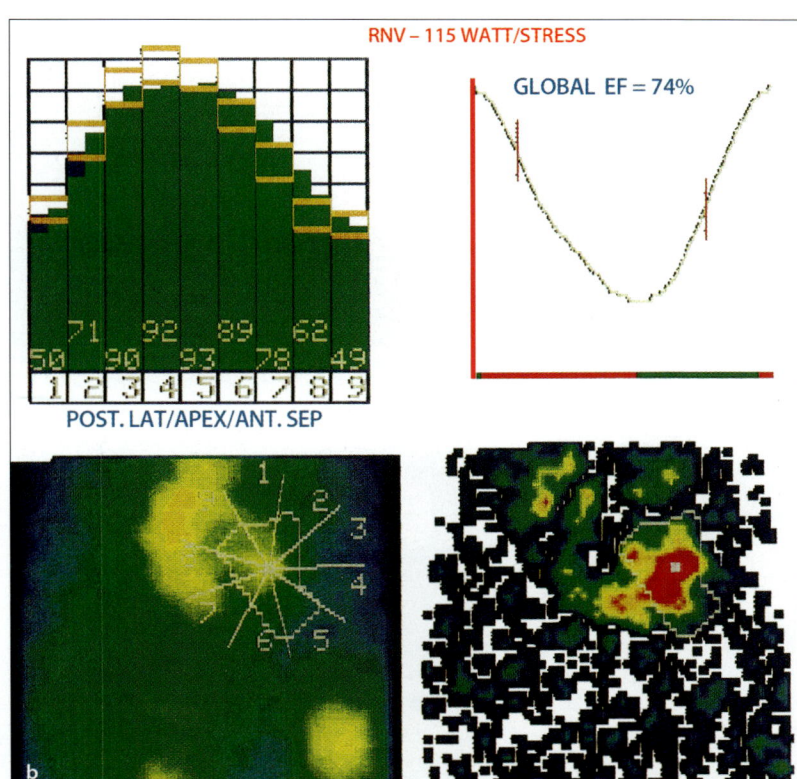

RNV – 115 WATT/STRESS

GLOBAL EF = 74%

POST. LAT/APEX/ANT. SEP

Fig. 2.86 b. *Continued*

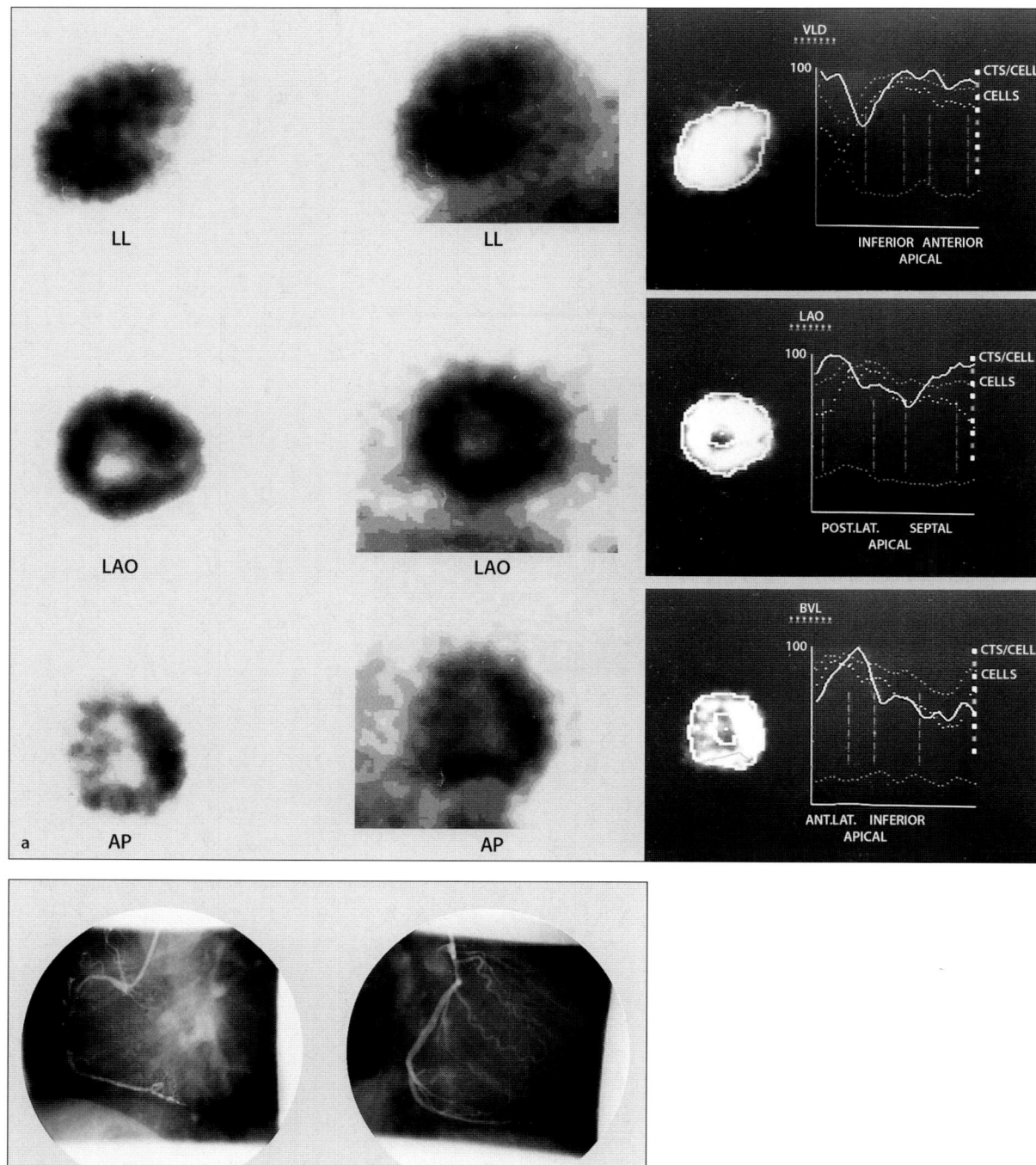

Fig. 2.87 a,b. Man 57 years of age with a long history of angina pectoris and mild exertional dyspnea. **a** Rest myocardial perfusion scan shows moderate hypoperfusion of the descending branch in the left myocardium and septal region. There is an overall decrease in tracer uptake. **b** Coronary angiography shows subtotal stenosis of the RCA, a low-grade stenosis of the LCX, and occlusion of the LAD with retrograde opacification. The coronary supply is good, with collateral flow providing relatively good preservation of viable myocardial tissue

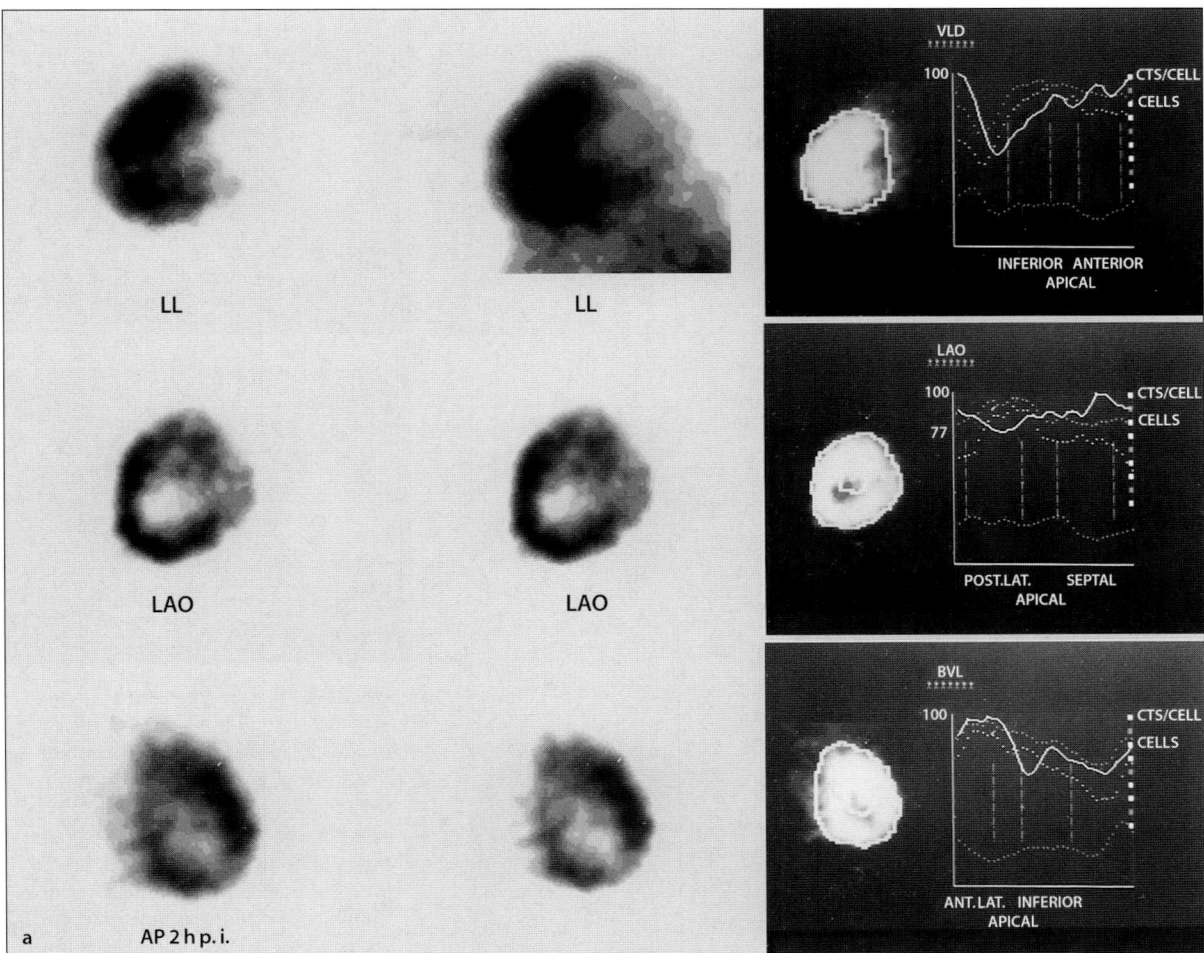

Fig. 2.88 a,b. A 57-year-old woman was evaluated for a two-year history of exertional dyspnea and burning retrosternal pain. **a** Myocardial perfusion scan at rest shows apical hypoperfusion with extension to the posterior wall. The defect is more conspicuous during exercise. Findings indicate multivessel disease with poststenotic viable tissue. **b** Coronary angiography shows subtotal stenosis of the LAD, occlusion of the LCX at its origin with retrograde opacification, and central occlusion of the RCA. Note: good collateral supply maintains tissue viability despite triple-vessel disease

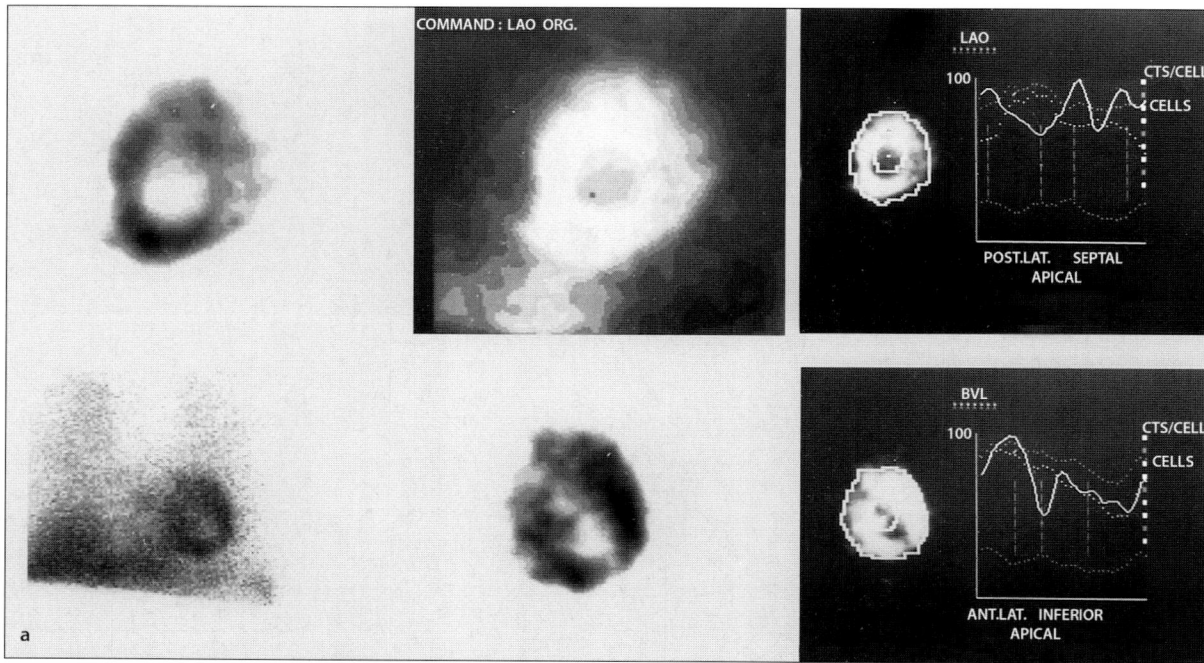

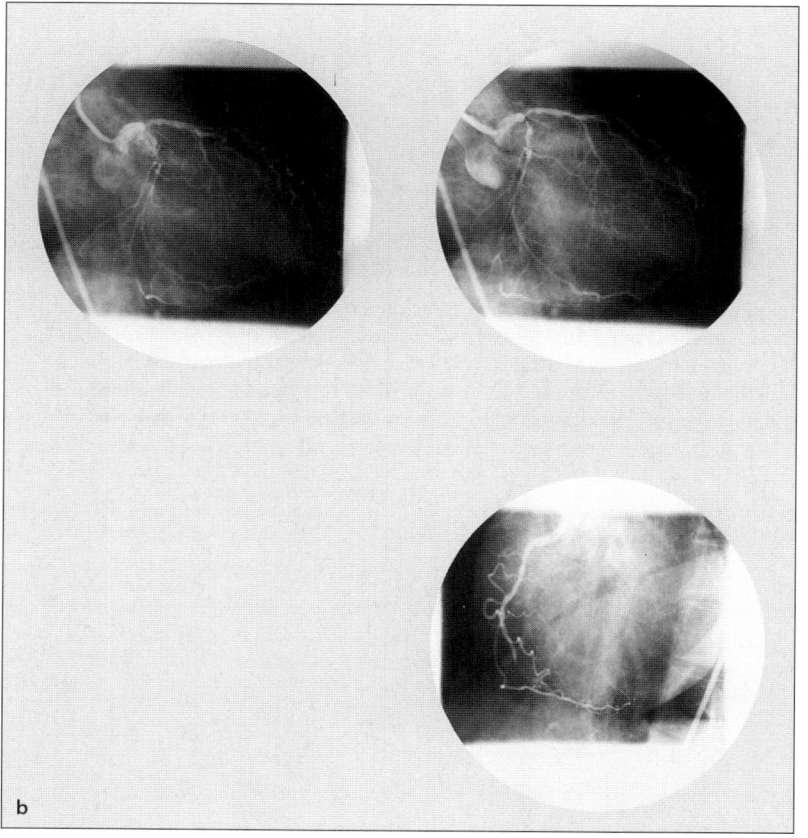

Fig. 2.88 a,b. A 57-year-old woman was evaluated for a two-year history of exertional dyspnea and burning retrosternal pain. **a** Myocardial perfusion scan at rest shows apical hypoperfusion with extension to the posterior wall. The defect is more conspicuous during exercise. Findings indicate multivessel disease with poststenotic viable tissue. **b** Coronary angiography shows subtotal stenosis of the LAD, occlusion of the LCX at its origin with retrograde opacification, and central occlusion of the RCA. Note: good collateral supply maintains tissue viability despite triple-vessel disease

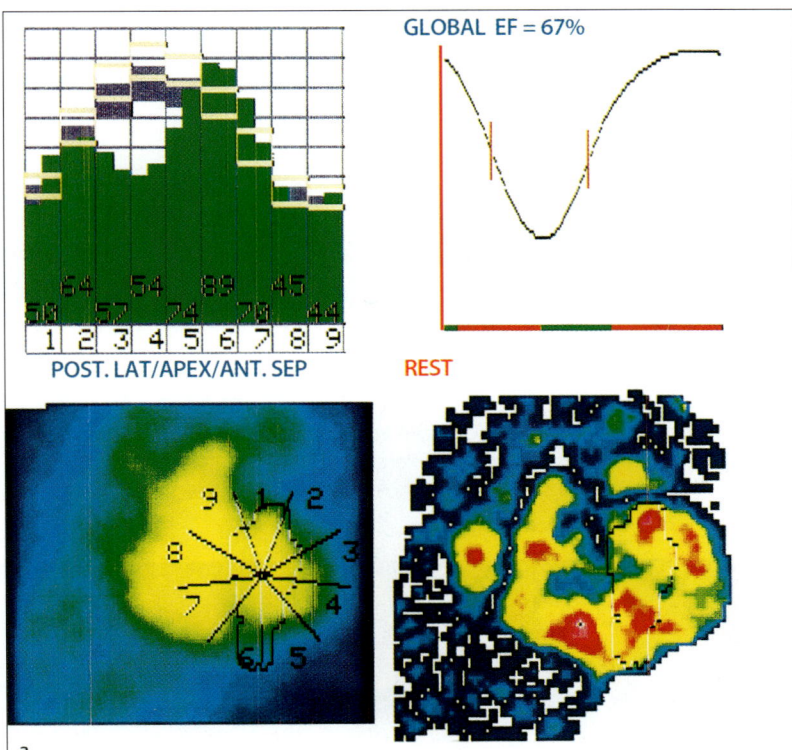

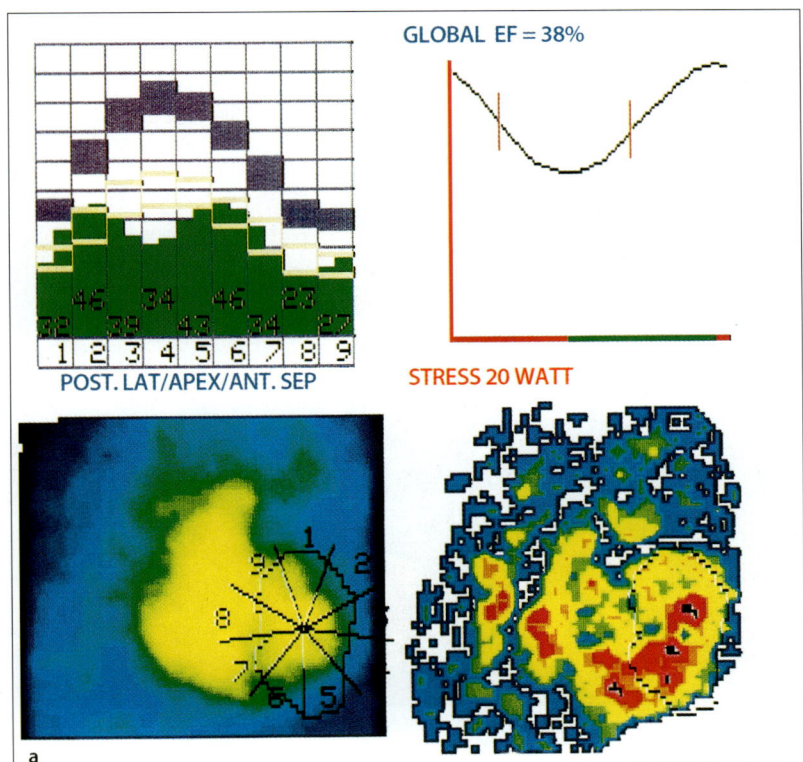

Fig. 2.89 a–c. A 43-year-old man underwent quintuple coronary bypass surgery one year before with internal thoracic artery bypass to the LAD, single vein grafts on the right posterior descending branch, and sequential grafts on the marginal branch, posterior lateral branch, and diagonal branch for treatment of triple-vessel disease. **a** Radionuclide ventriculography at rest shows a defect associated with anterior wall akinesis. On exercise at 20 W, significant restriction is seen throughout the left myocardium. **b** Exercise ^{201}Tl myocardial scan at 30 W shows multiple hypoperfused zones. Heart failure

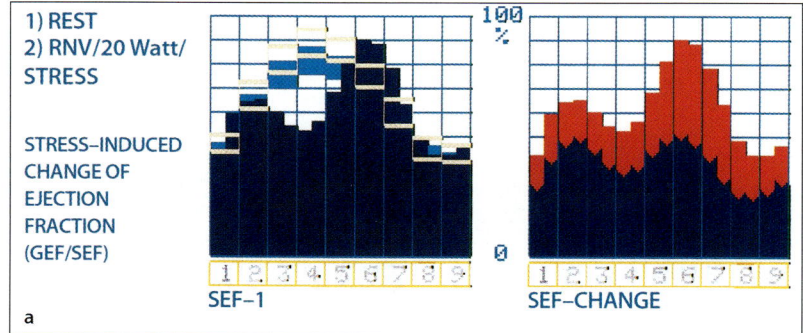

Fig. 2.89 a–c. A 43-year-old man underwent quintuple coronary bypass surgery one year before with internal thoracic artery bypass to the LAD, single vein grafts on the right posterior descending branch, and sequential grafts on the marginal branch, posterior lateral branch, and diagonal branch for treatment of triple-vessel disease. a Radionuclide ventriculography at rest shows a defect associated with anterior wall akinesis. On exercise at 20 W, significant restriction is seen throughout the left myocardium. b Exercise ^{201}Tl myocardial scan at 30 W shows multiple hypoperfused zones. Heart failure

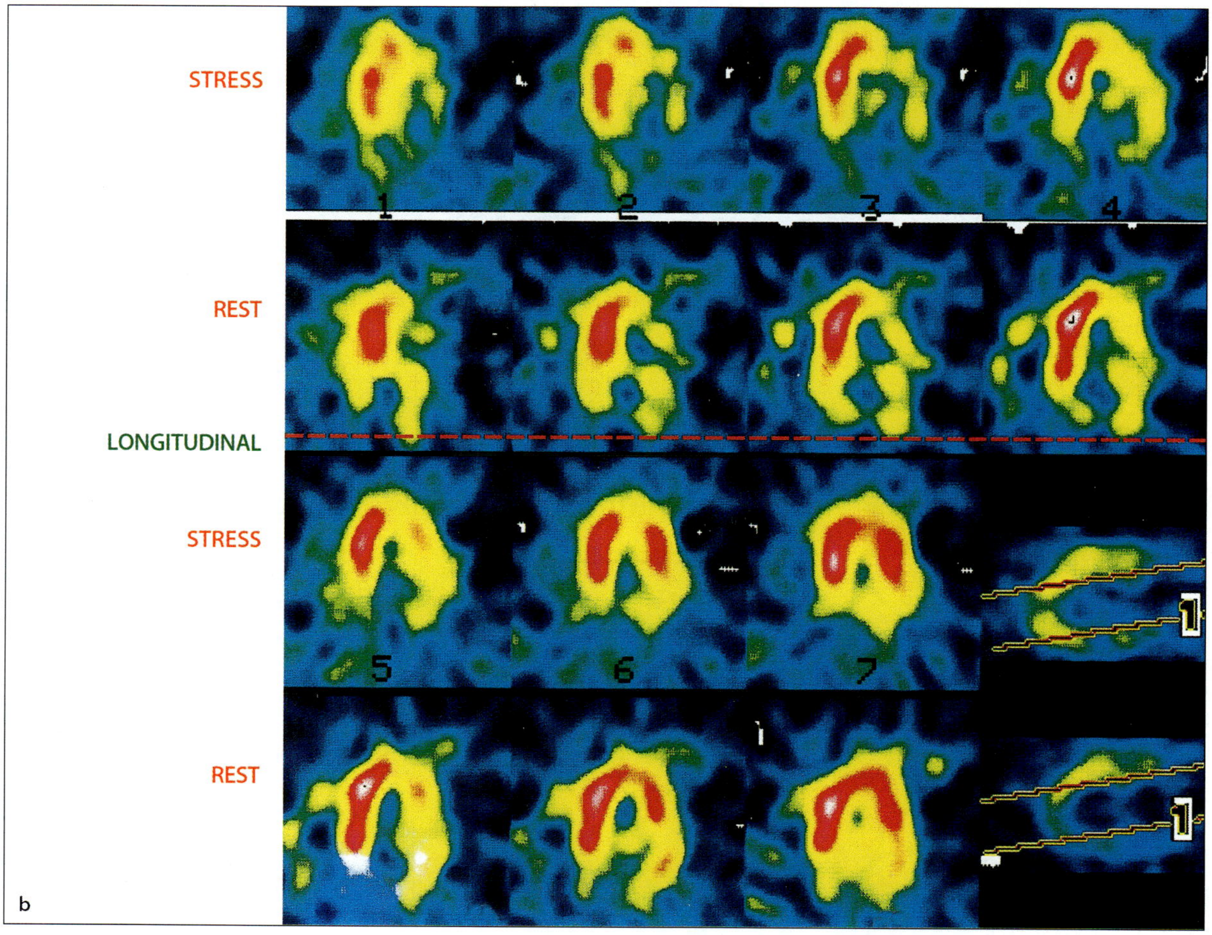

Fig. 2.89 b

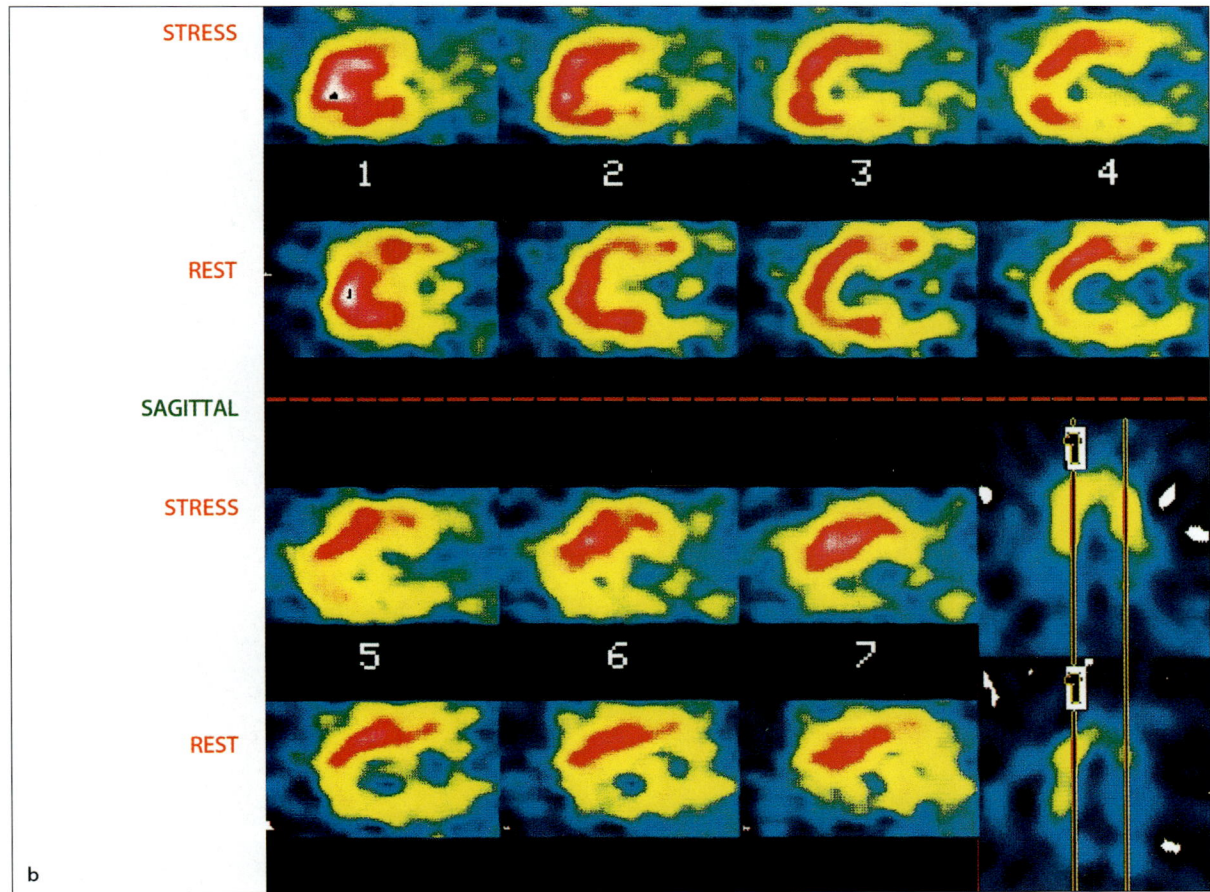

Fig. 2.89 b. *Continued*

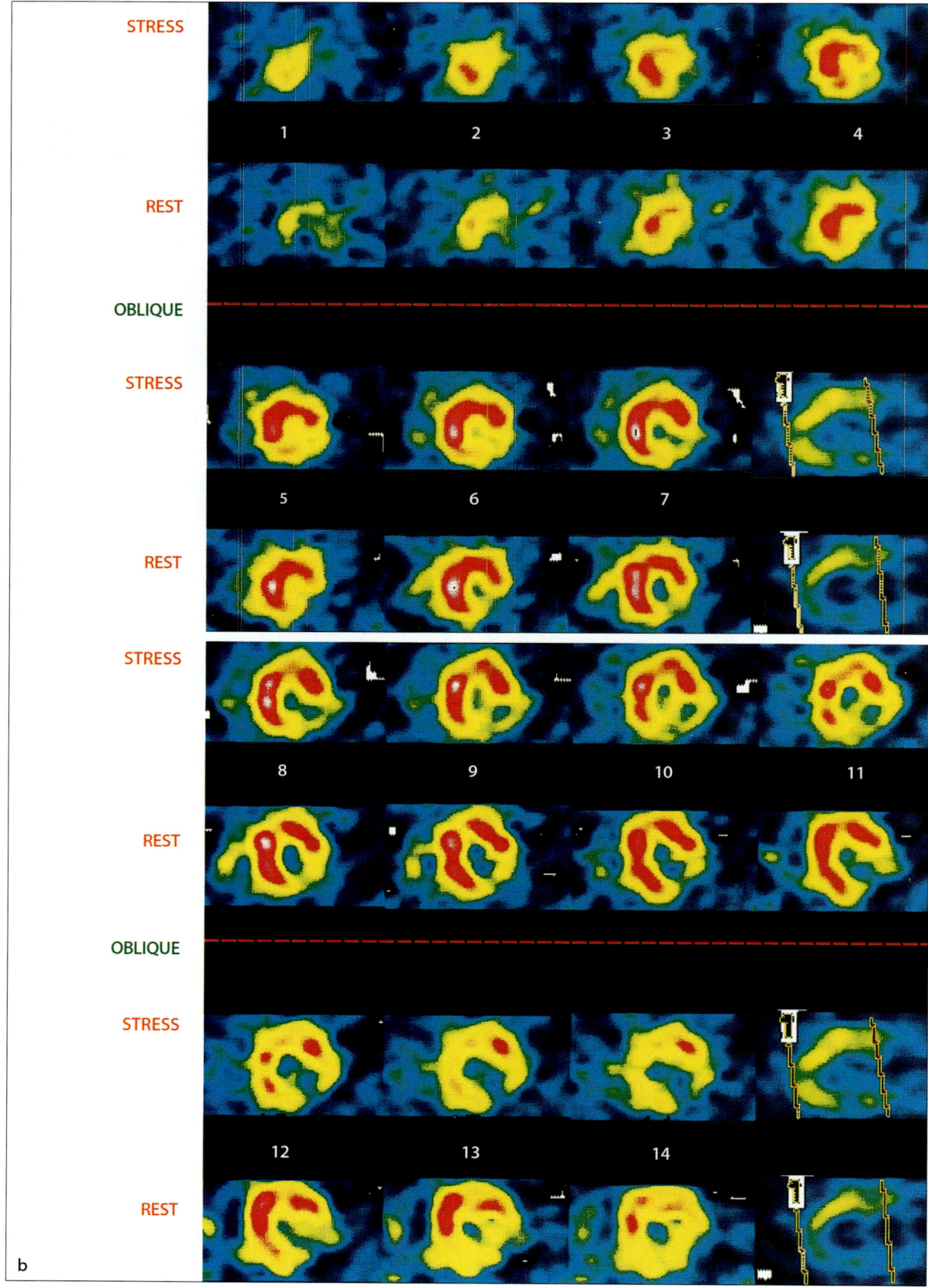

Fig. 2.89 b. *Continued*

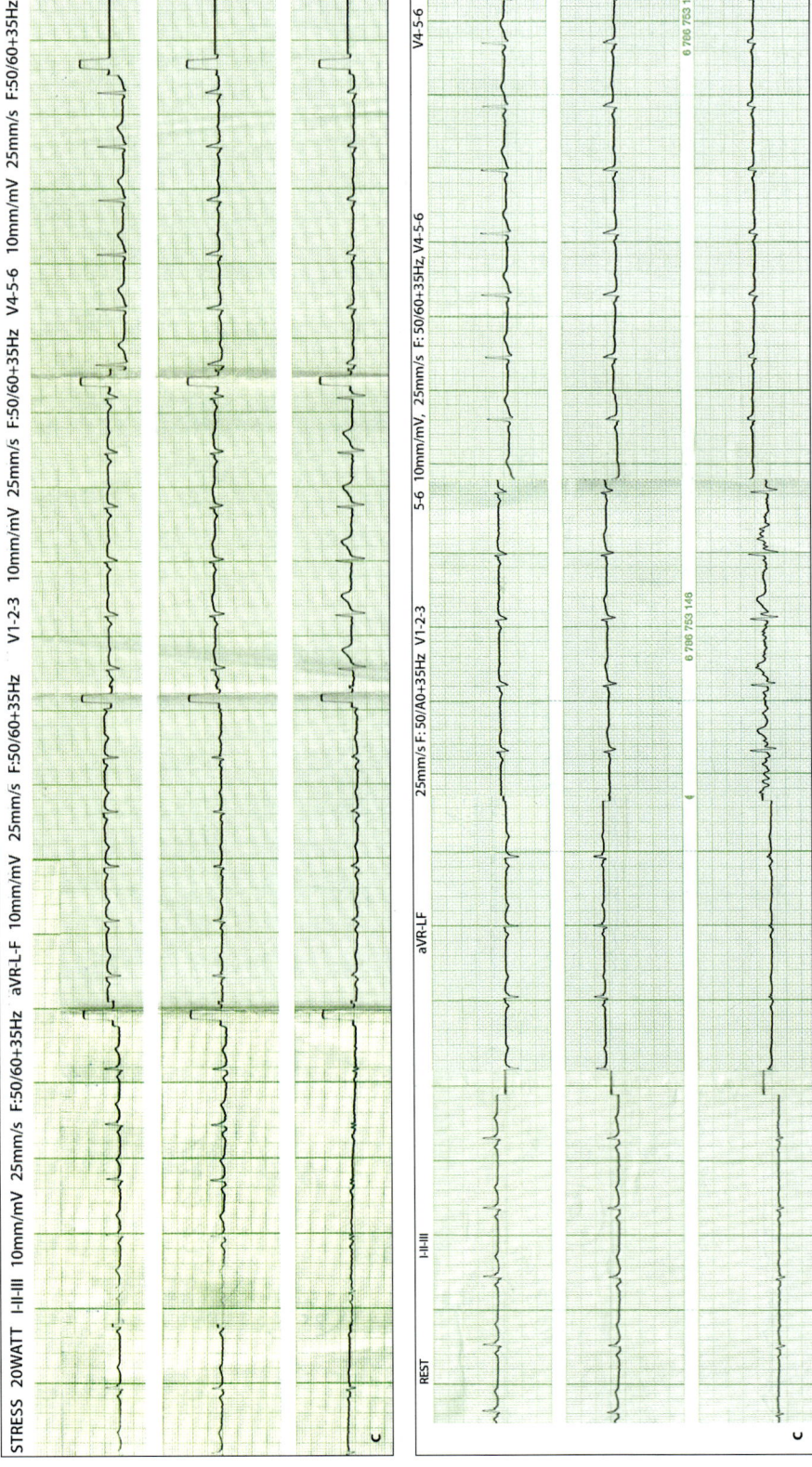

Fig. 2.89 a–c. A 43-year-old man underwent quintuple coronary bypass surgery one year before with internal thoracic artery bypass to the LAD, single vein grafts on the right posterior descending branch, and sequential grafts on the marginal branch, posterior lateral branch, and diagonal branch for treatment of triple-vessel disease. **a** Radionuclide ventriculography at rest shows a defect associated with anterior wall akinesis. On exercise at 20 W, significant restriction is seen throughout the left myocardium. **b** Exercise ^{201}Tl myocardial scan at 30 W shows multiple hypoperfused zones. Heart failure

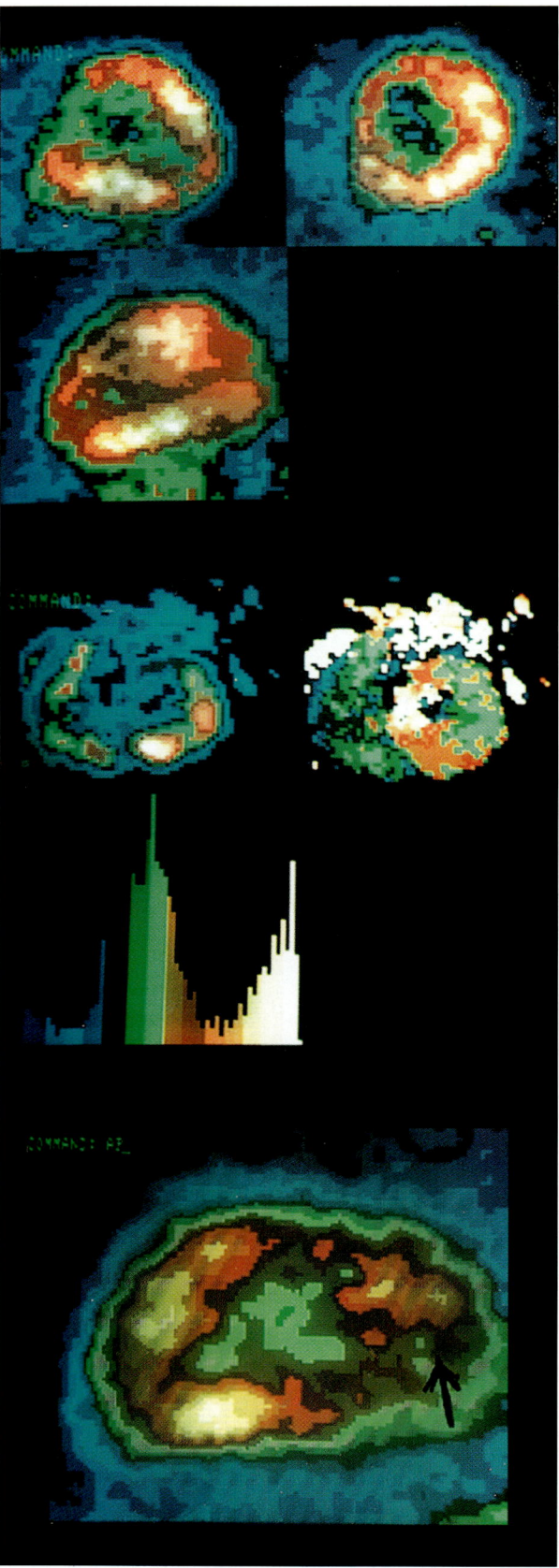

Fig. 2.90. Woman 60 years of age presented with dyspnea and a long history of retrosternal pain. Planar nuclear medicine imaging and radionuclide ventriculography show hypoperfusion in the anterior wall and septal region with extension to the posterior wall. Amplitude and phase analysis indicate an aneurysm involving the apex and anterior wall with markedly diminished amplitudes and out-of-phase motion (cor bovinum). At the base of the heart is an enlarged lymph node (*arrow*) showing thallium uptake

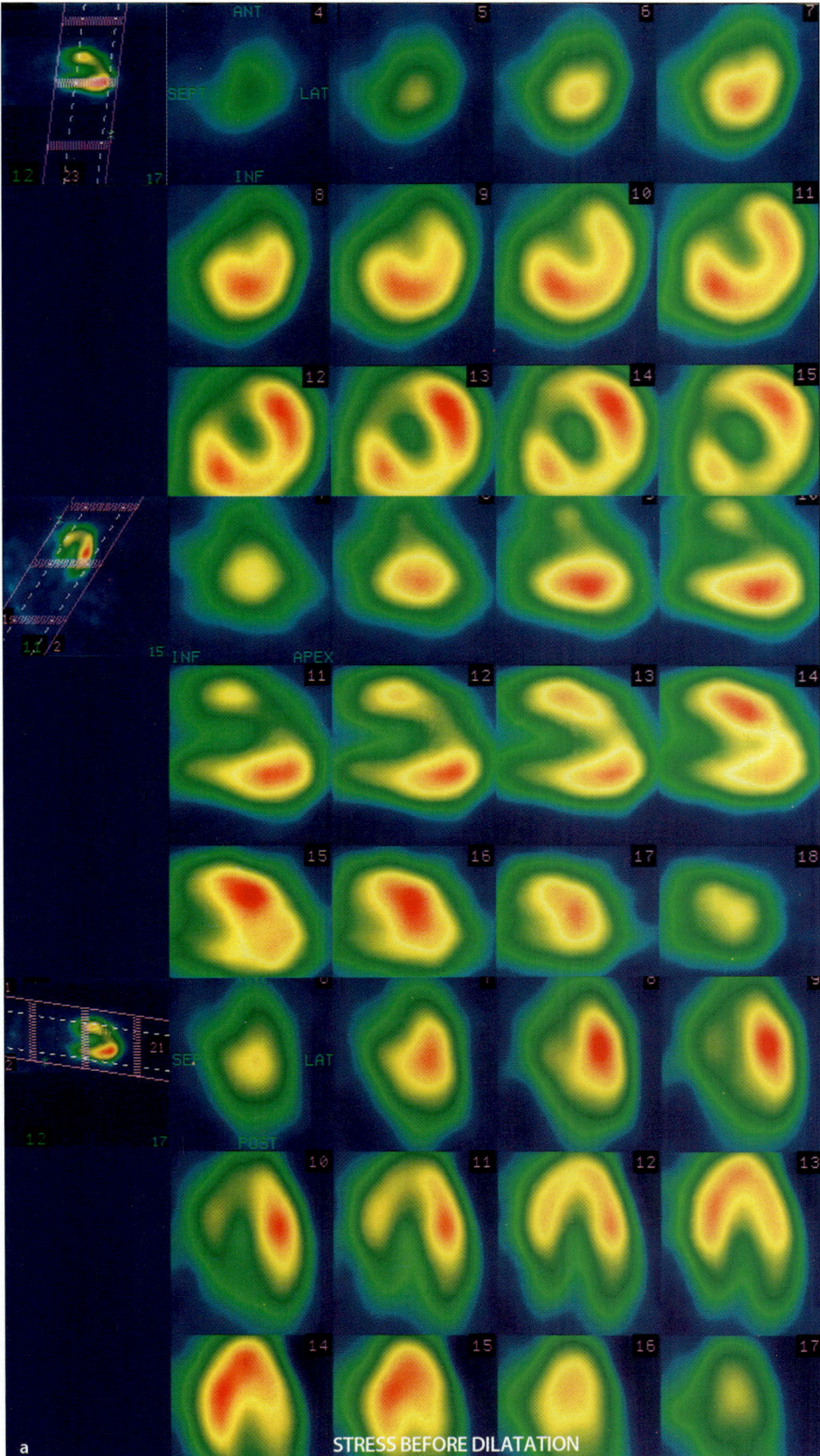

a STRESS BEFORE DILATATION

Fig. 2.91 a–d. Man 50 years of age with a long history of retrosternal pain.
a Myocardial perfusion scan with exercise to 175 W shows hypoperfusion in the anterior wall region and basal portion of the posterior wall.

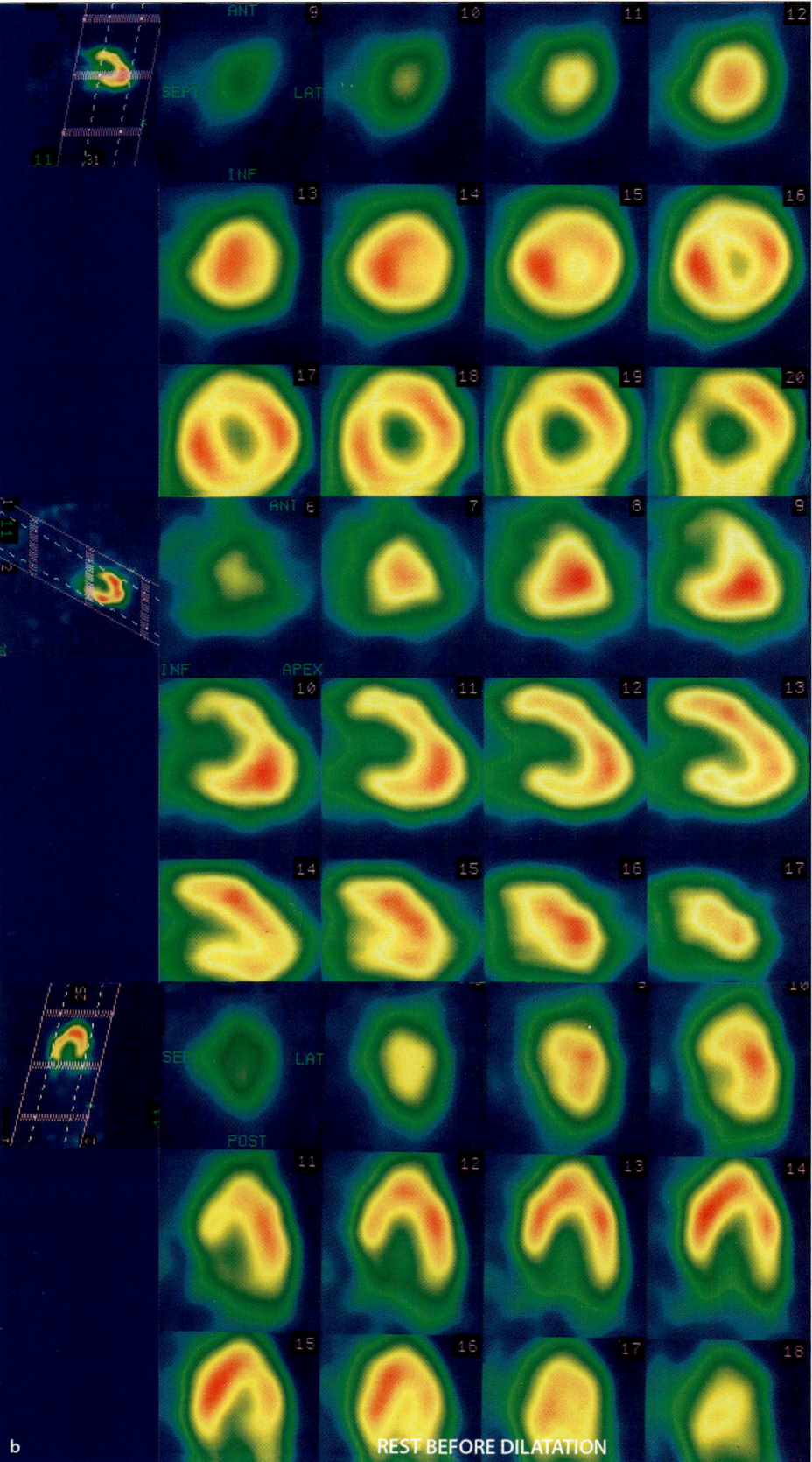

b

REST BEFORE DILATATION

Fig. 2.91 a–d. Man 50 years of age with a long history of retrosternal pain.
b Recovery scan at rest shows reperfusion of the anterior wall but continued slight redistribution in the posterior wall region.

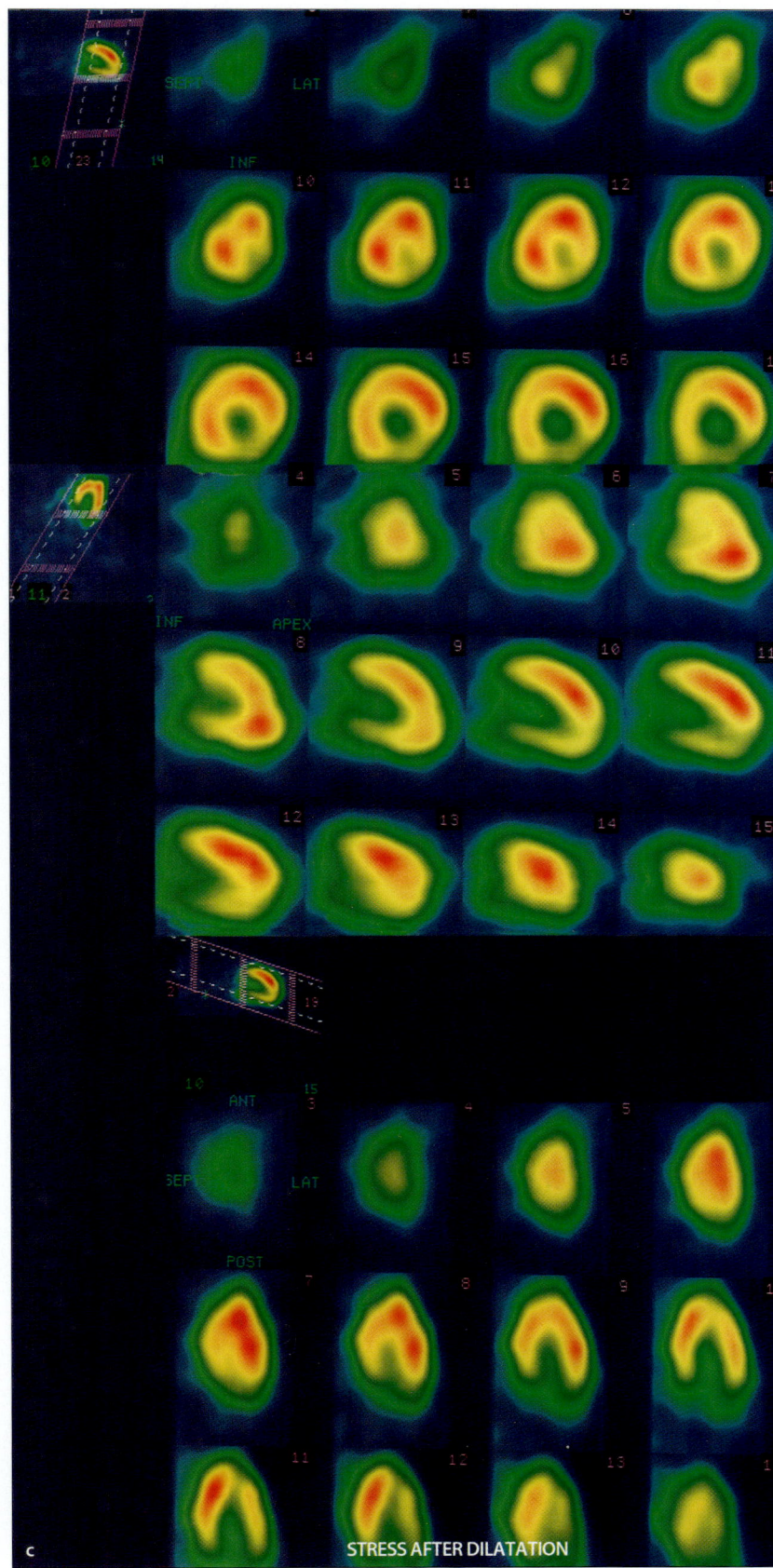

Fig. 2.91 a–d. Man 50 years of age with a long history of retrosternal pain.
c Repeat scan after dilatation shows good anterior wall perfusion and complete recanalization with persistence of mild hypoperfusion in the posterior wall

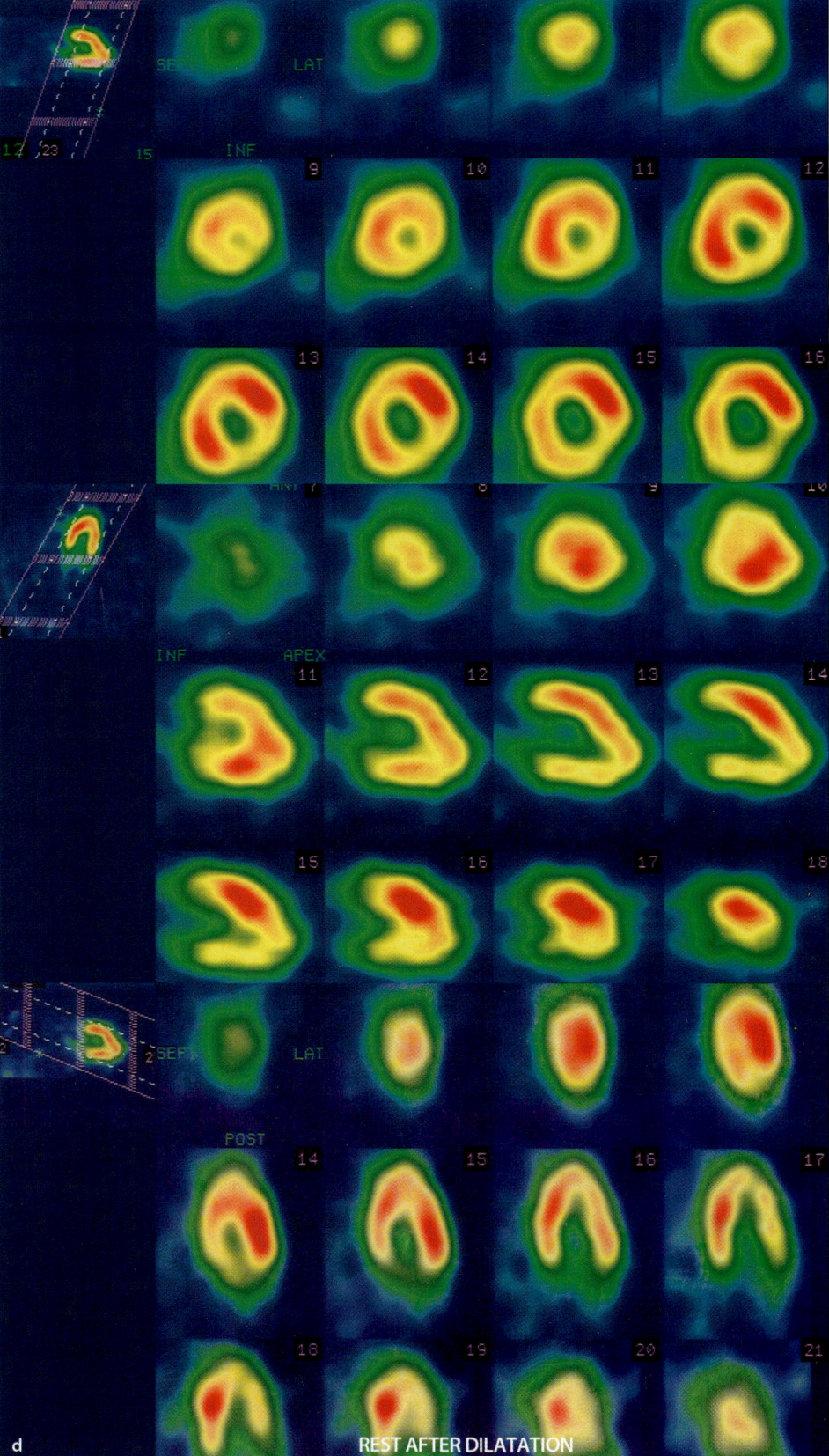

Fig. 2.91 a–d. Man 50 years of age with a long history of retrosternal pain. **d** Repeat scan after dilatation shows good anterior wall perfusion and complete recanalization with persistence of mild hypoperfusion in the posterior wall

REST AFTER DILATATION

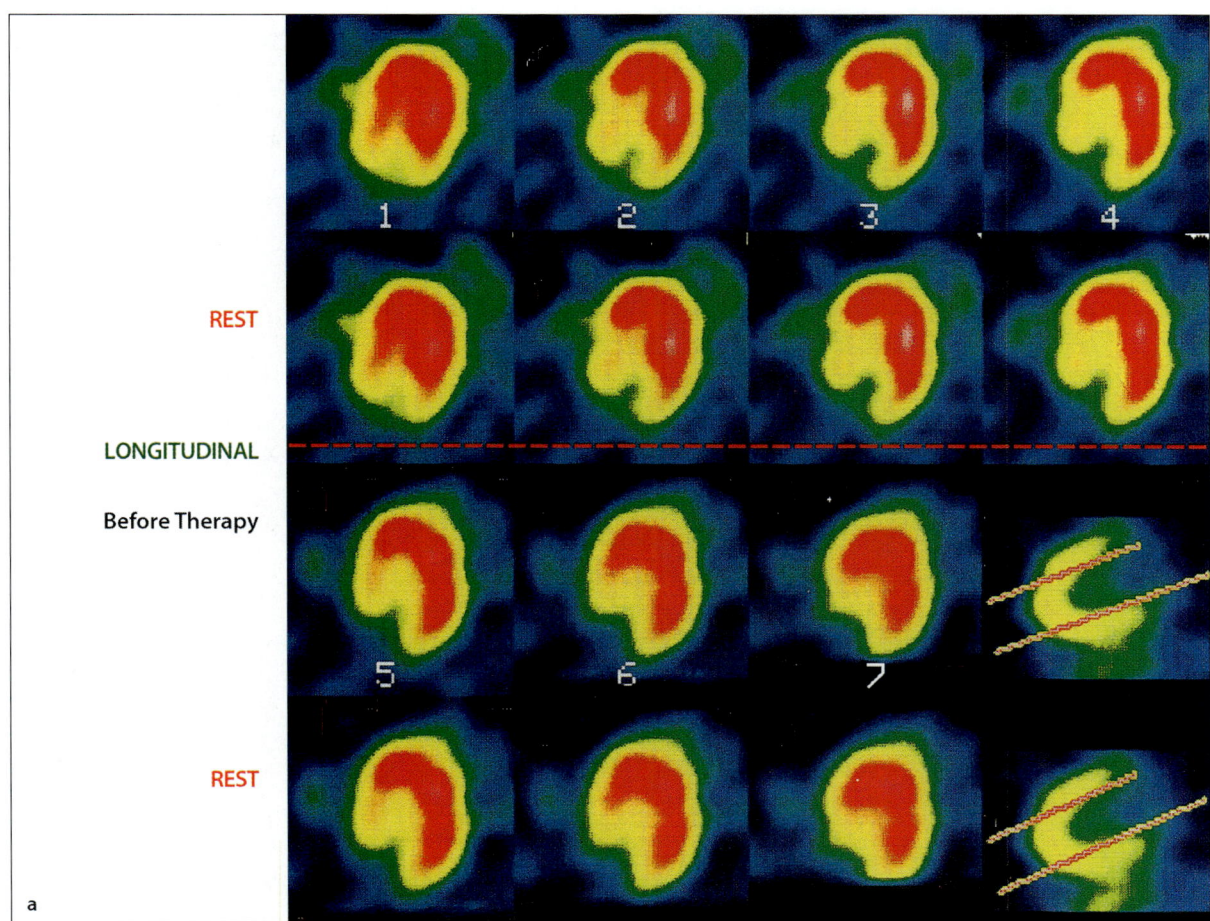

REST

LONGITUDINAL

Before Therapy

REST

a

Fig. 2.92 a,b. Woman 64 years of age, a heavy smoker, was evaluated for sudden retrosternal pain. **a** Myocardial perfusion scan at rest shows abnormal perfusion in the anterior wall, which was treated immediately with streptokinase. **b** Follow-up at 8 weeks shows good anterior wall perfusion. This case illustrates the immediate, successful treatment of myocardial infarction (MI). It is noteworthy that ECG was negative for MI in this patient. A positive blood study was obtained 6 hours after the event

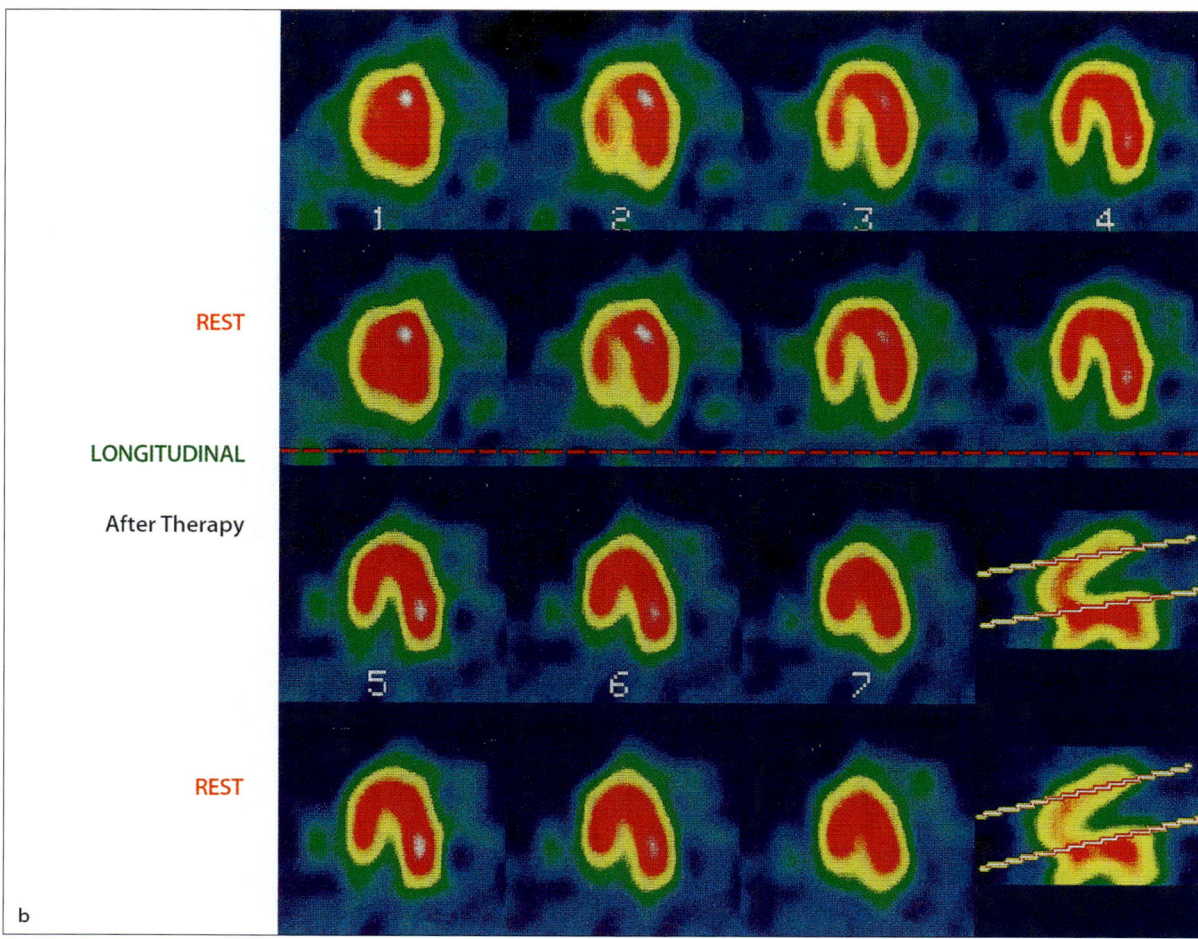

b

Fig. 2.92 a,b. Woman 64 years of age, a heavy smoker, was evaluated for sudden retrosternal pain. **a** Myocardial perfusion scan at rest shows abnormal perfusion in the anterior wall, which was treated immediately with streptokinase. **b** Follow-up at 8 weeks shows good anterior wall perfusion. This case illustrates the immediate, successful treatment of myocardial infarction (MI). It is noteworthy that ECG was negative for MI in this patient. A positive blood study was obtained 6 hours after the event

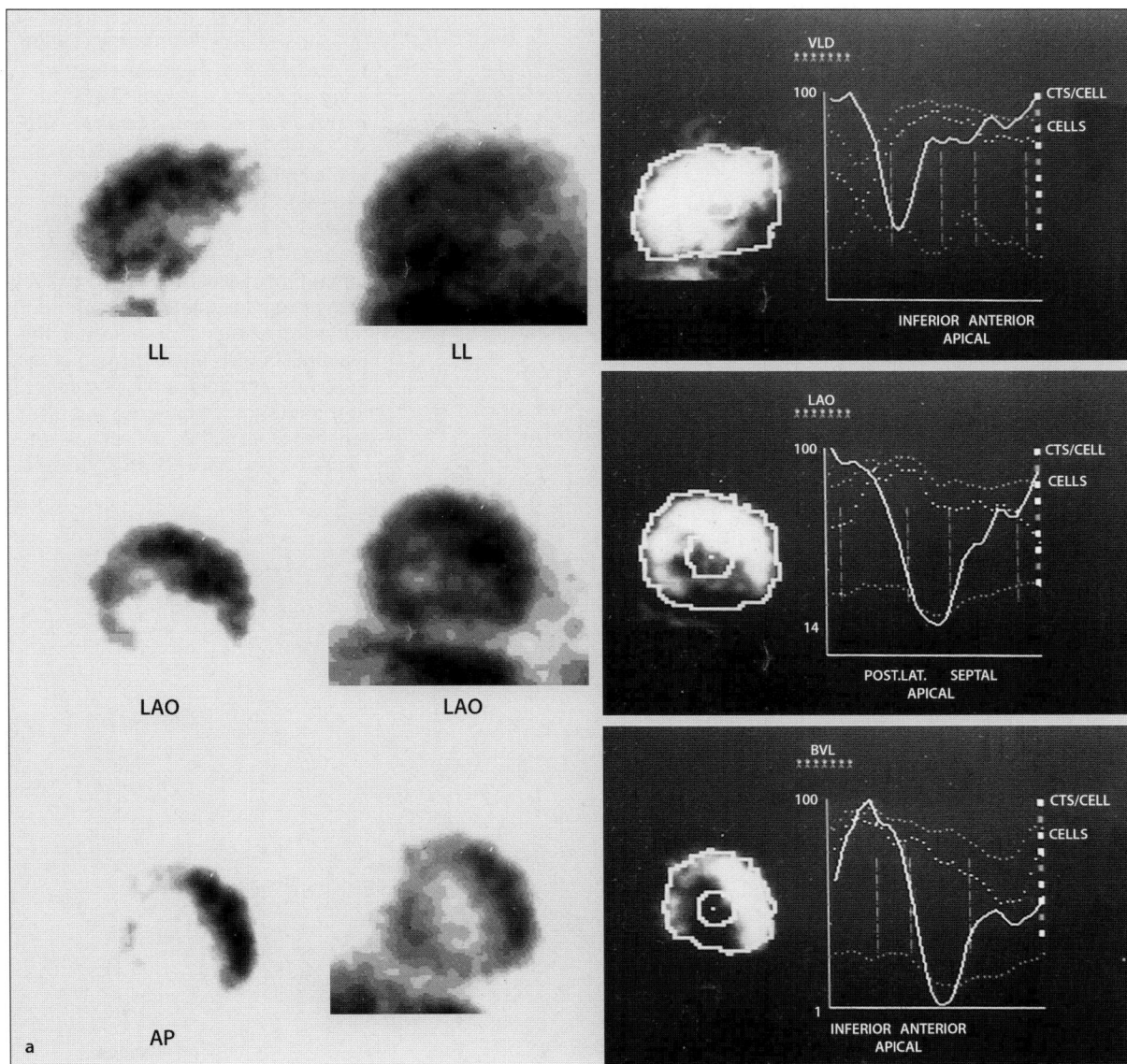

Fig. 2.93 a,b. A 59-year-old man suffered a posterolateral MI years before; he presented now with intermittent angina pectoris. **a** Myocardial perfusion scan at rest, with myocardial profile, shows significant hypoperfusion in the apical region with inferior extension. **b** Coronary angiography shows an occlusion in the upper third of the LAD with retrograde opacification, a proximal occlusion of the LCX with retrograde opacification through the marginal branch, a stenosis in the diagonal branch, and occlusion of the RCA with retrograde opacification. Rest scan shows relatively good maintenance of viable tissue owing to retrograde filling of the coronary vessels

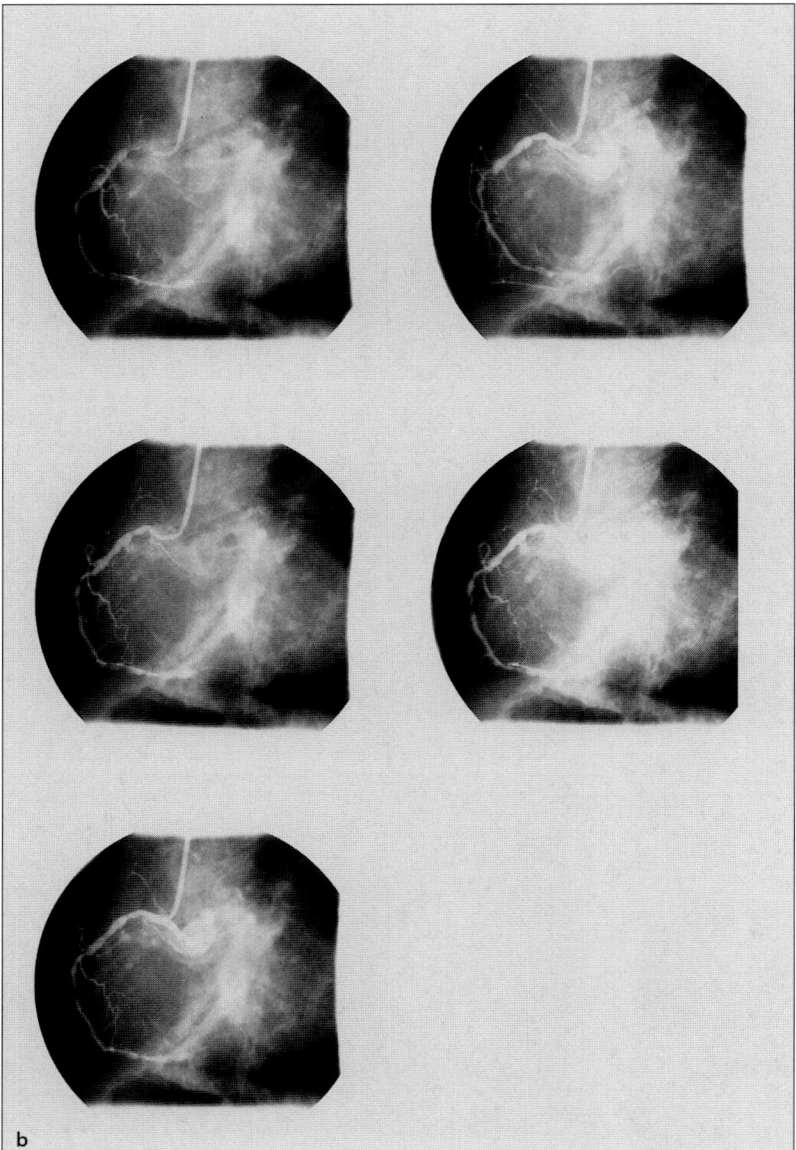

b

Fig. 2.93 a,b. A 59-year-old man suffered a posterolateral MI years before; he presented now with intermittent angina pectoris. **a** Myocardial perfusion scan at rest, with myocardial profile, shows significant hypoperfusion in the apical region with inferior extension. **b** Coronary angiography shows an occlusion in the upper third of the LAD with retrograde opacification, a proximal occlusion of the LCX with retrograde opacification through the marginal branch, a stenosis in the diagonal branch, and occlusion of the RCA with retrograde opacification. Rest scan shows relatively good maintenance of viable tissue owing to retrograde filling of the coronary vessels

Fig. 2.94 a,b. A 68-year-old woman was diagnosed two years earlier with MI. She now complained of chest tightness and vertigo on three consecutive days along with transient, mild retrosternal pain. She was hospitalized, and a posterior wall infarction was diagnosed by ECG. The patient was exercised to 100 W for stress ^{201}Tl perfusion scanning; this was the highest level tolerated due to dyspnea. The stress scan shows hypoperfusion on the LCX (oblique 12–13, sagittal 5–6) and of the posterior descending branch of the RCA. Rest scan shows redistribution in the LCX but no redistribution in the posterior branch. This indicates scarring of the posterior wall and a hemodynamically significant lesion of the LCA. The stenosis is also clearly demonstrated in the bull's-eye profile

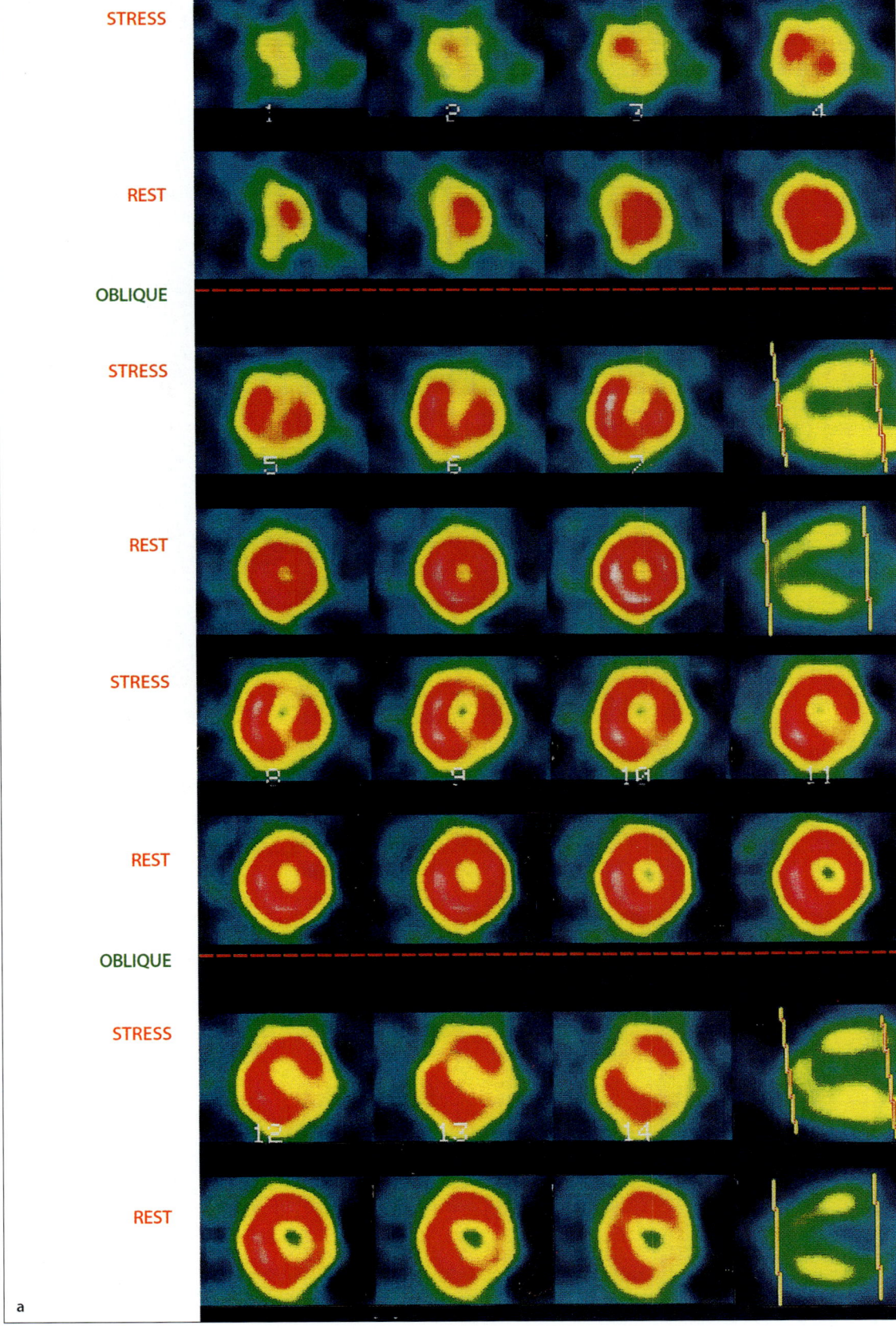

STRESS

REST

OBLIQUE

STRESS

REST

STRESS

REST

OBLIQUE

STRESS

REST

a

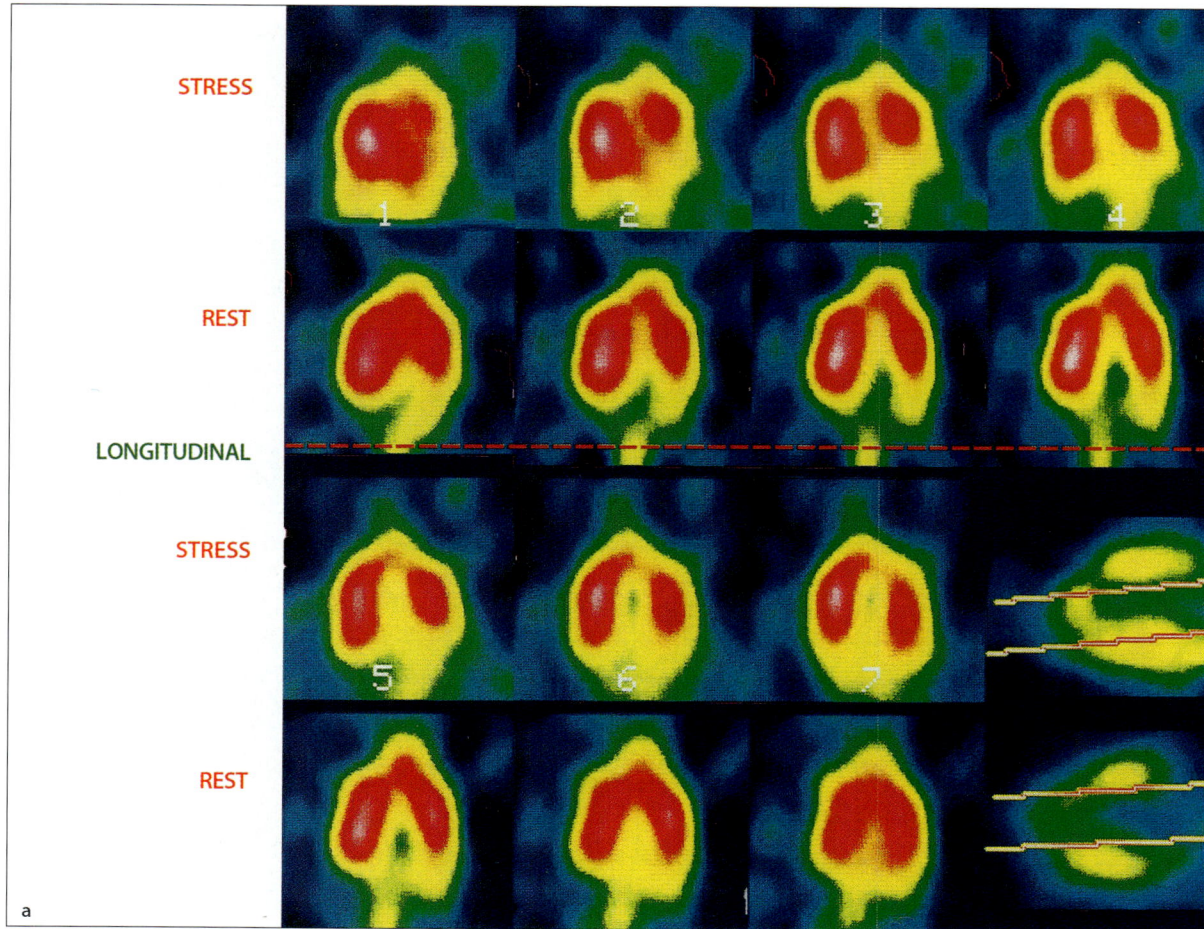

Fig. 2.94 a,b. A 68-year-old woman was diagnosed two years earlier with MI. She now complained of chest tightness and vertigo on three consecutive days along with transient, mild retrosternal pain. She was hospitalized, and a posterior wall infarction was diagnosed by ECG. The patient was exercised to 100 W for stress ^{201}Tl perfusion scanning; this was the highest level tolerated due to dyspnea. The stress scan shows hypoperfusion on the LCX (oblique 12–13, sagittal 5–6) and of the posterior descending branch of the RCA. Rest scan shows redistribution in the LCX but no redistribution in the posterior branch. This indicates scarring of the posterior wall and a hemodynamically significant lesion of the LCA. The stenosis is also clearly demonstrated in the bull's-eye profile

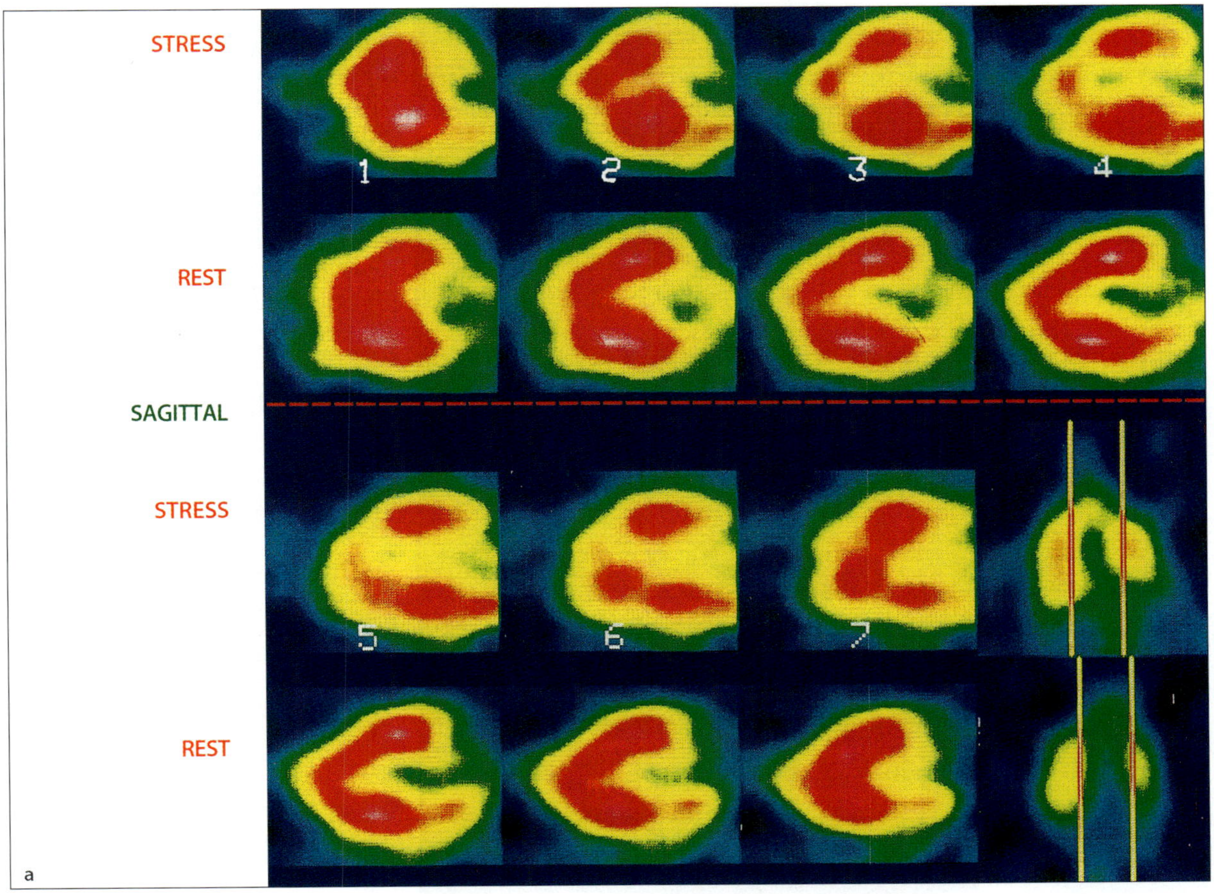

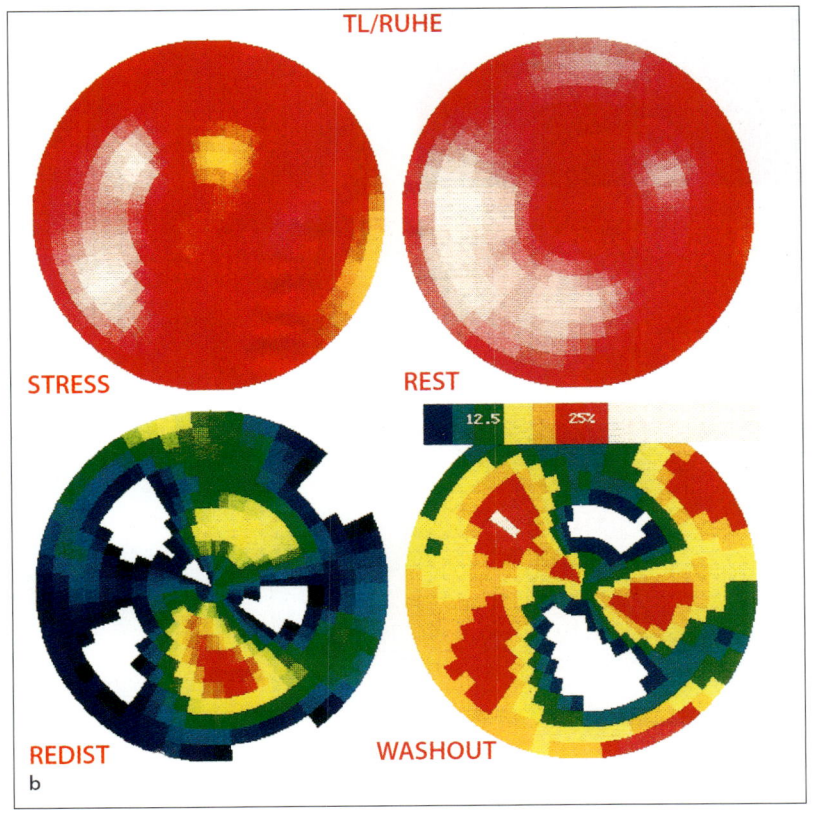

Fig. 2.94 a. *Continued*

Fig. 2.94 b

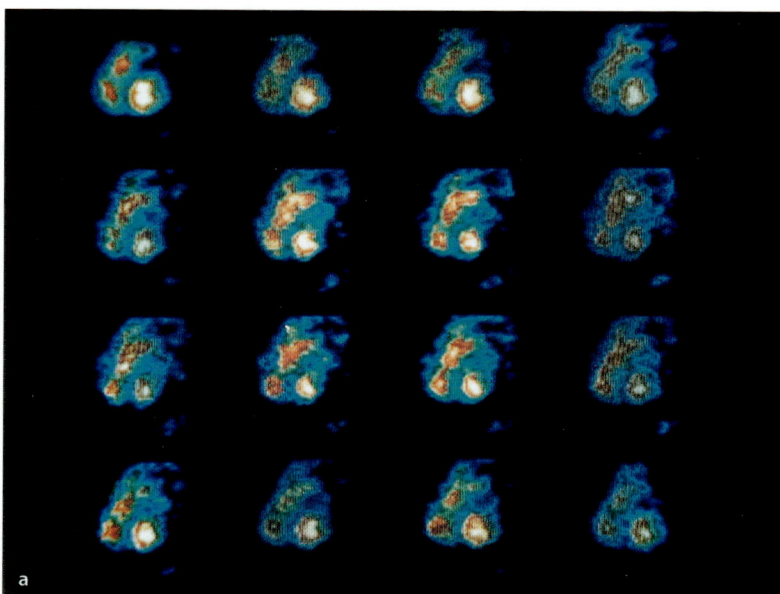

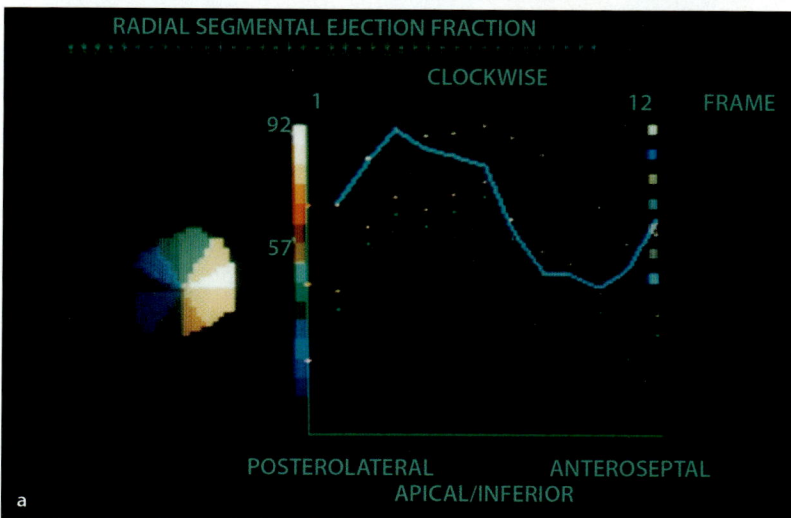

Fig. 2.95 a,b. Man 60 years of age with intermittent angina pectoris and a suspected anterior wall infarction eight years before. **a** Radionuclide ventriculography with amplitude and phase analysis and sector wall motion shows significant hypokinesis in the anterior wall and septal region and diminished amplitudes. **b** Coronary angiography demonstrates a grade-III stenosis in the proximal LAD, an occlusion in the initial third of the anterior interventricular branch, and multiple stenoses in the LCX

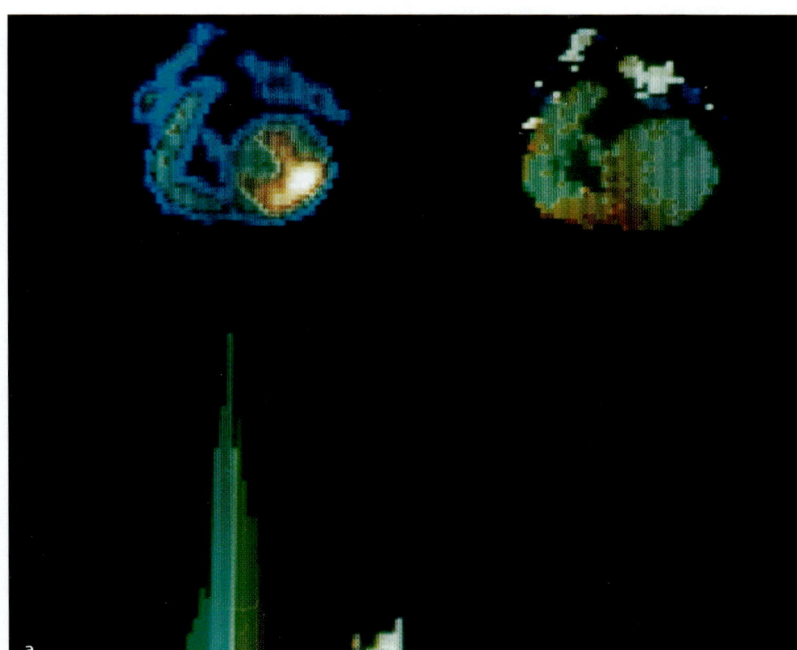

Fig. 2.95 a. *Continued*

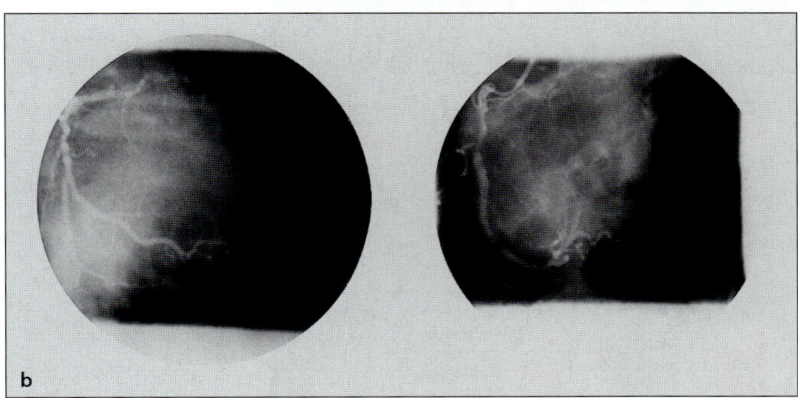

Fig. 2.95 b. Coronary angiography demonstrates a grade-III stenosis in the proximal LAD, an occlusion in the initial third of the anterior interventricular branch, and multiple stenoses in the LCX

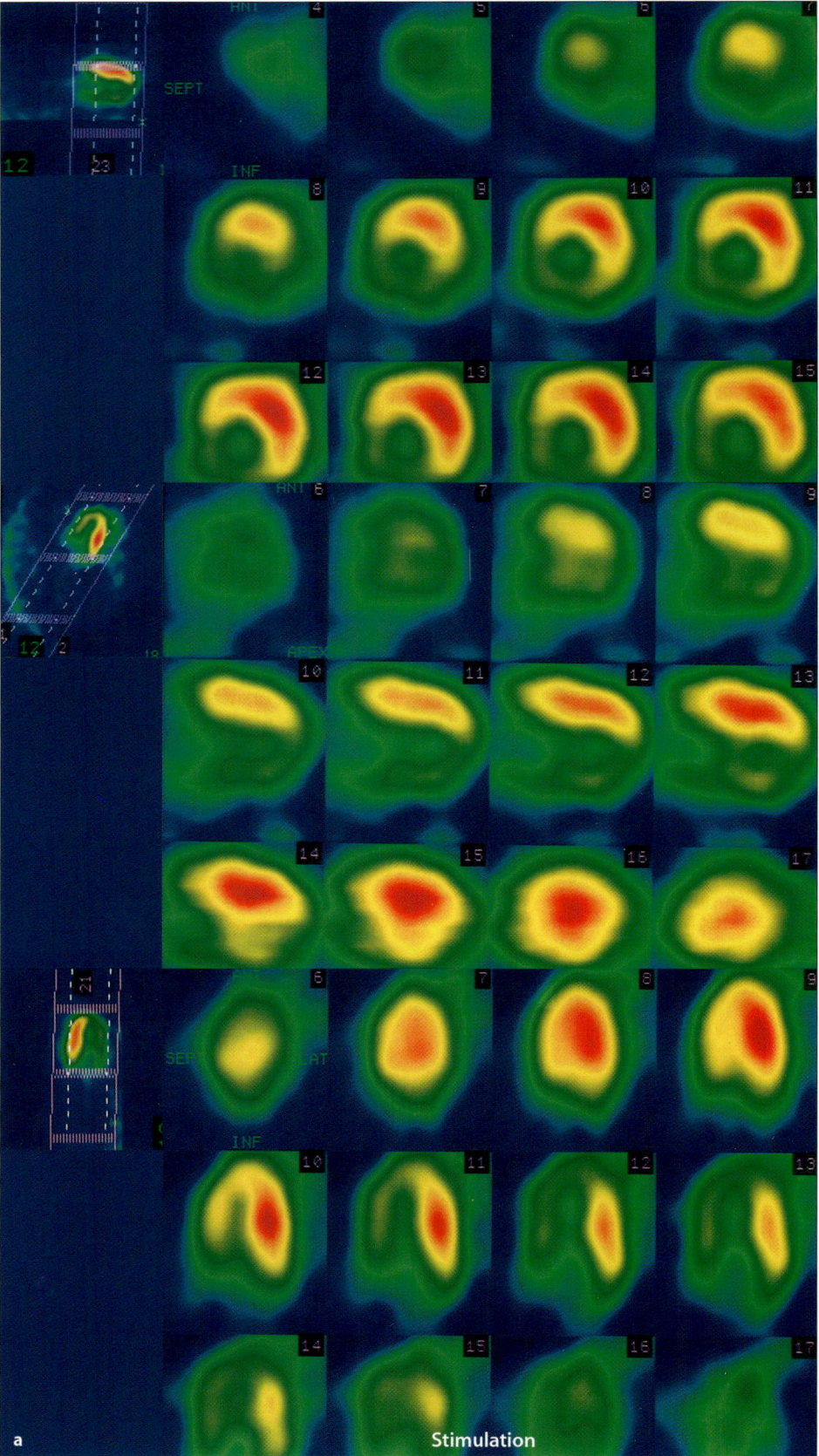

Fig. 2.96 a–d. Follow-up stress study in a 74-year-old woman with a pacemaker. Stress was induced by means of a Guidant dual-chamber (DDD) pacing system with atrioventricular leads, producing a heart rate of 124 bps. Stress scan shows hypoperfusion in the posterior wall, septum, and portions of the anterior wall. Subsequent rest scan shows redistribution in the anterior wall and apical portion of the posterior wall with a persistent perfusion defect in the septal region

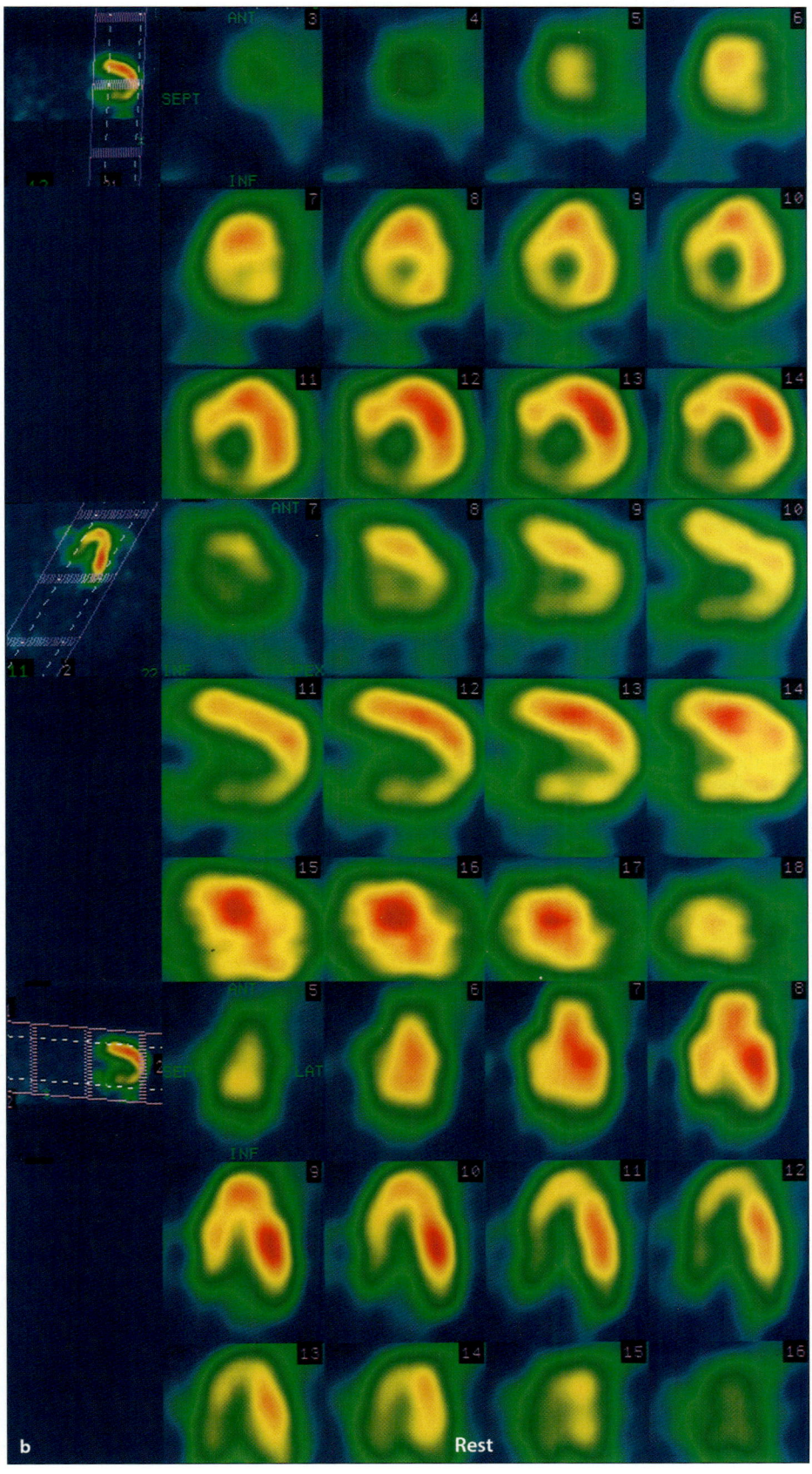

Fig. 2.96 b

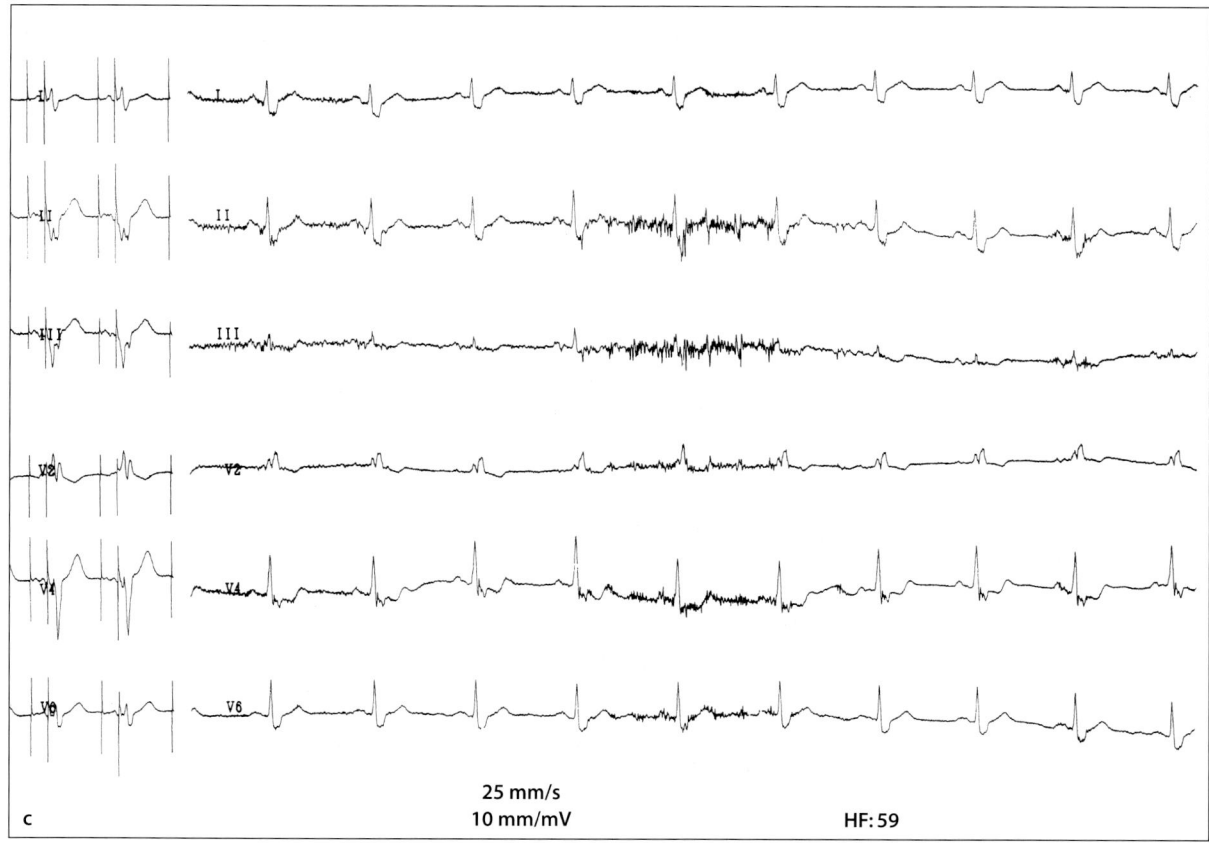

25 mm/s
10 mm/mV   HF: 59

c

Fig. 2.96 a–d. Follow-up stress study in a 74-year-old woman with a pacemaker. Stress was induced by means of a Guidant dual-chamber (DDD) pacing system with atrioventricular leads, producing a heart rate of 124 bps. Stress scan shows hypoperfusion in the posterior wall, septum, and portions of the anterior wall. Subsequent rest scan shows redistribution in the anterior wall and apical portion of the posterior wall with a persistent perfusion defect in the septal region

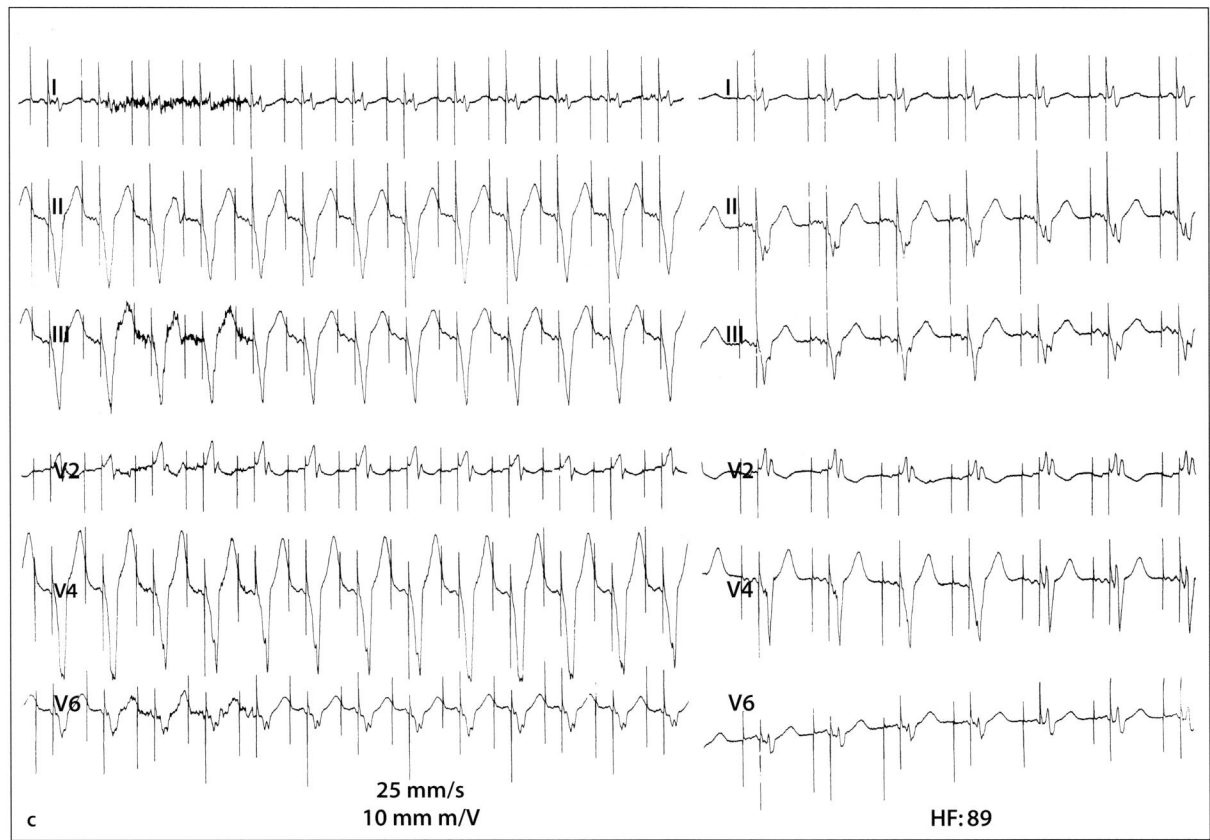

Fig. 2.96 c. *Continued*

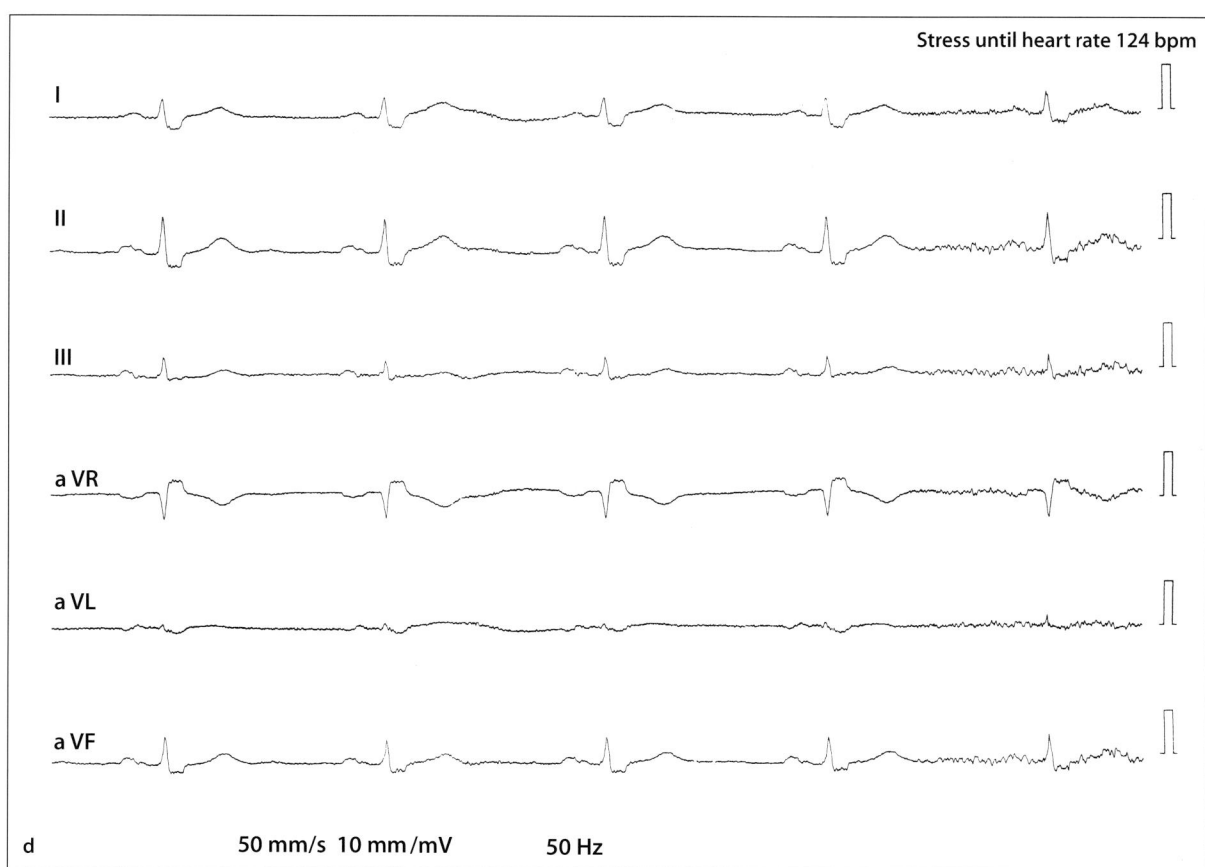

Stress until heart rate 124 bpm

I

II

III

a VR

a VL

a VF

d   50 mm/s 10 mm/mV   50 Hz

Fig. 2.96 a–d. Follow-up stress study in a 74-year-old woman with a pacemaker. Stress was induced by means of a Guidant dual-chamber (DDD) pacing system with atrioventricular leads, producing a heart rate of 124 bps. Stress scan shows hypoperfusion in the posterior wall, septum, and portions of the anterior wall. Subsequent rest scan shows redistribution in the anterior wall and apical portion of the posterior wall with a persistent perfusion defect in the septal region

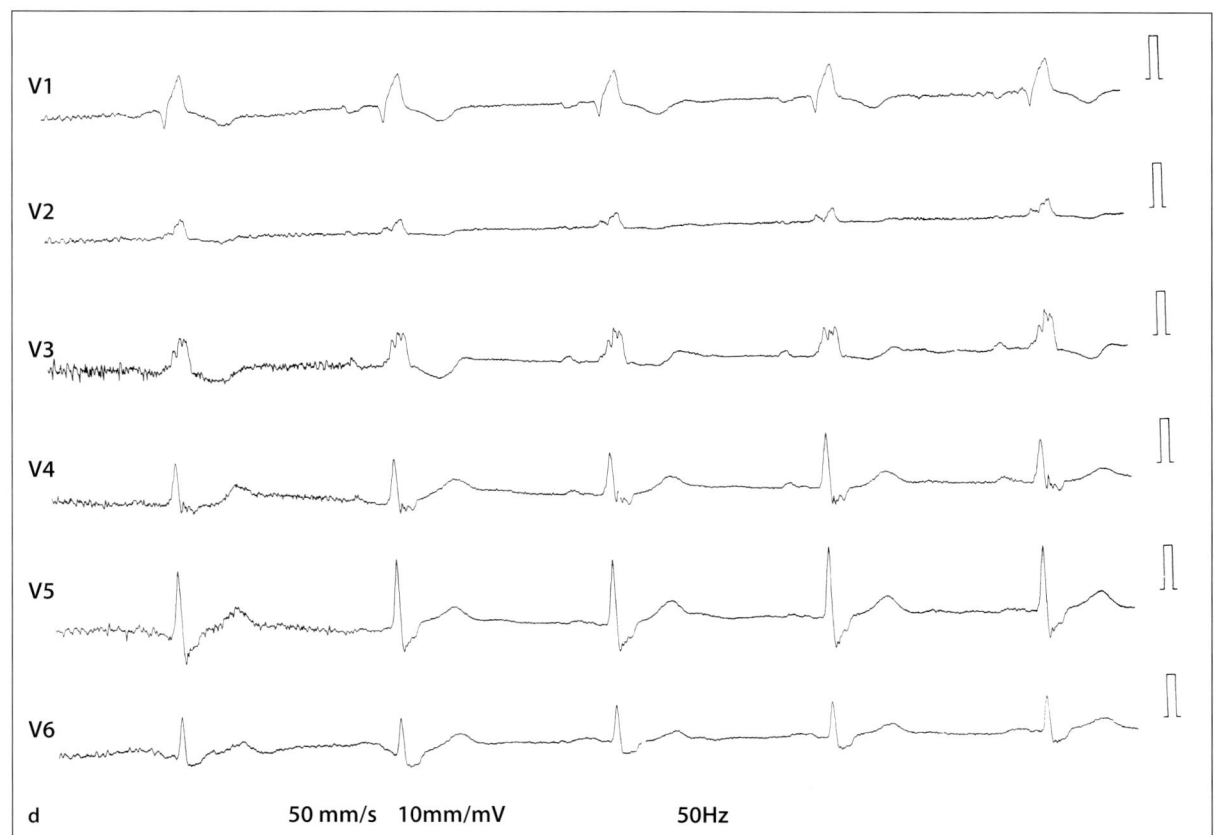

V1

V2

V3

V4

V5

V6

d   50 mm/s   10mm/mV   50Hz

Fig. 2.96 d. *Continued*

3 Abdomen

Despite technical and methodologic advances, nuclear medicine has not gained an established role in the clinical diagnosis of gastric disorders. This is because even when a gamma camera specially designed for this type of examination is used, the nuclear medicine physician still must rely on the results of other specialties. Nuclear medicine examinations of the stomach can be distorted by several factors, particularly the gastric contents and blood clots. Carcinomas arising from the cardia or pylorus may produce a positive scan only after they have infiltrated the stomach.

The domain of nuclear medicine is in the diagnosis of gastrointestinal tract bleeding and Meckel's diverticulum in pediatric patients and adults. Nuclear medicine is a helpful tool in the diagnosis of inflammatory conditions such as appendicitis, Crohn's disease, and diffuse colitis. Gallium-67 imaging can provide specific information and often an accurate diagnosis in patients with unexplained abdominal symptoms.

Technical advances in radionuclide imaging and improvements in radiopharmaceuticals have gained nuclear medicine an established place in studies of the liver and hepatobiliary system. Hepatobiliary and hepatocyte-specific radiopharmaceuticals have become indispensable for these investigations. Despite improvements in equipment resolution and motion correction techniques, the accuracy of radionuclide imaging has improved very little in the diagnosis of focal lesions. One problem has been the motion of the liver caused by respiratory excursions. Studies at our center using a liver phantom have shown that with a respiratory excursion of 2 cm, a cold nodule 2.3 cm in diameter cannot be detected either visually or with profile techniques (see Figs 3.19–3.21). Respiratory triggering is of major importance in eliminating this problem on liver scans.

The subtraction method (el Helou 1981) has become important in hepatobiliary function studies, as it can eliminate loss of information due to superimposed structures.

Considerable research has been done on the functional interaction of the duodenal papilla and common bile duct in controlling biliary flow ("cocktail shaker" mechanism, Hand 1973; "active milking," Hallenbeck 1967). A study done by the author under physiologic conditions in healthy subjects and gender-mixed patients with various types of biliary tract disease (el Helou 1982) showed that, regardless of underlying disease, gender, and age, the time-activity curve displays the same shape over the common bile duct and over the horizontal part of the duodenum. This finding may serve as an impetus for further functional investigations of the choledochoduodenal junction.

3.2
Kidneys

Because nuclear medicine examinations are essentially functional studies and because functional changes generally precede changes in morphology, nuclear medicine imaging is very useful for the early detection of renal disease. Indeed, radionuclide imaging is considered to have a primary role in a number of areas: the differential diagnosis of urinary tract diseases, renal transplant evaluation, assessing residual kidney function after surgery, diagnosing perfusion abnormalities (e.g., renal embolism) and evaluating their response to therapy, investigating renal hypertension, and determining whether a kidney affected by neoplastic or other unilateral disease is worth salvaging. Nuclear medicine also provides a noninvasive, well-tolerated, time-saving tool for emergency diagnosis that can provide management guidelines for the treating physician. Information on renal function is also valuable in following the course of diabetic neuropathy, pyelo- and glomerulonephritis, shock, nephrotoxicity, and anuria.

The simple renogram can provide quantitative orientation in the form of T_{max} (time to reach peak activity), $T_{1/2}$ (fall of the curve to one-half peak) (see Figs. 3.66–3.68), and the triphasic shape of the renogram curve.

The availability of SPECT imaging has significantly improved the diagnosis of mass lesions (see Fig. 3.69). The data from a SPECT acquisition can be processed to yield multiple image slices or a moving cine display.

3.3
Adrenals

Due to the lack of organ-specific, economical, low-dosimetry radiopharmaceuticals, along with the technical complexity of the scan protocol and the high background activity of the liver, radionuclide imaging of the adrenal glands has been unable to establish itself as a routine clinical study.

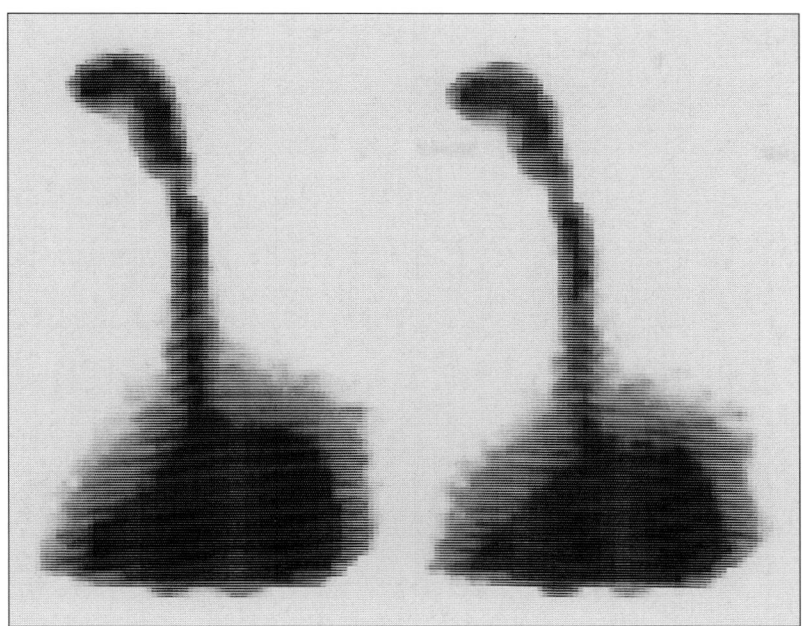

Fig. 3.1. Normal sequential and static radionuclide images of the esophagus

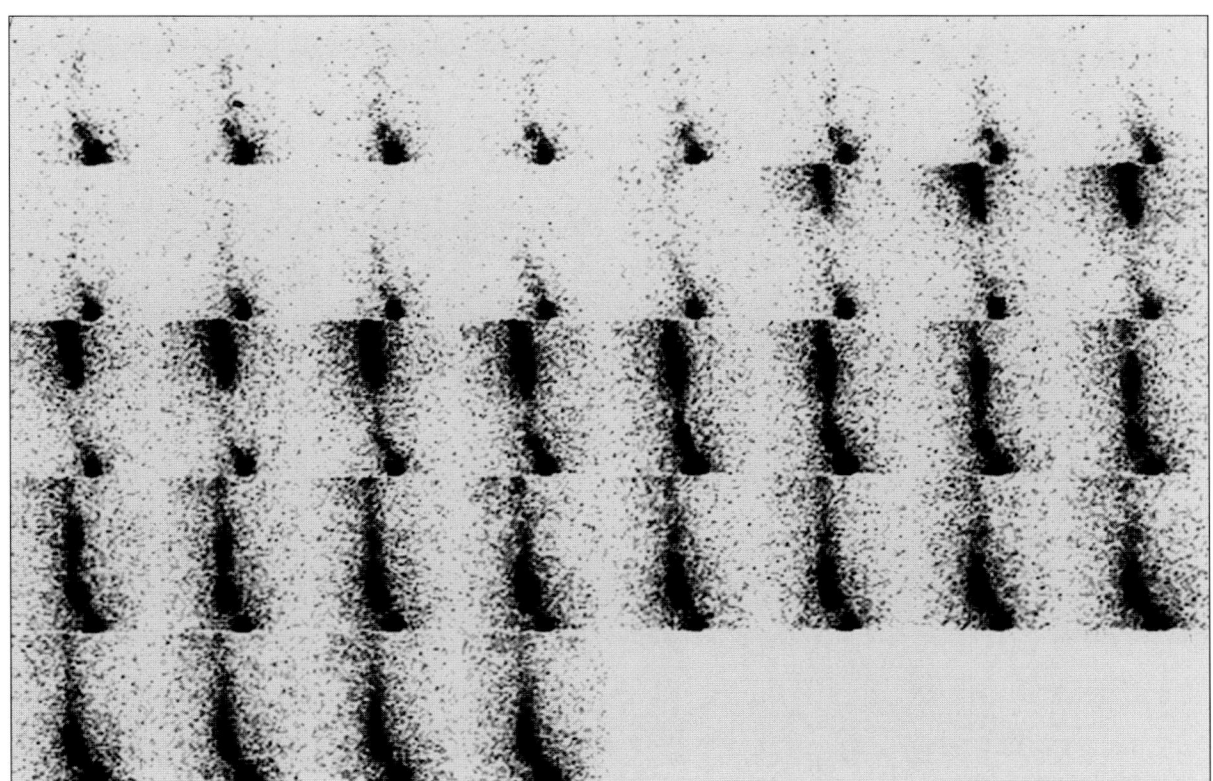

Fig. 3.2. Esophagitis in a female alcoholic who complained of retrosternal burning

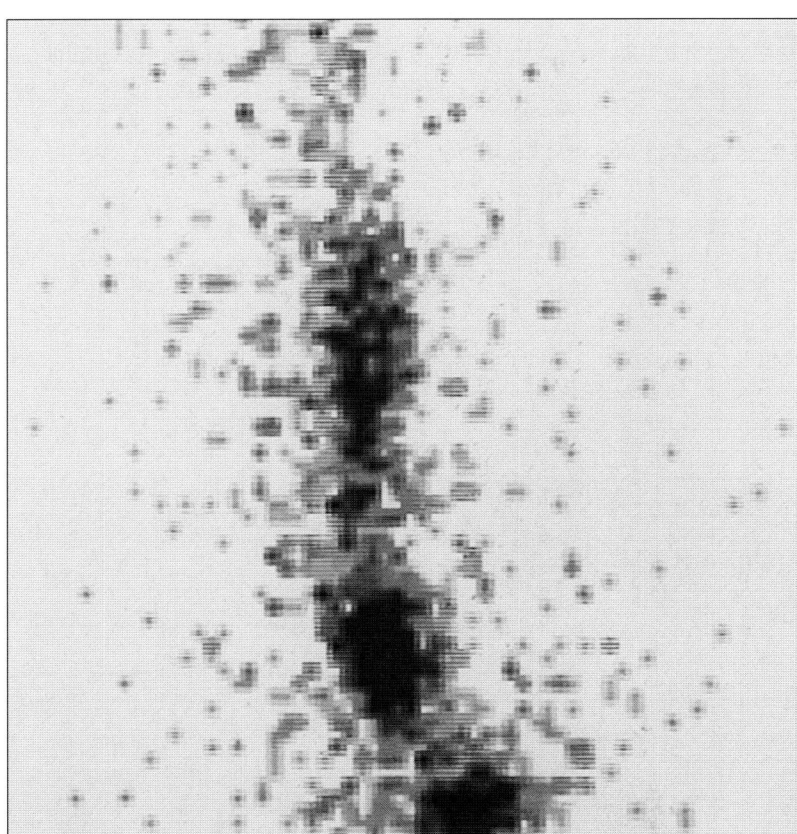

Fig. 3.2. *Continued*

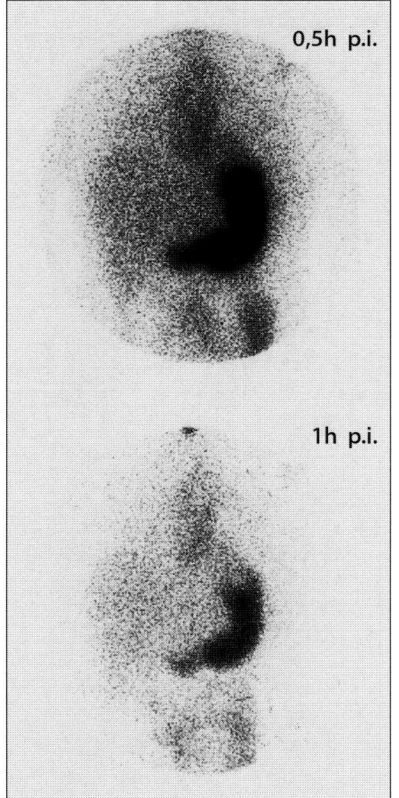

0,5h p.i.

1h p.i.

Fig. 3.3. Normal appearance of a gastric scintigram

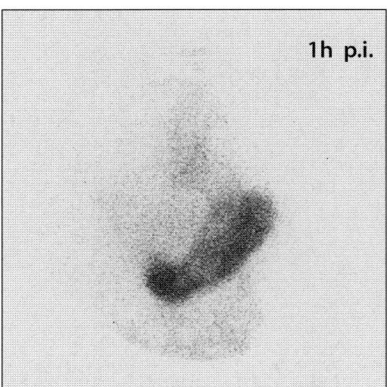

1h p.i.

Fig. 3.4. Food residues in the stomach appear as multiple cold defects that may have a rounded shape

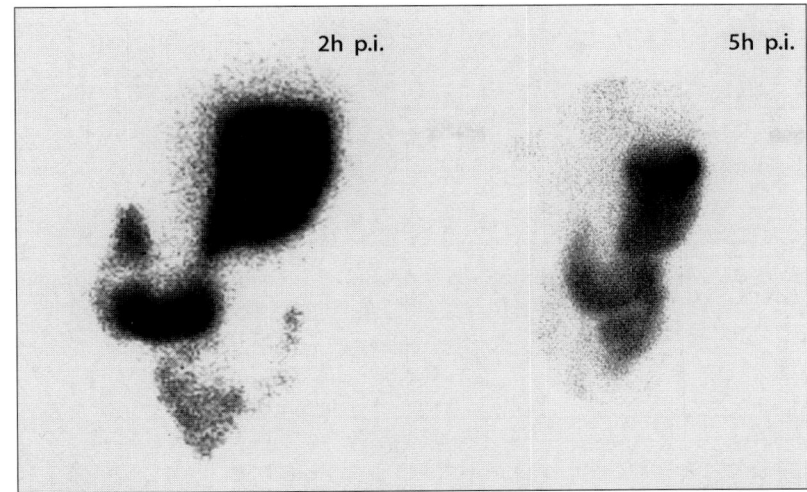

Fig. 3.5. Pyloric stenosis

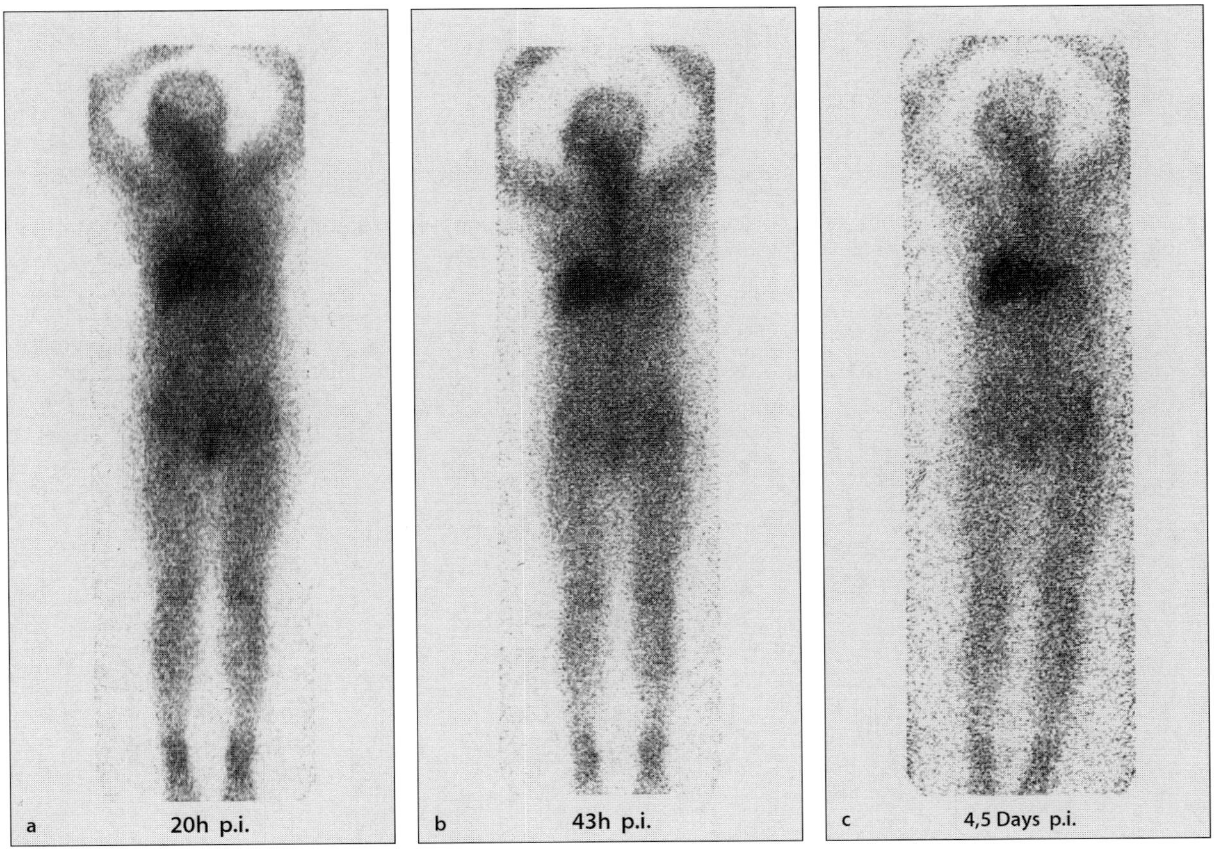

2h p.i.

5h p.i.

a   20h p.i.

b   43h p.i.

c   4,5 Days p.i.

Fig. 3.6 a–c. Normal ^{67}Ga whole-body scan in a patient screened for tumors or inflammatory disease

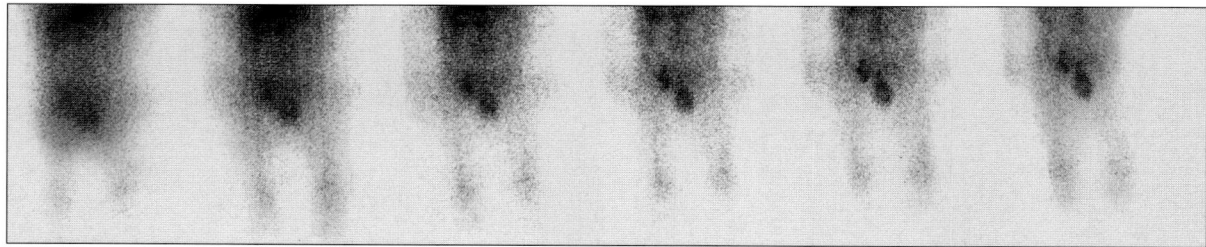

Fig. 3.7. This patient presented with unexplained lower abdominal symptoms and fever, which had been present for several days. ^{67}Ga whole-body scan is suspicious for encapsulated perforated appendicitis. Surgery confirmed the radionuclide diagnosis

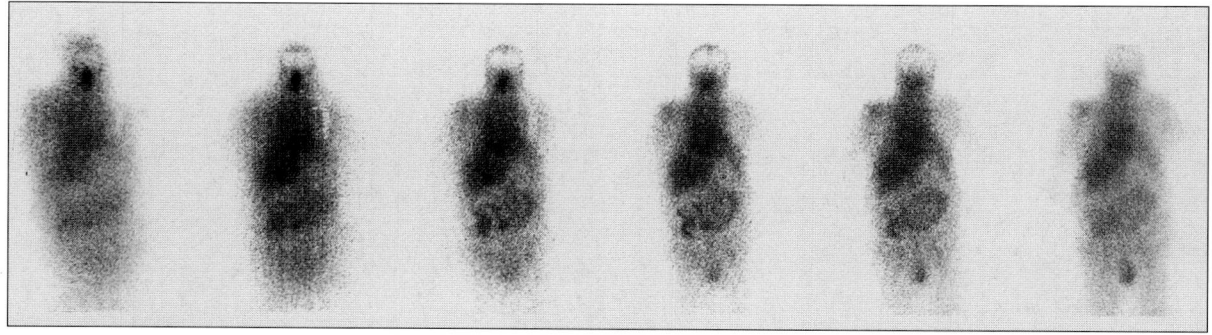

Fig. 3.8. Woman with lower abdominal complaints. Gynecologic disease was suspected, but findings were equivocal. Whole-body scan (Phocon technique) suggests appendicitis, which was confirmed surgically

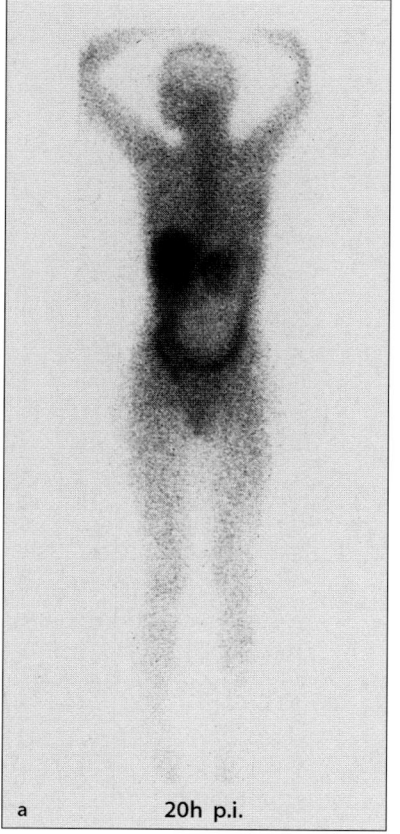
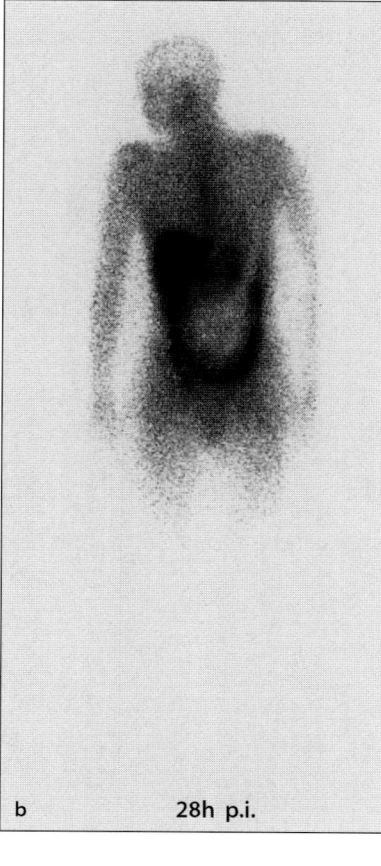

Fig. 3.9 a,b. Tumor screen in an emaciated patient with chronic constipation. ^{67}Ga whole-body scan shows a sagging transverse colon with no evidence of neoplastic disease

a   20h p.i.

b   28h p.i.

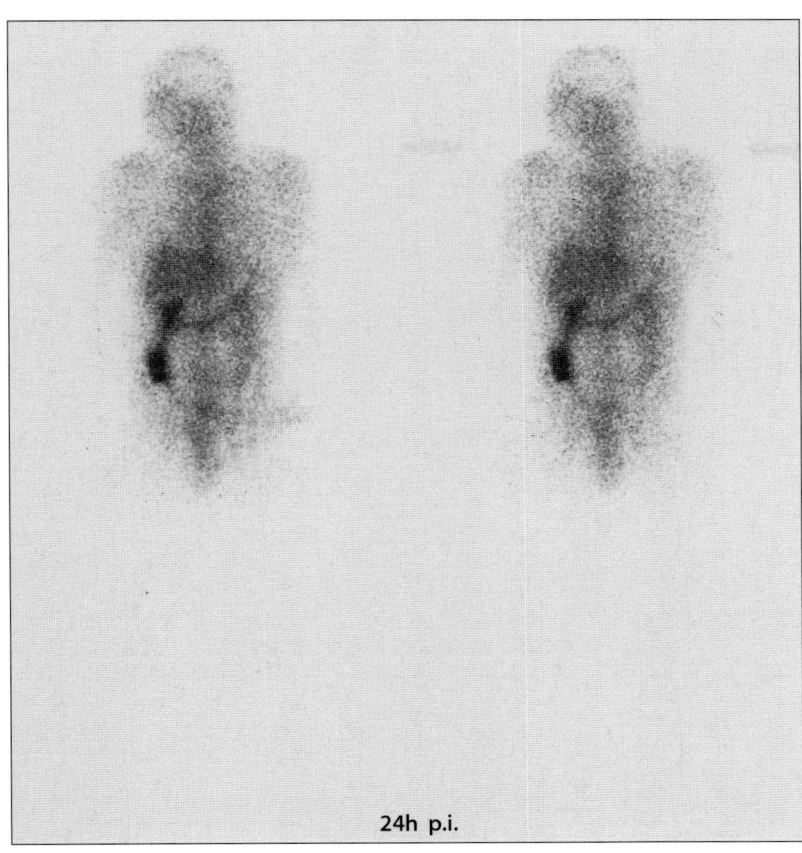

24h p.i.

Fig. 3.10. Woman with intermittent lower abdominal pain and blood in the stool. ⁶⁷Ga scan raises urgent suspicion of Crohn's disease, which was confirmed histologically

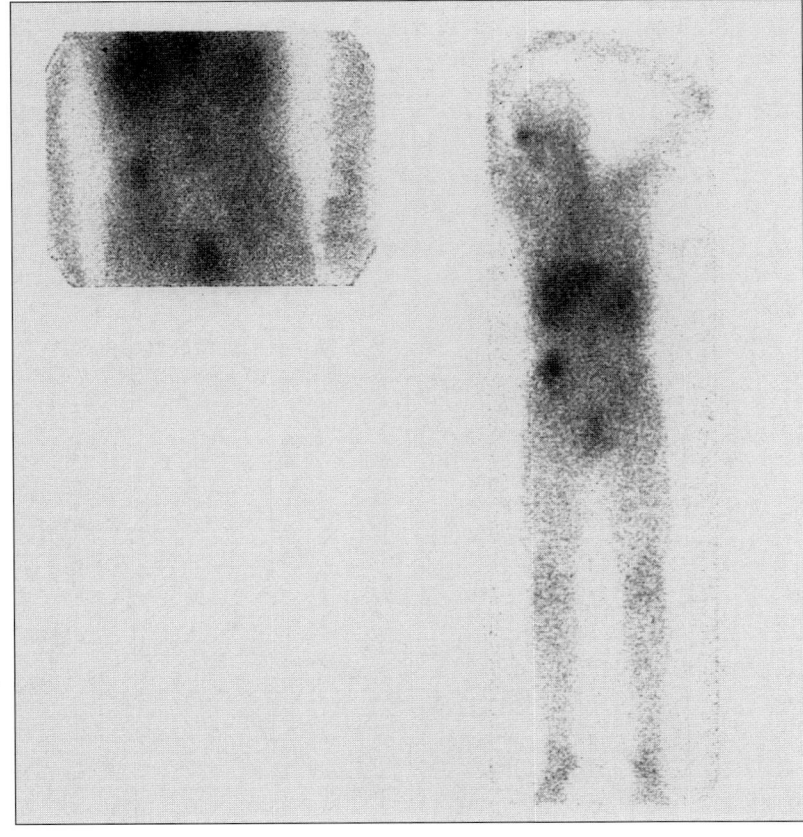

Fig. 3.11. ⁶⁷Ga scan in a patient with right-sided abdominal tenderness shows a focal abnormality in the central portion of the ascending colon. The lesion is an inflamed polyp

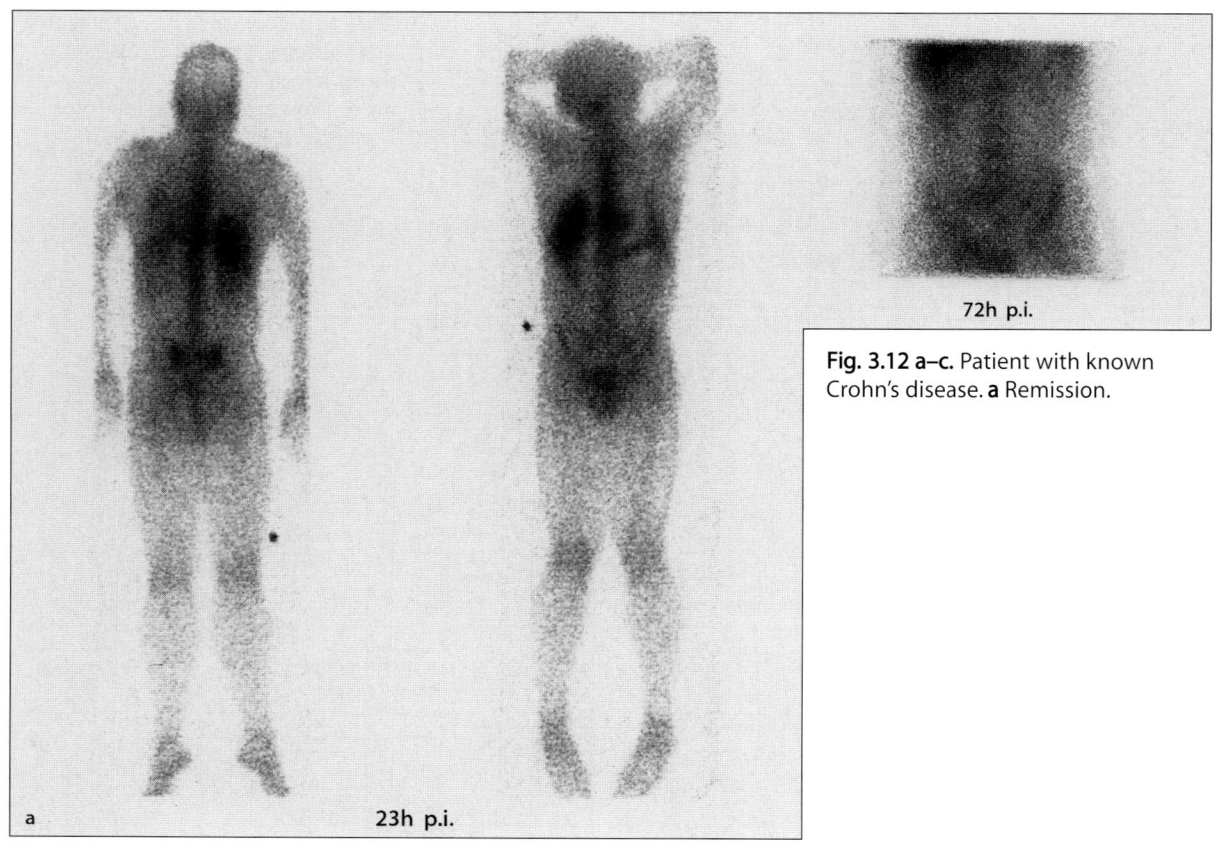

24h p.i.   82h p.i.

Fig. 3.11. *Continued*

72h p.i.

Fig. 3.12 a–c. Patient with known Crohn's disease. **a** Remission.

a   23h p.i.

Fig. 3.12 b. Recrudescence.

24h p.i.

b   72h p.i.

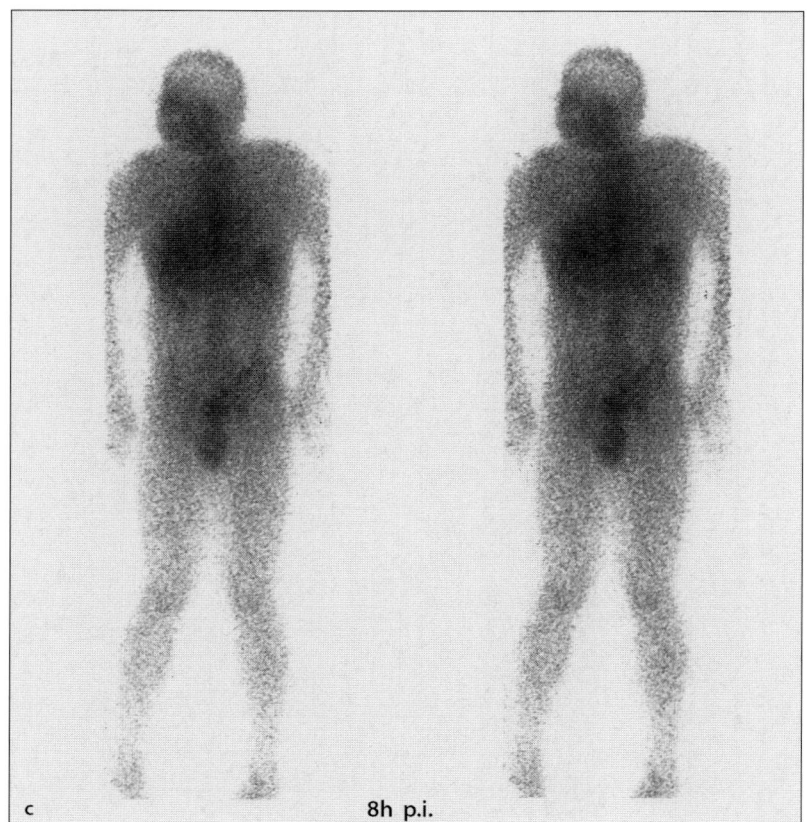

Fig. 3.12 c. Slight regression

c   8h p.i.

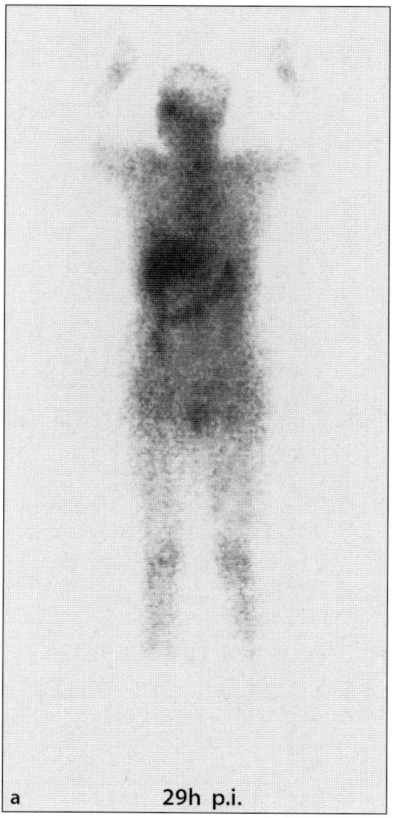

Fig. 3.13 a,b. Woman with known colonic diverticulosis and abdominal complaints. [67]Ga scan indicates diverticulitis

a   29h p.i.   b   43h p.i.

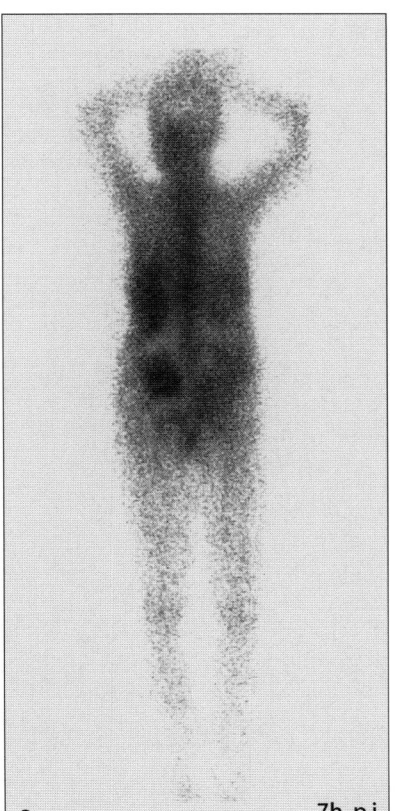
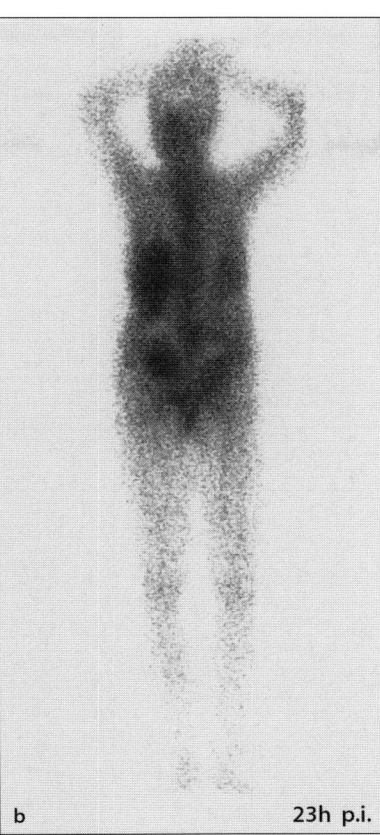

a   7h p.i.

b   23h p.i.

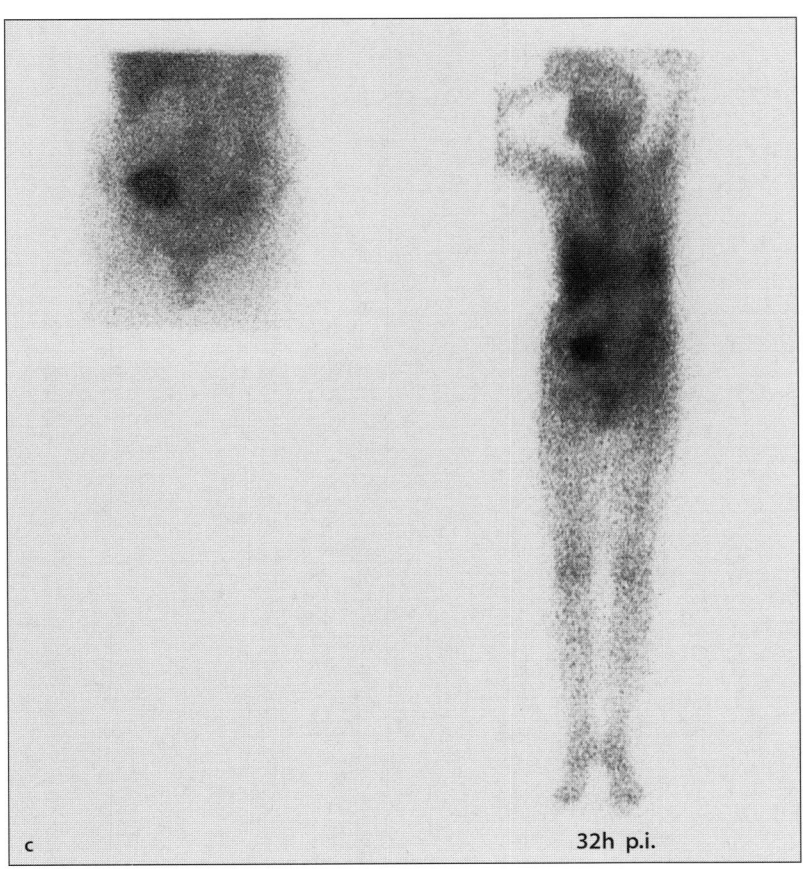

c

32h p.i.

Fig. 3.14 a–d. Woman with blood in the stool was treated for hemorrhoids by her family doctor. ^{67}Ga scan demonstrates a colonic mass. At surgery, an ulcerated adenocarcinoma 8 cm in diameter, with accompanying carcinomatous lymphangitis, was removed from the lower end of the cecum

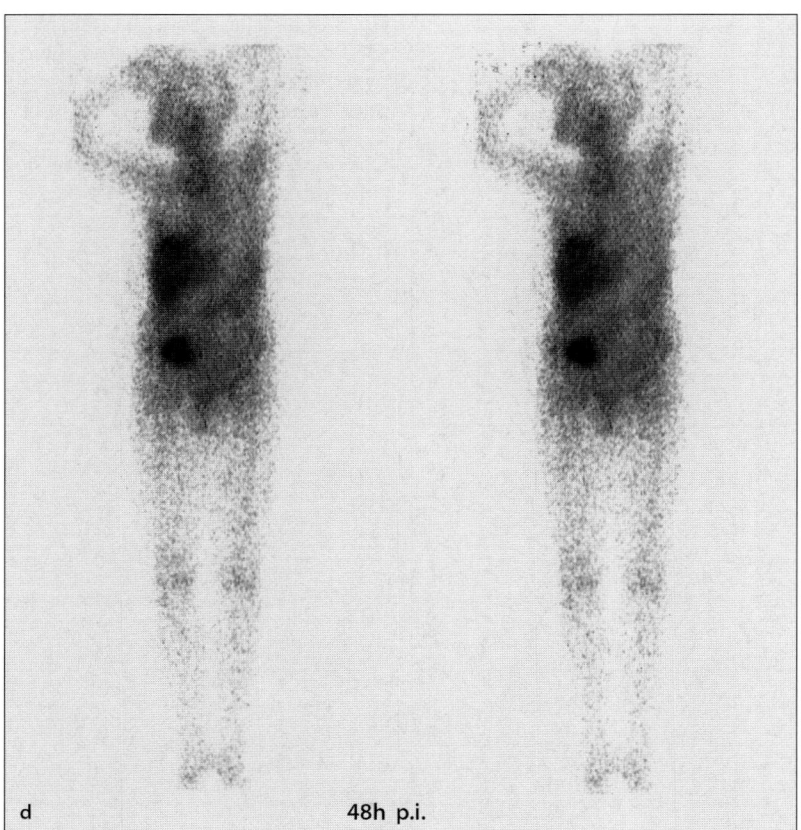

d   48h p.i.

Fig. 3.14 a–d. Woman with blood in the stool was treated for hemorrhoids by her family doctor. ^{67}Ga scan demonstrates a colonic mass. At surgery, an ulcerated adenocarcinoma 8 cm in diameter, with accompanying carcinomatous lymphangitis, was removed from the lower end of the cecum

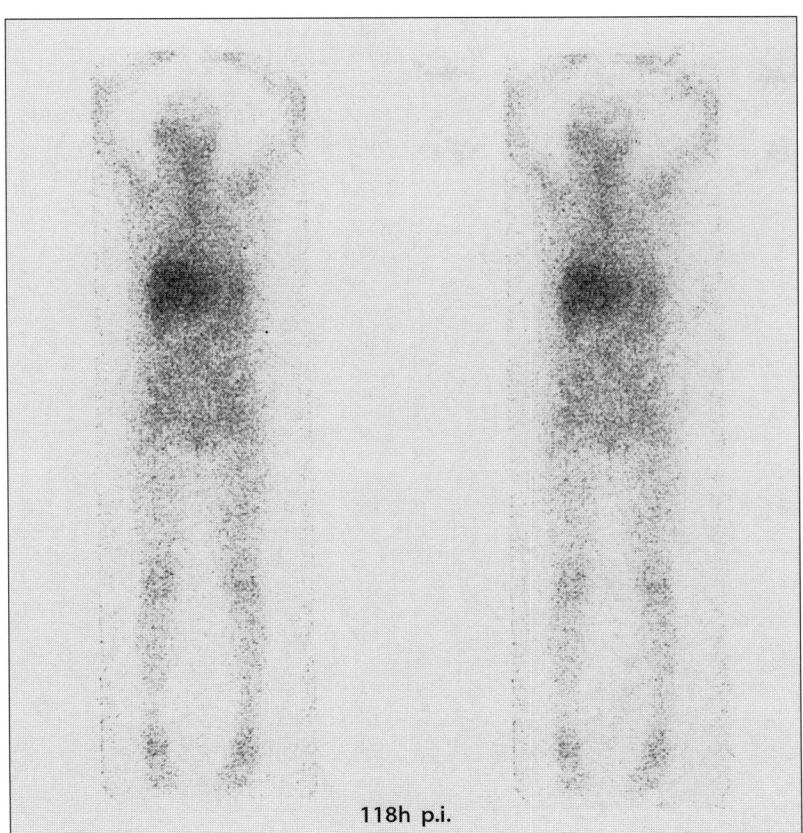

118h p.i.

Fig. 3.15. Status post-hemicolectomy for malignant tumor. ^{67}Ga scan shows no evidence of tumor recurrence

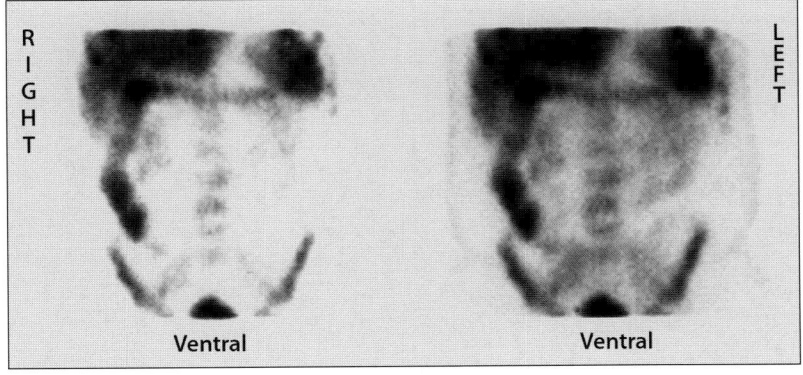

R I G H T

L E F T

Ventral

Ventral

Fig. 3.16. Scan with radiolabeled leukocytes confirms suspicion of colitis in the ascending colon and part of the transverse colon

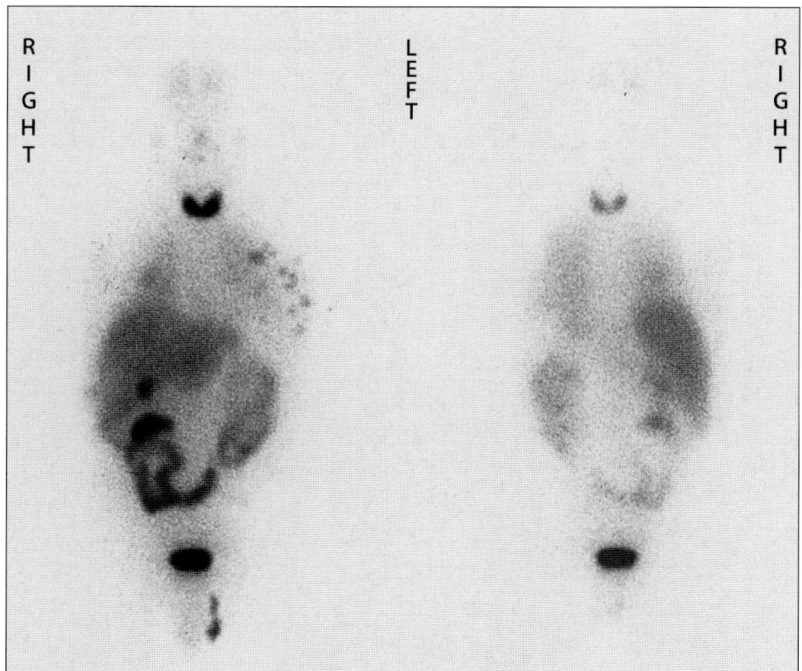

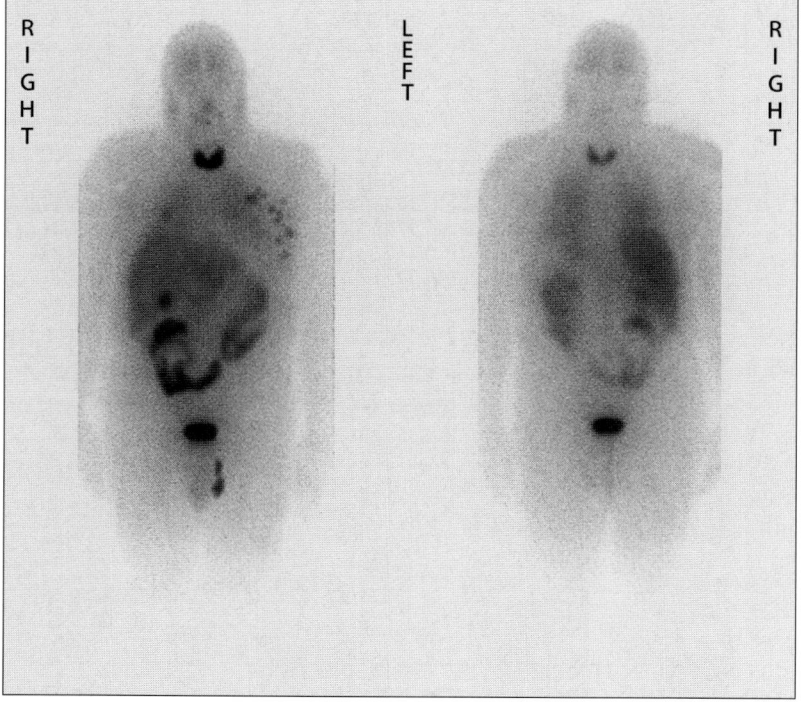

Fig. 3.17. Metastasis screen in a patient with known melanoma. Whole-body scan with iodobenzamide (IBZM) demonstrates cutaneous, pulmonary, and hepatic metastases from the malignant melanoma

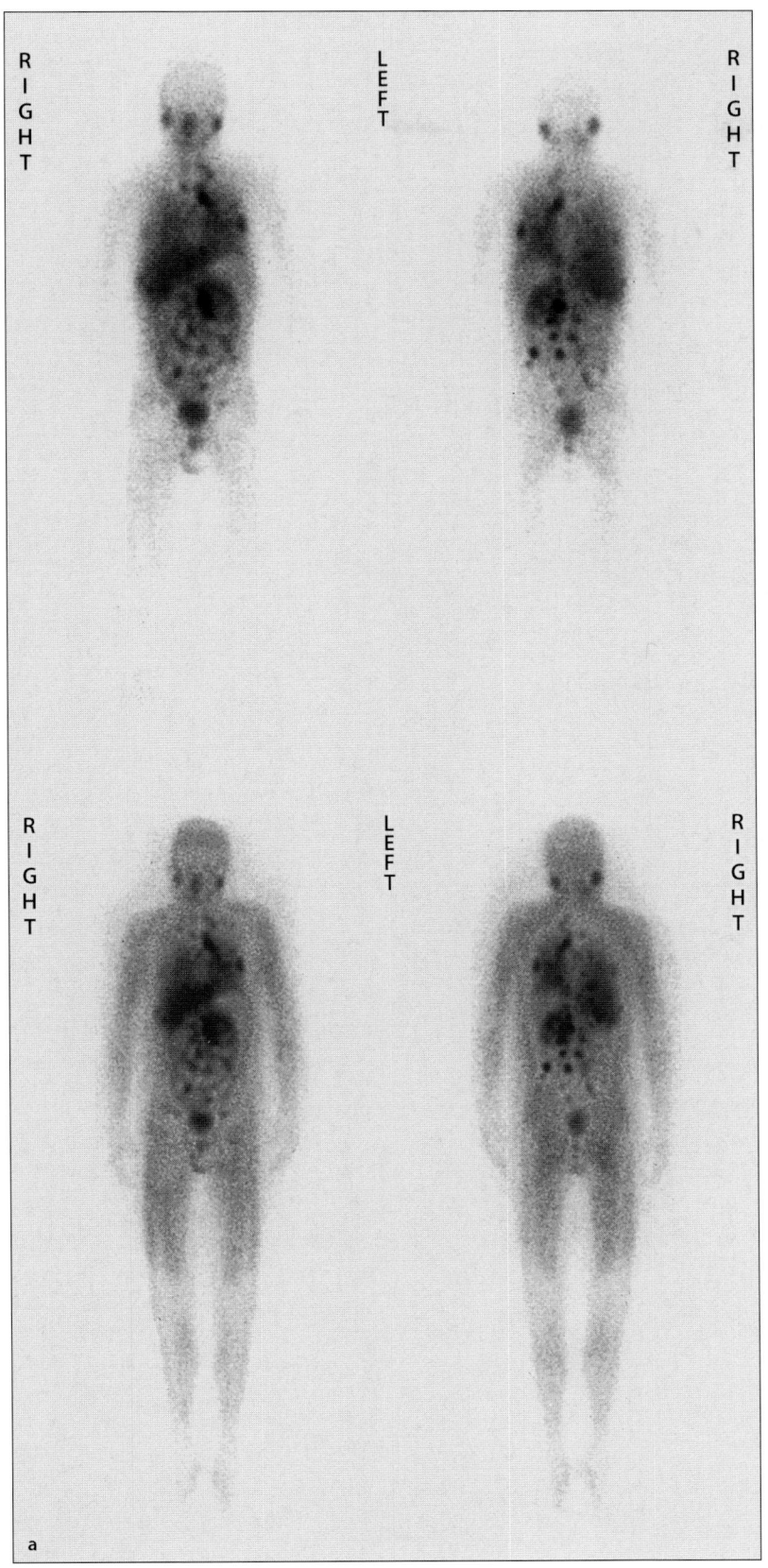

Fig. 3.18 a,b. Metastasis screen in a patient previously operated for neuroblastoma. [123]I meta-iodobenzyl-guanidine (MIBG) scan demonstrates multiple metastases

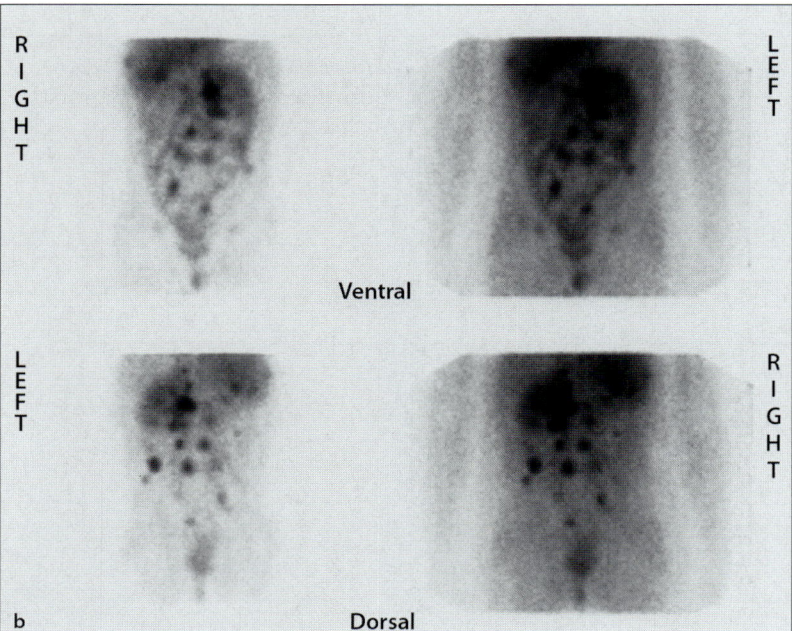

Fig. 3.18 b

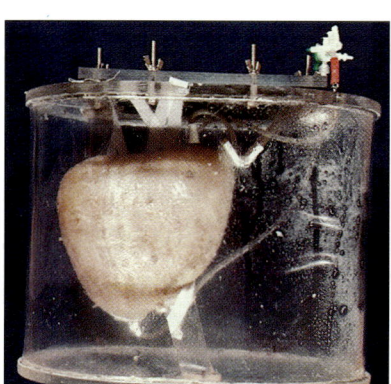

Fig. 3.19. Liver phantom

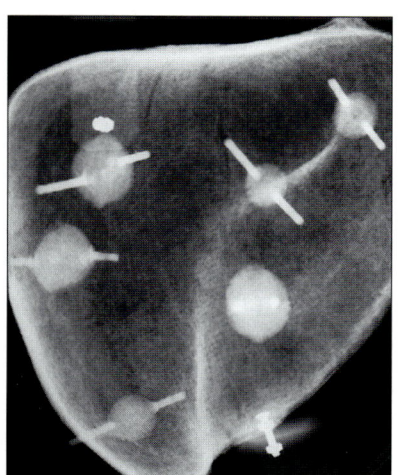

Fig. 3.20. Radiographic image of the liver phantom

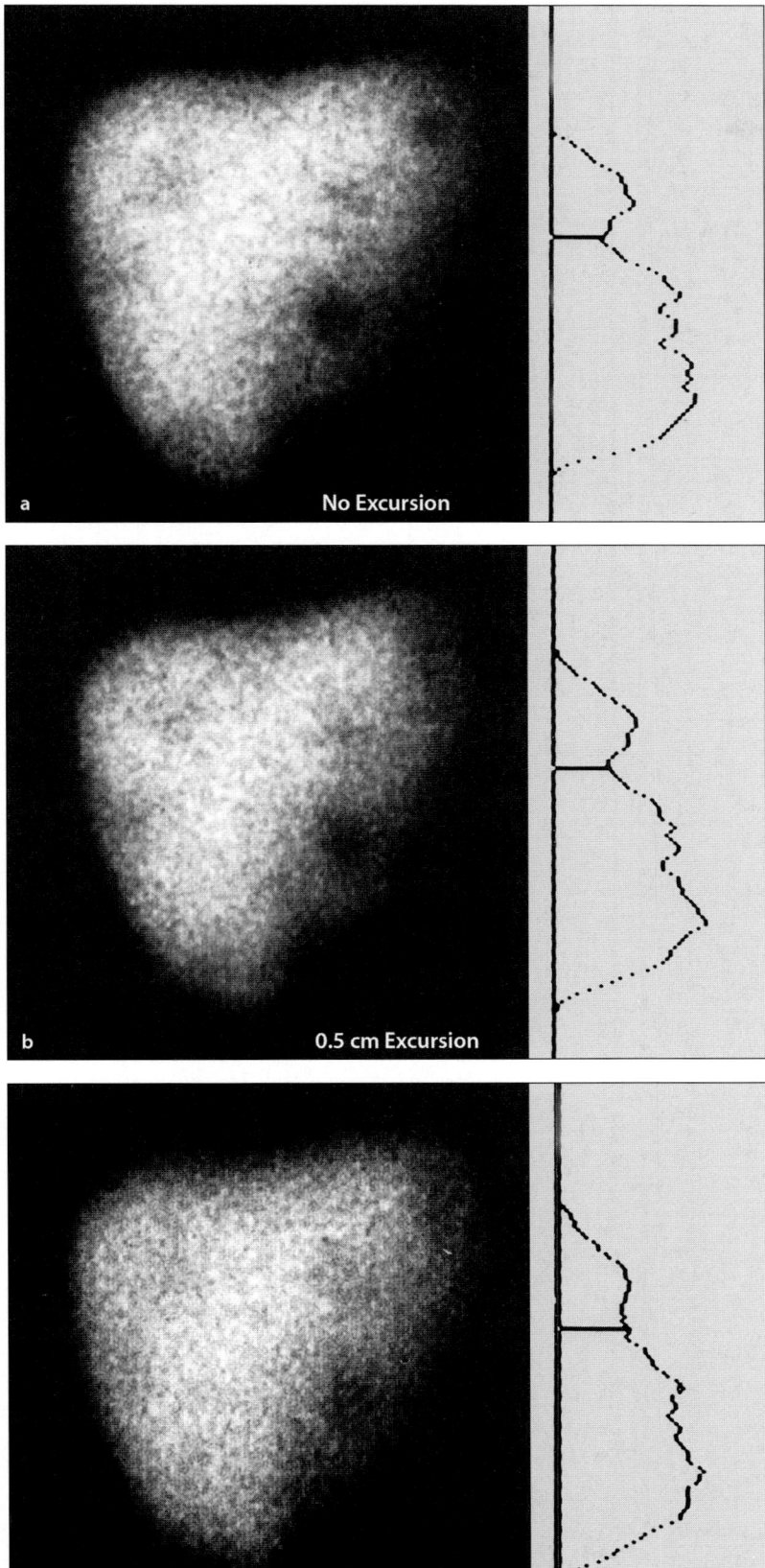

a   No Excursion

b   0.5 cm Excursion

c   1 cm Excursion

Fig. 3.21 a–g. Radionuclide images of the liver phantom at various respiratory excursions (*a1–f1*) and the corresponding profile curves (*a2–f2, g*) of a nodule with breath held. *Key to figure labels (top to bottom, left to right)*: AP view of the liver phantom in various degrees of excursion: no excursion; 0.5 cm excursion; 1 cm excursion; 1.5 cm excursion; 2 cm excursion; 3 cm excursion

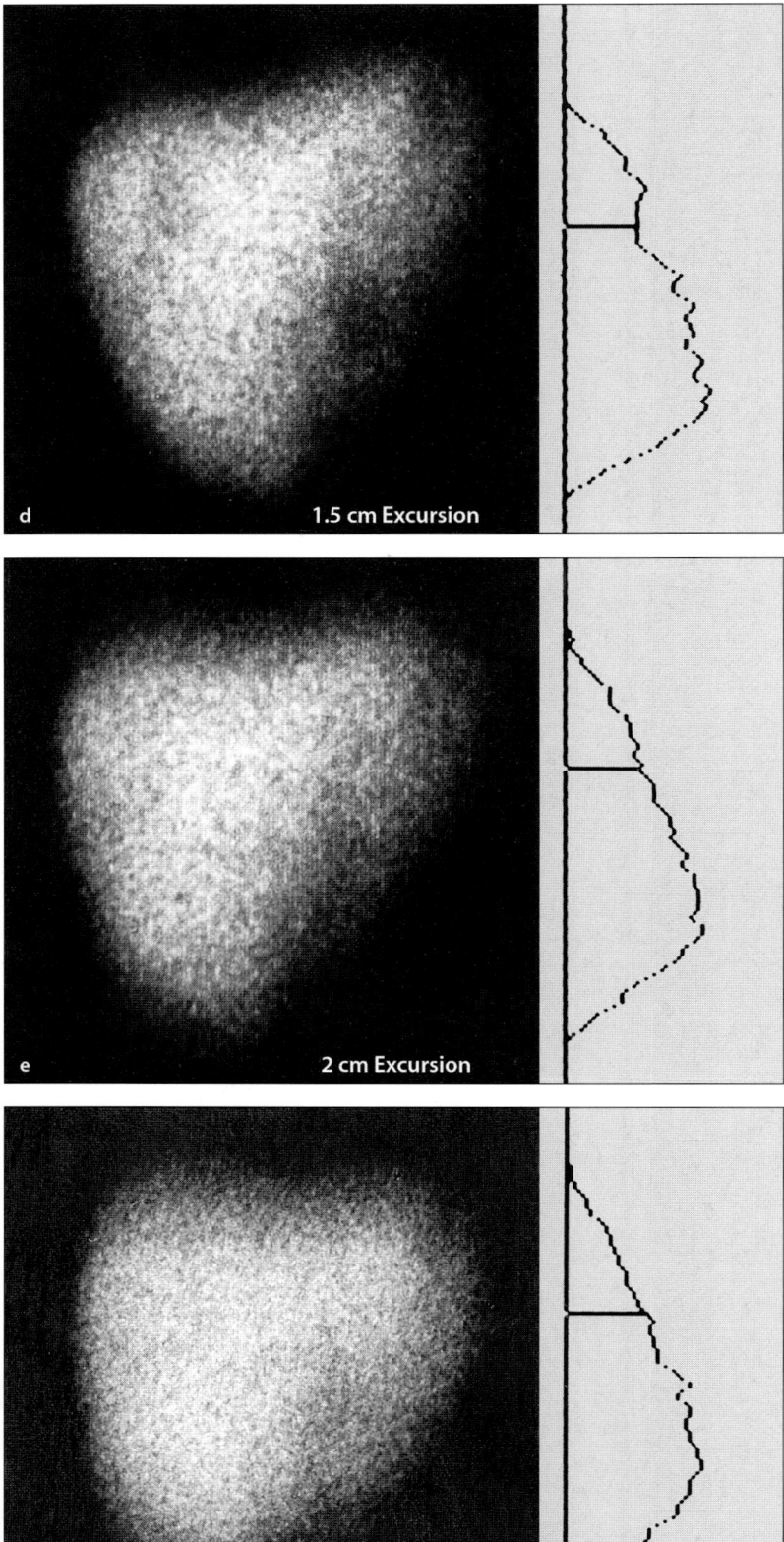

Fig. 3.21 a–g. Radionuclide images of the liver phantom at various respiratory excursions (*a1–f1*) and the corresponding profile curves (*a2–f2, g*) of a nodule with breath held. *Key to figure labels (top to bottom, left to right):* AP view of the liver phantom in various degrees of excursion: no excursion; 0.5 cm excursion; 1 cm excursion; 1.5 cm excursion; 2 cm excursion; 3 cm excursion

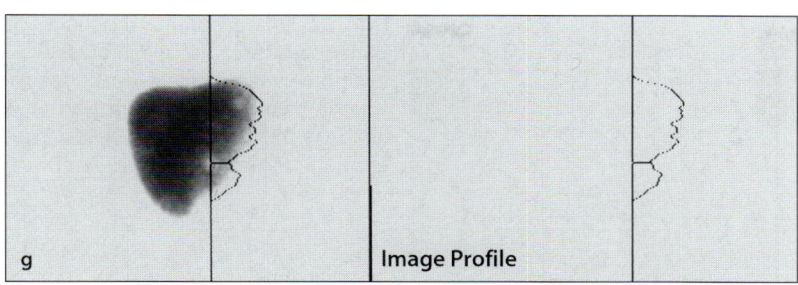

Fig. 3.21 g

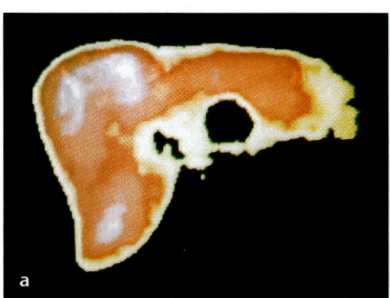
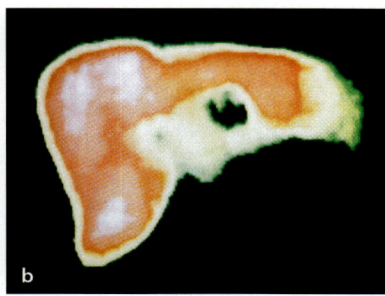

Fig. 3.22 a,b. Liver scan was obtained in a 65-year-old woman hospitalized with elevated transaminase and bilirubin levels. **a** Scan without respiratory triggering shows a perihilar mass with smooth margins. **b** Scan with respiratory triggering gives better edge definition of the villous carcinoma margin and shows central liquefaction

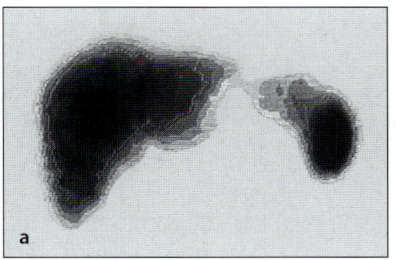
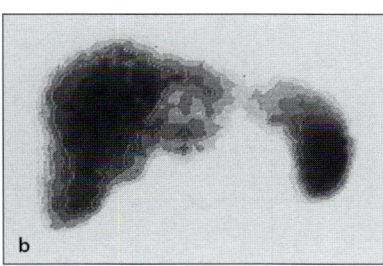

Fig. 3.23 a,b. Liver scan was obtained in a 45-year-old woman hospitalized for upper abdominal complaints, low-grade fever, and mildly elevated transaminase levels. **a** Scan without respiratory triggering shows no abnormality. **b** Scan with respiratory triggering demonstrates an abscess in the left lobe of the liver

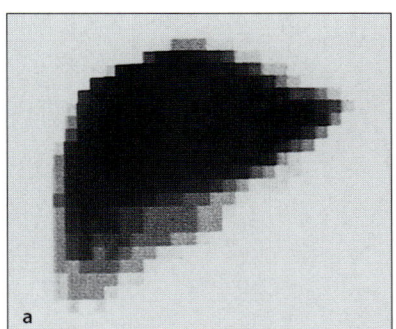
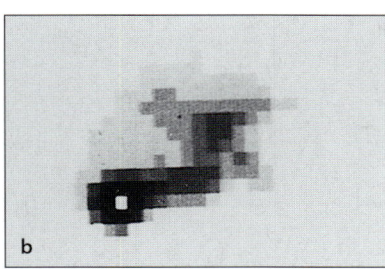
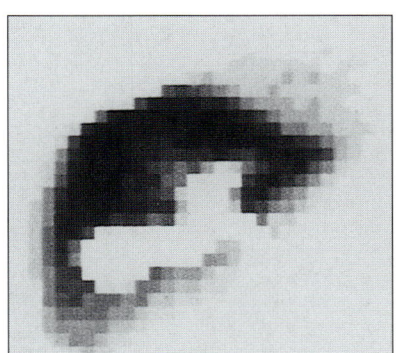
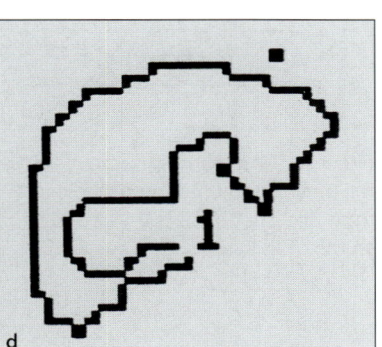

Fig. 3.24 a–d. Use of the subtraction method for evaluating damage to the hepatic parenchyma. **a** Liver. **b** Bile ducts and bile. **c** Subtraction image (*a–b*)

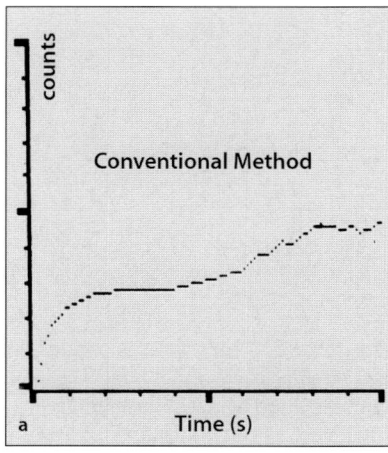

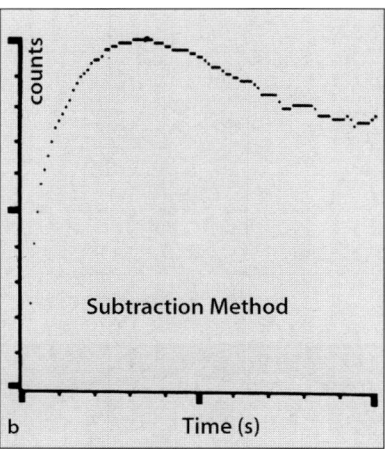

Fig. 3.2.5. a Conventional scan in a patient with an atypical gallbladder location gives a spurious result due to superimposed bile. **b** Subtraction image in the same patient yields an accurate result

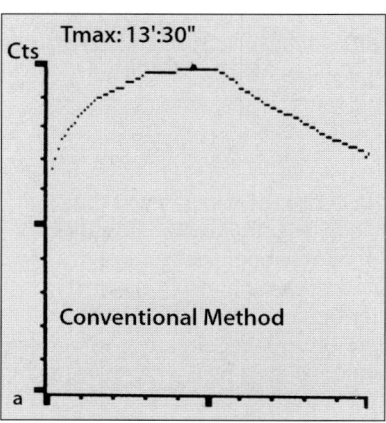

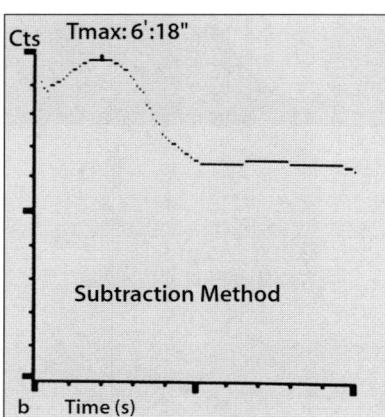

Fig. 3.26. a Spurious results with a conventional scan ($T_{max} = 13.3$ min). **b** Subtraction method yields more accurate results ($T_{max} = 6.6$ min)

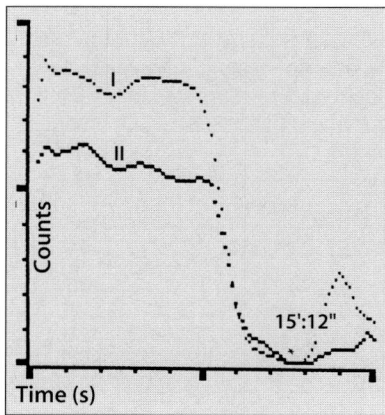

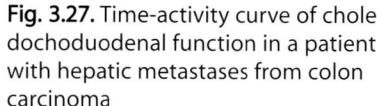

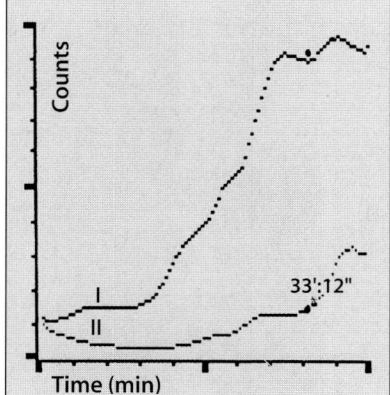

Fig. 3.27. Time-activity curve of choledochoduodenal function in a patient with hepatic metastases from colon carcinoma

Fig. 3.28. Time-activity curve of a partial outflow obstruction of the common bile duct. Note the stepped shape of the curve

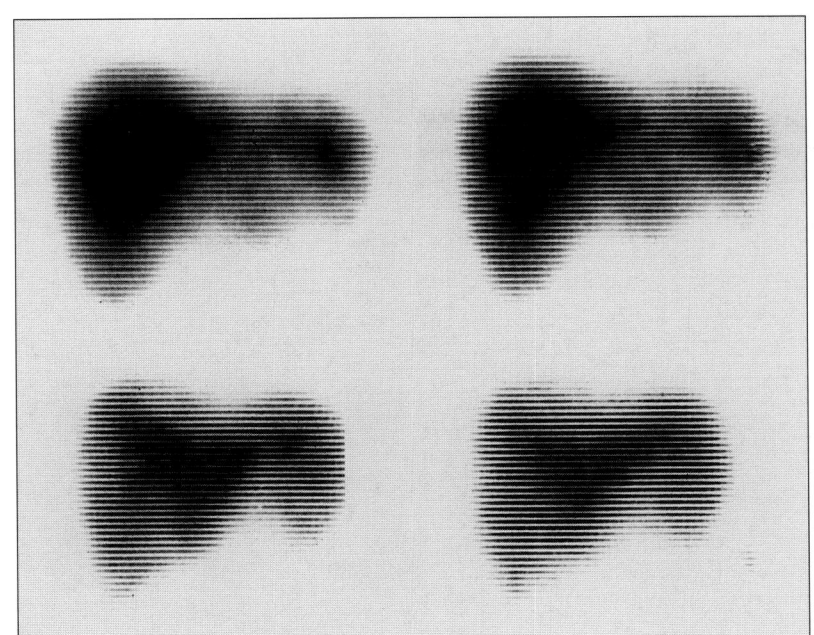

Fig. 3.29. Normal SPECT liver-spleen scan

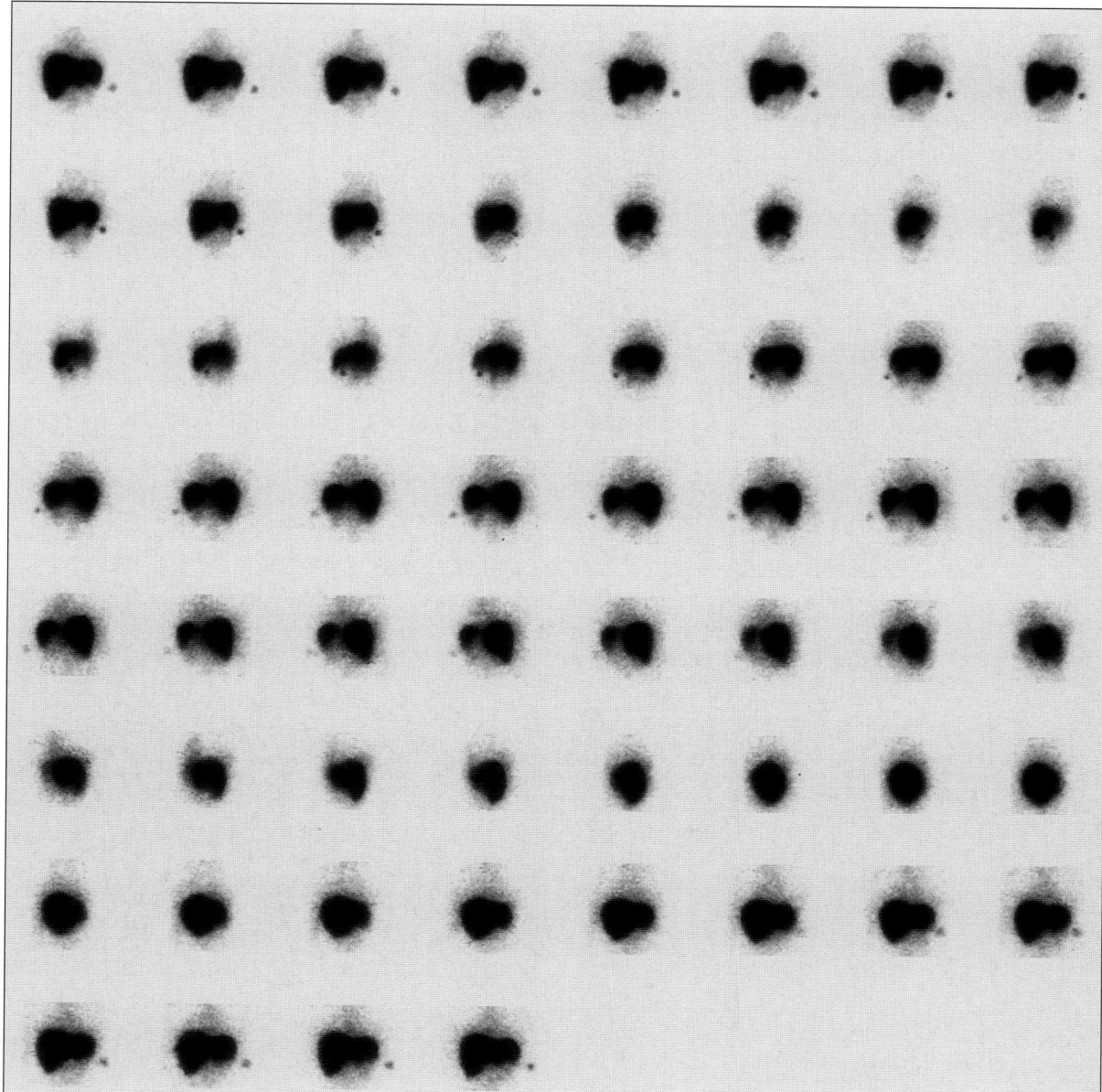

Fig. 3.29. Normal SPECT liver-spleen scan

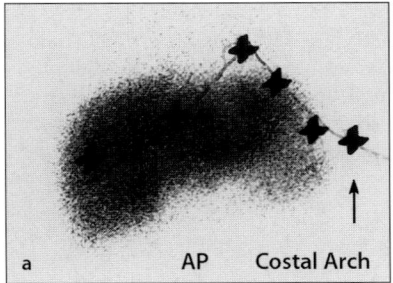

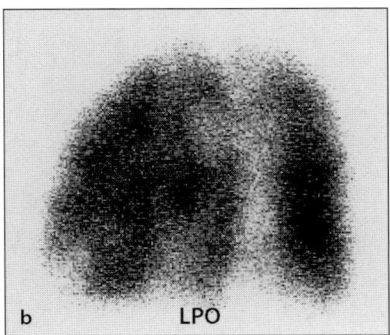

Fig. 3.30 a,b. A low position of the liver was noted clinically in a 65-year-old man with respiratory distress. Radionuclide scan shows a normal-size liver. Displacement of the diaphragm due to bullous emphysema gave a false clinical impression of hepatomegaly

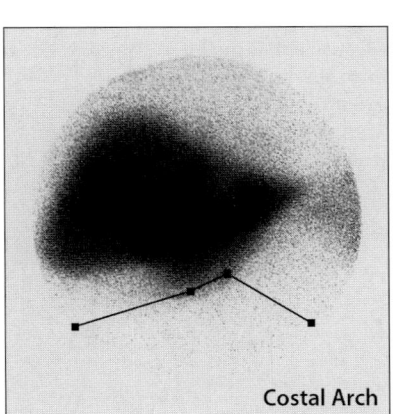

Fig. 3.31. This patient complained of pressure in the lower right hemithorax, which had been present for months. Physical examination revealed dullness in the lower hemithorax and restriction of diaphragmatic motion. The liver could not be palpated on deep inspiration. Liver scanning was requested to determine the cause. The scan shows a slightly enlarged liver with accentuation of the dome. The liver has been displaced upward due to diaphragmatic hernia

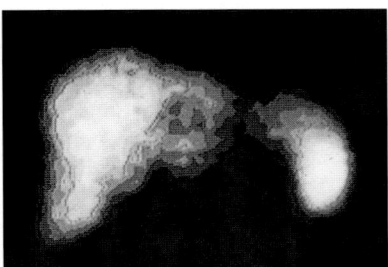

Fig. 3.32. A 36-year-old woman presented with fever, epigastric tenderness, slightly elevated transaminase levels, and a normal-size liver. Radionuclide scan shows an abscess directly adjacent to the round ligament of the liver. The lesion showed good regression with antibiotic treatment

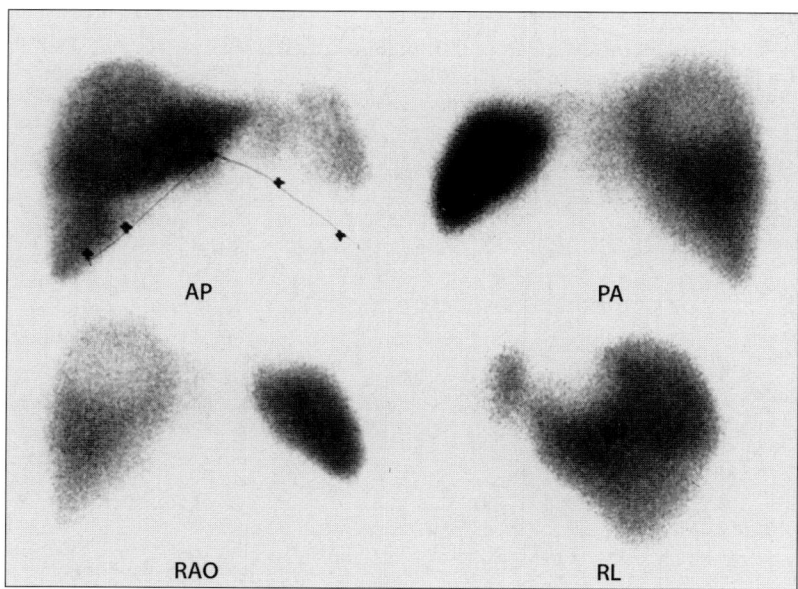

Fig. 3.33. This patient was admitted with high fever and severe RUQ pain. Her transaminase levels were slightly high. Radionuclide scan shows a cold defect with rounded margins below the diaphragm. Subphrenic abscess

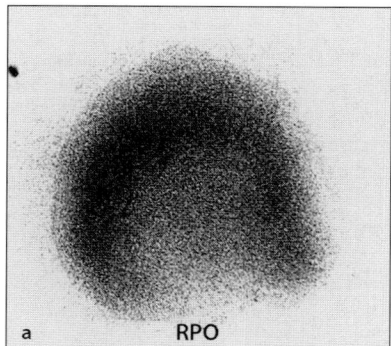

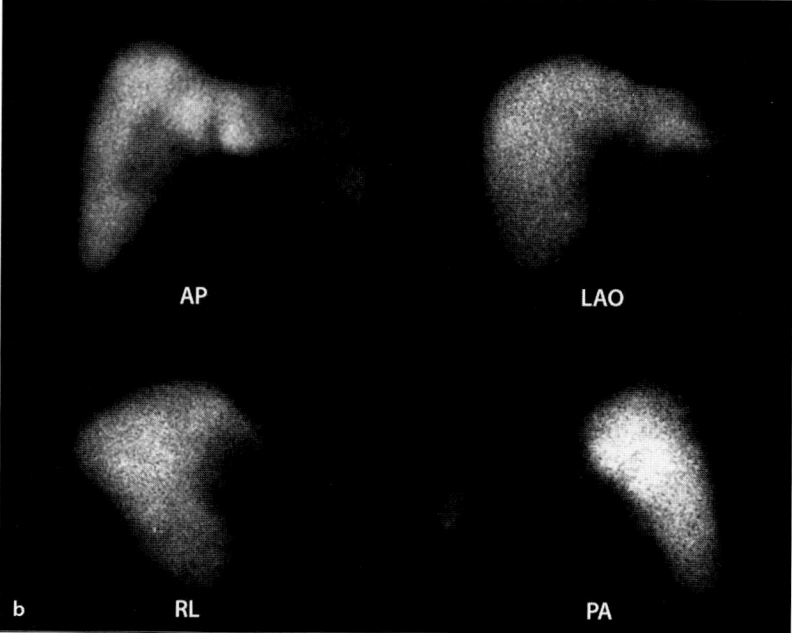

Fig. 3.34 a,b. This patient presented clinically with high fever, marked tenderness below the right costal arch, yellow sclerae, and elevated transaminase and bilirubin levels. **a** Radionuclide scan shows a curvilinear defect in the central portion of the inferior hepatic border, consistent with gallbladder hydrops. The patient was treated surgically. After a period of remission, fever recurred. **b** Repeat scan demonstrates an abscess at the operative site. The lesion was surgically evacuated

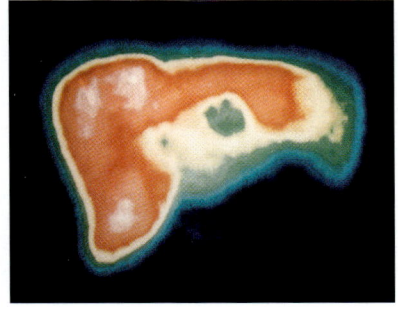

Fig. 3.35. A 70-year-old woman was admitted with cachexia and elevated transaminase and bilirubin levels. Liver scan shows a photopenic area with a central cold spot in the left lobe, raising suspicion of a malignant tumor with central necrosis. The lesion was diagnosed by ultrasound, CT, and ERCP as a primary hepatic carcinoma. Autopsy revealed a primary bile duct carcinoma

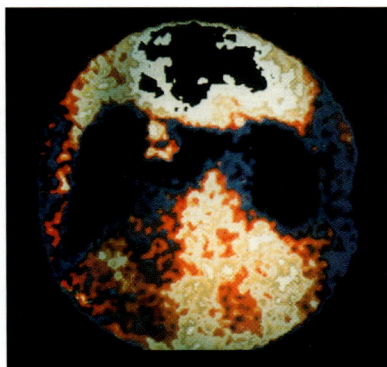

Fig. 3.36. ^{67}Ga colloid liver scan (subtraction image) of hepatocellular carcinoma

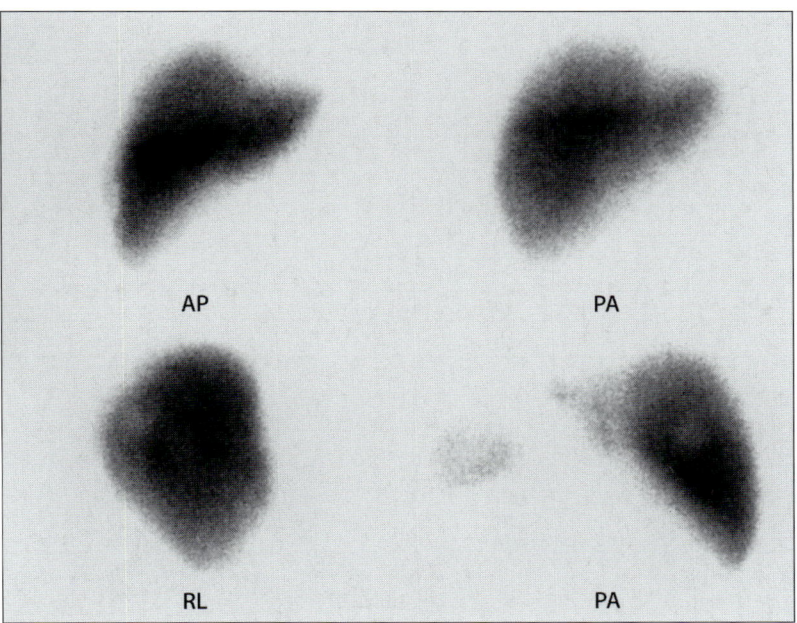

Fig. 3.37. Follow-up scan in a young patient with non-Hodgkin's lymphoma demonstrates a solitary hepatic metastasis

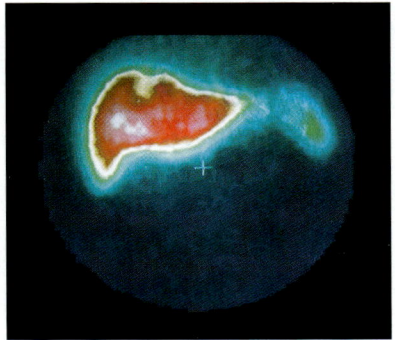

Fig. 3.38. Woman with breast carcinoma and slightly elevated transaminases and tumor markers. Ultrasound findings were normal. Radionuclide scan clearly demonstrates a metastasis located near the diaphragm

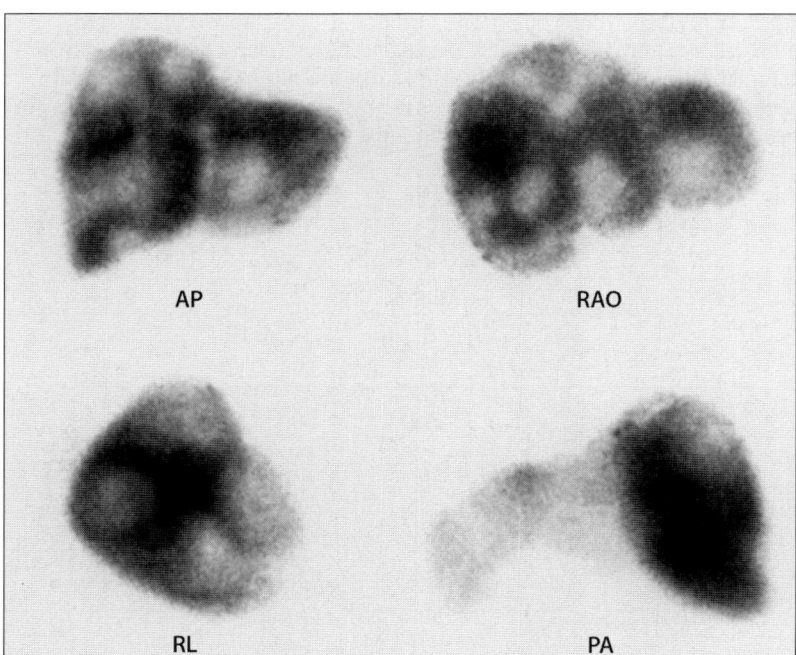

Fig. 3.39. Follow-up of a patient previously operated for colon carcinoma. Radionuclide scan shows multiple metastases

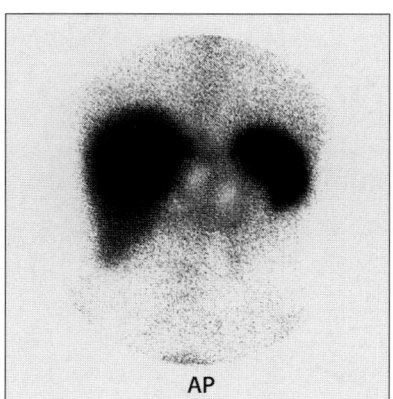

Fig. 3.40. Follow-up examination in an elderly man with colon carcinoma and slight tumor marker elevation. Radionuclide scan demonstrates metastases in the left lobe of the liver

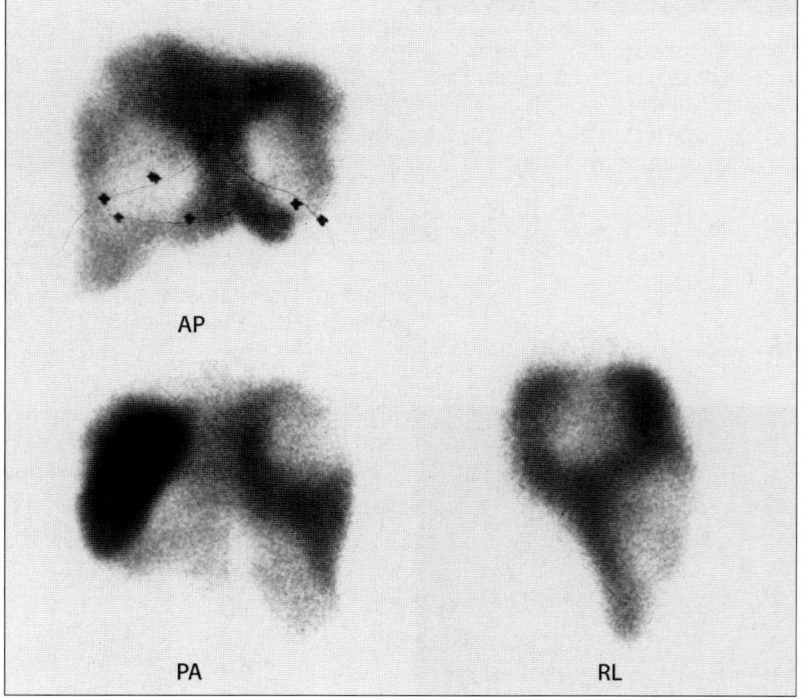

Fig. 3.41. Man 44 years of age underwent previous surgery for hypernephroma. Physical examination revealed a very large intraabdominal mass. Radionuclide scan shows significant enlargement of the liver, which is permeated by multiple metastases with central necrotic foci

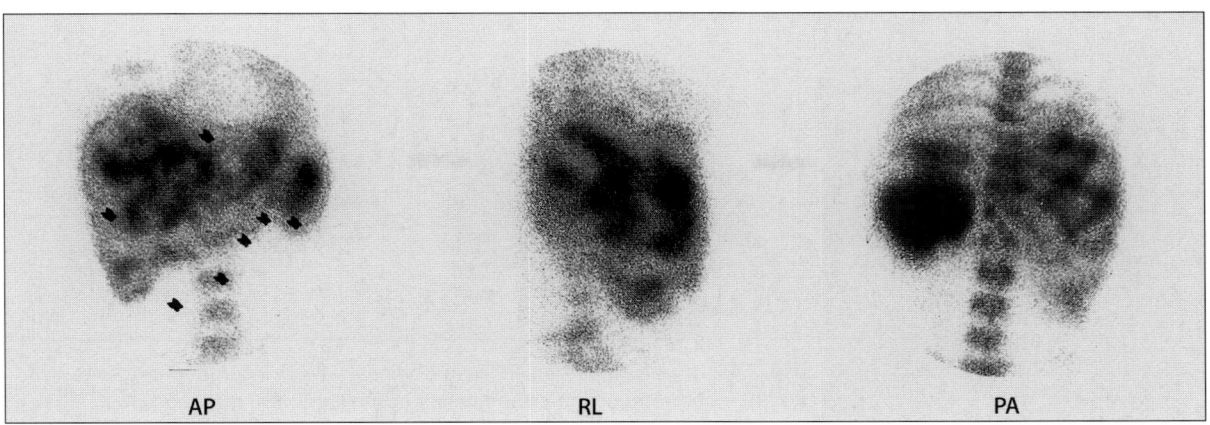

Fig. 3.42. Alcoholic 42 years of age with a tarry stool. On physical examination the liver was hard, nodulated, and markedly enlarged. Liver-spleen scan shows hepatosplenomegaly and patchy, nonhomogeneous tracer uptake, also phagocytosis of the tracer in the vertebral column and ribs. The patient has advanced hepatic cirrhosis based on fatty liver degeneration with portal hypertension. Endoscopy showed marked varicosity of the esophagus and cardia

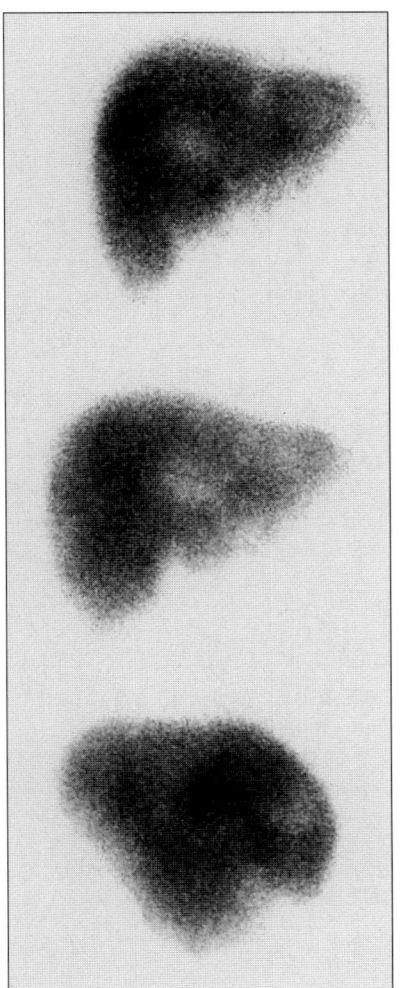

Fig. 3.43. A young woman presented clinically with low-grade fever, epigastric pressure, and slight hepatic tenderness. Liver scan shows nonhomogeneous uptake with several cold spots resembling hepatic metastases. These changes represent involvement of the liver by actinomycosis

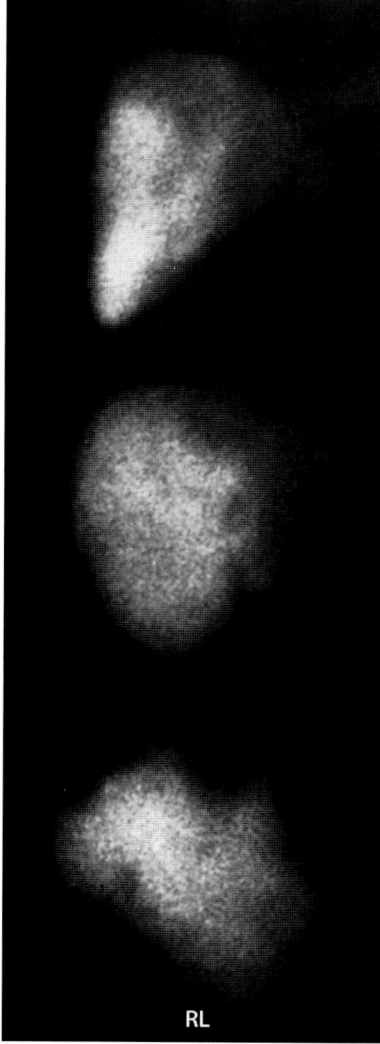

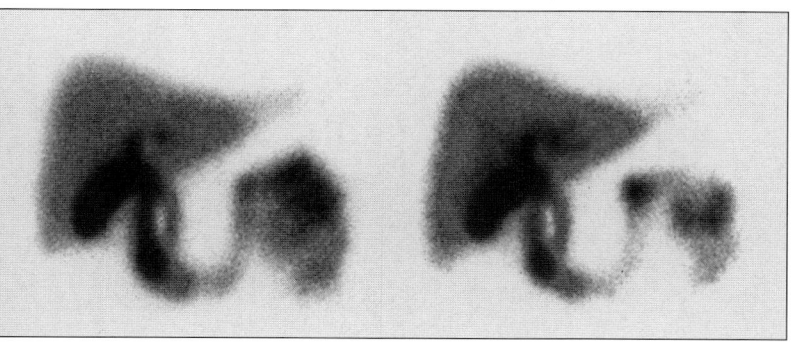

Fig. 3.45. Normal hepatobiliary scan demonstrates the intrahepatic ducts, gallbladder, common bile duct, and biliary outflow into the duodenum

Fig. 3.44. This patient presented with upper abdominal pain, constant nausea, occasional vomiting, and intermittent fever. For some time the patient had malaise and slightly elevated liver values. Liver scan shows multiple well-defined, multilacunar cold spots in the liver representing hydatid cysts

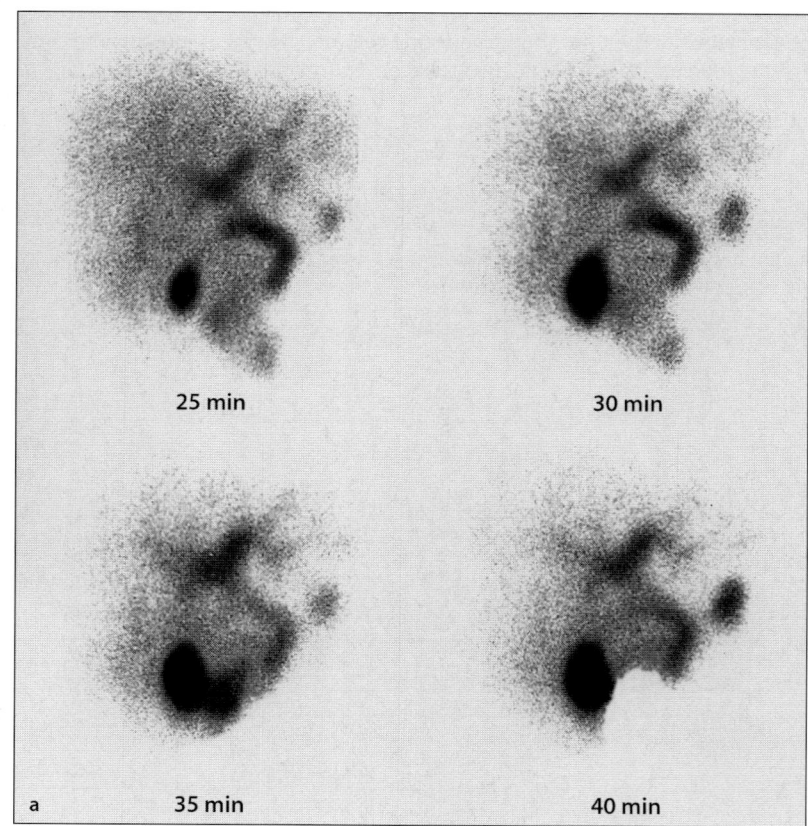

a   25 min   30 min

    35 min   40 min

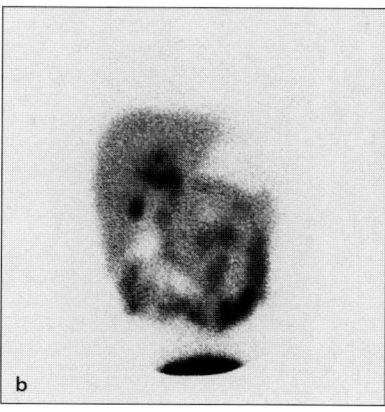

b

Fig. 3.46 a,b. Woman 46 years of age with a bloated feeling after meals. Clinical examination was normal. Hepatobiliary function scan (**a**) shows slightly delayed emptying of the gallbladder, but reasonably good emptying occurred after stimulation (**b**). Gallbladder atony

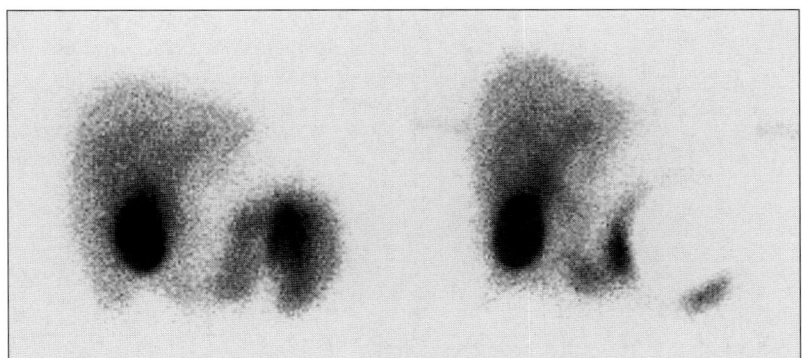

Fig. 3.47. Gallbladder atony

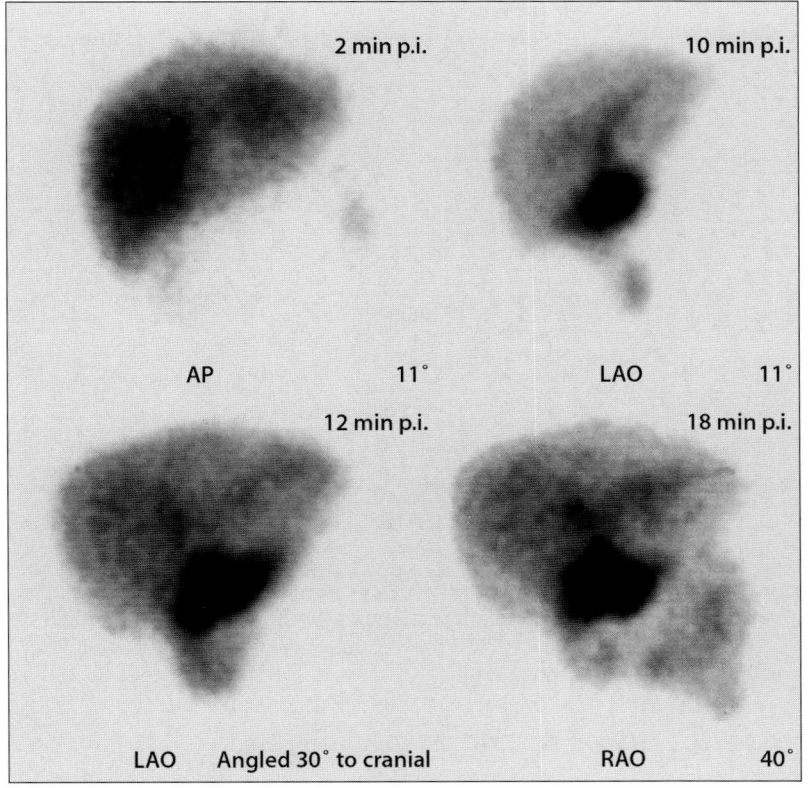

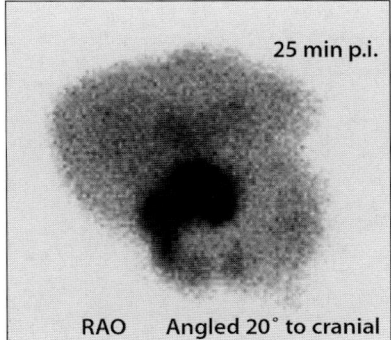

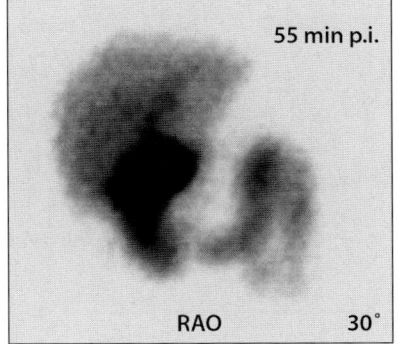

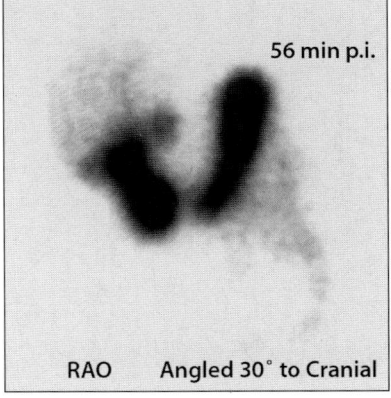

Fig. 3.48. Complaints recurred in a patient who previously underwent choledo-choduodenostomy. Hepatobiliary function scan shows a partial outflow obstruction and significant reflux, prompting surgical reintervention

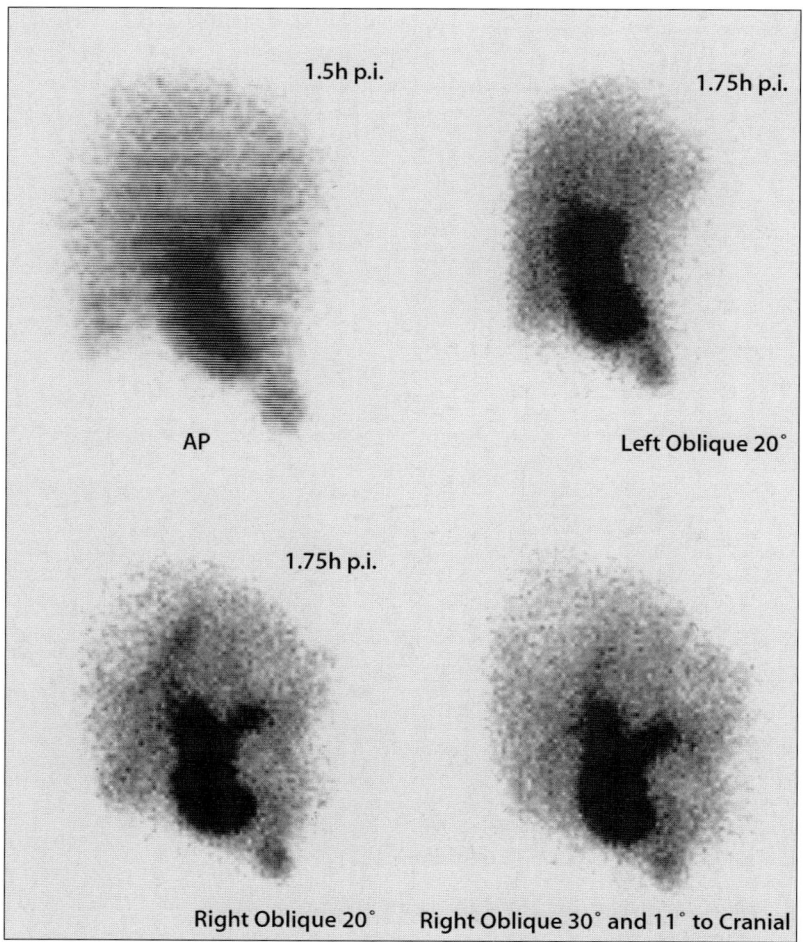

Fig. 3.49. Patient who underwent cholecystectomy for gallstones presented with a recurrence of biliary colic and elevated bilirubin. Scan shows outflow obstruction with retrograde obstruction of the intrahepatic ducts

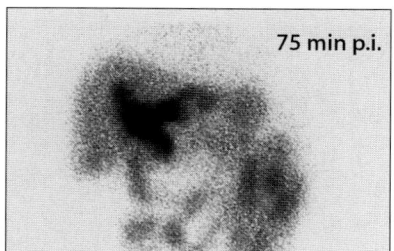

Fig. 3.50. This patient presented with RUQ pressure that was most pronounced after meals. Hepatobiliary function scan shows dilatation of the intrahepatic ducts and common bile duct. ERCP showed sclerosis of the duodenal papilla, creating a partial biliary obstruction

Fig. 3.51. This patient complained of intermittent, colicky epigastric pain that had become constant on the previous day. Clinically, a painful mass was palpable on the hepatic border. Hepatobiliary scan shows common bile duct obstruction with gallbladder hydrops. The obstructing stone was surgically removed

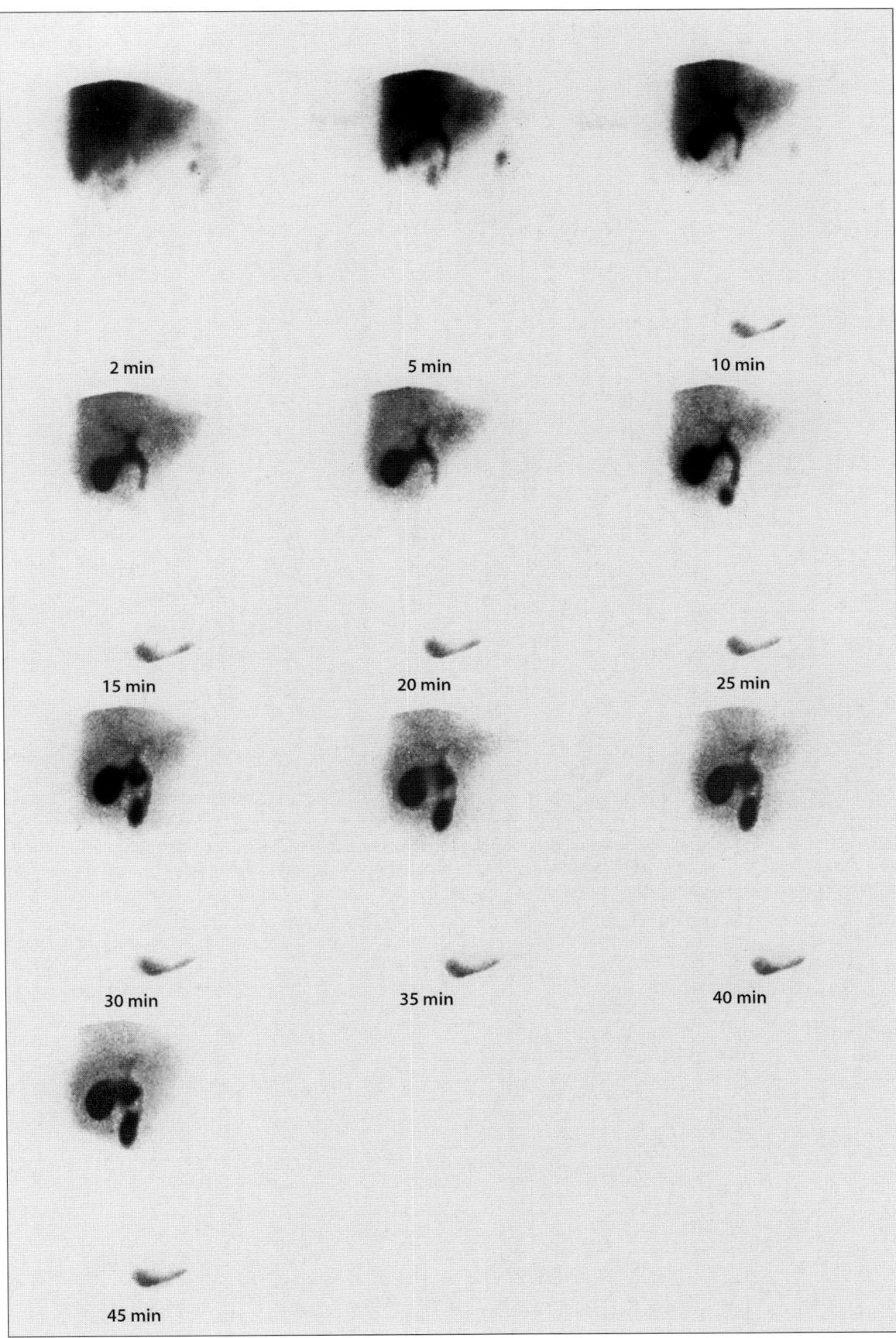

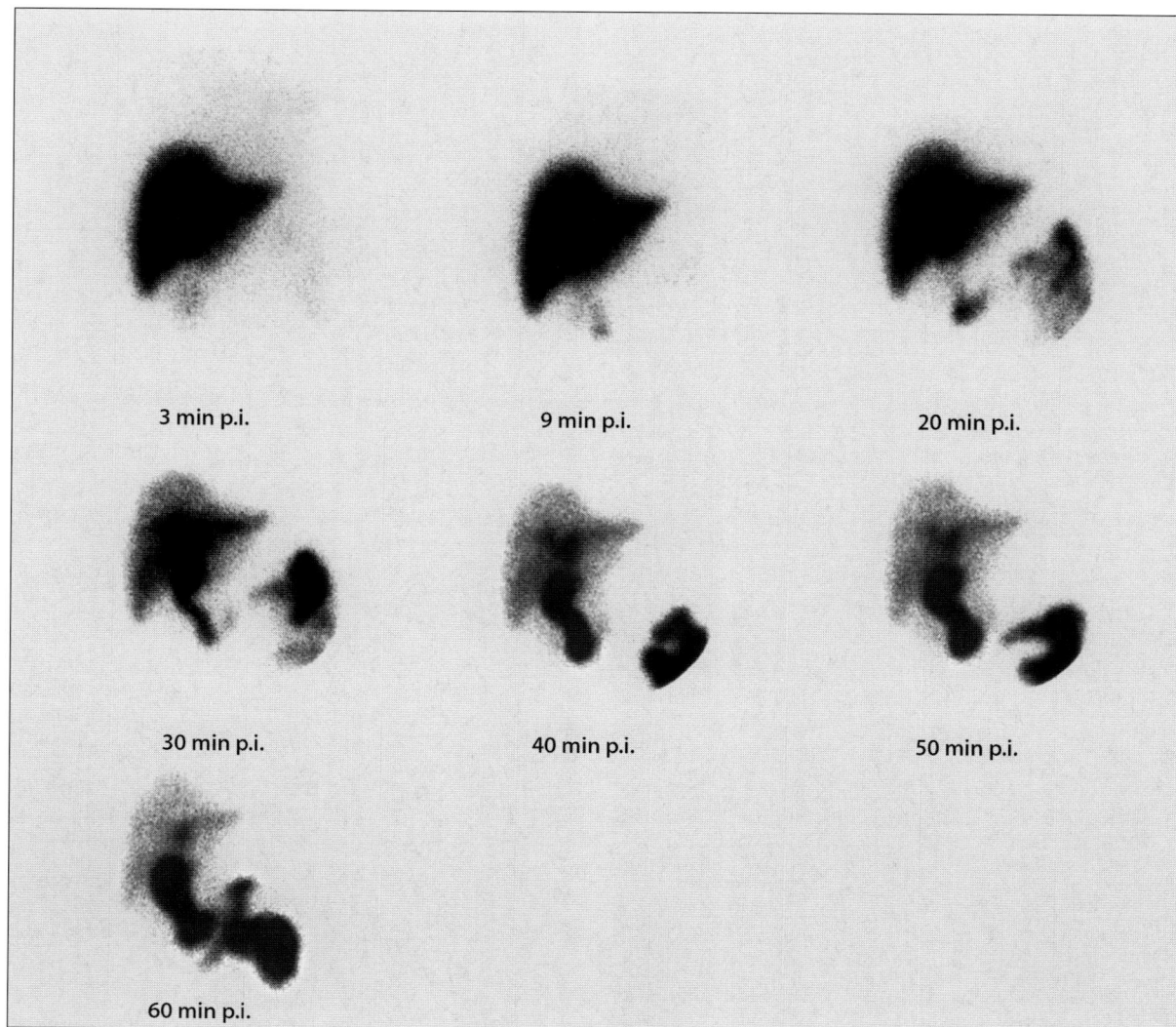

3 min p.i.   9 min p.i.   20 min p.i.

30 min p.i.   40 min p.i.   50 min p.i.

60 min p.i.

Fig. 3.52. Patient who underwent previous choledochoduodenostomy presented with severe epigastric complaints and elevated transaminase and bilirubin levels. Scan demonstrates anastomotic obstruction. At surgery, the anastomosis was found to be encased by dense adhesions

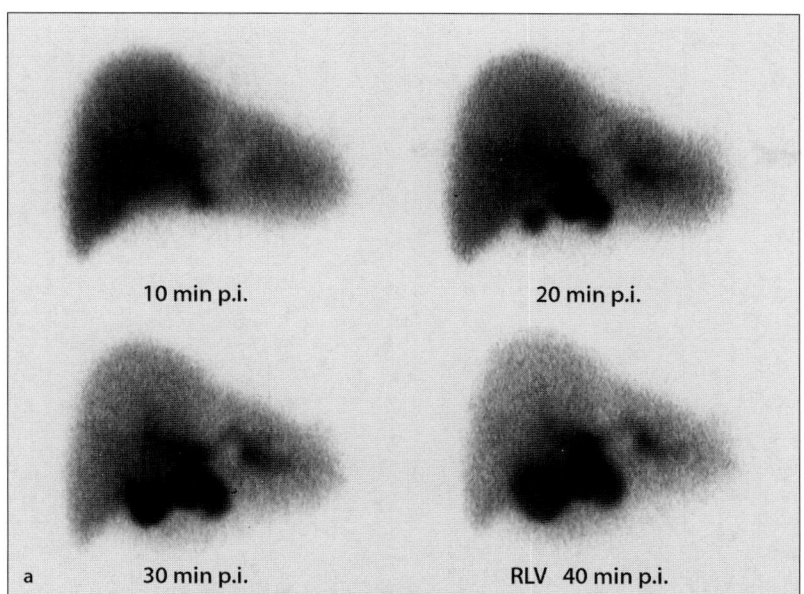

10 min p.i.   20 min p.i.

30 min p.i.   RLV 40 min p.i.

a

Fig. 3.53 a,b. Avascular tumor in the left hepatic lobe produces a curvilinear impression but does not obstruct outflow from the left hepatic duct

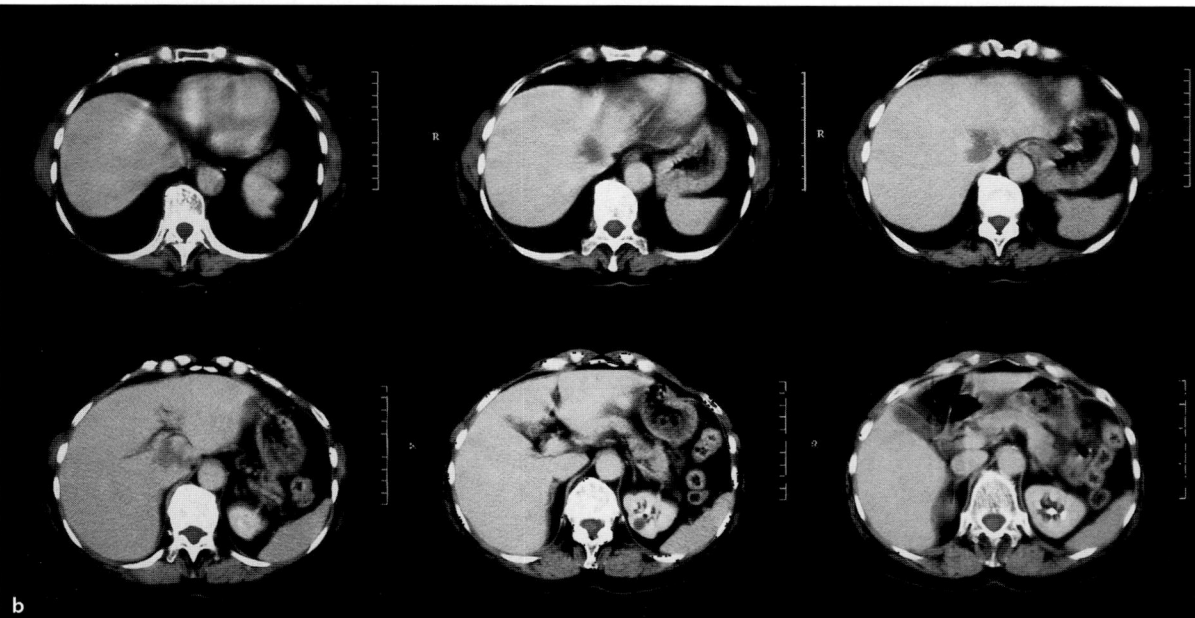

b

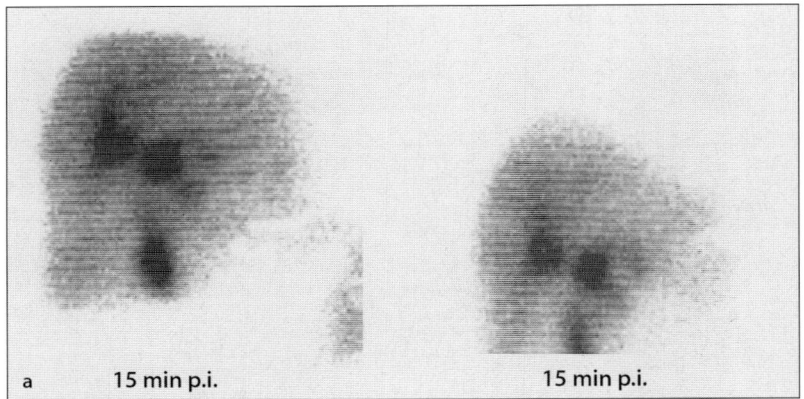

a   15 min p.i.   15 min p.i.

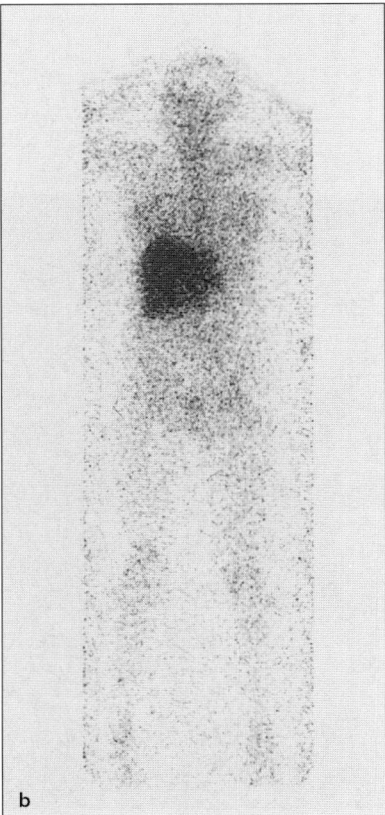

b

Fig. 3.54 a,b. This woman presented with unexplained epigastric complaints that were most pronounced after a full meal. Hepatobiliary function scan shows two well-defined bile-filled structures in the course of the right hepatic duct and at the junction of the right and left hepatic ducts. These structures, which do not take up ^{67}Ga, are bile duct cysts

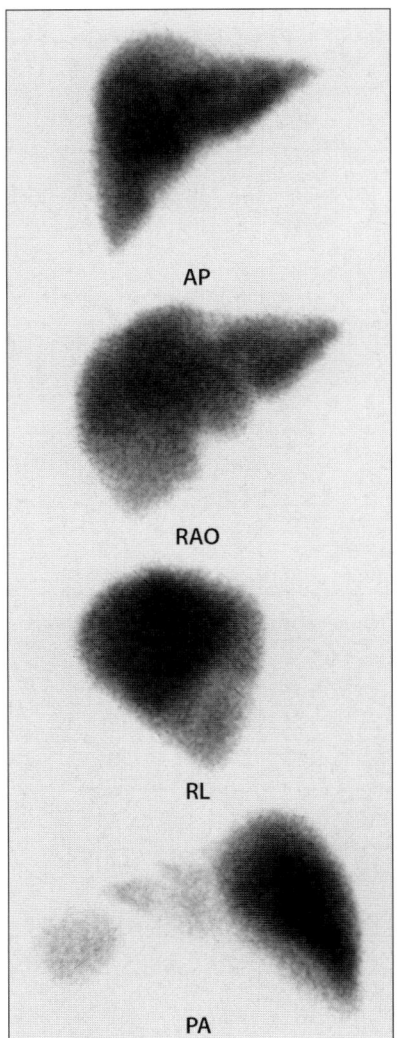

AP

RAO

RL

PA

Fig. 3.55. Normal-size spleen located in a normal position

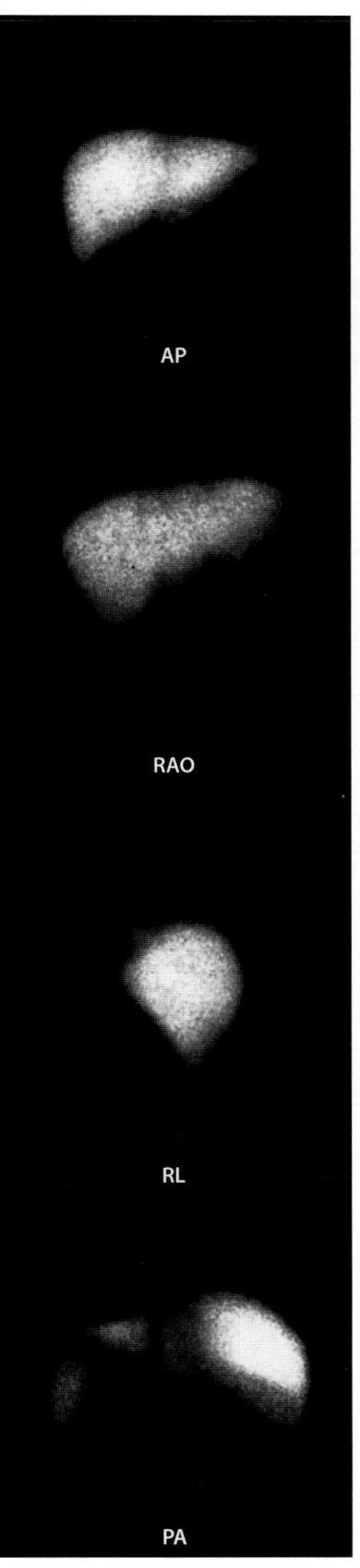

AP

RAO

RL

PA

Fig. 3.56. Patient with known chronic hepatitis was evaluated for portal hypertension. The scan shows a normal-appearing spleen with nonhomogeneous tracer uptake in the liver

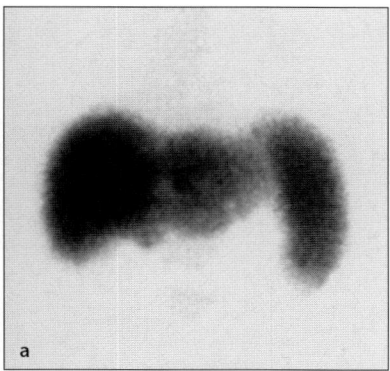

a

Fig. 3.57 a,b. Patient with known chronic hepatitis was evaluated for incipient portal hypertension. The scan shows a large left hepatic lobe, moderate splenomegaly, and an initial reversal of hepatic blood flow consistent with incipient portal hypertension

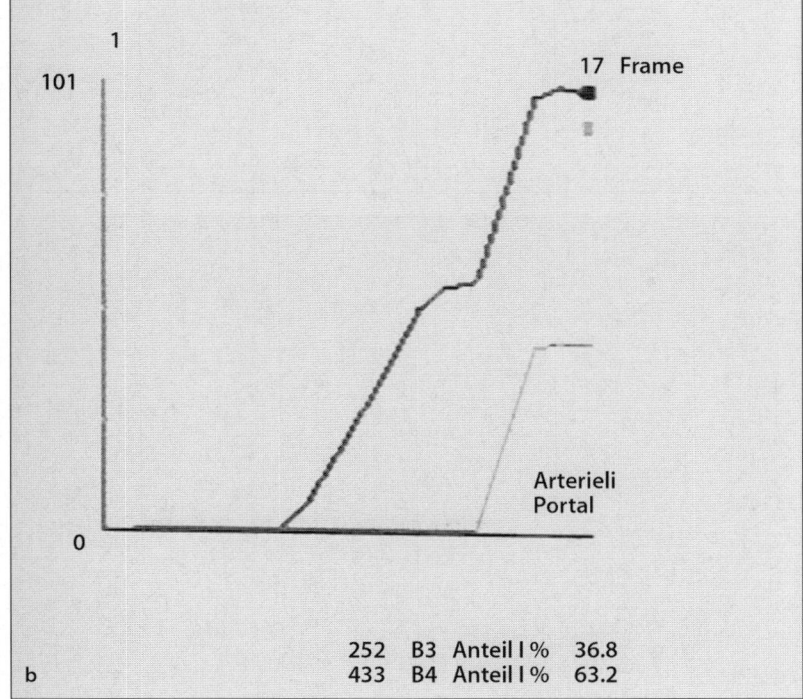

b

252	B3	Anteil l %	36.8
433	B4	Anteil l %	63.2

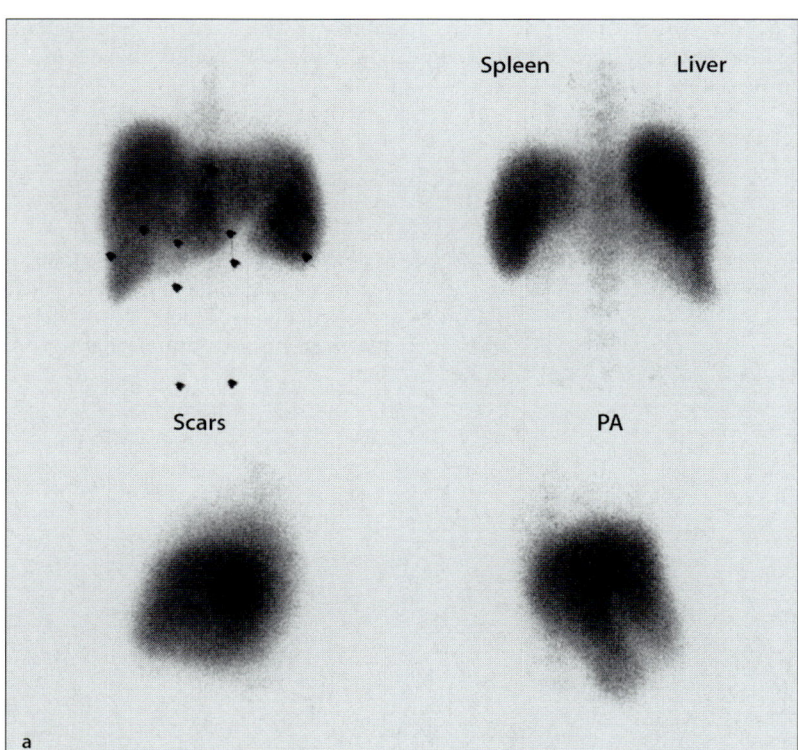

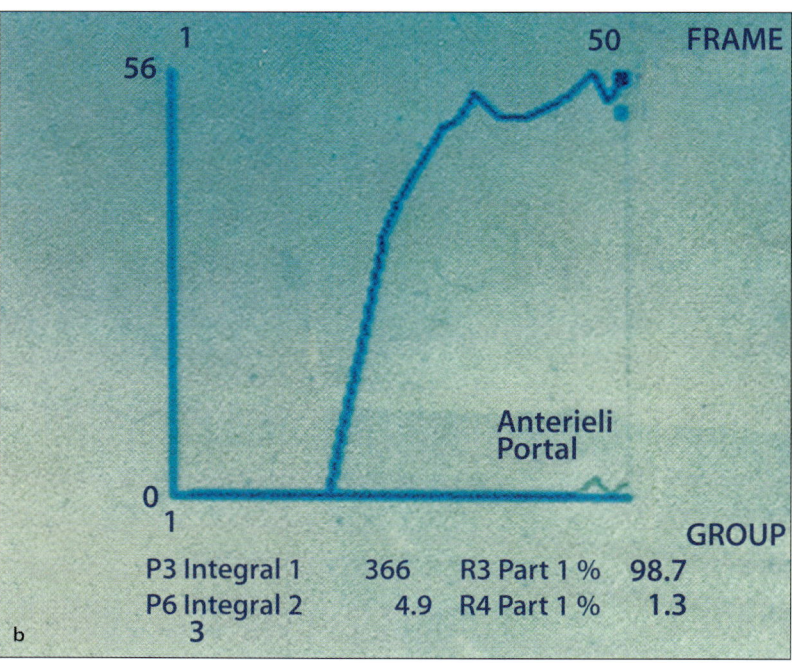

Fig. 3.58 a,b. Patient with a fatty, cirrhotic liver was evaluated for portal hypertension. The scan shows marked hepatosplenomegaly and a reversal of hepatic blood flow indicating significant portal hypertension

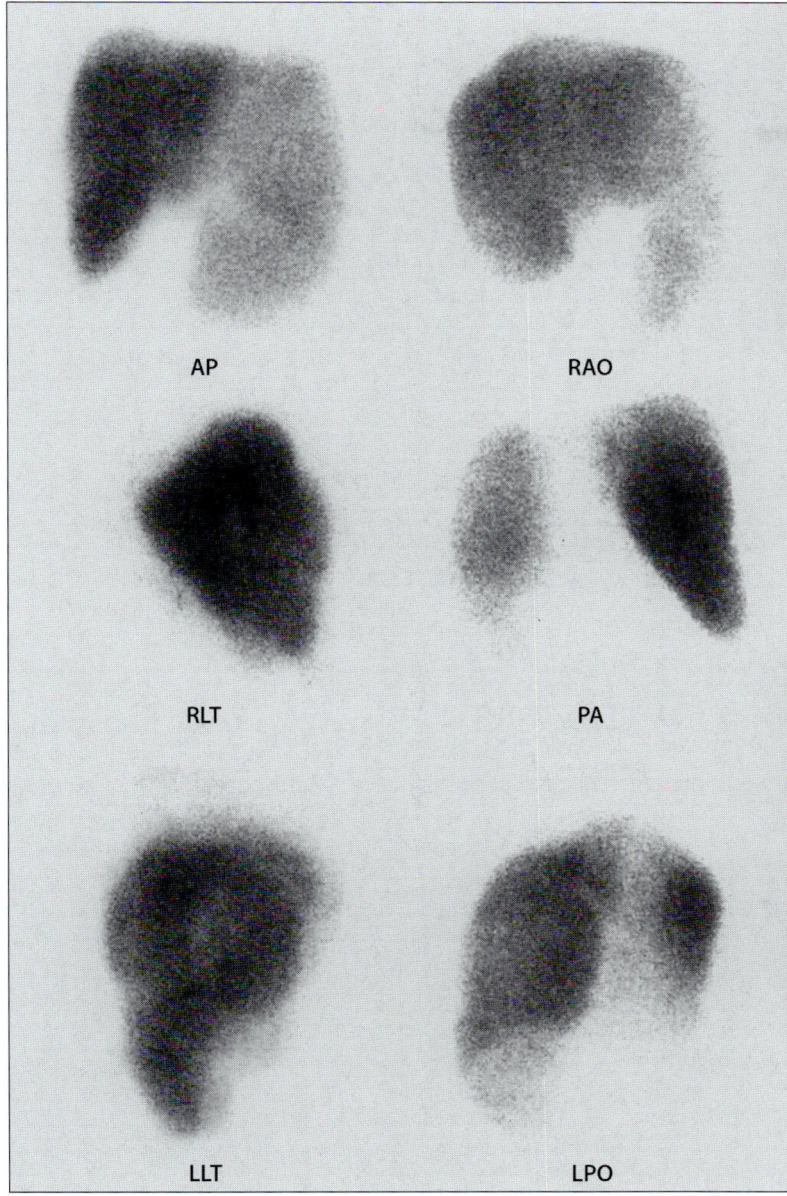

AP

RAO

RLT

PA

LLT

LPO

Fig. 3.59. Hepatosplenomegaly in osteomyelosclerosis

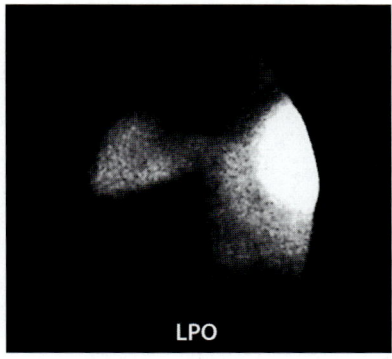

LPO

Fig. 3.60. This patient reported sudden, excruciating pain in the lower left hemithorax, but he was free of complaints on admission. Scan shows a wedge-shaped cold defect in the upper pole of the spleen. Splenic infarction

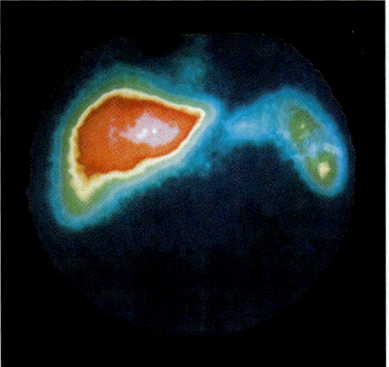

Fig. 3.61. Young patient presented with low-grade fever and dull pain in the left upper chest radiating to the back. Scan shows a small cold-to-photopenic defect in the central portion of the spleen. Splenic abscess

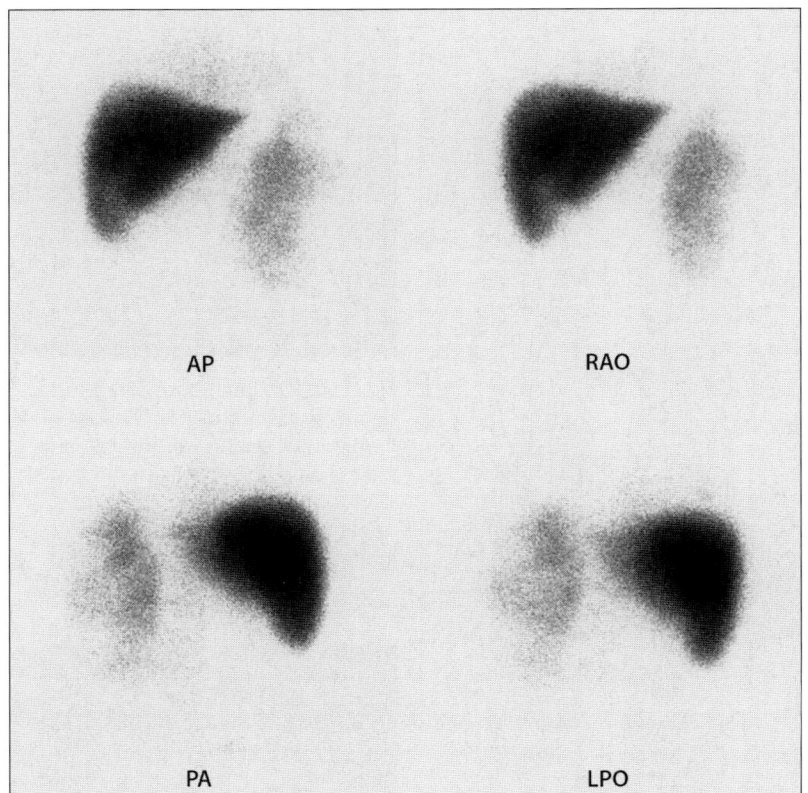

Fig. 3.62. Patient with known poly-cythemia vera presented with splenomegaly after prior embolization of the splenic artery. Follow-up scan shows considerable residual splenic parenchyma, indicating a moderately successful embolization

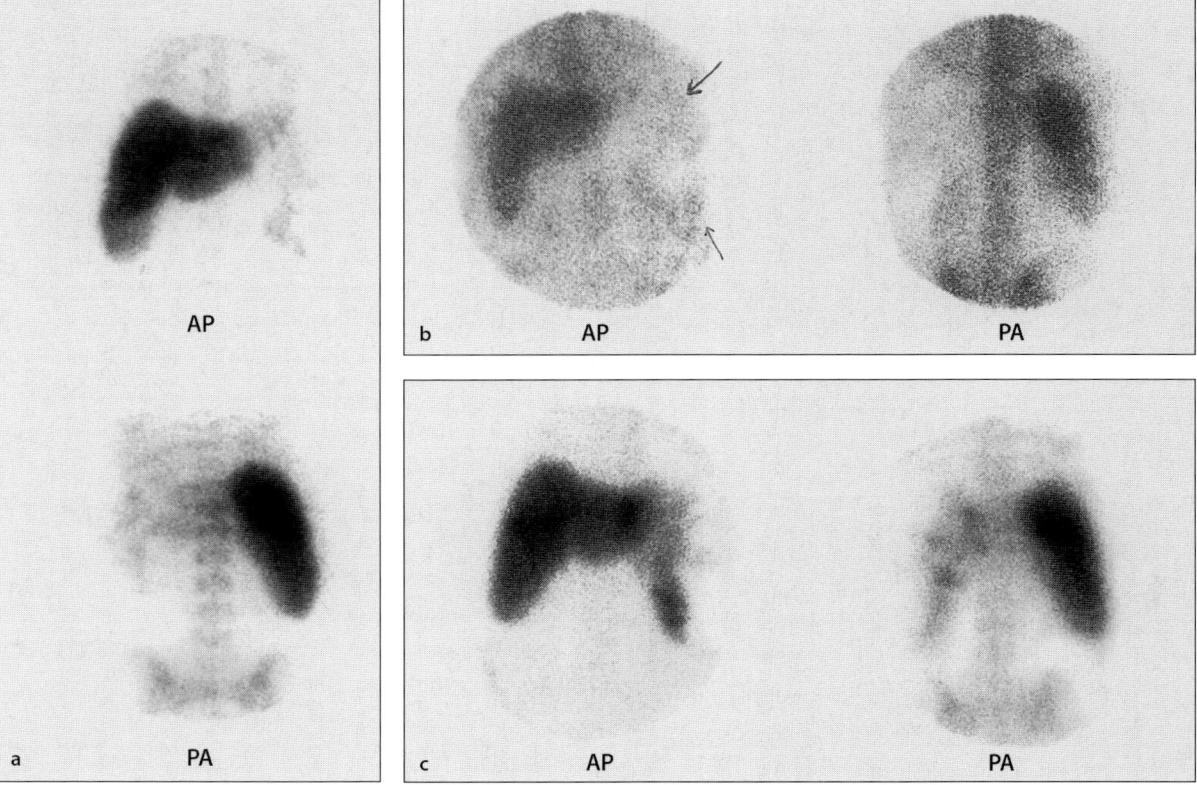

Fig. 3.63 a–d. Status post embolization of the splenic artery. **a** Embolization produced an excellent initial result. **b** Follow-up at approximately three weeks still indicates a successful procedure. **c** Follow-up at 34 days shows incipient recanalization. **d** Perfusion scan at 46 days demonstrates blood flow to a small island of splenic tissue in the inferomedial part of the spleen

Fig. 3.63 d

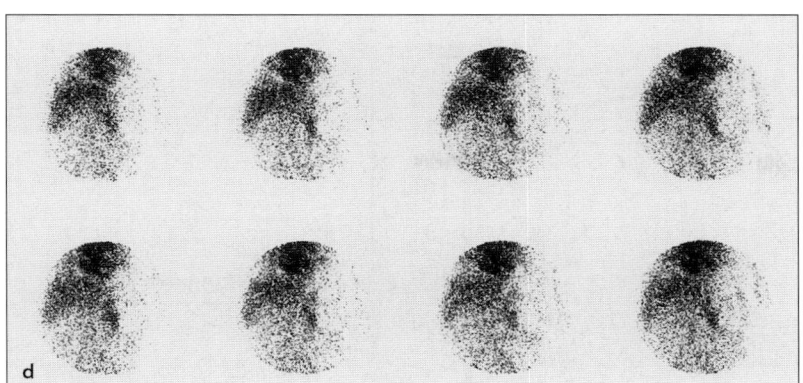

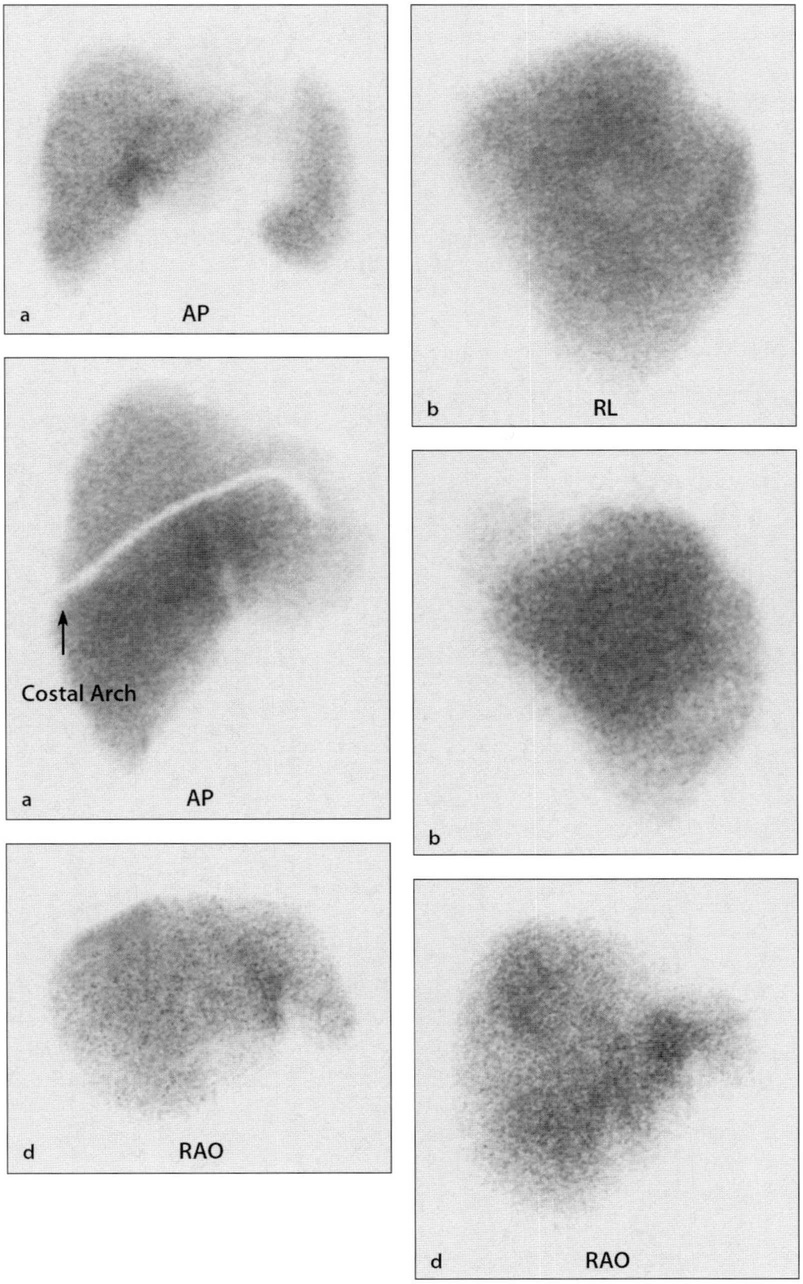

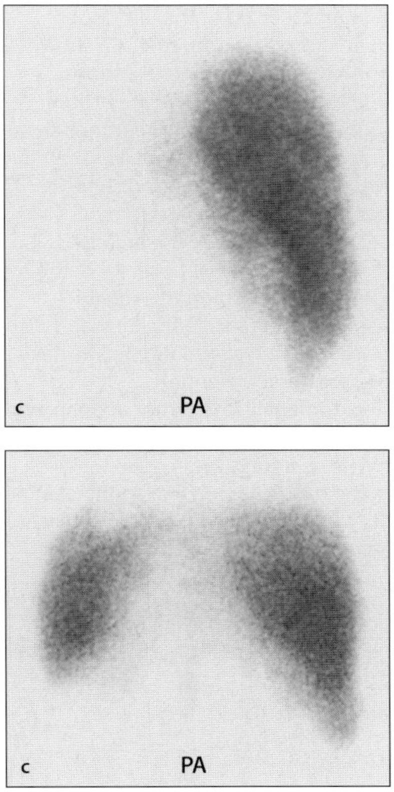

a   AP

b   RL

c   PA

a   AP

Costal Arch

b

c   PA

d   RAO

d   RAO

Fig. 3.64 a–d. Follow-up scans at one year (*a1–d1*) and three years (*a2–d2*) after splenic vein thrombosis indicate a proliferative syndrome

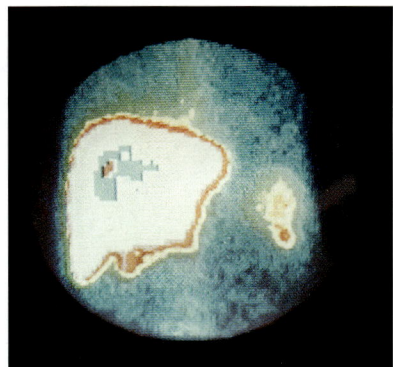

Fig. 3.65. A 66-year-old man was hospitalized for investigation of a clinically palpable mass in the left upper quadrant of the abdomen. CT showed a 15-cm tumor apparently arising from the tail of the pancreas. Ultrasound suggested that the tumor arose from the spleen. Radionuclide scan with respiratory triggering shows a nonhomogeneous pattern of decreased uptake in the enlarged medial and superior portions of the spleen. In this region the spleen appears to extend to the liver and displace it. Relatively good tracer uptake is seen in the lower pole. Hepatomegaly. The tumor appears to originate from the spleen. A splenic tumor weighing 2 kg and extending to the gastric lumen was found at surgery. It was identified histologically as hemangiopericytoma

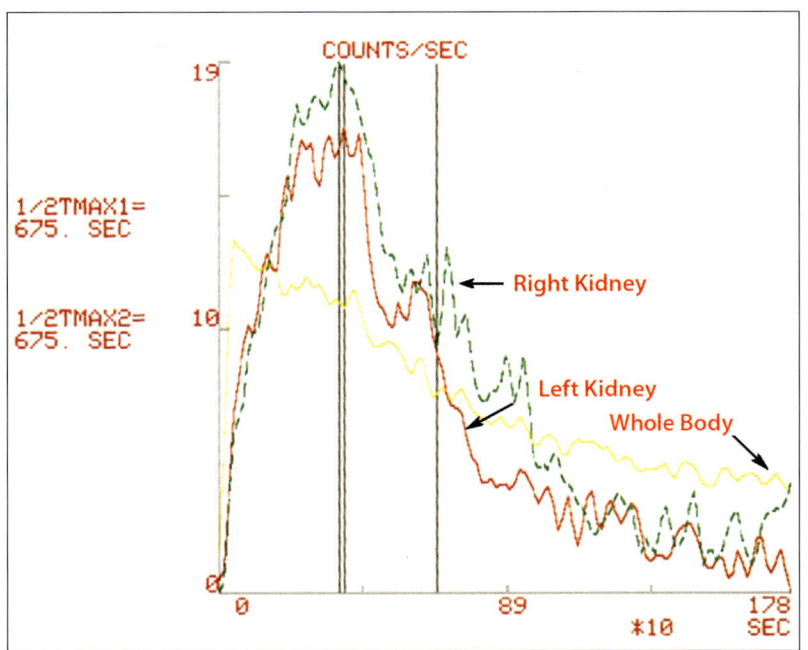

Fig. 3.66. T_{max} and $T_{1/2}$ in this renogram are within normal limits. There is no sign of parenchymal damage or outflow obstruction

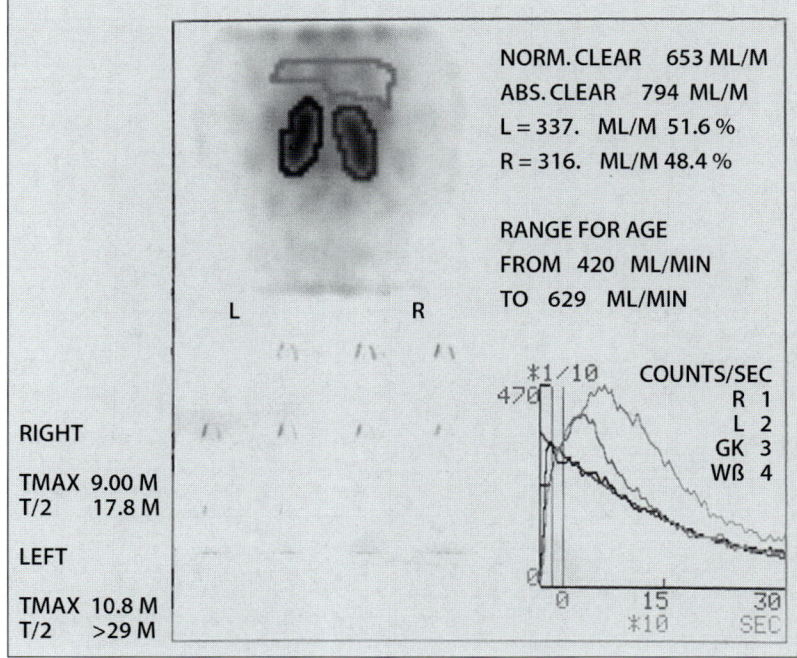

Fig. 3.67. The $T_{1/2}$ in the left kidney is slightly prolonged, indicating a prolonged intrarenal transit time

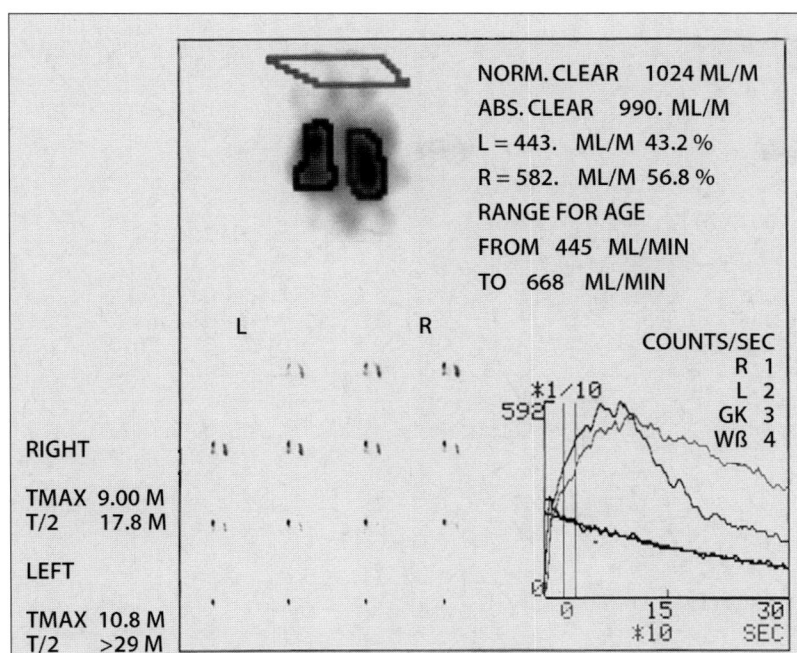

Fig. 3.68. Both the right and left renograms indicate a prolonged intrarenal transit time

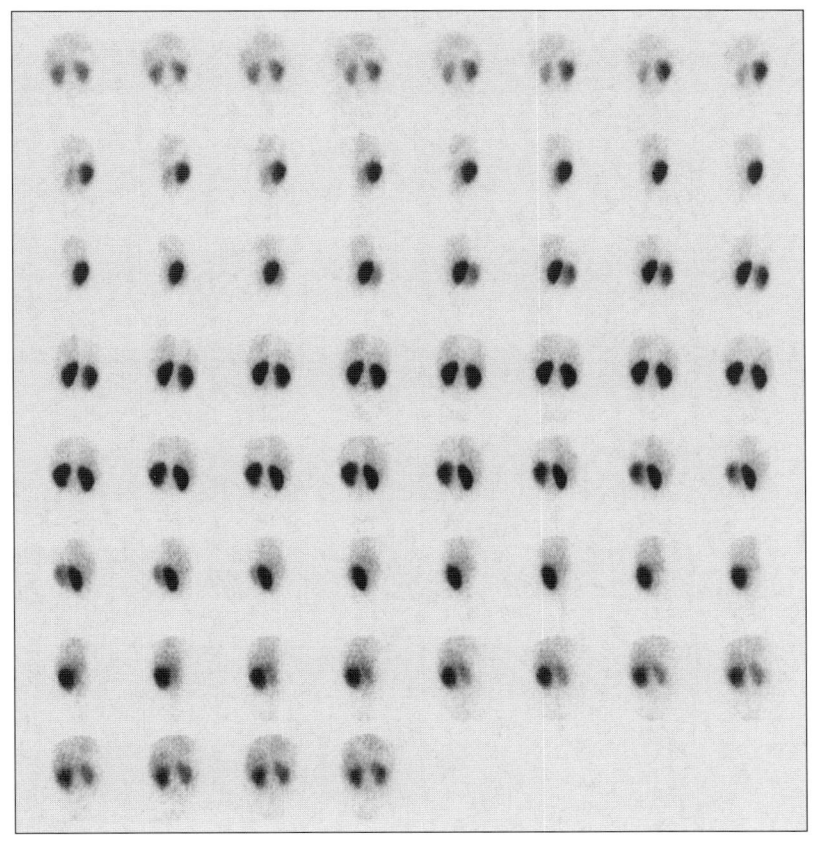

Fig. 3.69. SPECT renal image demonstrates a mass lesion in the right kidney that was not appreciated in the static view

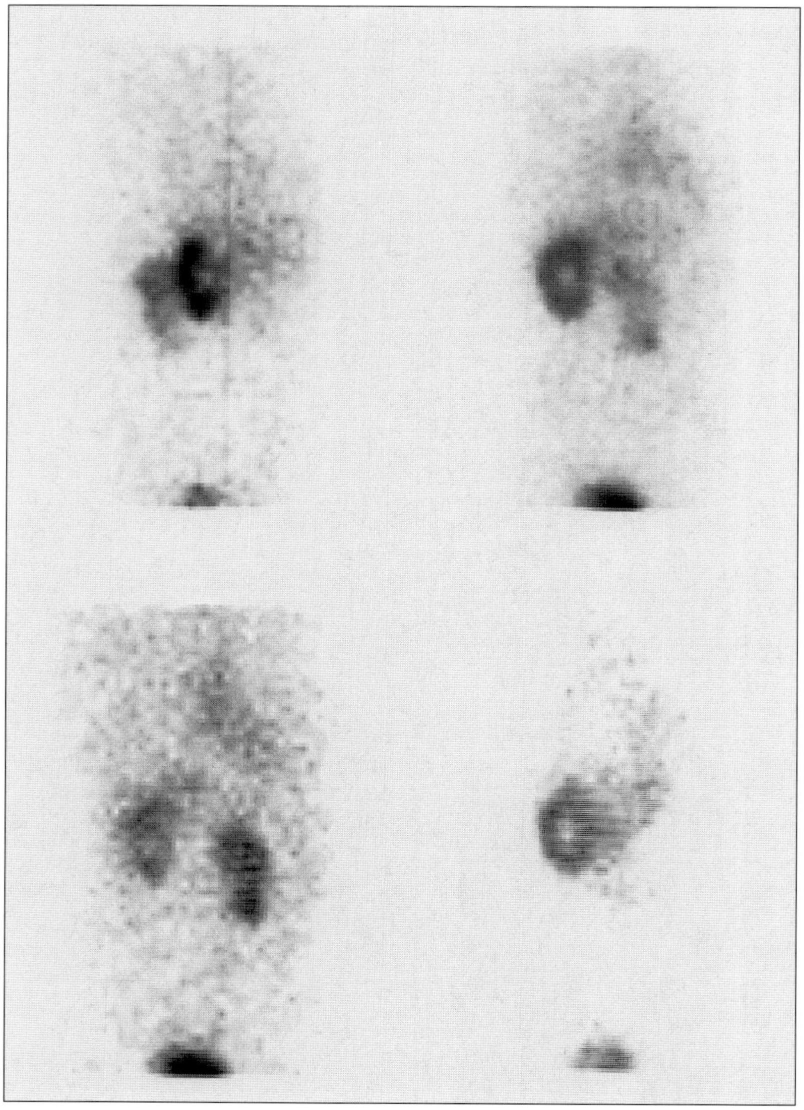

Fig. 3.69. SPECT renal image demonstrates a mass lesion in the right kidney that was not appreciated in the static view

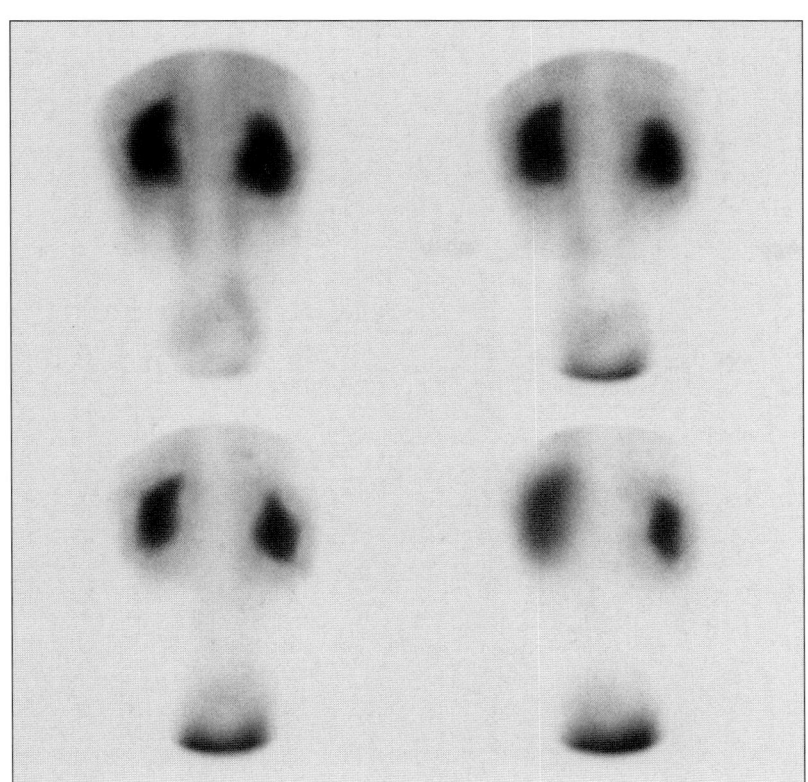

Fig. 3.70. Static summation images from a renal series show normal-appearing, normally positioned kidneys with no sign of a mass lesion or outflow obstruction

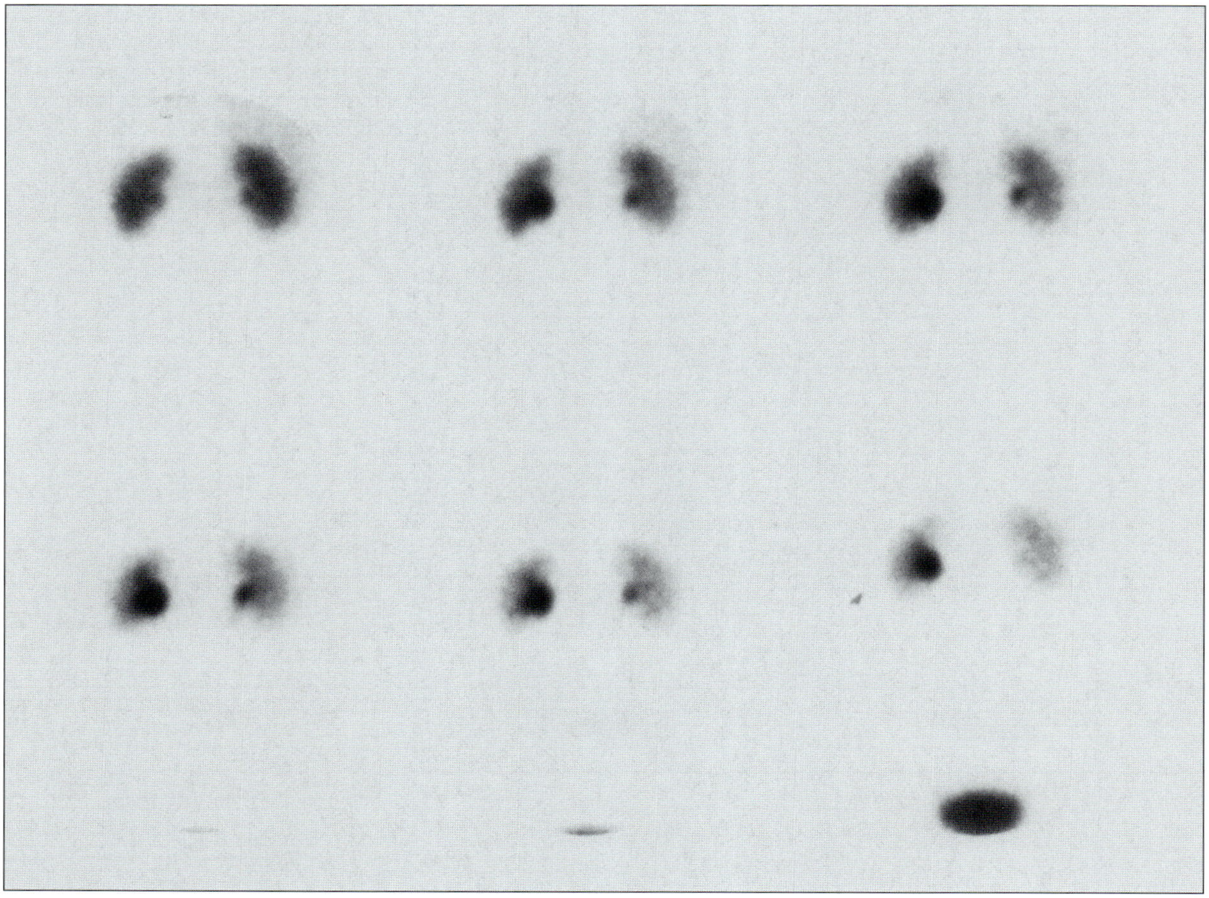

Fig. 3.71. Normally positioned, smooth-bordered kidneys with prolonged retention of the radiotracer in the right renal pelvis. An ampullary pelvis is the most likely cause

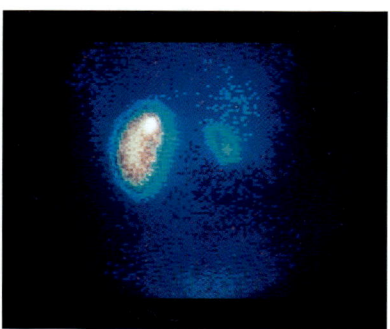

Fig. 3.72. Static renal images show a very small left kidney with smooth contours, probably a congenital variant. The presence of clinical symptoms would warrant further investigation. The right kidney is relatively large and also has smooth contours. Both kidneys are normally positioned

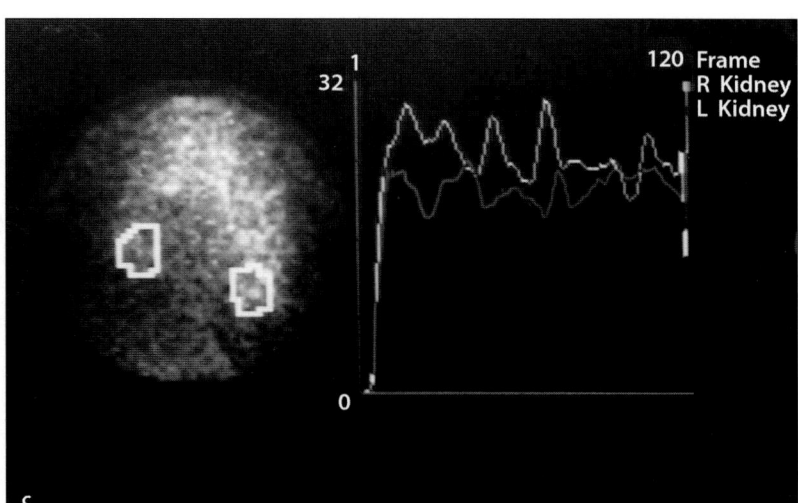

Fig. 3.76 c

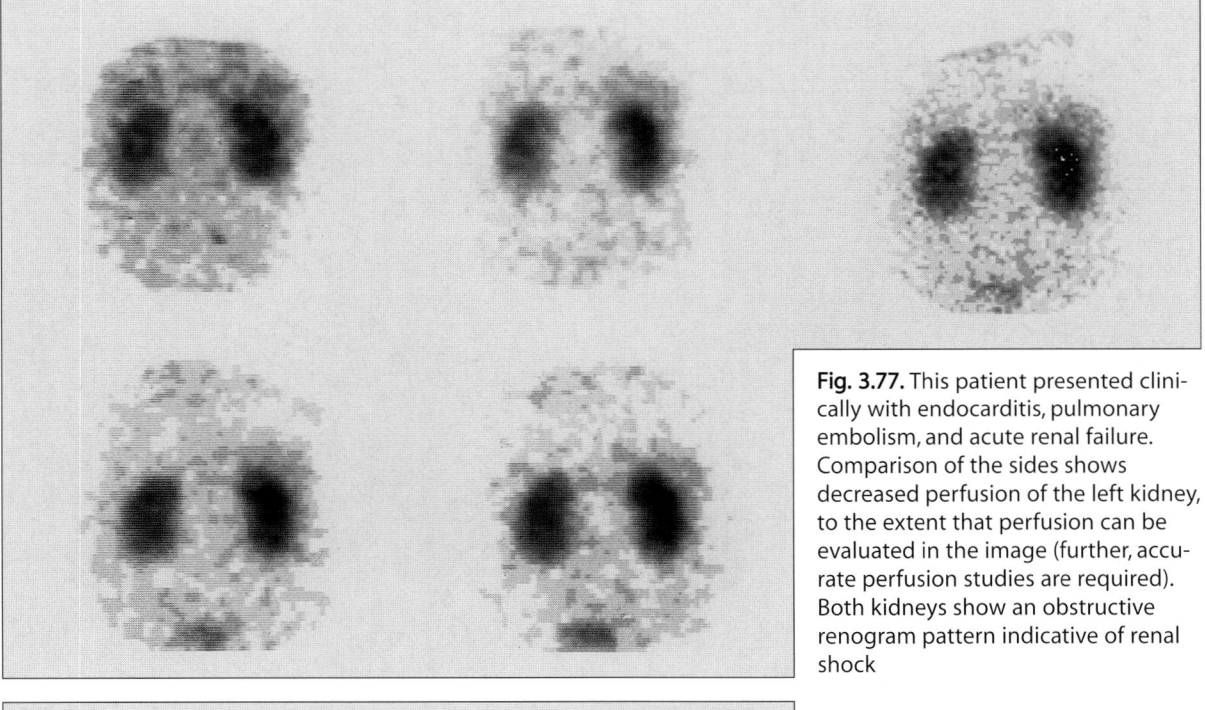

Fig. 3.77. This patient presented clinically with endocarditis, pulmonary embolism, and acute renal failure. Comparison of the sides shows decreased perfusion of the left kidney, to the extent that perfusion can be evaluated in the image (further, accurate perfusion studies are required). Both kidneys show an obstructive renogram pattern indicative of renal shock

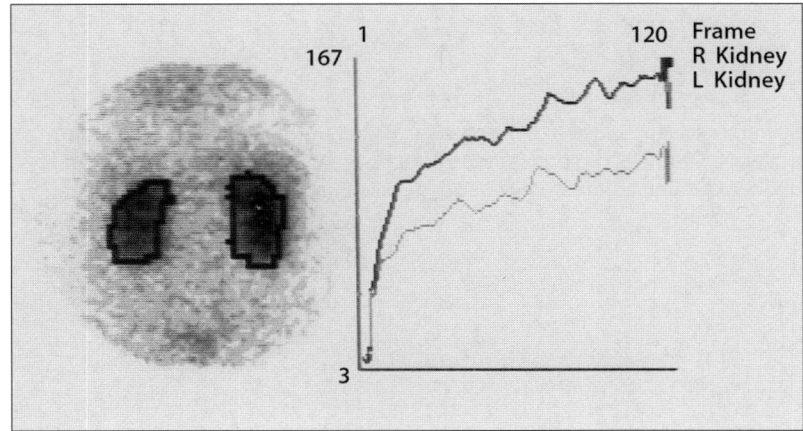

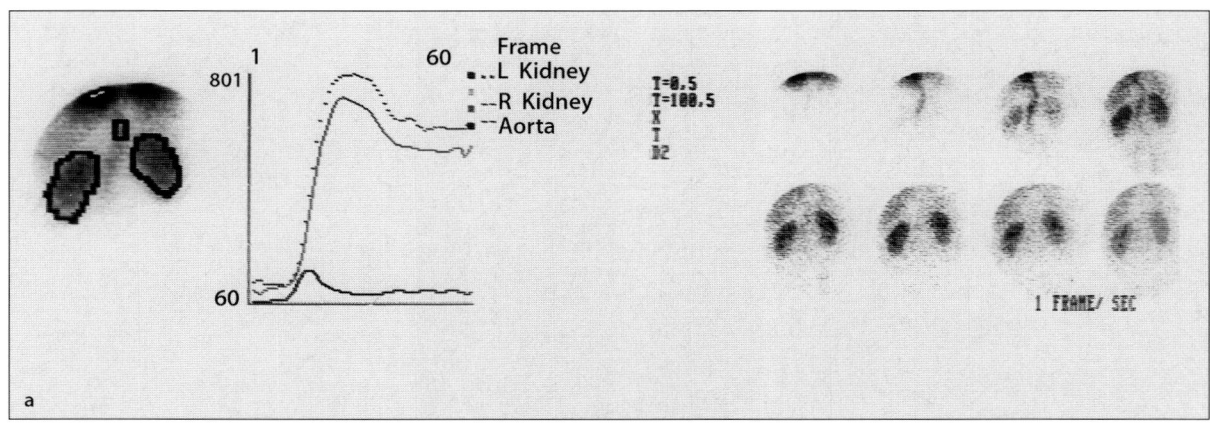

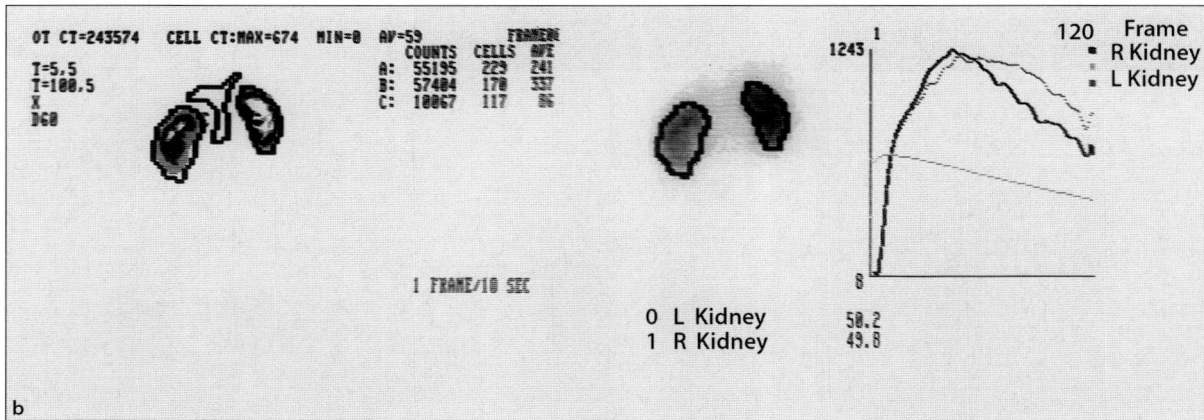

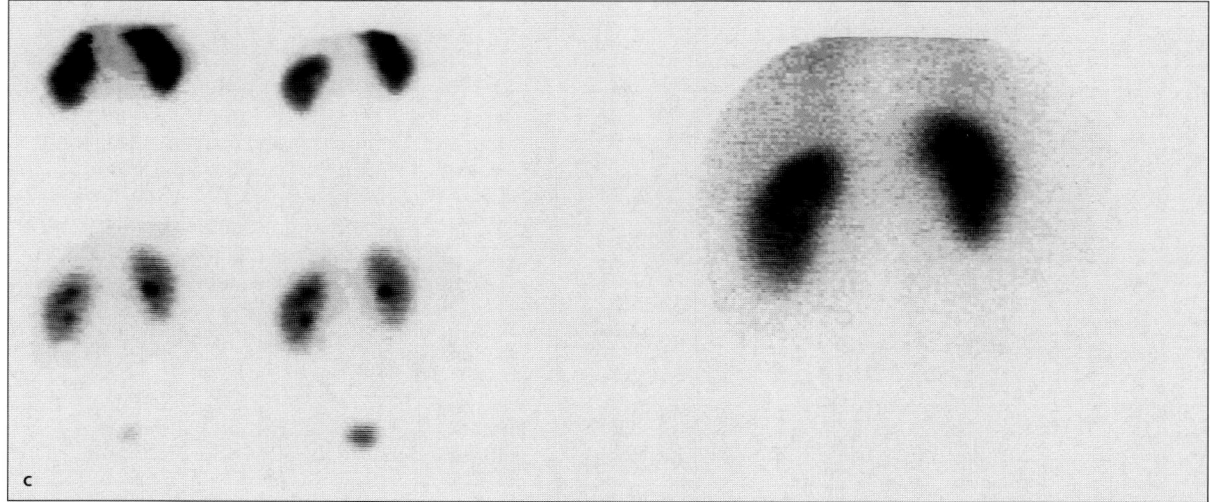

Fig. 3.78 a–c. Renal perfusion is asymmetric in this patient, but the discrepancy is within normal limits and the kidneys have approximately equal function. Intrarenal transit time is prolonged in both kidneys, which are of normal size, have smooth contours, and are normally positioned. Assuming adequate hydration, the scan findings indicate early-stage parenchymal damage

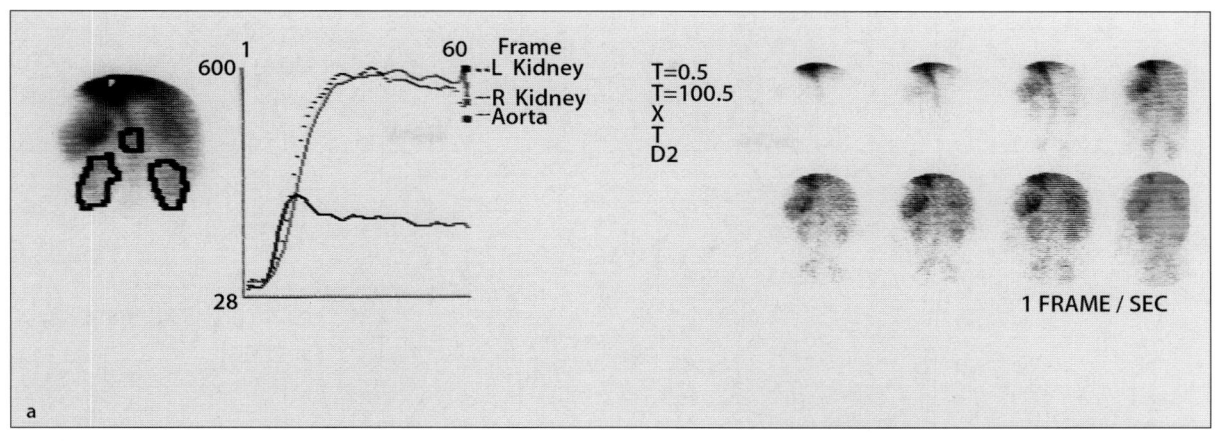

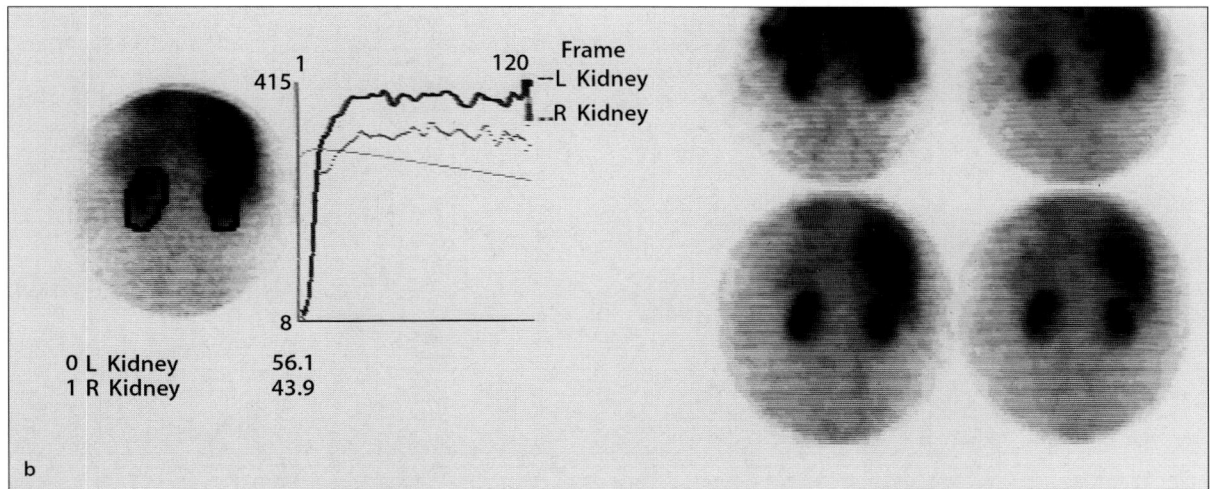

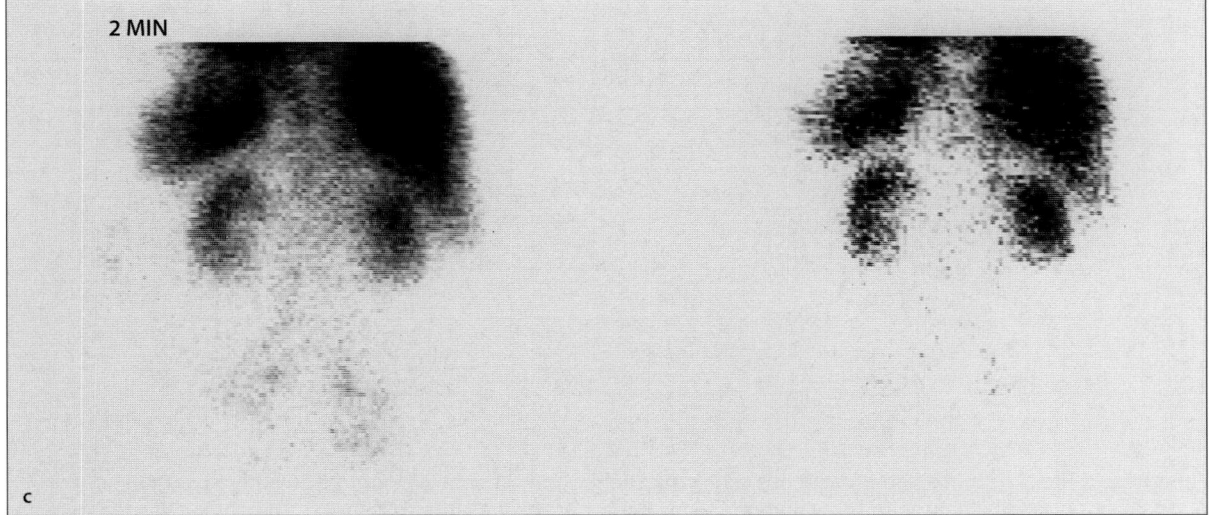

Fig. 3.79 a–c. Renal scan in a hypertensive patient shows symmetrical but slightly delayed perfusion of the small, normally positioned kidneys. There is nonhomogeneous uptake with significant functional impairment. The patient has bilateral renal failure, probably based on chronic perfusion abnormalities

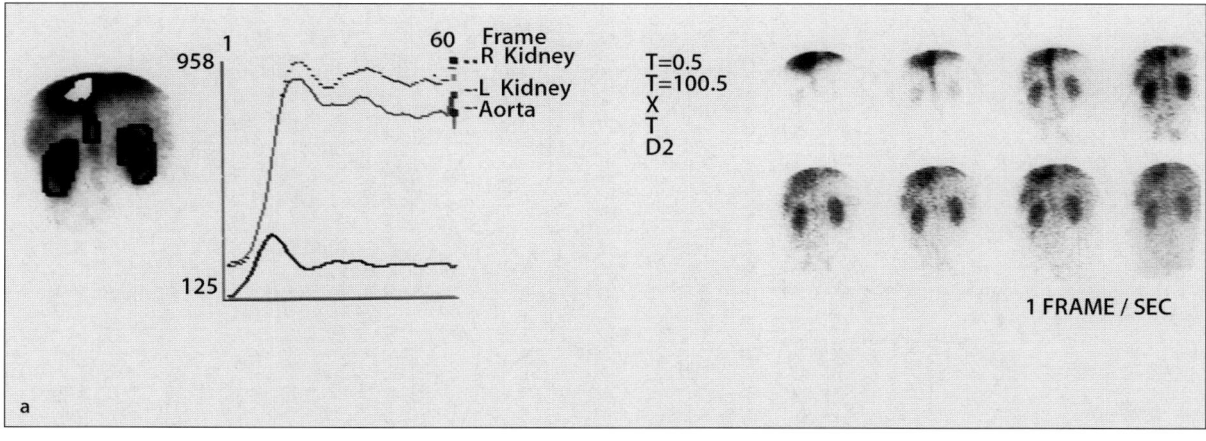

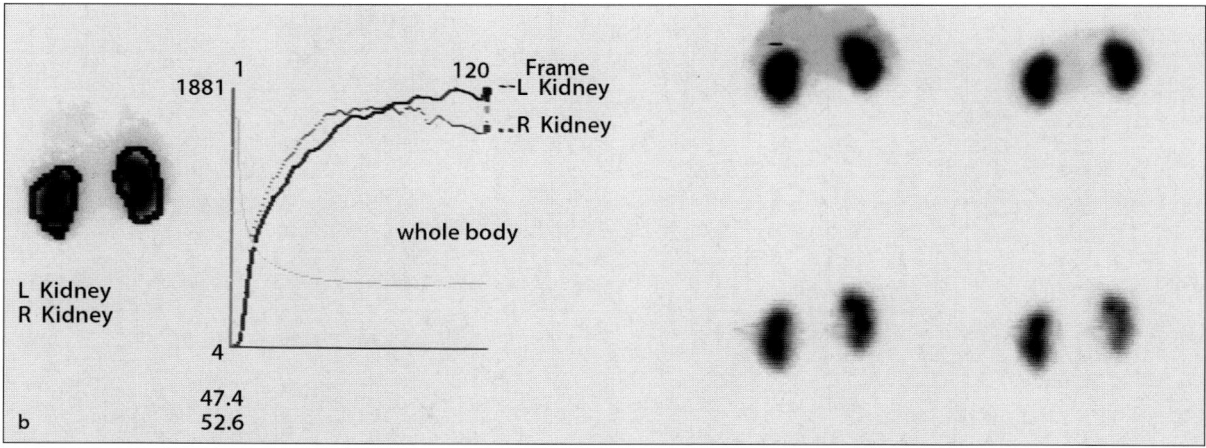

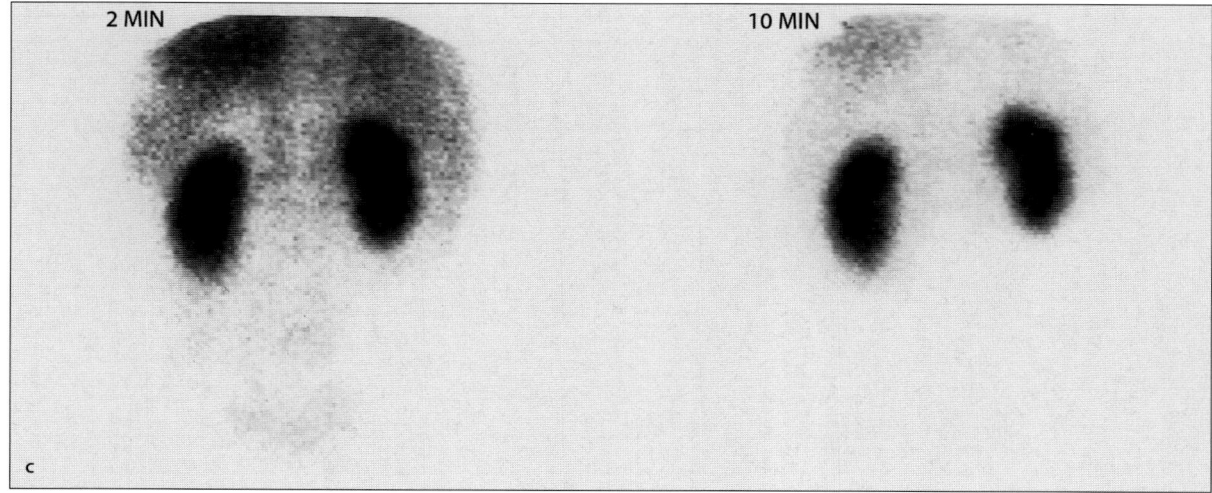

Fig. 3.80 a–c. Renal scan in a patient with posttraumatic anuria shows symmetrical perfusion and visualization of the normally positioned kidneys, with show homogeneous tracer uptake and smooth contours. The obstructive renogram pattern is indicative of renal shock

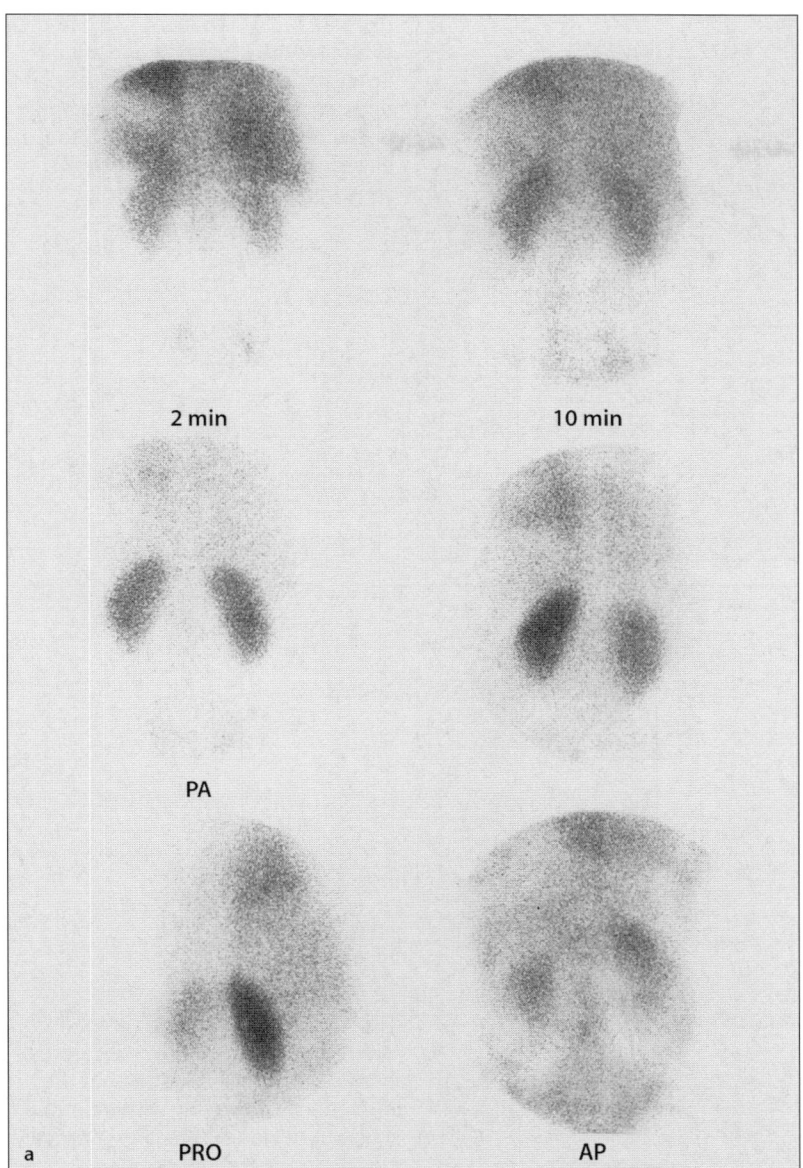

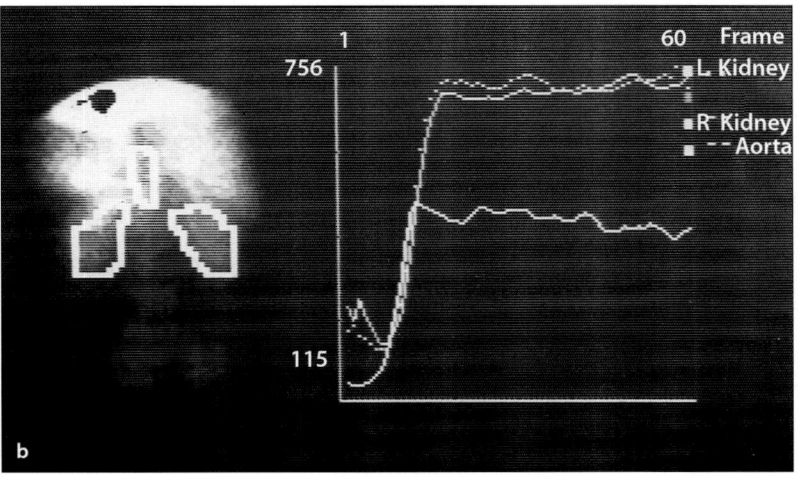

Fig. 3.81 a–c. This patient presented clinically with eclampsia and anuria. Scintigraphy shows symmetrical, delayed renal perfusion and homogeneous but decreased uptake in the enlarged kidneys. The renogram shows an obstructive pattern

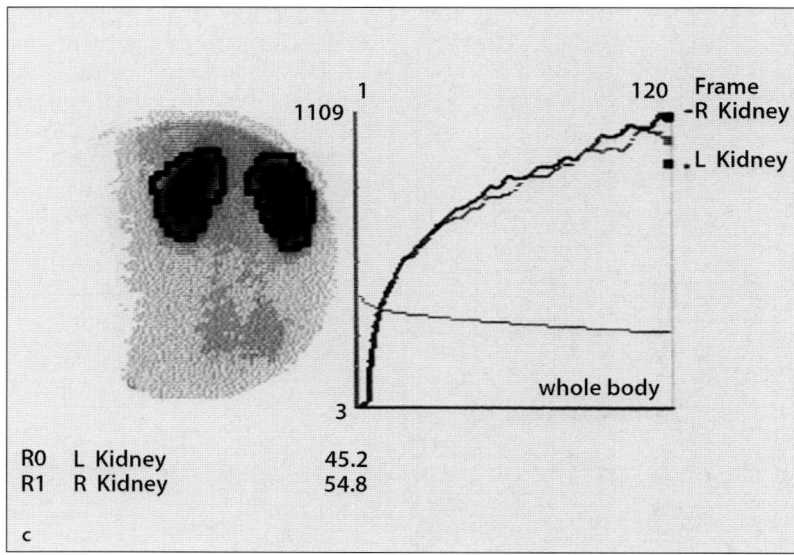

Fig. 3.81 a–c. This patient presented clinically with eclampsia and anuria. Scintigraphy shows symmetrical, delayed renal perfusion and homogeneous but decreased uptake in the enlarged kidneys. The renogram shows an obstructive pattern

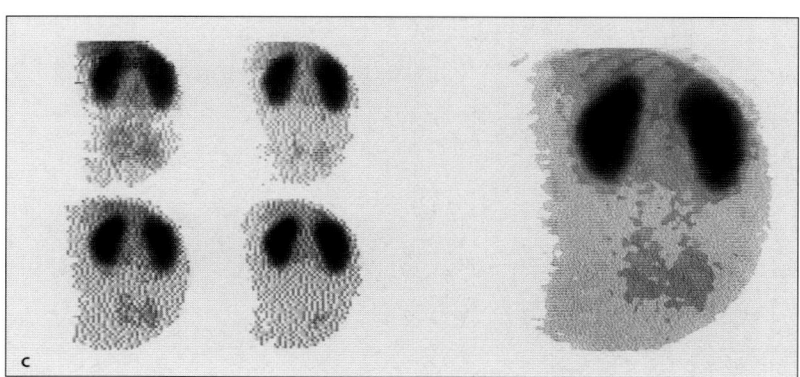

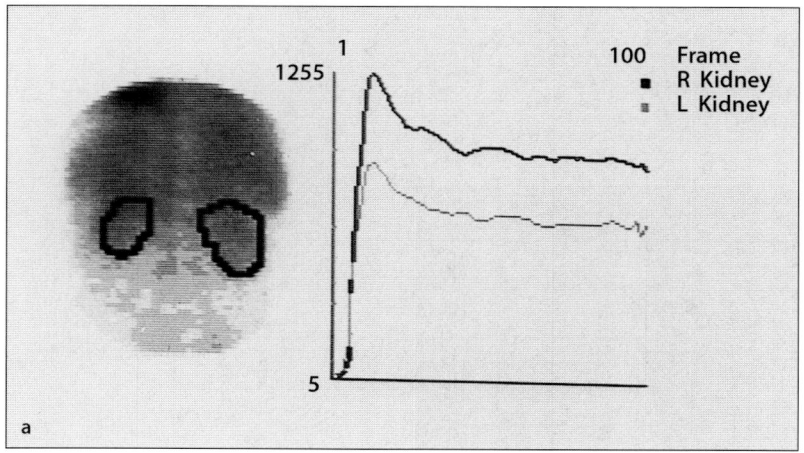

Fig. 3.82 a,b. Side-to-side comparison of the renal images shows decreased perfusion of the left kidney, but the discrepancy is roughly within normal limits. Both kidneys are large, normally positioned, and show decreased, homogeneous uptake. Renogram shows an obstructive pattern. The clinical presentation suggests toxicity-related changes

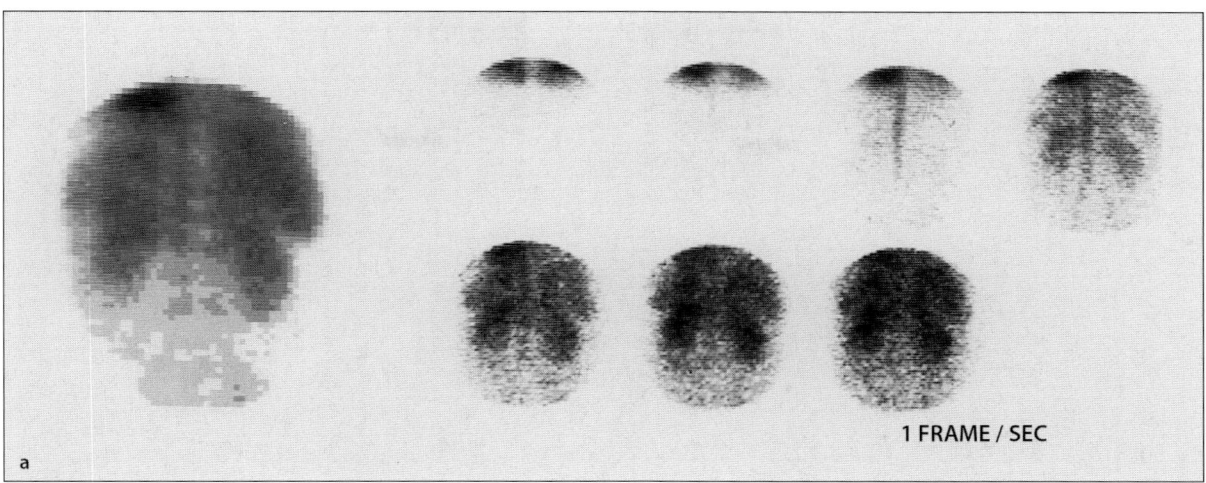

1 FRAME / SEC

Fig. 3.82 a. *Continued*

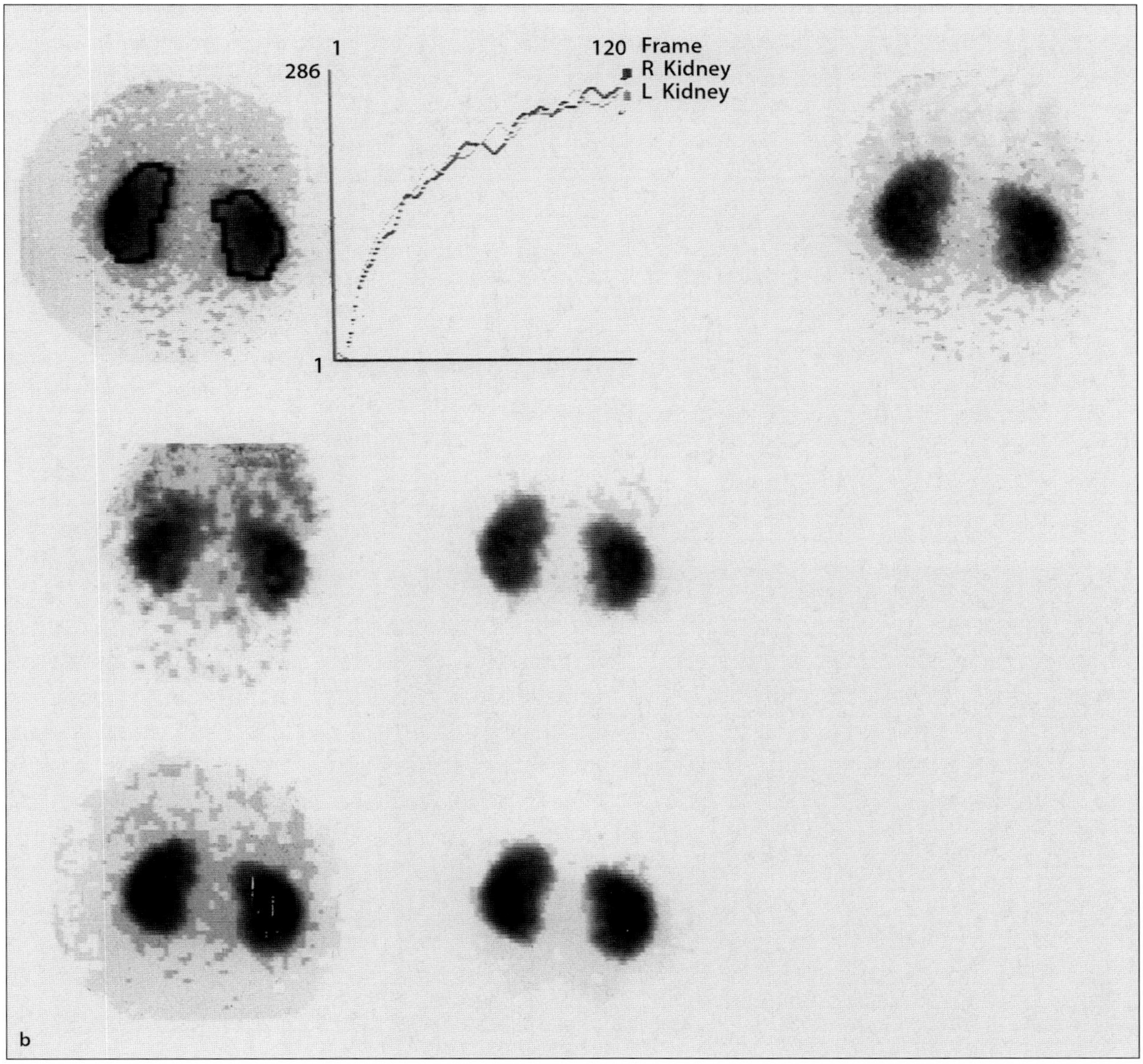

Fig. 3.82 b

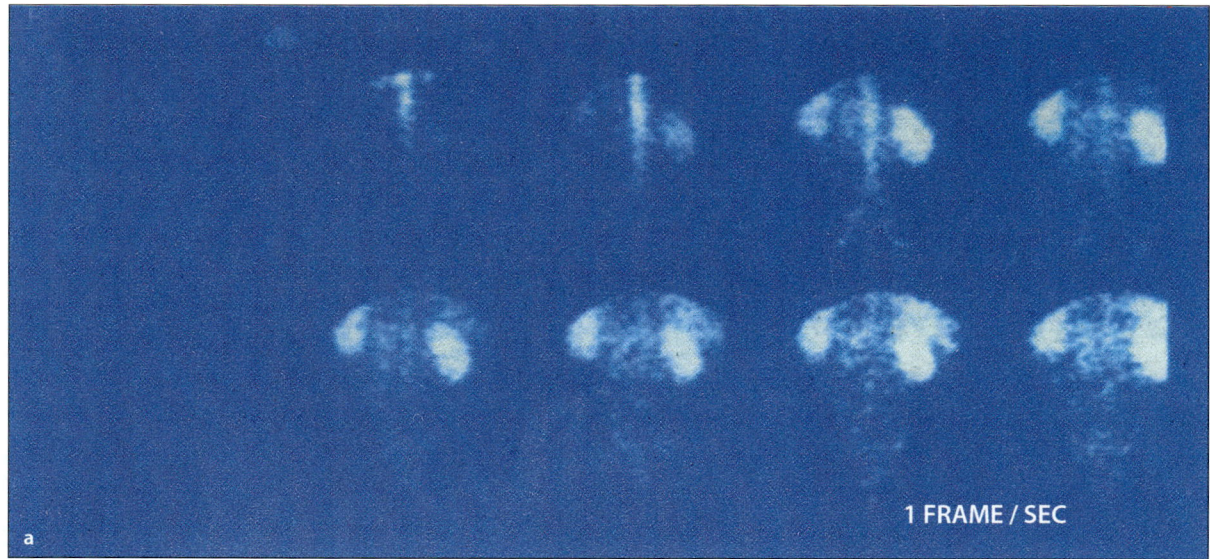

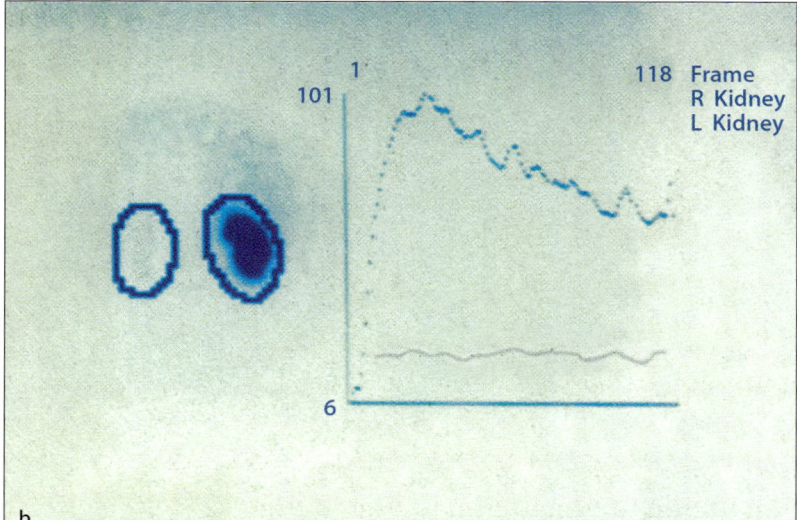

Fig. 3.83 a–c. Acute abdomen with predominantly left-sided pain of sudden onset. Renal scan shows absence of perfusion and nonvisualization of the left kidney. Ultrasound demonstrated a left kidney of normal size. The right kidney shows good excretory function with a slight delay in $T_{1/2}$, probably caused by dehydration. Correlation with the ultrasound findings suggests an embolism of the left renal artery, which was confirmed by angiography

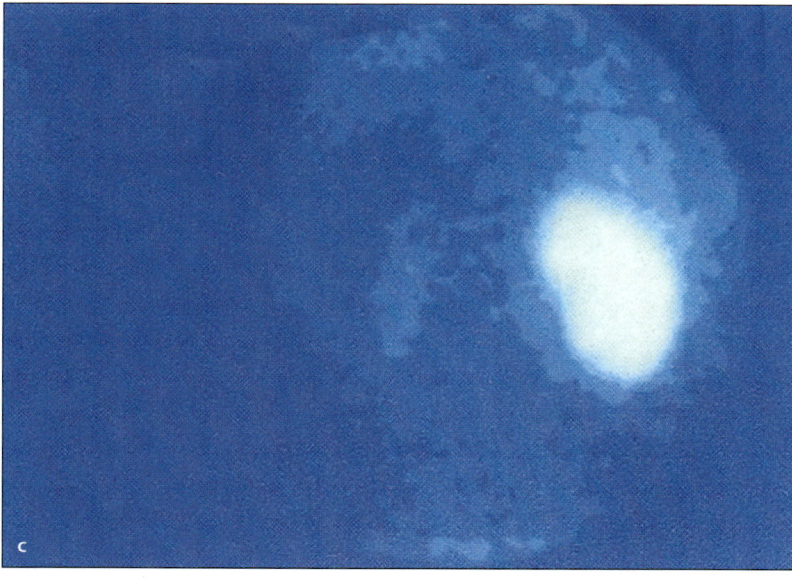

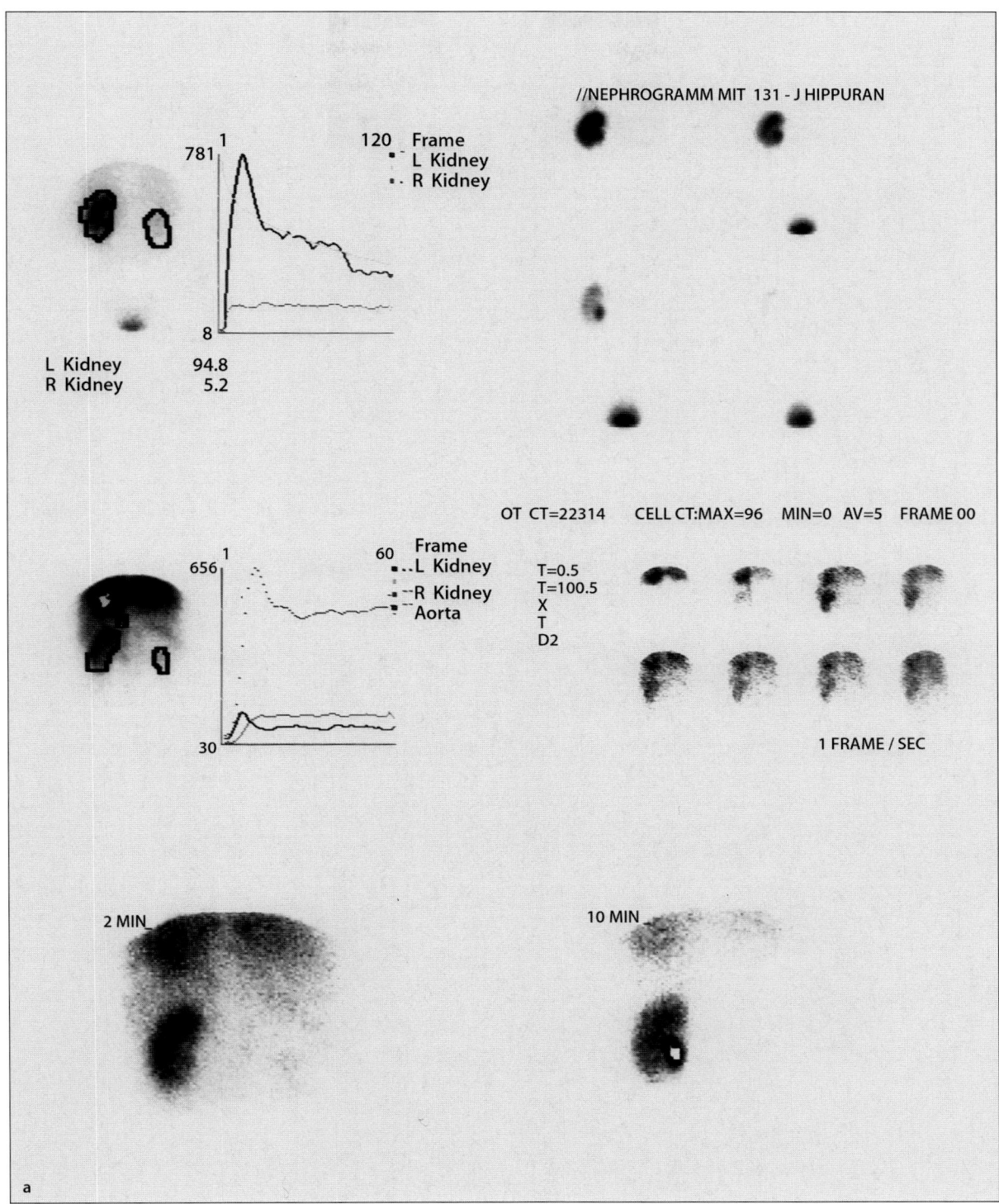

Fig. 3.84 a,b. Right-sided embolism (**a**). Follow-up during thrombolytic therapy (**b**) demonstrates initial reperfusion

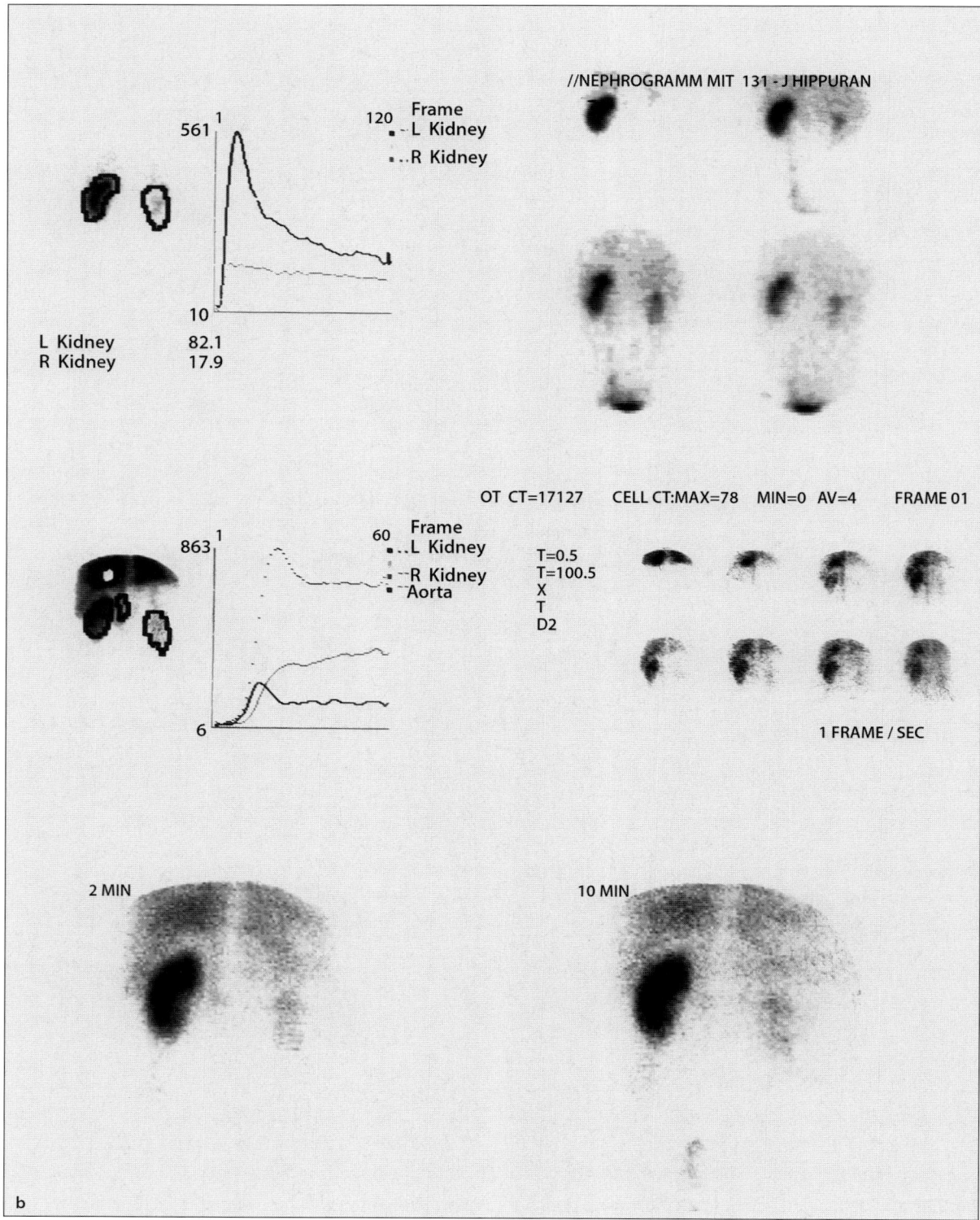

Fig. 3.84 a,b. Right-sided embolism (**a**). Follow-up during thrombolytic therapy (**b**) demonstrates initial reperfusion

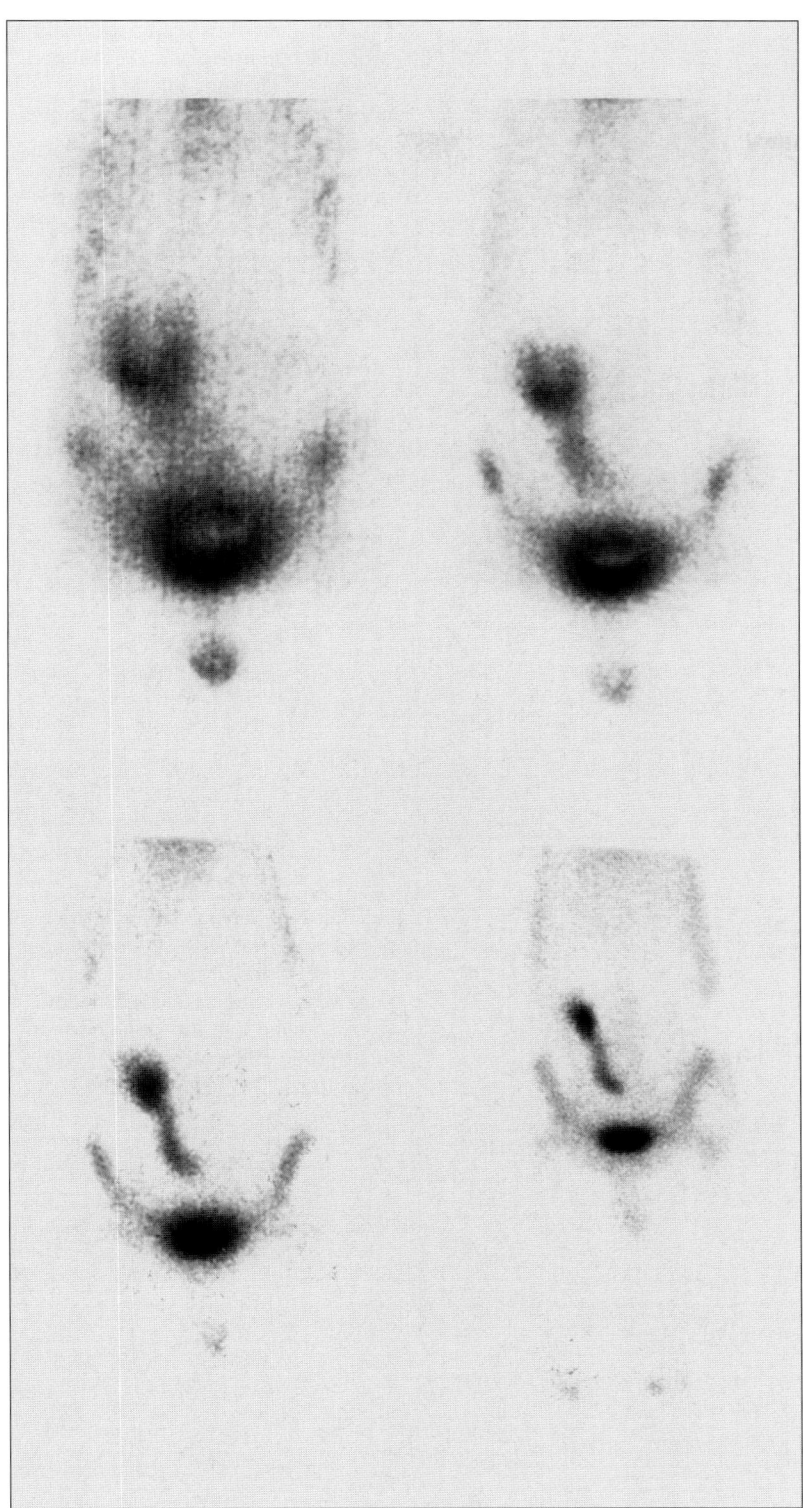

Fig. 3.85. Patient with back pain and prostatic hypertrophy was evaluated for skeletal changes. Whole-body bone scan (Photon technique) shows no skeletal changes that could account for the complaints, but incidental note is made of a congested kidney with a prevesical urinary outflow obstruction. Urologic workup revealed a ureteral stone

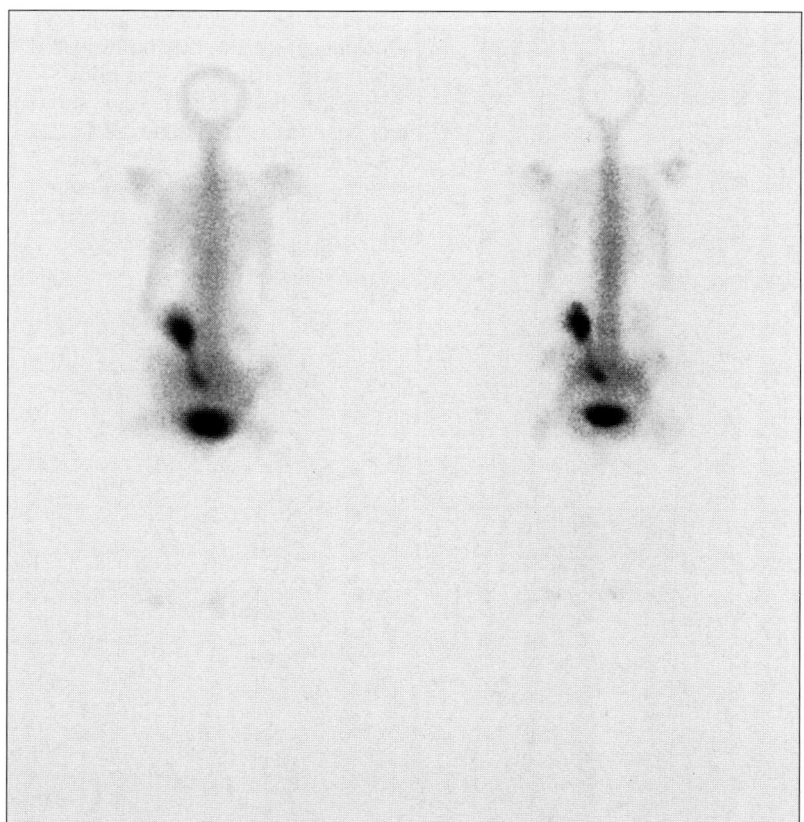

Fig. 3.85. Patient with back pain and prostatic hypertrophy was evaluated for skeletal changes. Whole-body bone scan (Photon technique) shows no skeletal changes that could account for the complaints, but incidental note is made of a congested kidney with a prevesical urinary outflow obstruction. Urologic workup revealed a ureteral stone

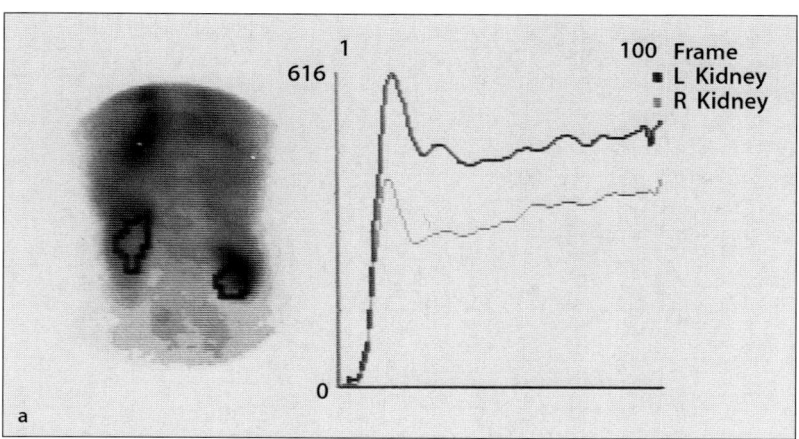

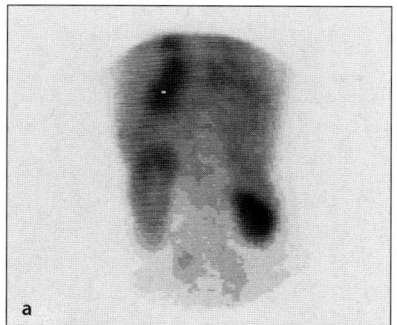

Fig. 3.86 a–c. Salvageability of the right kidney was assessed in a patient with right-sided ureteropelvic junction stenosis. Radionuclide function study showed that the kidney was still functioning efficiently and was worth salvaging

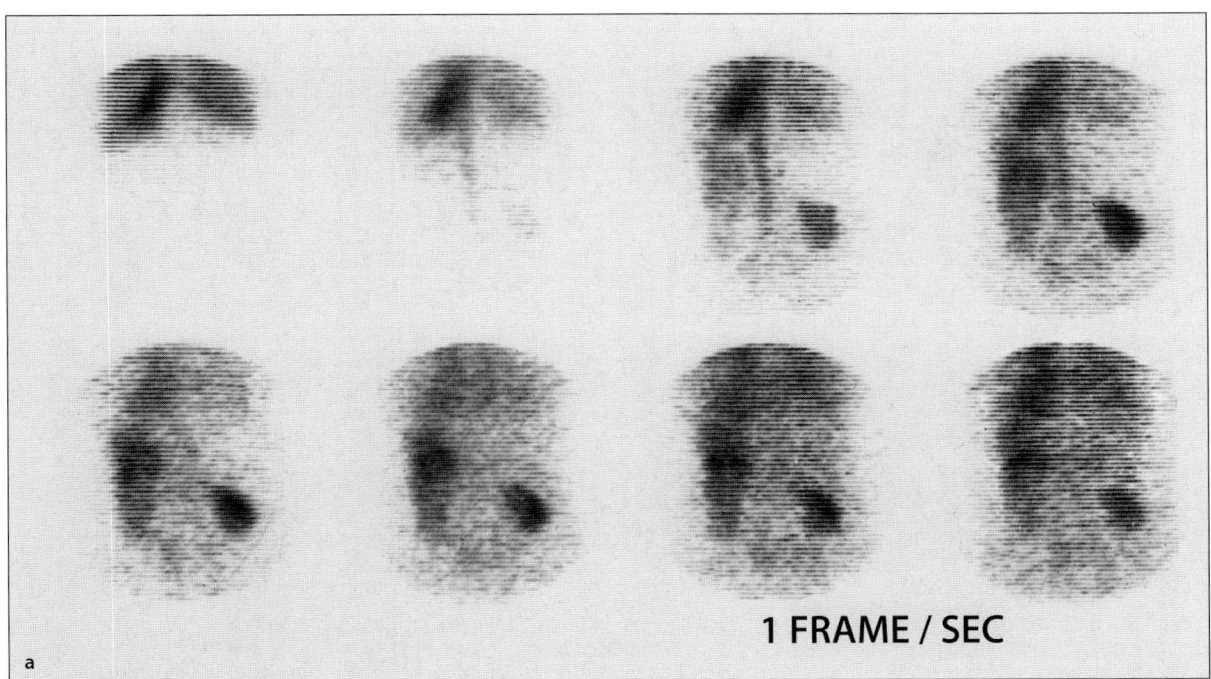

Fig. 3.86 a. *Continued*

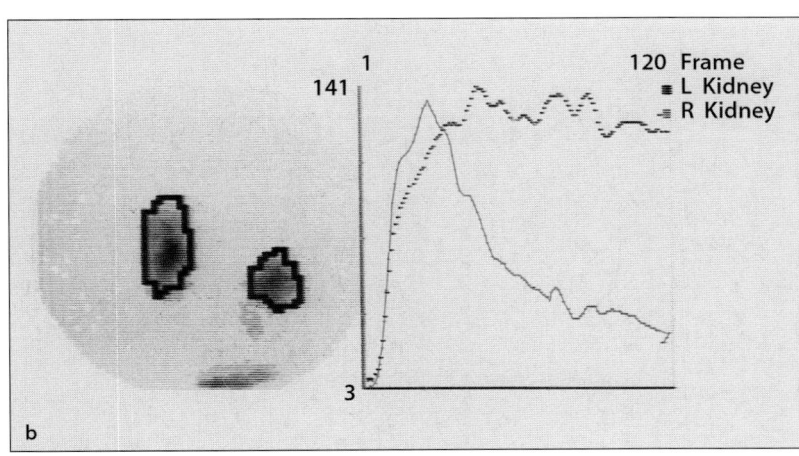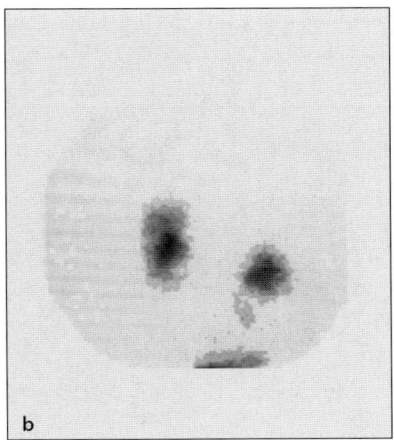

Fig. 3.86 b

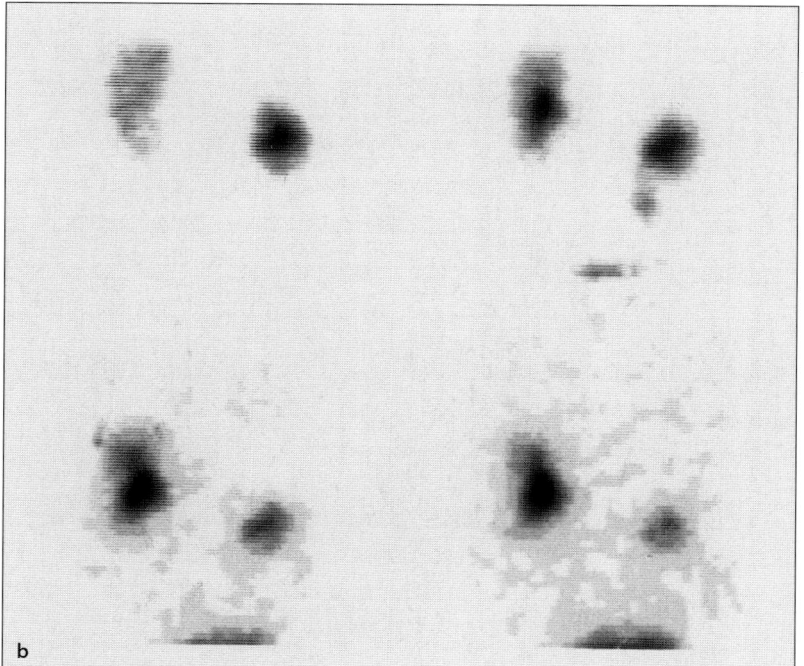

Fig. 3.86 a–c. Salvageability of the right kidney was assessed in a patient with right-sided ureteropelvic junction stenosis. Radionuclide function study showed that the kidney was still functioning efficiently and was worth salvaging

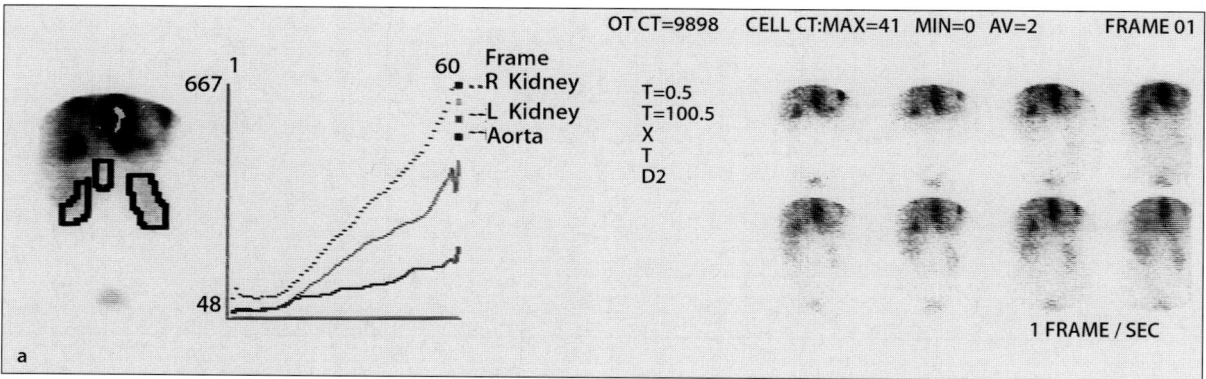

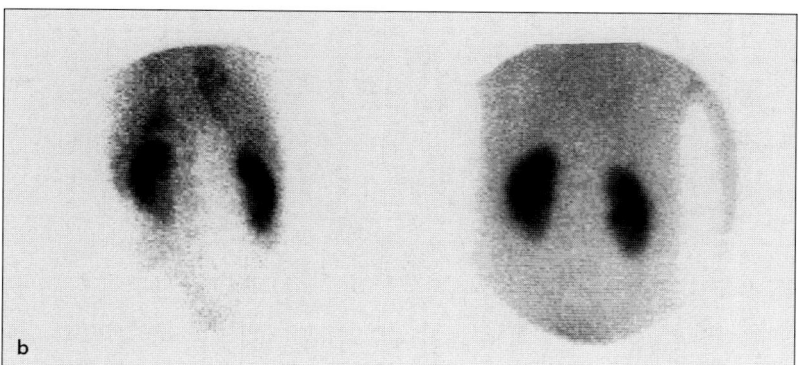

Fig. 3.87 a,b. This patient was admitted with sudden abdominal pain radiating to the back. The same symptoms had occurred some time before. Sequential renal scan shows a perfusion cutoff above the kidneys, whose complete visualization is greatly delayed. This finding suggests a suprarenal obstruction. Contrast angiography confirmed a suprarenal obstruction with a collateral supply

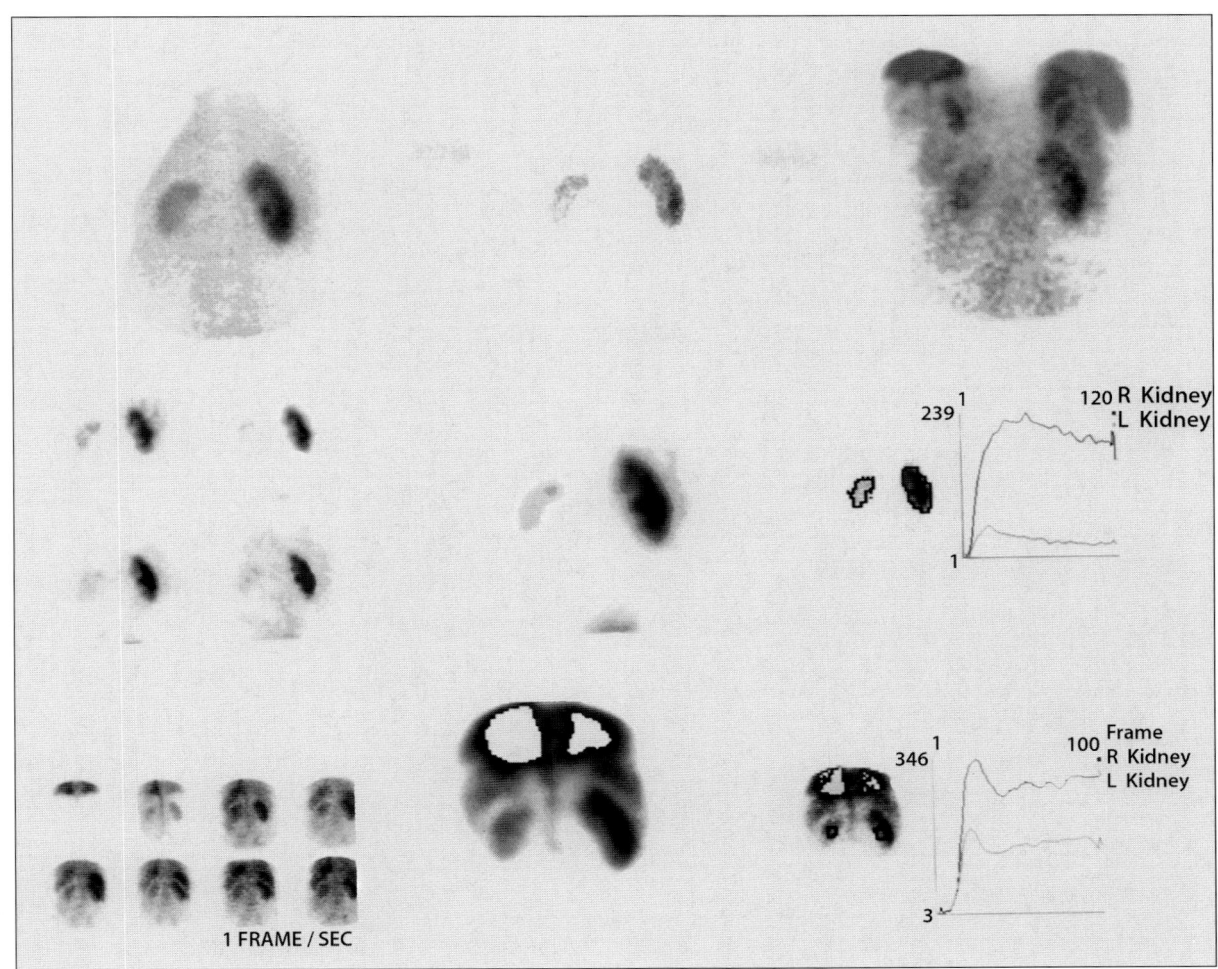

Fig. 3.88. Evaluation of a renal artery stenosis bypass shows persistence of the stenosis with significant functional impairment of the left kidney

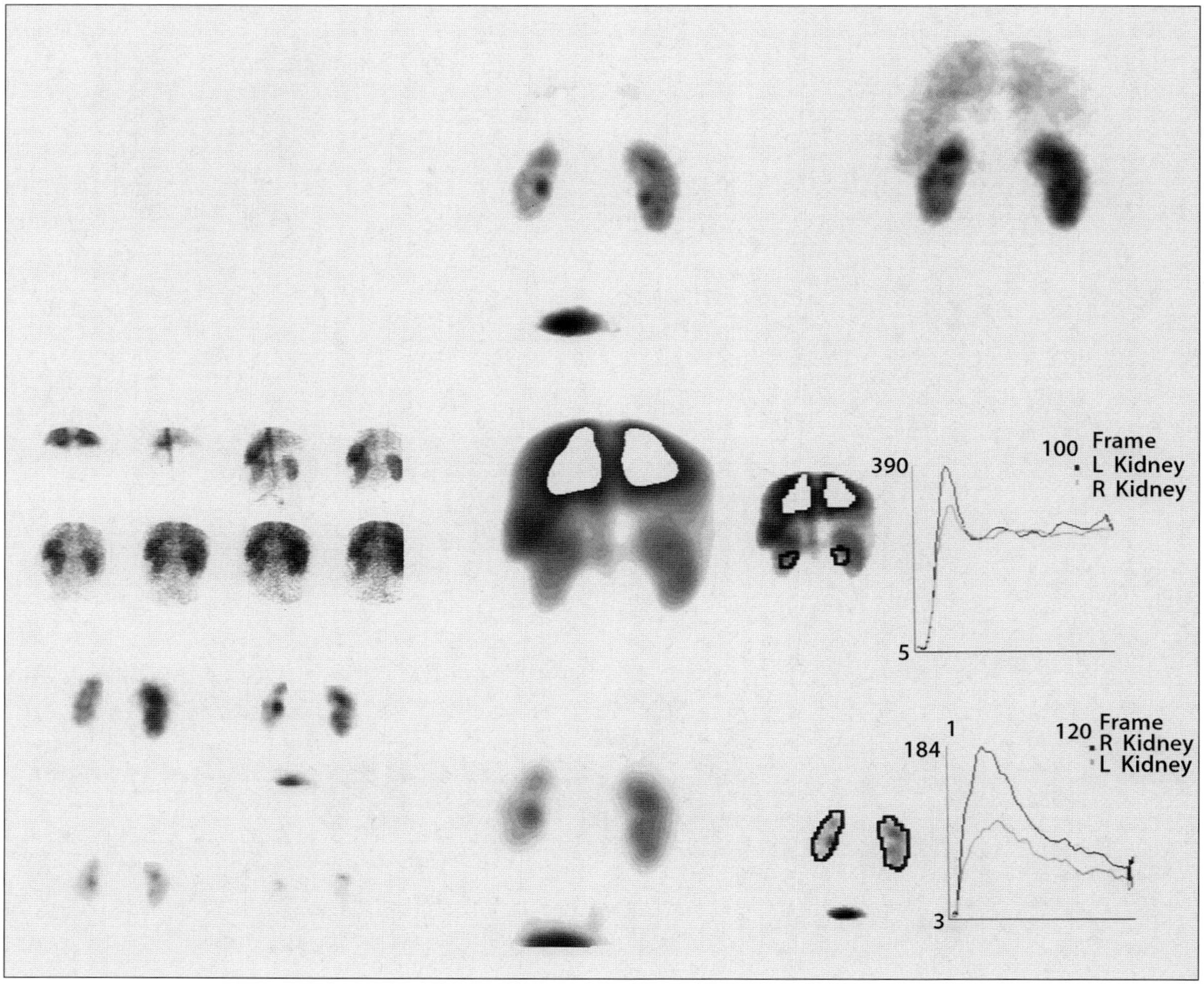

Fig. 3.89. Follow-up in a patient who underwent dilatation of renal artery stenosis. The side-to-side difference in renal perfusion is within normal limits. The result of the dilatation is good, but functional recovery is not yet complete

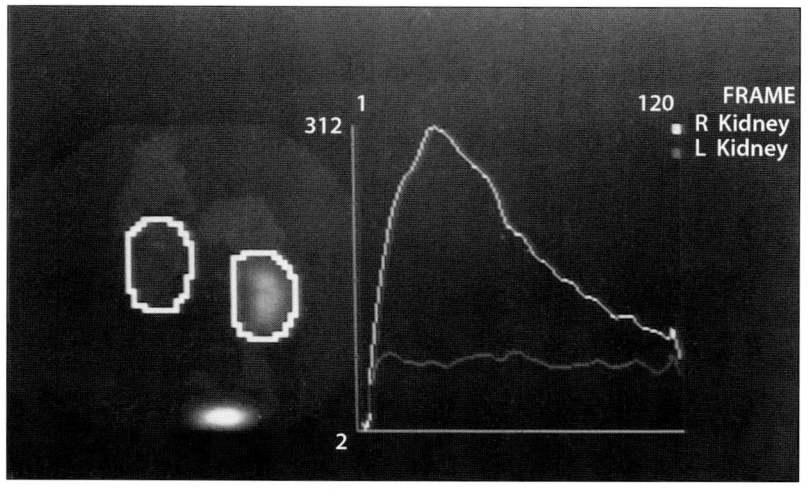

Fig. 3.90. Patient with left renal artery stenosis was scanned to evaluate left renal function and determine whether dilatation was worthwhile. The scan demonstrates a complete absence of perfusion and function on the affected side. The renogram shows an isosthenuric pattern

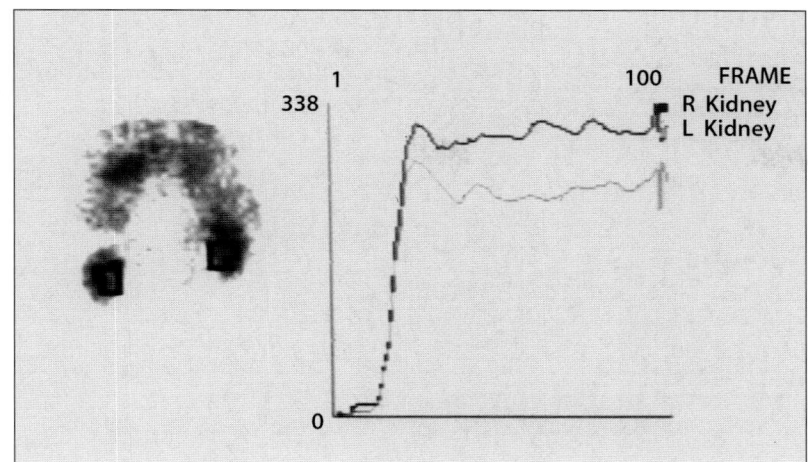

Fig. 3.91. Hypertensive patient who underwent percutaneous transluminal dilatation (PTD) was evaluated for symmetry of renal perfusion. Radionuclide scan shows good, symmetrical visualization of the kidneys

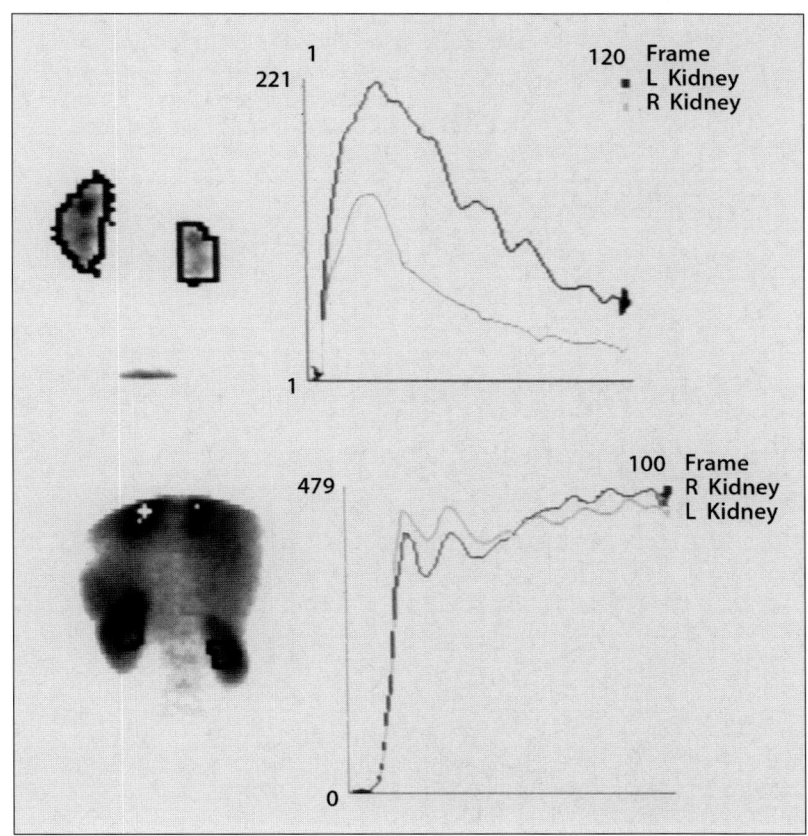

Fig. 3.92. Follow-up scan confirms successful dilatation of the right renal artery

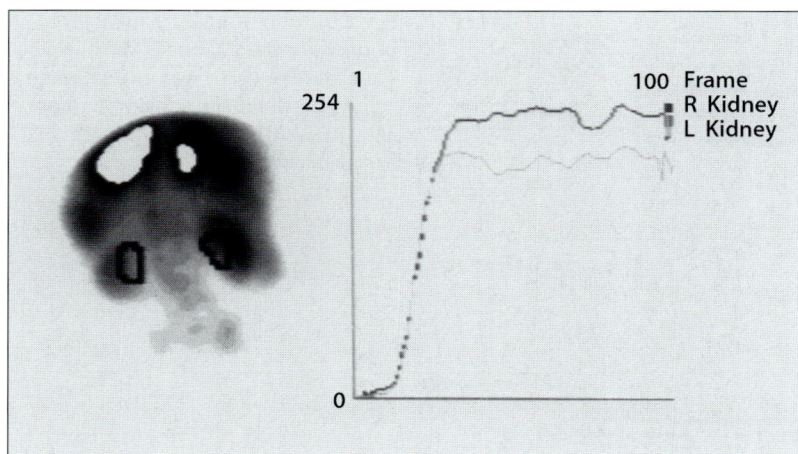

Fig. 3.93. Post-dilatation follow-up scan of a hypertensive patient confirms a successful dilatation with symmetrical renal perfusion

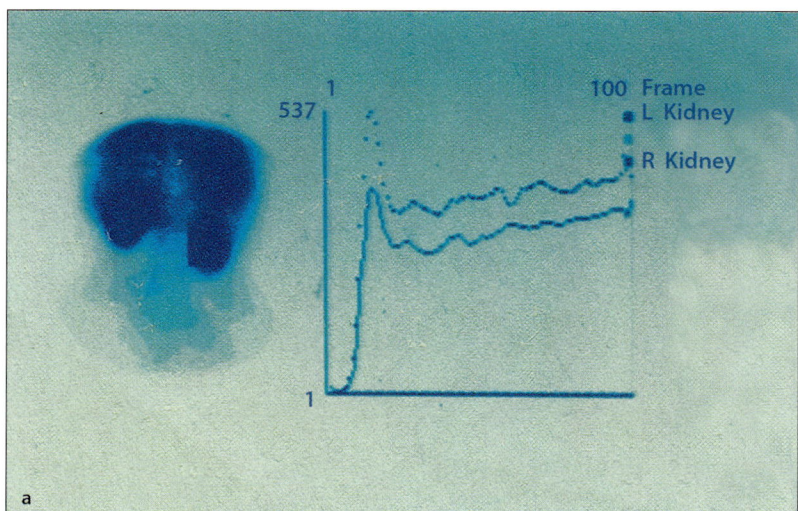

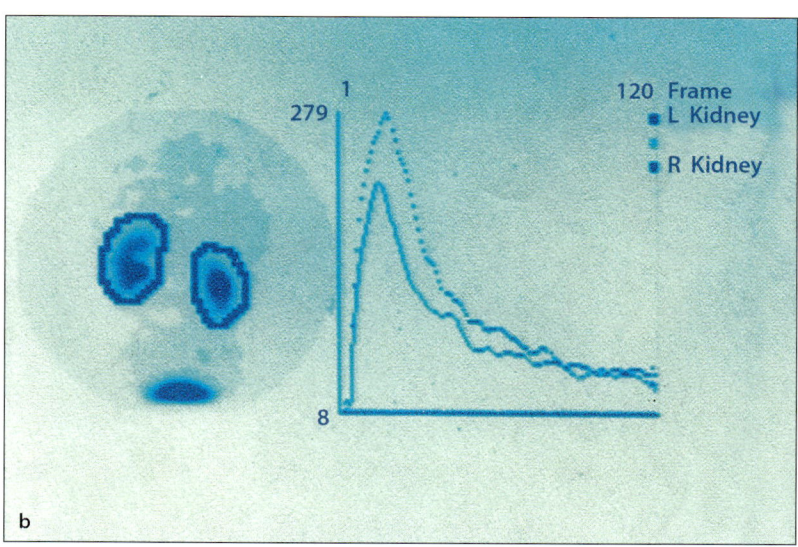

Fig. 3.94 a,b. Follow-up in a patient who underwent PTD for renal artery stenosis confirms a successful outcome with good recovery of tubular and excretory function and good clearance

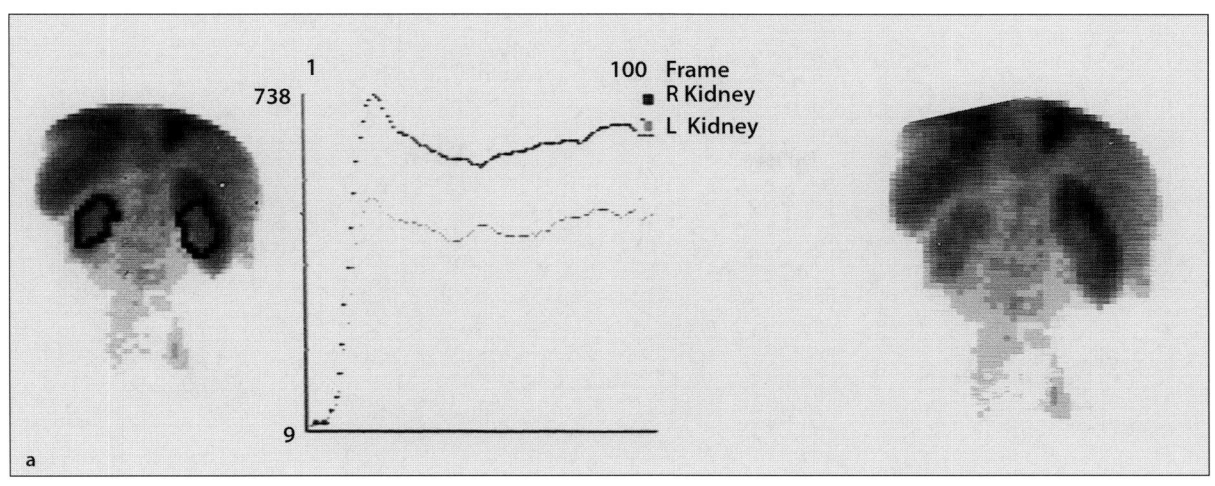

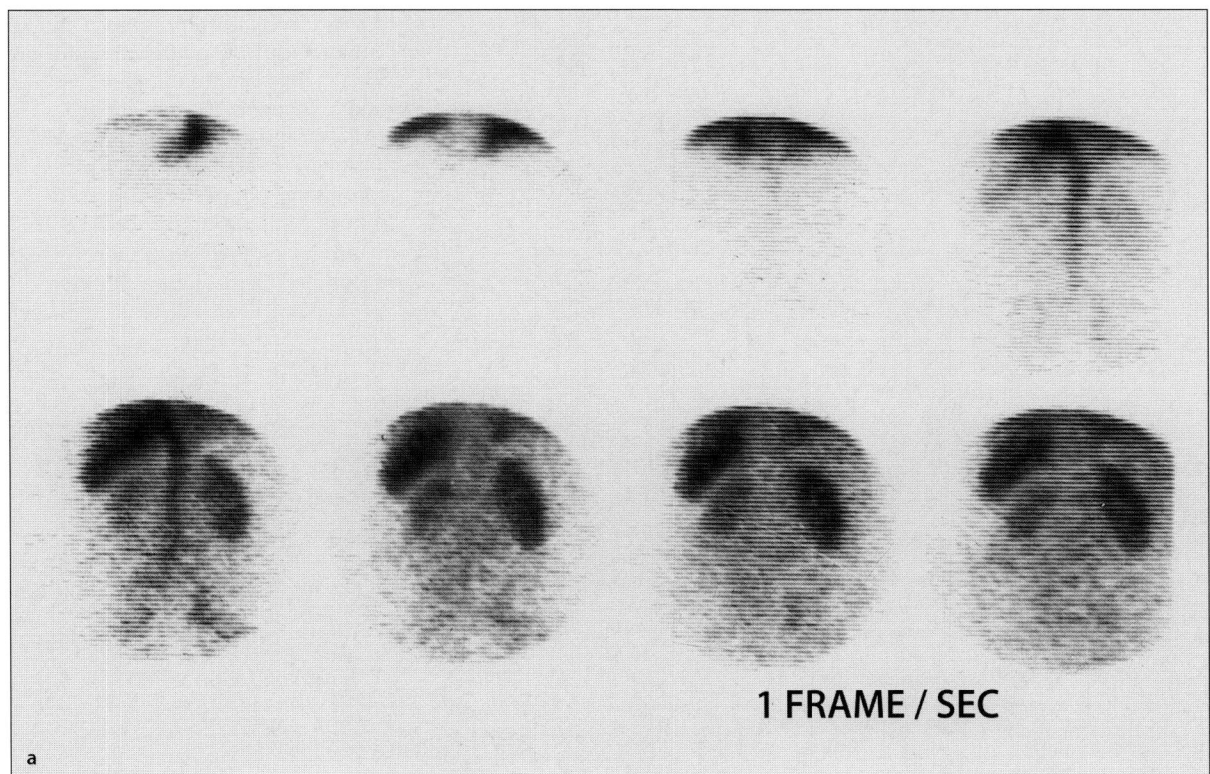

Fig. 3.95 a,b. Renal perfusion study in a hypertensive patient with a history of bilateral renal artery stenosis shows slightly decreased perfusion of the left kidney with significant impairment of tubular function. The left kidney is small and has irregular contours with no sign of outflow obstruction. The right kidney is relatively large with smooth contours (compensatory enlargement) and displays good tubular function

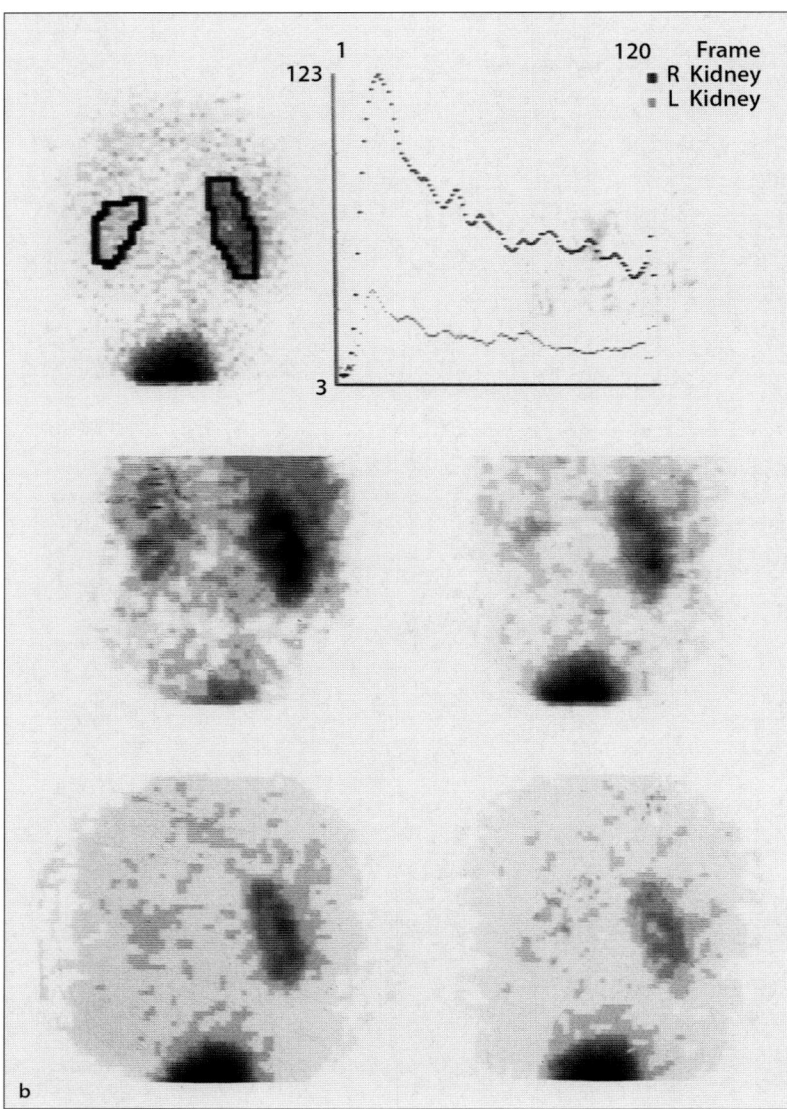

Fig. 3.95 a,b. Renal perfusion study in a hypertensive patient with a history of bilateral renal artery stenosis shows slightly decreased perfusion of the left kidney with significant impairment of tubular function. The left kidney is small and has irregular contours with no sign of outflow obstruction. The right kidney is relatively large with smooth contours (compensatory enlargement) and displays good tubular function

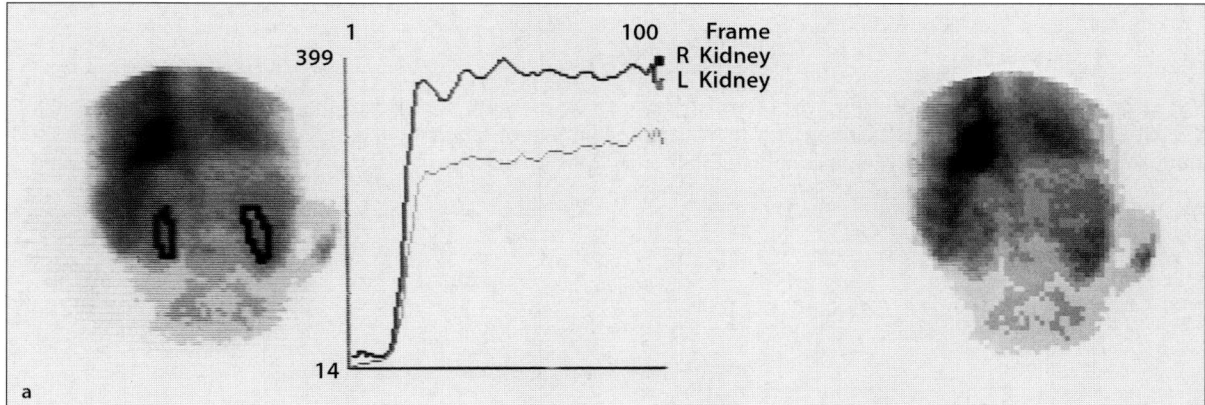

Fig. 3.96 a,b. Right-sided hypernephroma and left renal artery stenosis, leading to nonvisualization of the upper and central portions of the right kidney and delayed visualization of the left kidney. The kidneys are equivalent in tubular function and intrarenal transit time

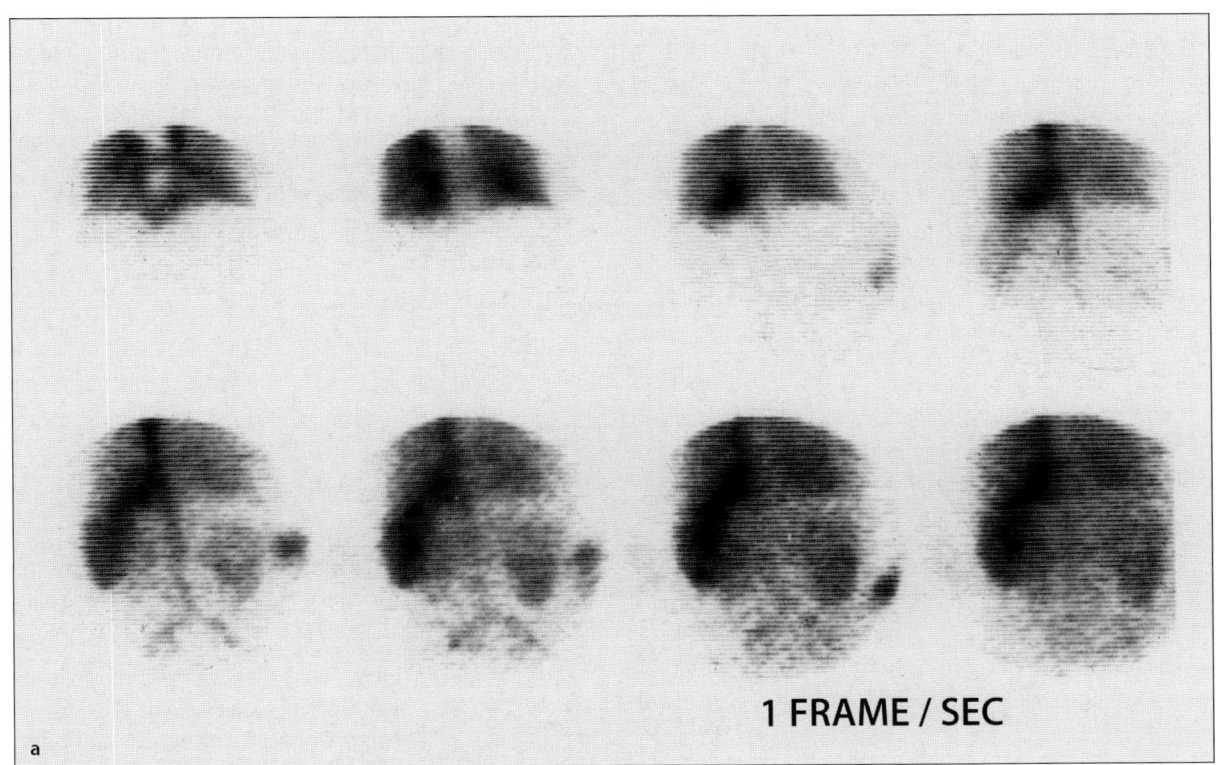

1 FRAME / SEC

Fig. 3.96 a. *Continued*

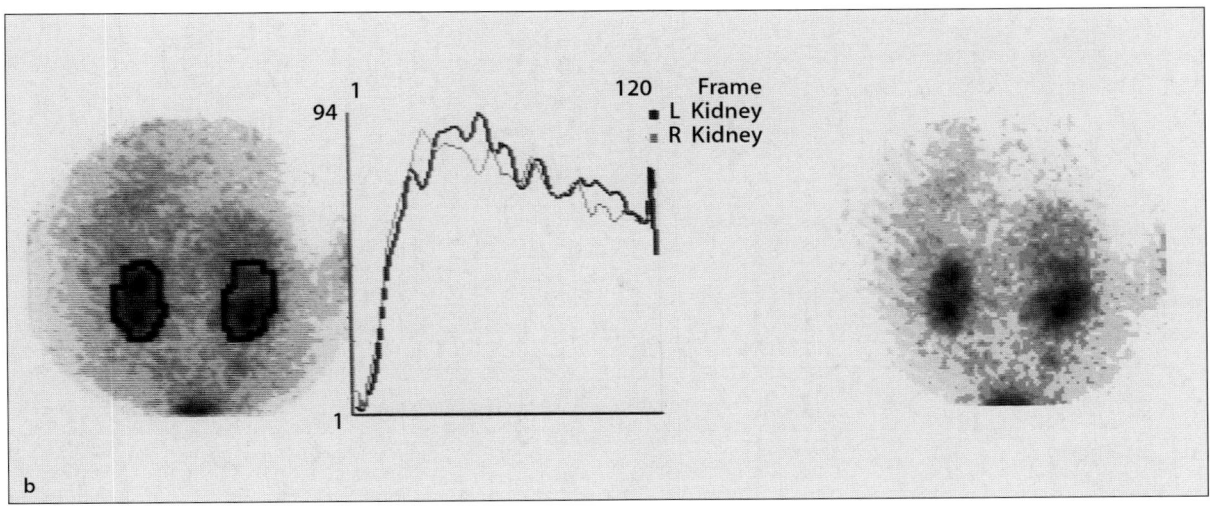

Fig. 3.96 b

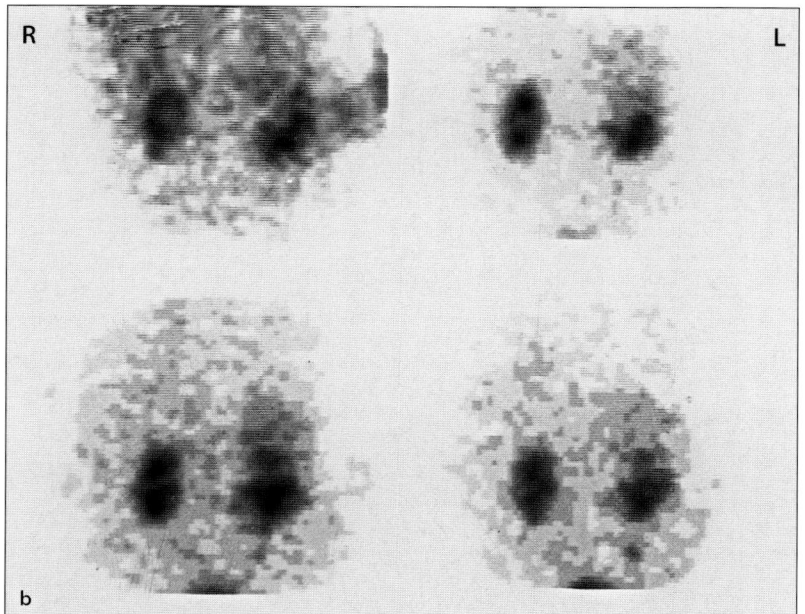

Fig. 3.96 a,b. Right-sided hyper-nephroma and left renal artery steno-sis, leading to nonvisualization of the upper and central portions of the right kidney and delayed visualization of the left kidney. The kidneys are equivalent in tubular function and intrarenal transit time

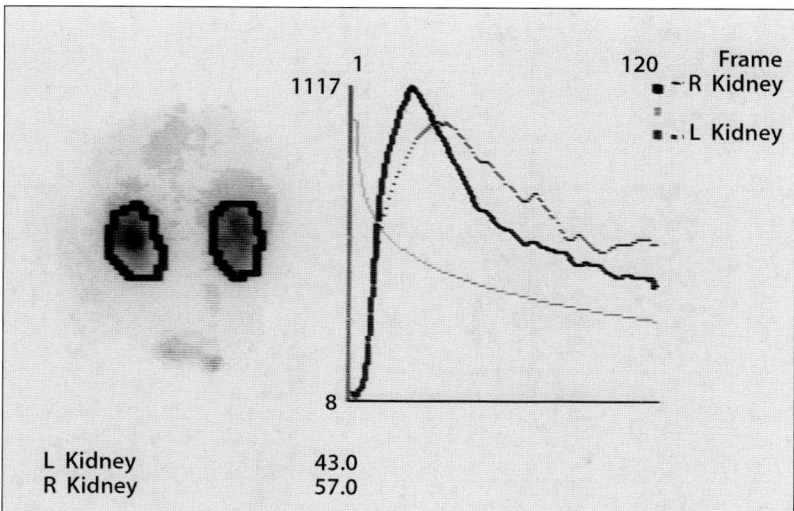

Fig. 3.97. Radionuclide study shows a hypervascular mass in the left kidney with symmetrical perfusion. Intrarenal transit time is slightly prolonged, and left renal clearance is 43% of total function

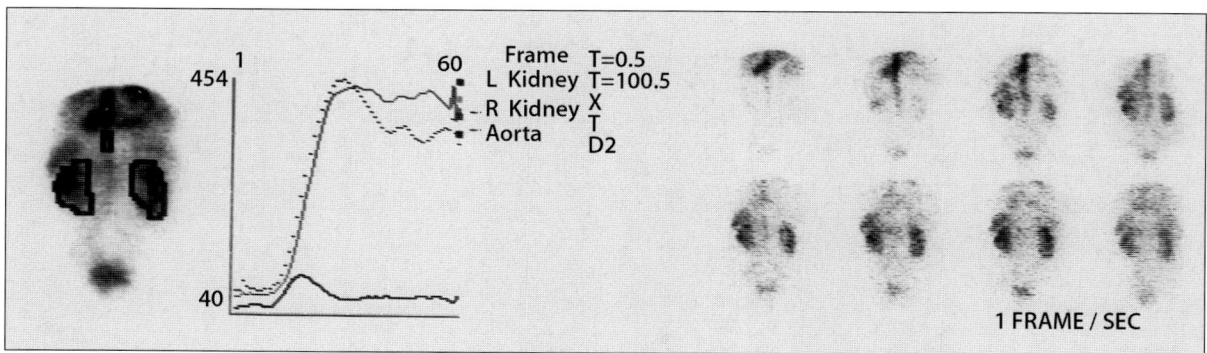

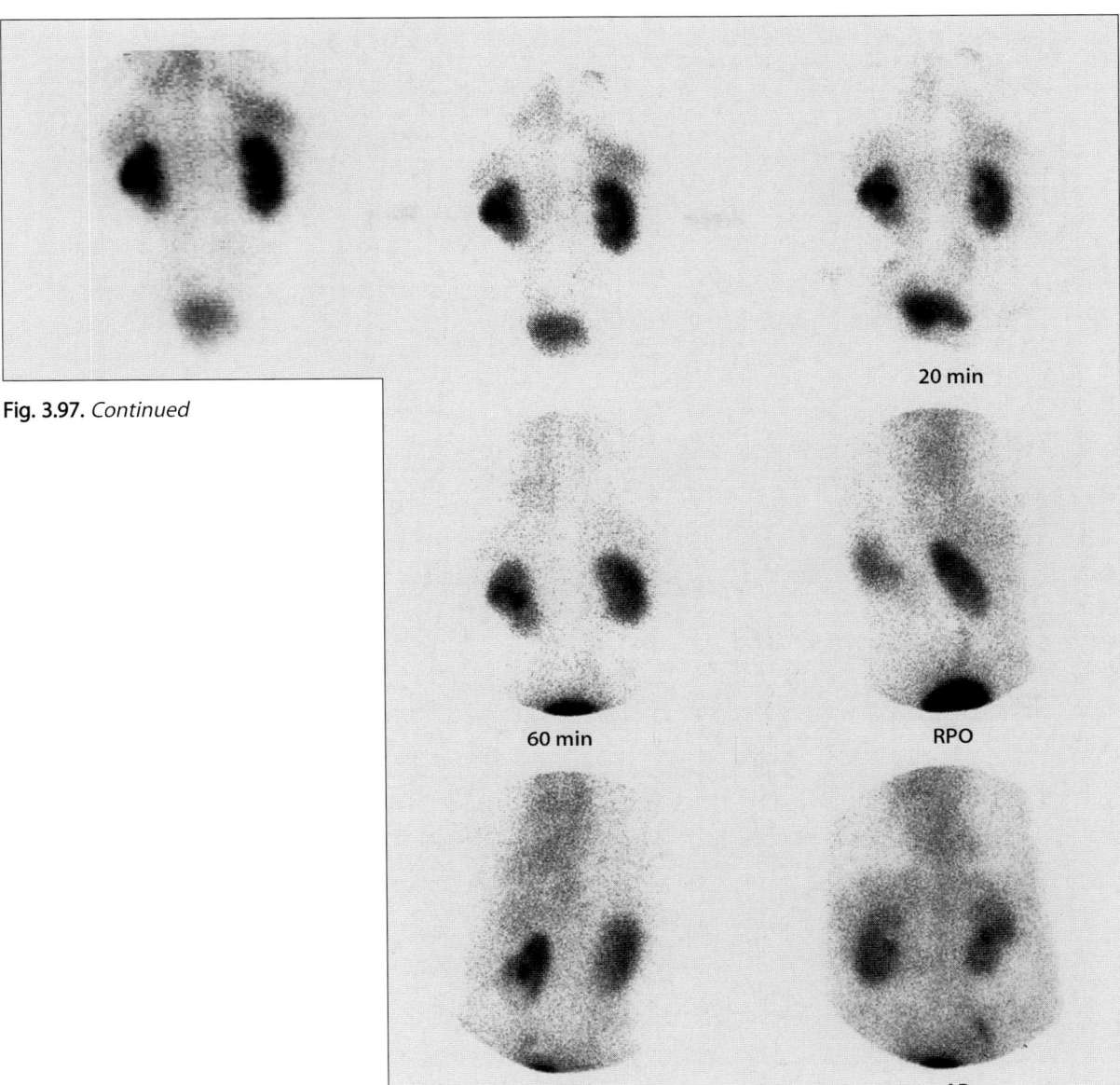

Fig. 3.97. *Continued*

20 min

60 min

RPO

LPO

AP

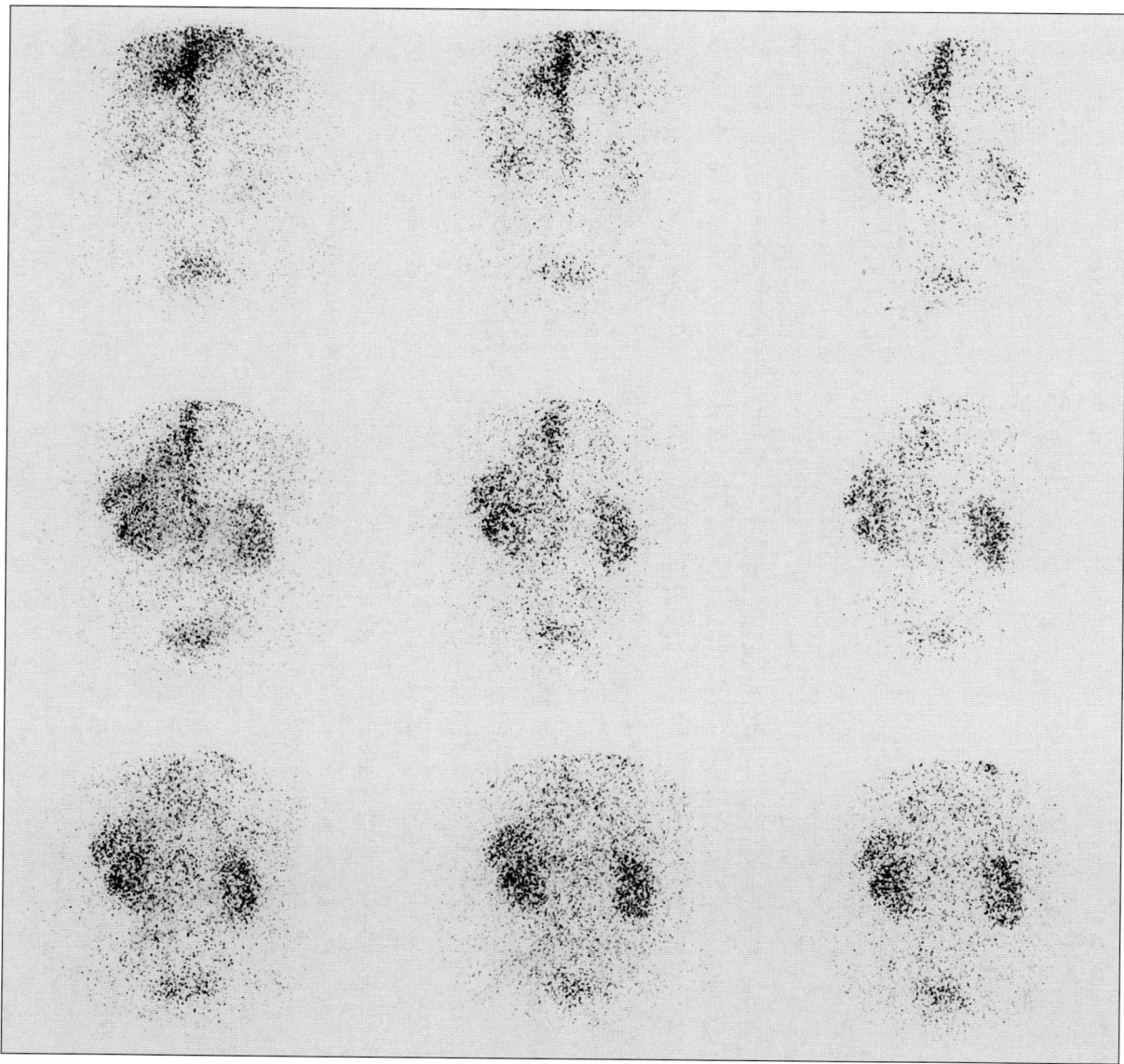

Fig. 3.97. Radionuclide study shows a hypervascular mass in the left kidney with symmetrical perfusion. Intrarenal transit time is slightly prolonged, and left renal clearance is 43% of total function

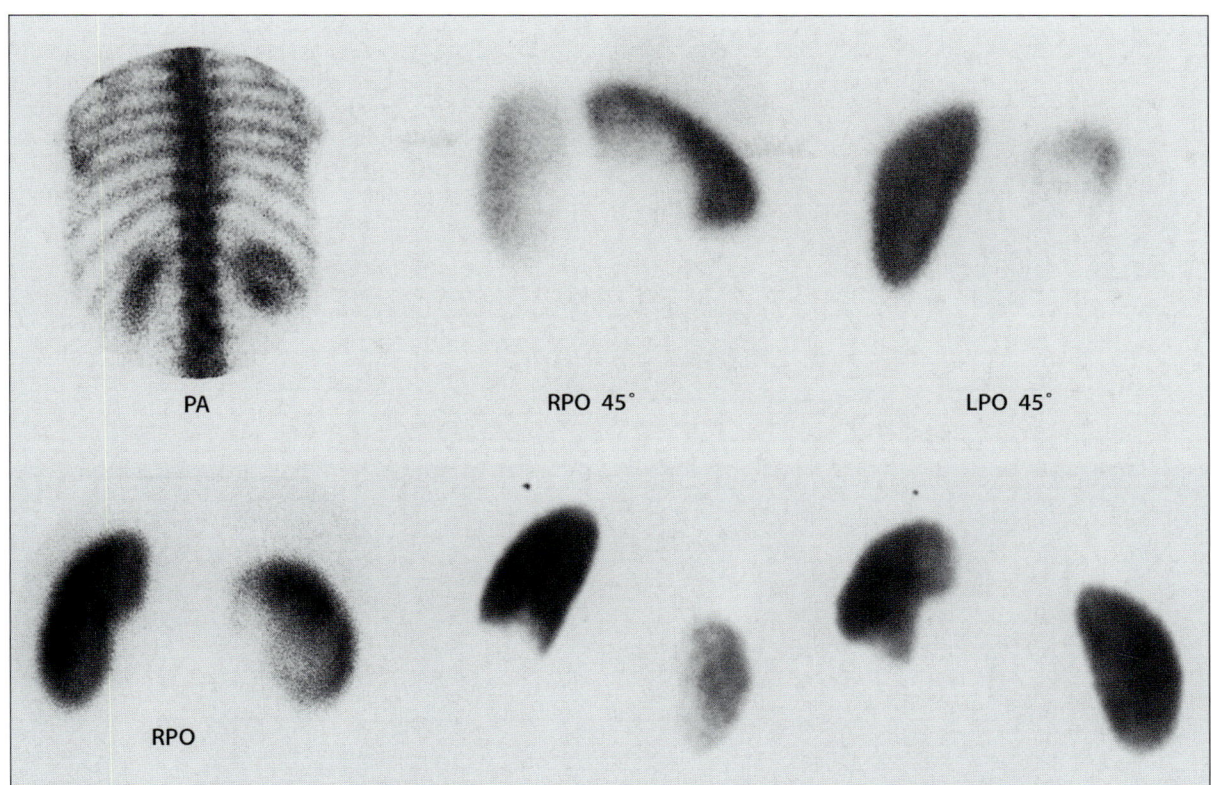

Fig. 3.98. Incidental finding in a patient with prostatic carcinoma who was screened for metastases. Scan shows accentuation of the right kidney with nonvisualization of the upper pole (various projections). Carcinoma of the right kidney

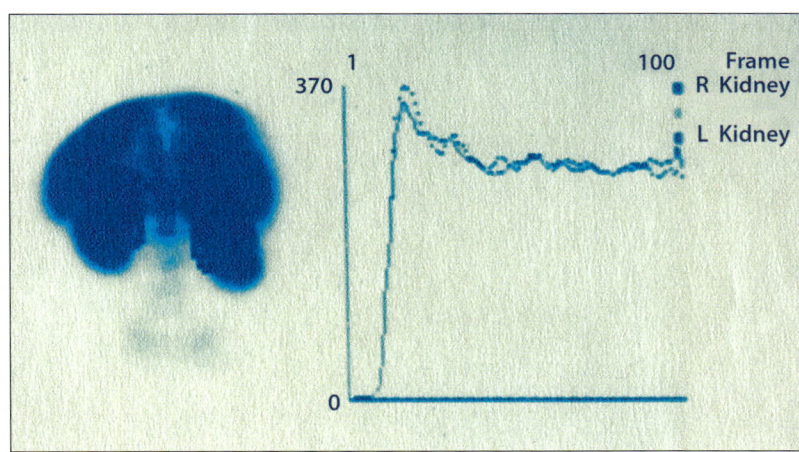

Fig. 3.99. Radionuclide scan in a young patient with high fever and back pain shows large, smooth-bordered kidneys with good uptake and good excretory function but significantly prolonged intrarenal transit times. This pattern is consistent with glomerulonephritis

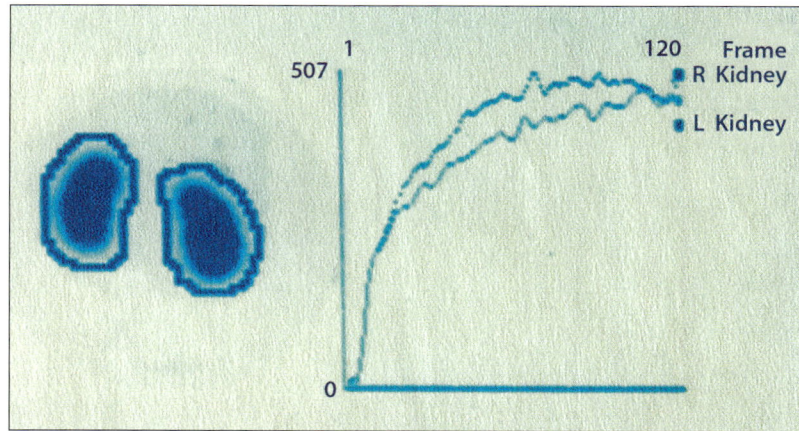

Fig. 3.99. Radionuclide scan in a young patient with high fever and back pain shows large, smooth-bordered kidneys with good uptake and good excretory function but significantly prolonged intrarenal transit times. This pattern is consistent with glomerulonephritis

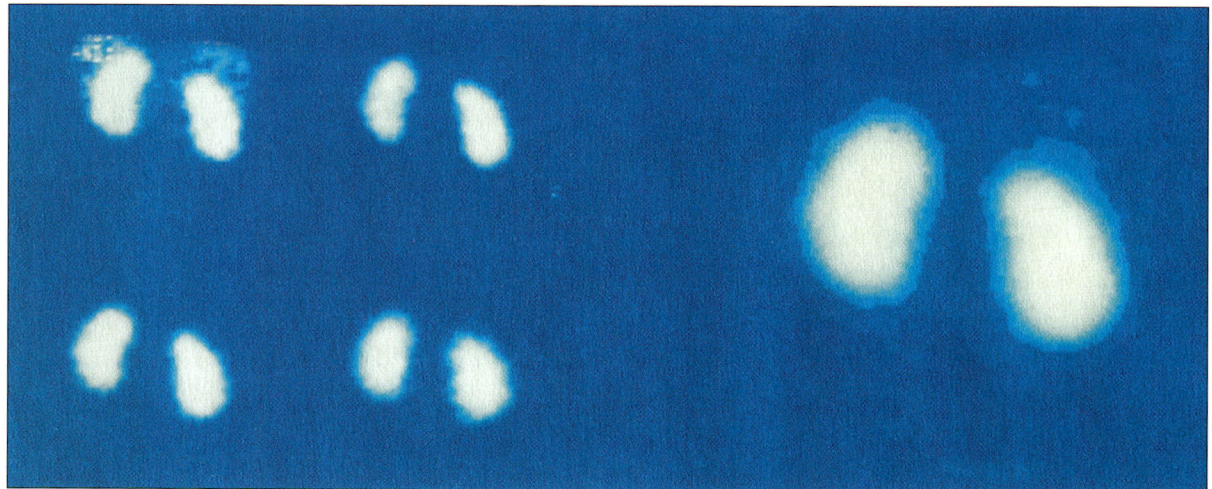

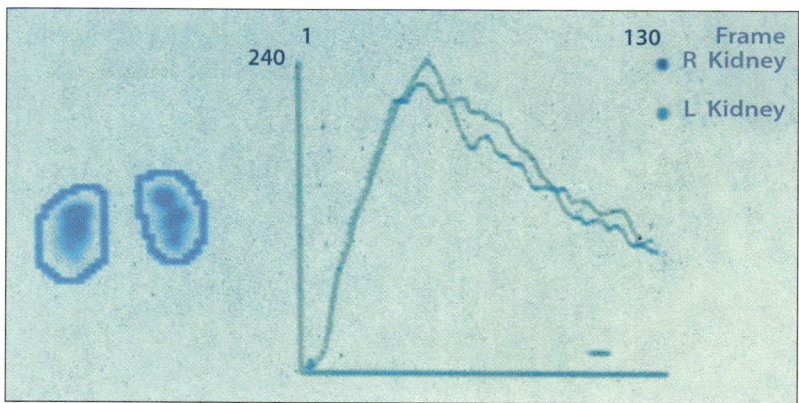

Fig. 3.100. Phenacetin abuse. Renogram indicates early-stage renal damage

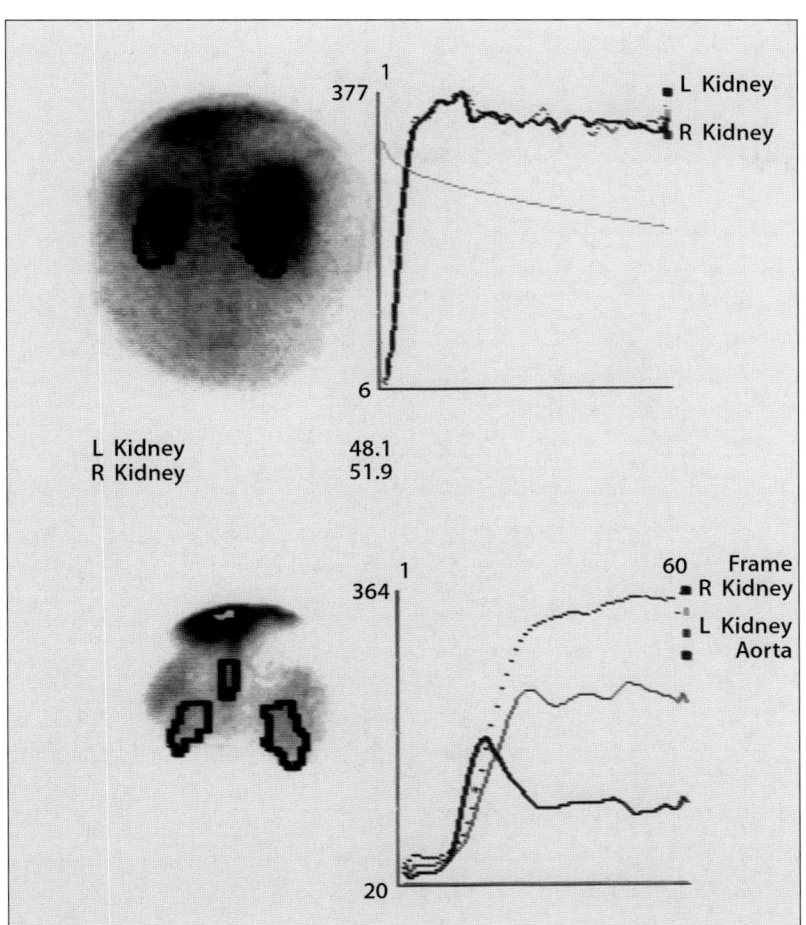

Fig. 3.101. Renogram in a patient with diabetes mellitus shows a delayed upstroke in both kidneys (left > right) with significant bilateral impairment of renal function. Klimmelstiel-Wilson syndrome

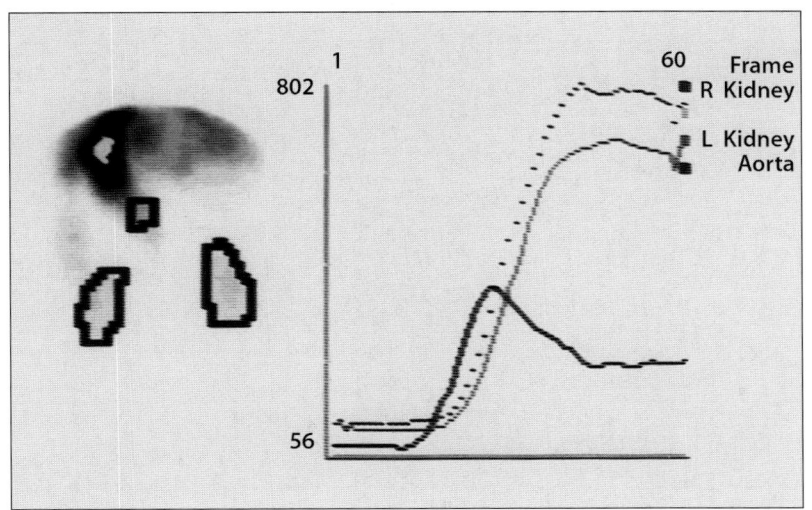

Fig. 3.102. Perfusion scan demonstrates a conical aortic stenosis at the prerenal level

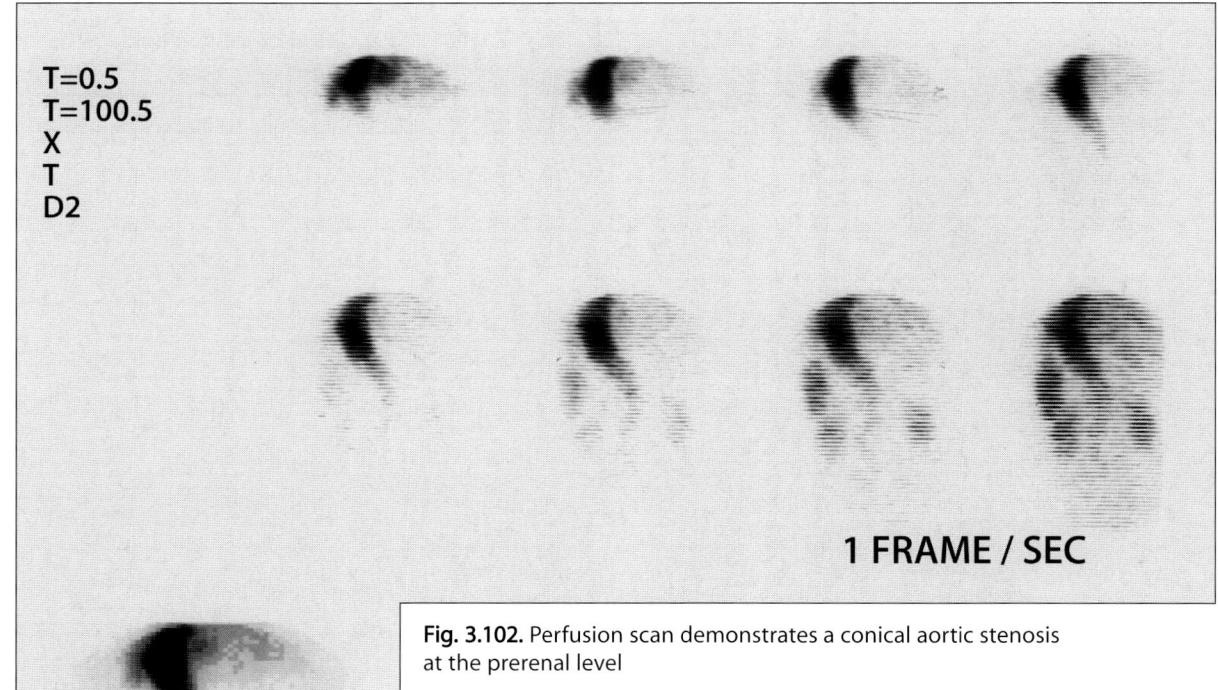

T=0.5
T=100.5
X
T
D2

1 FRAME / SEC

Fig. 3.102. Perfusion scan demonstrates a conical aortic stenosis at the prerenal level

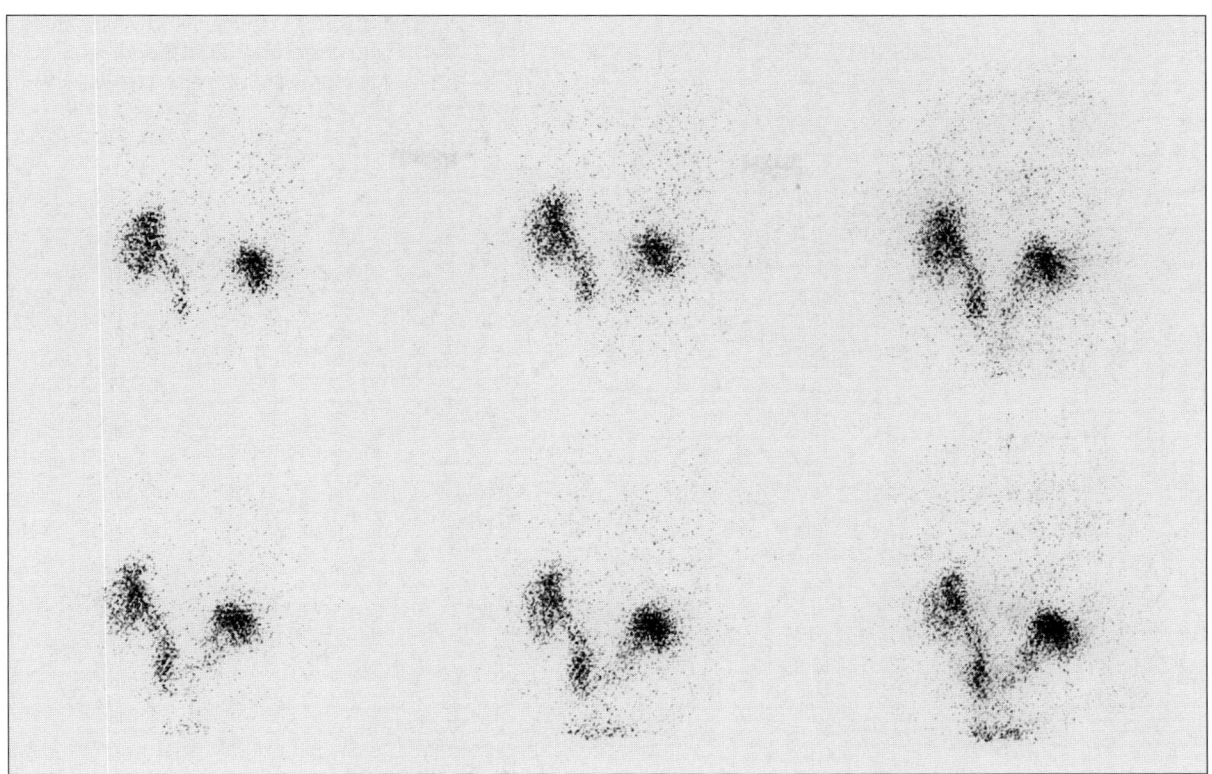

Fig. 3.103. Renal scan in a patient who underwent sacroabdominal proctectomy shows an area of activity in the lower abdomen outside the urinary tract. It was later identified as a ureteral-enteric fistula

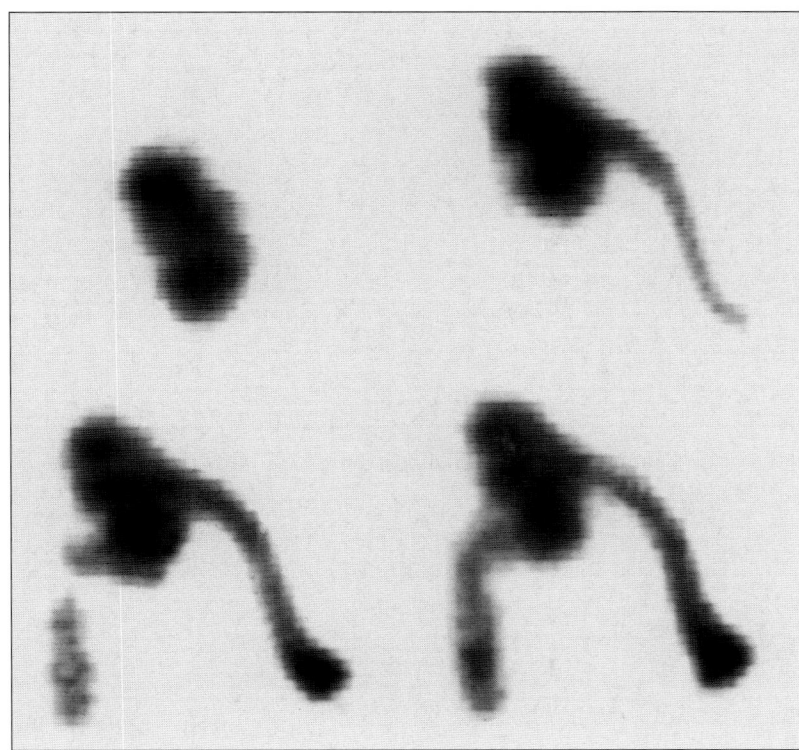

Fig. 3.104. Scan to evaluate renal drainage shows good excretory function

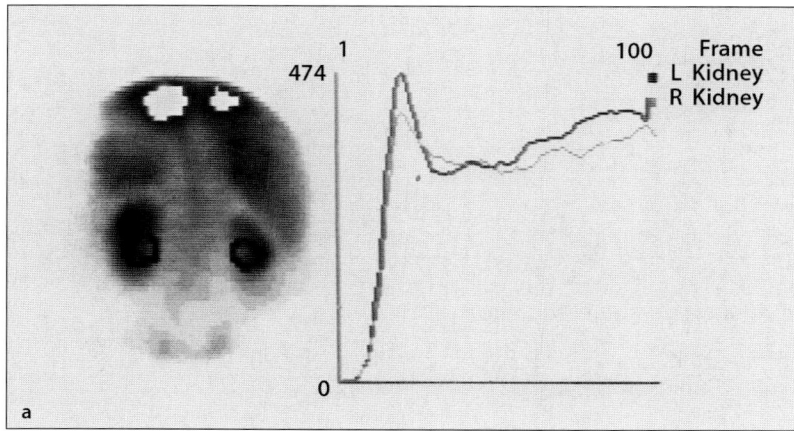

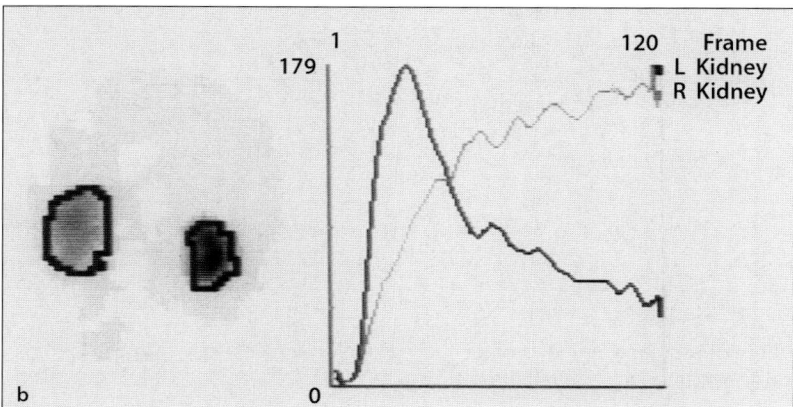

Fig. 3.105 a,b. Renal study in a patient who underwent right-sided hemicolectomy shows symmetrical perfusion and good function of the left kidney with right-sided renal shock (**b**)

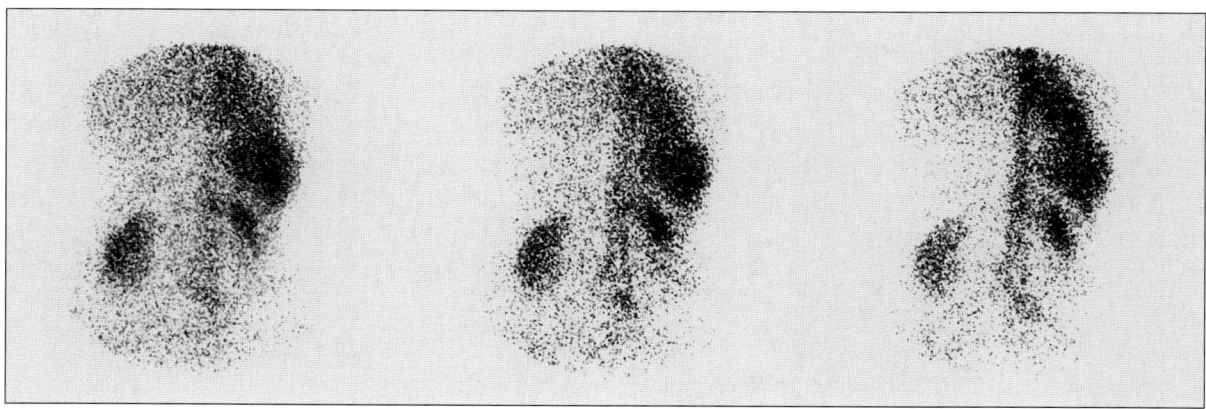

Fig. 3.106. Renal scan shows duplication of the distal abdominal aorta terminating in an area of activity. Angiography defined the lesion as a fistula between the aorta and ovarian artery

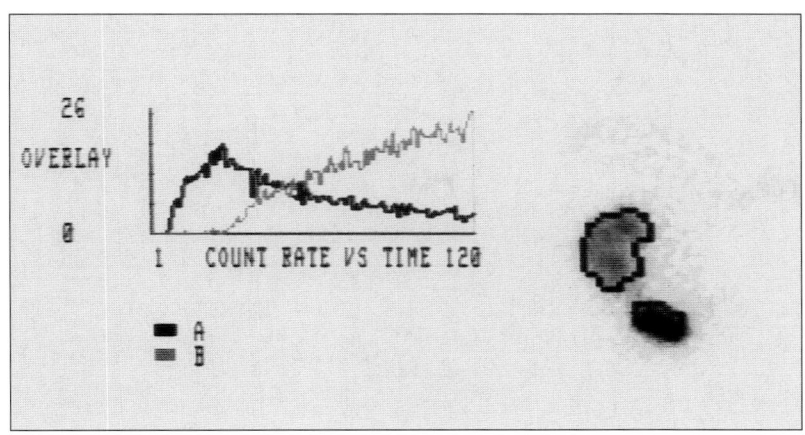

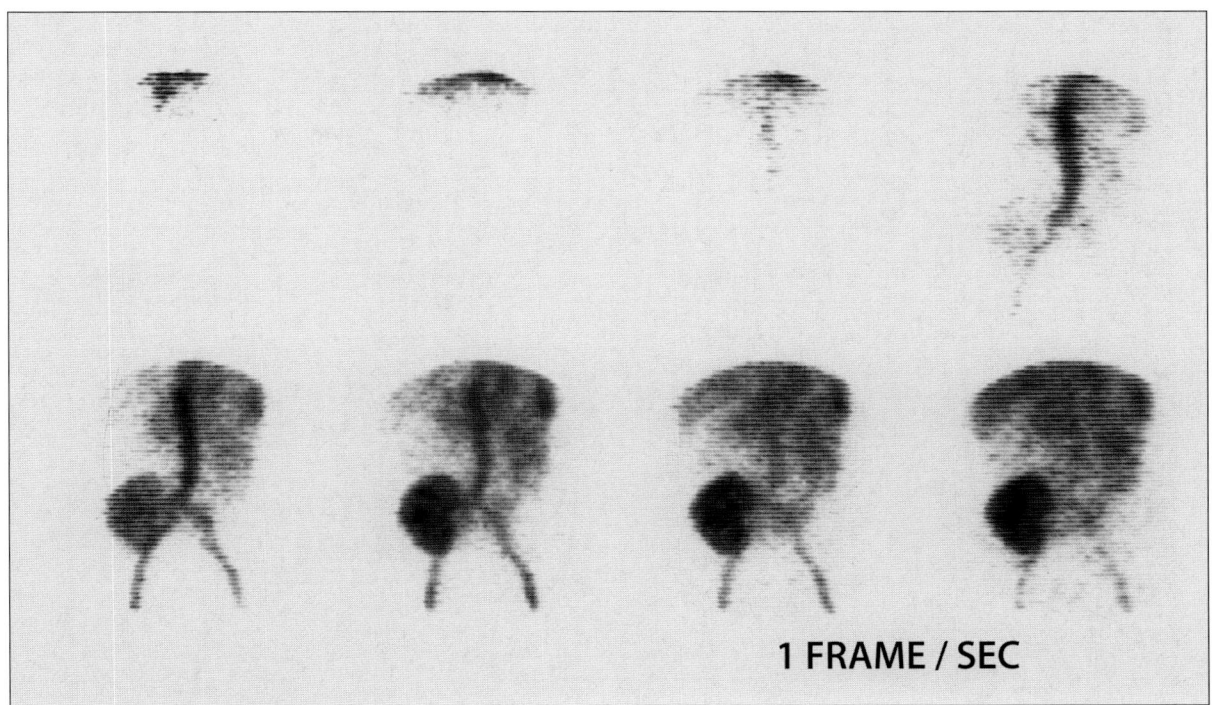

1 FRAME / SEC

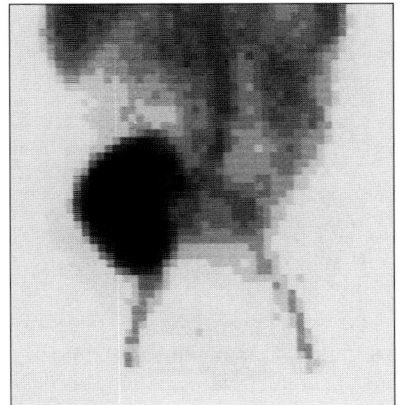

Fig. 3.107. Posttransplantation renal scan shows excellent perfusion of the graft with homogeneous uptake and good tubular and excretory function

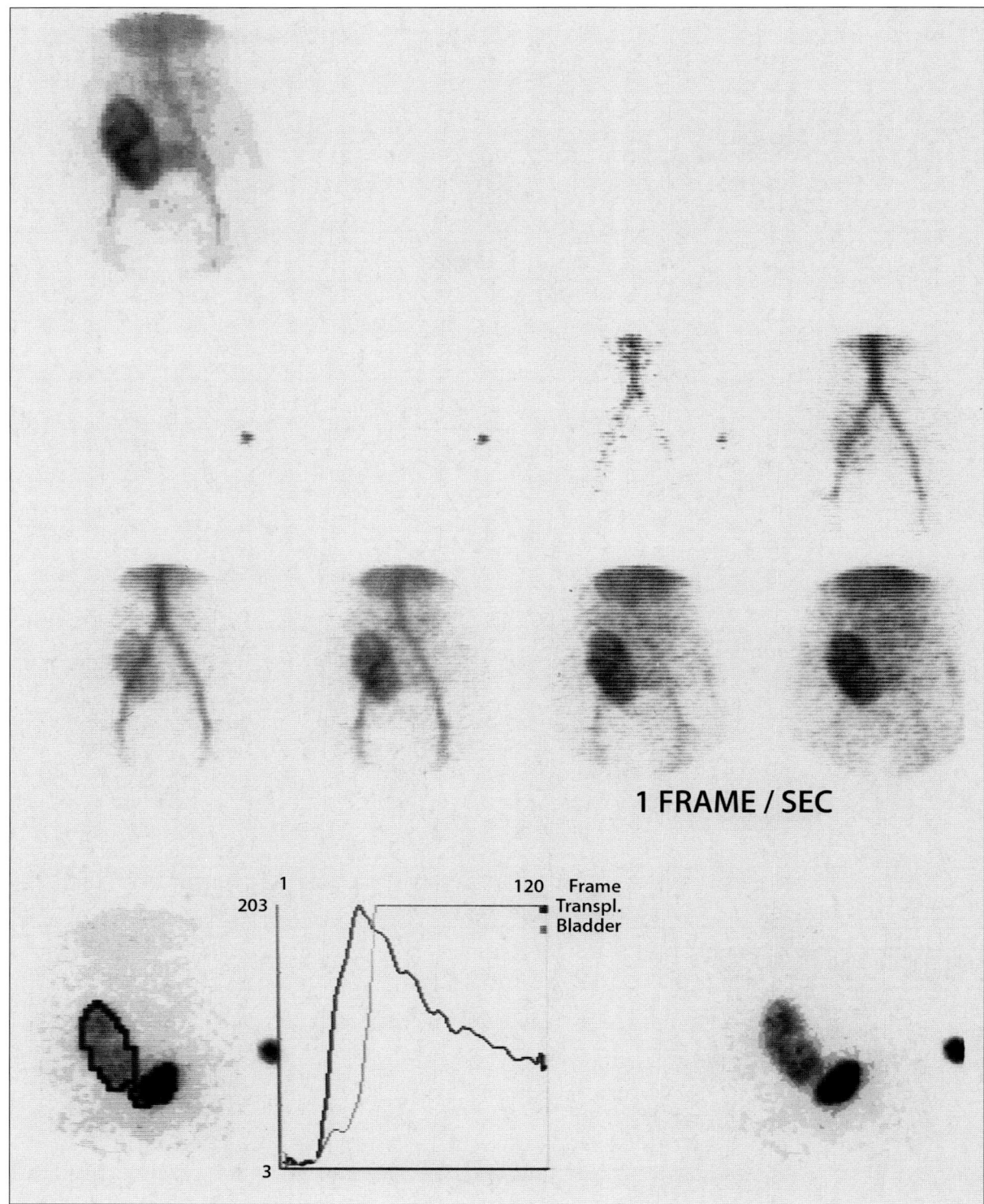

1 FRAME / SEC

Fig. 3.108. Examination 10 days after renal transplantation shows good tubular and excretory function but nonhomogeneous uptake. Close-interval follow-ups are necessary to monitor for acute rejection, but complete recovery may occur

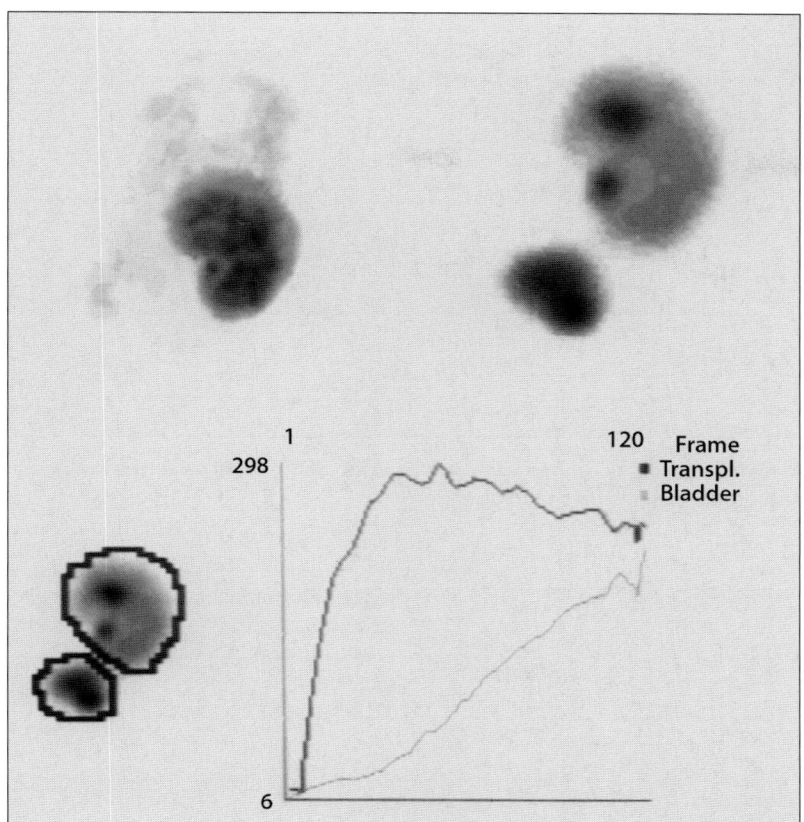

Fig. 3.109. Renal scan on the first post-operative day shows good perfusion and function of the graft, given the timing of the examination. The enlarged upper caliceal group requires follow-up attention

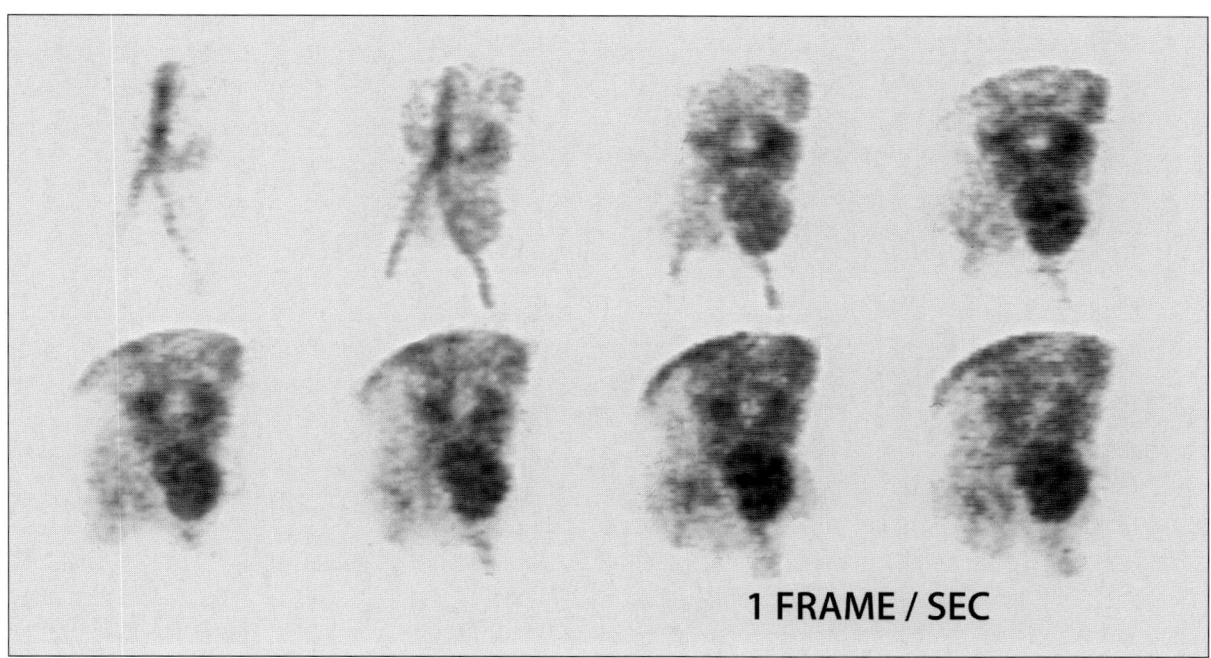

1 FRAME / SEC

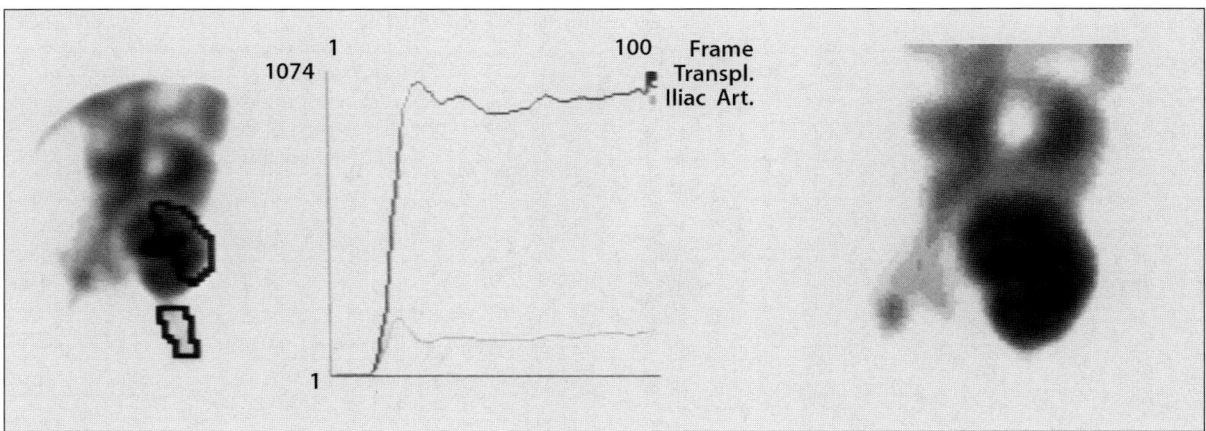

Fig. 3.109. Renal scan on the first postoperative day shows good perfusion and function of the graft, given the timing of the examination. The enlarged upper caliceal group requires follow-up attention

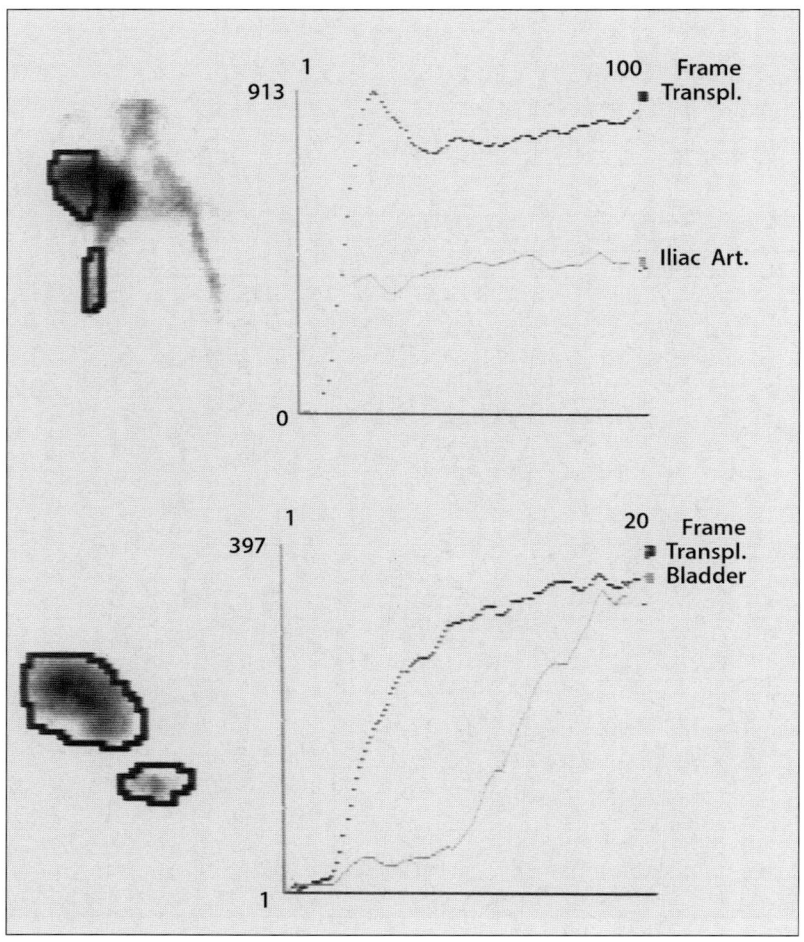

Fig. 3.110. Examination on the first postoperative day shows a good early result, but continued follow-ups are necessary

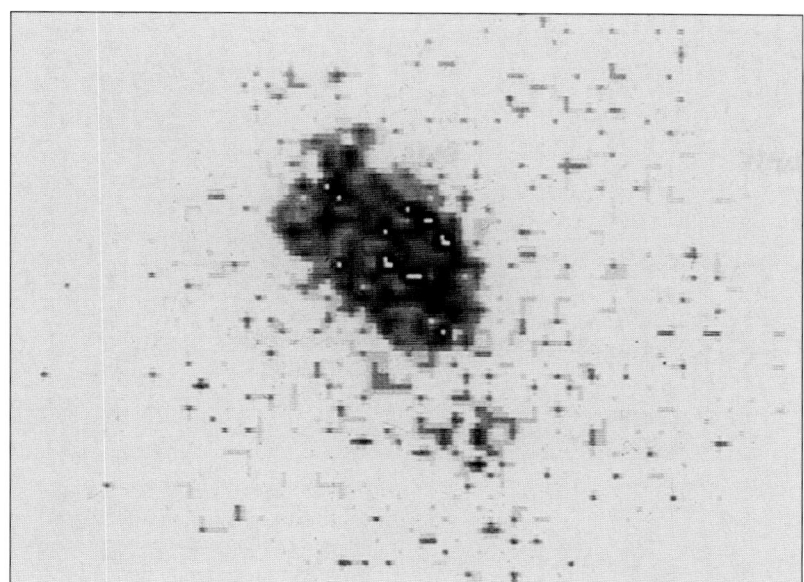

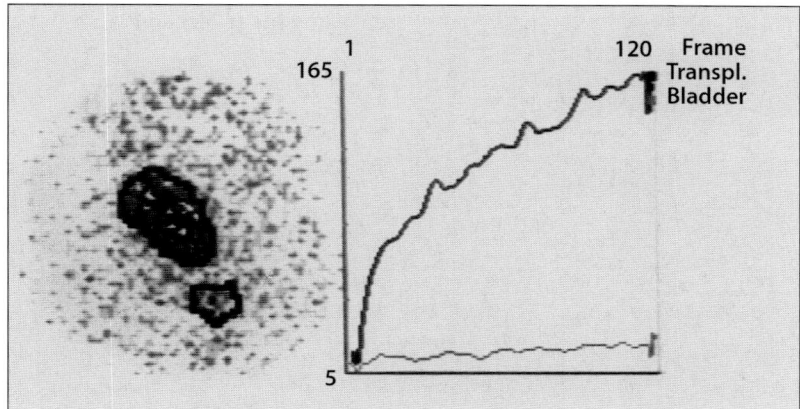

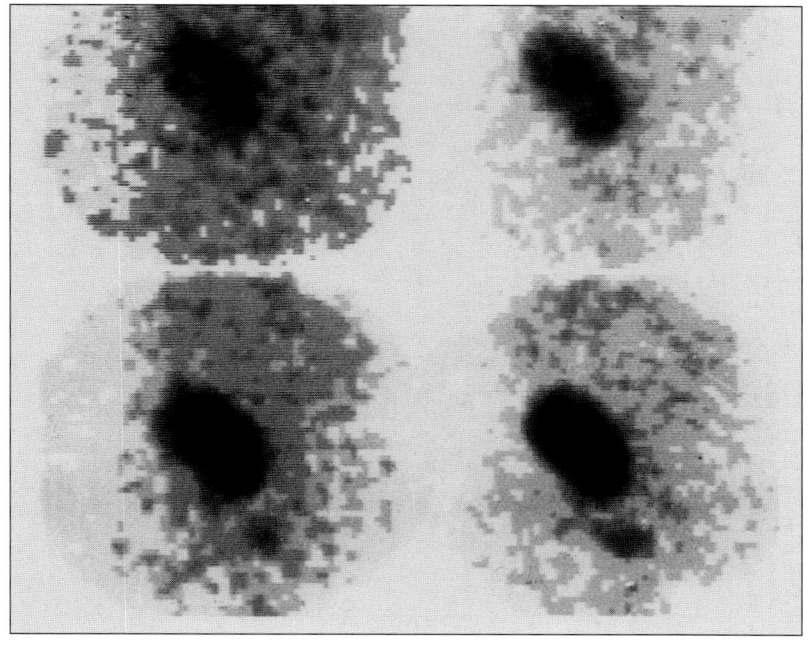

Fig. 3.111. Scan 3 weeks postoperatively shows patchy tracer uptake and almost no excretory function. Tubular secretion is still preserved

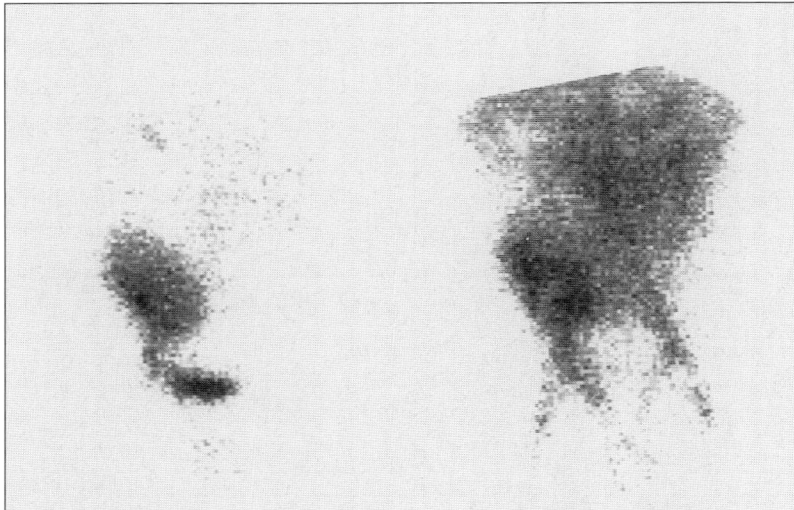

Fig. 3.112. Scan 3 weeks postoperatively shows delayed and decreased perfusion of the graft, homogeneous uptake, and moderately decreased excretion. These findings are consistent with clinical infection

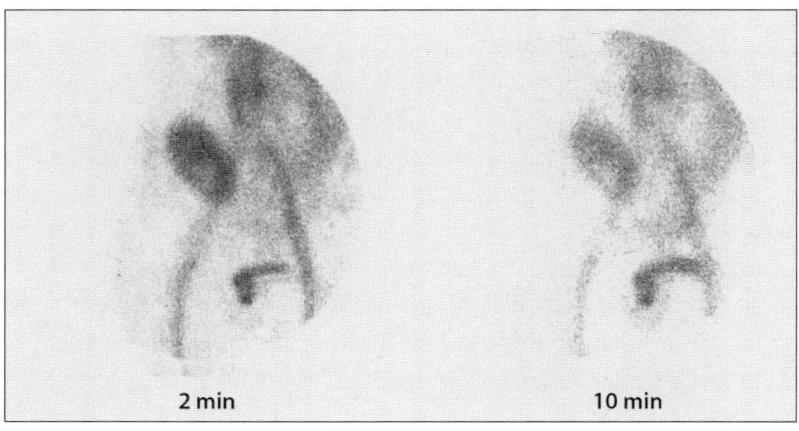

Fig. 3.113. Parapelvic and inferomedial renal mass, identified as an encapsulated hematoma

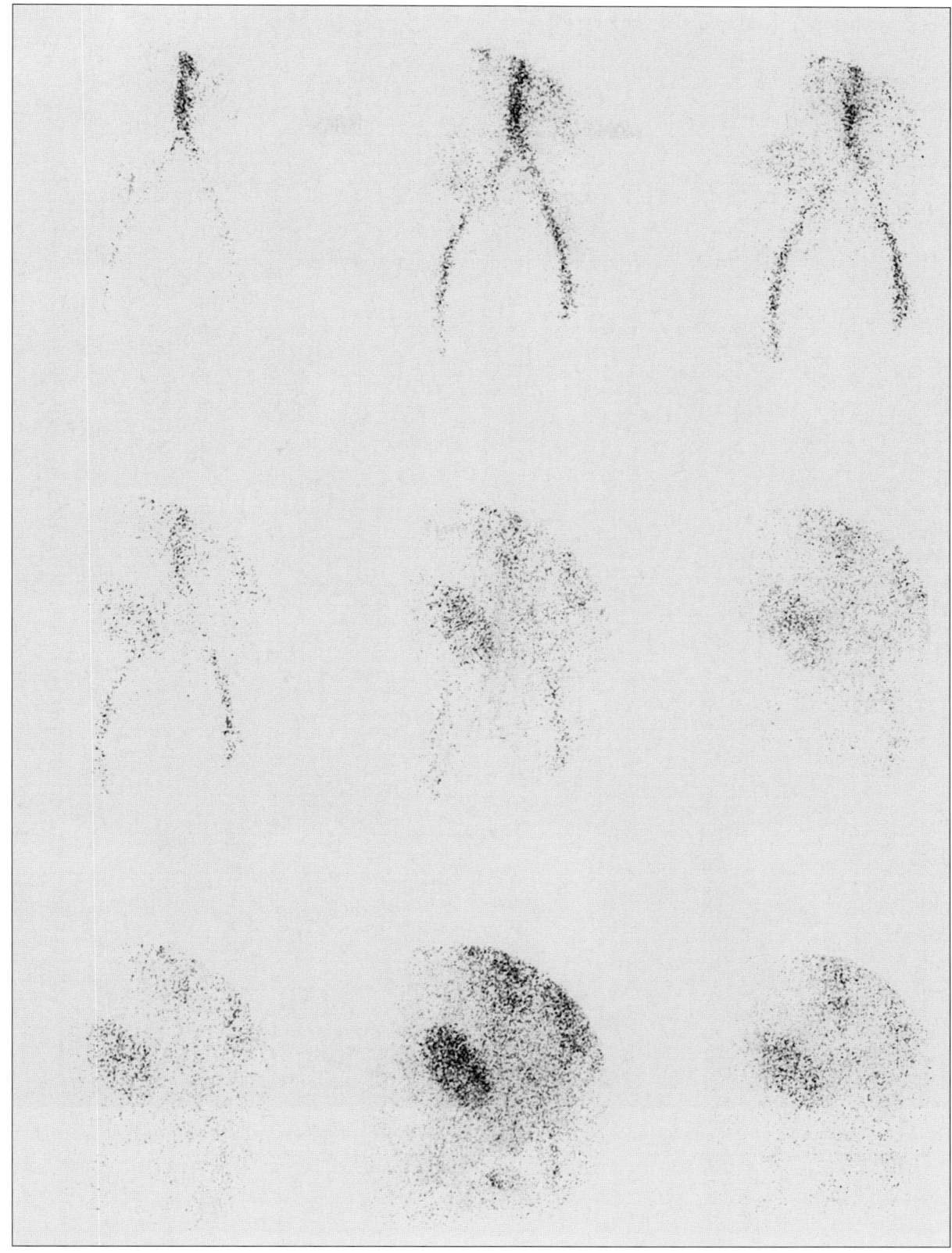

Fig. 3.113. *Continued*

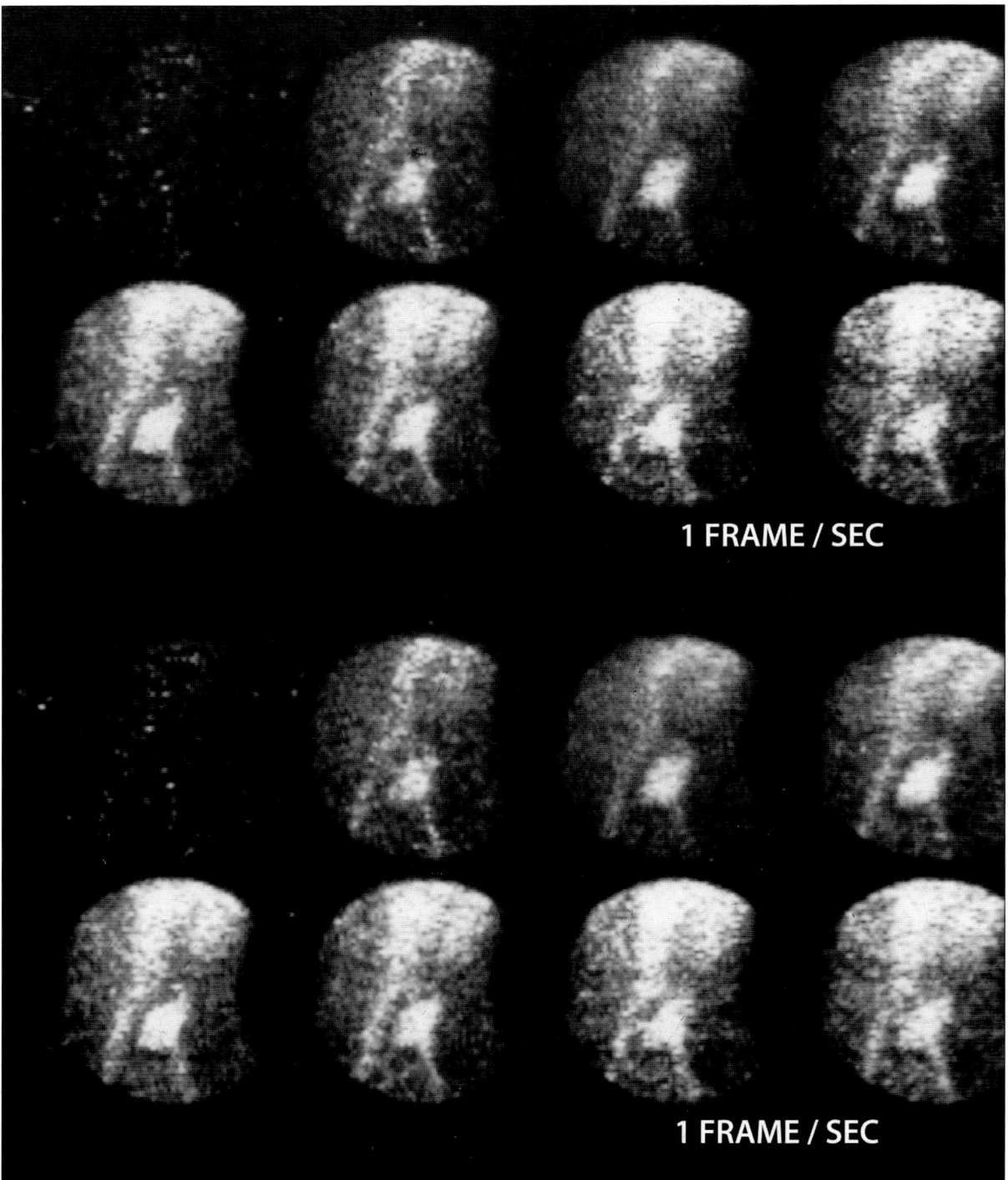

Fig. 3.114. The capsule on the superomedial portion of the graft was torn during the transplant surgery. Otherwise the graft appears normal for its age

Fig. 3.114. *Continued*

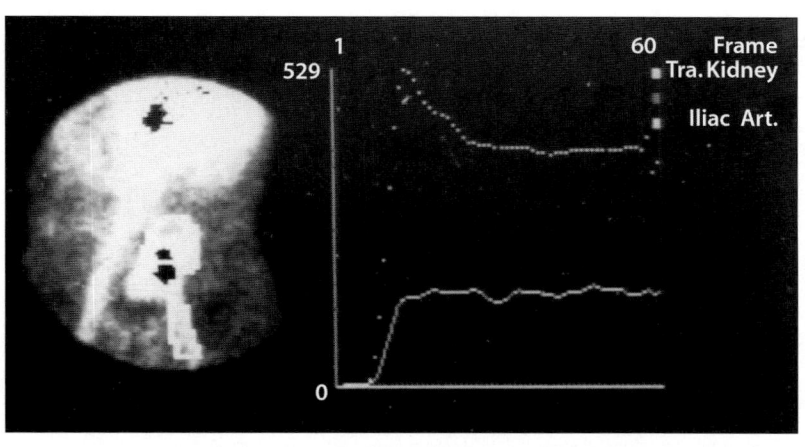

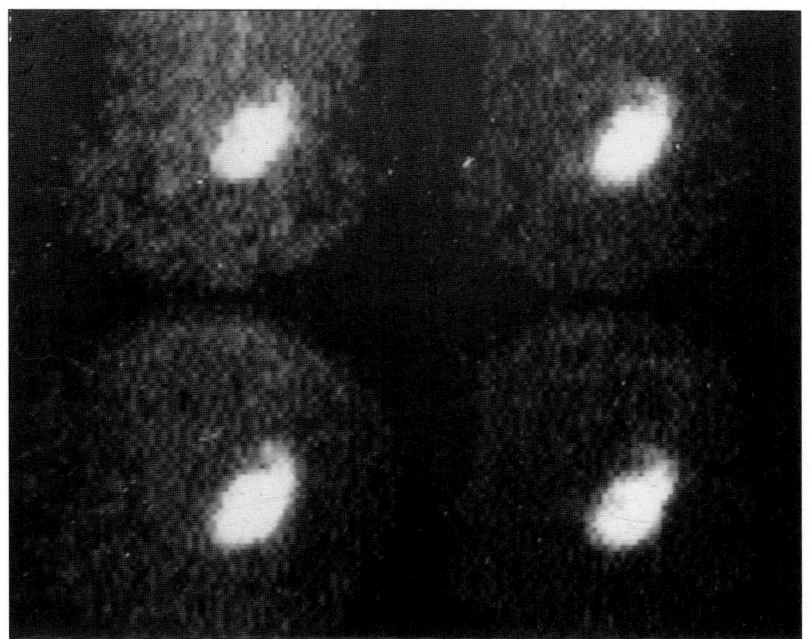

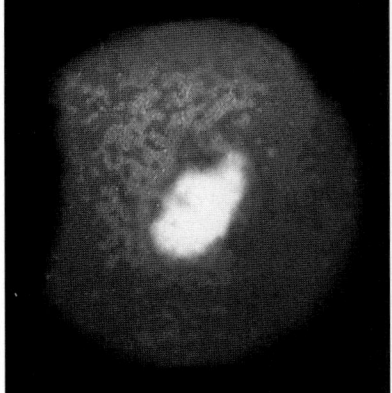
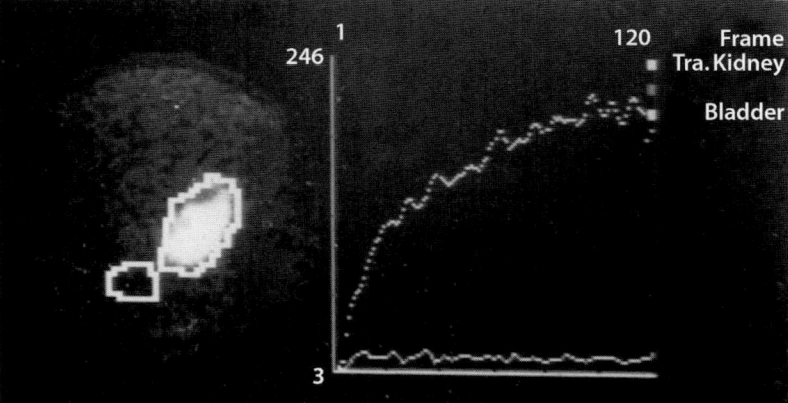

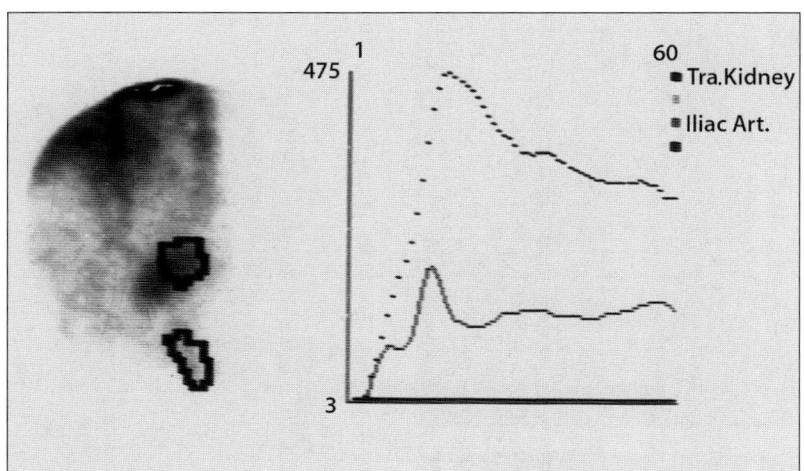

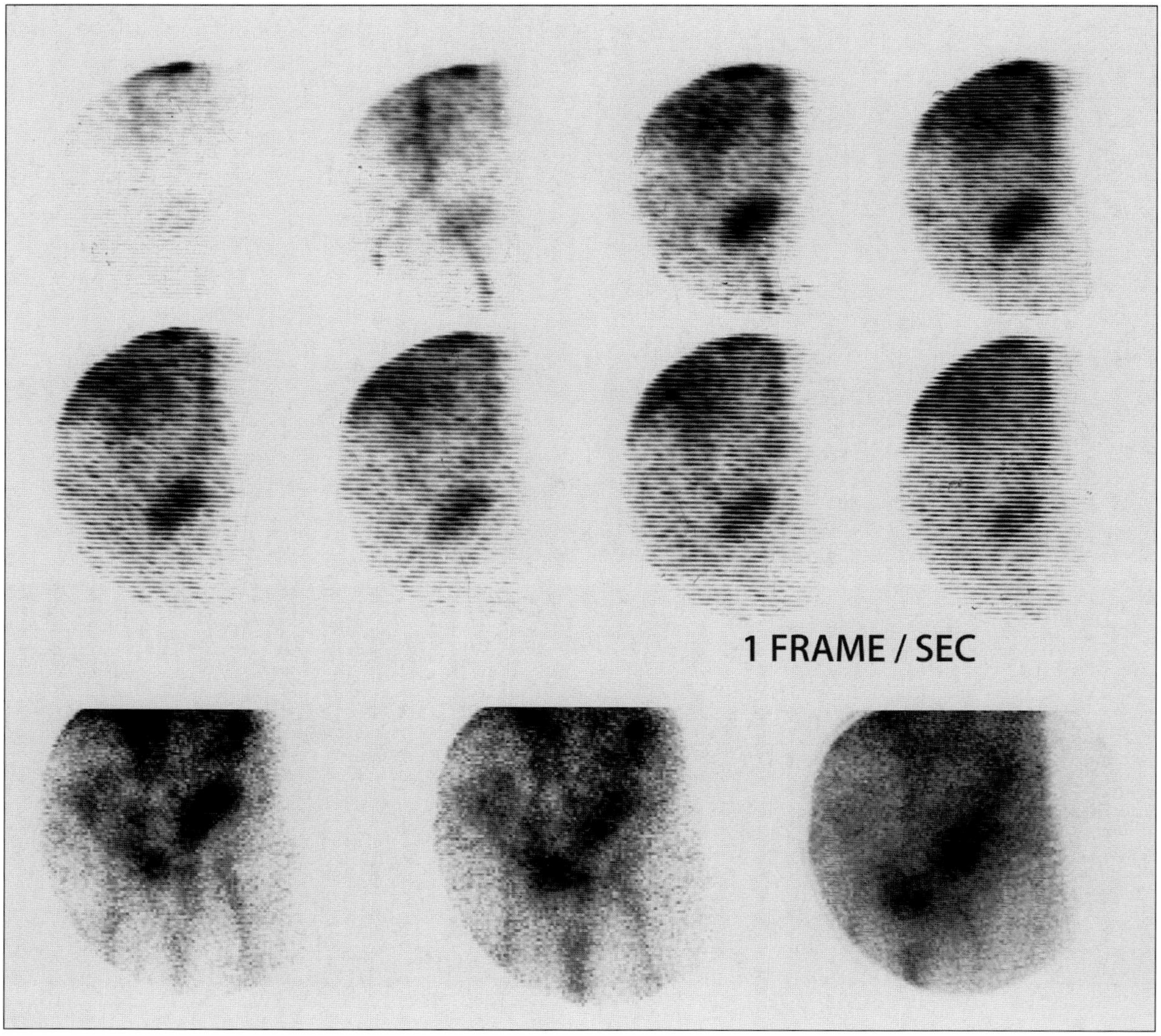

Fig. 3.115. Follow-up scan shows good graft perfusion with ectopic activity in the lesser pelvis caused by urinary extravasation

1 FRAME / SEC

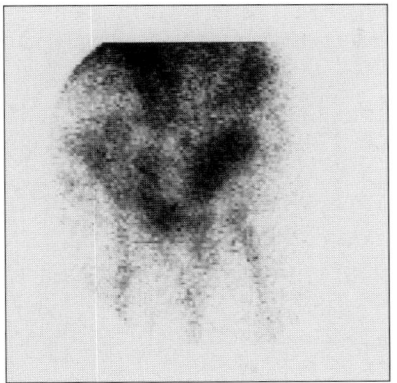

Fig. 3.115. *Continued*

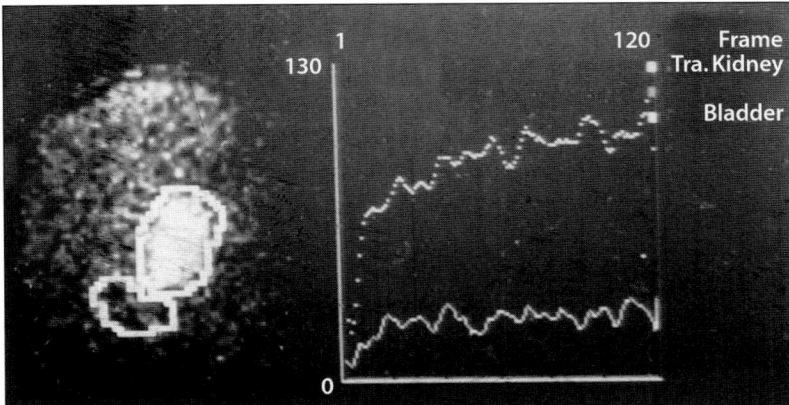

Fig. 3.116. Scan shows decreased, nonhomogeneous perfusion of the graft with activity in the lesser pelvis due to urinary extravasation. Impending rejection

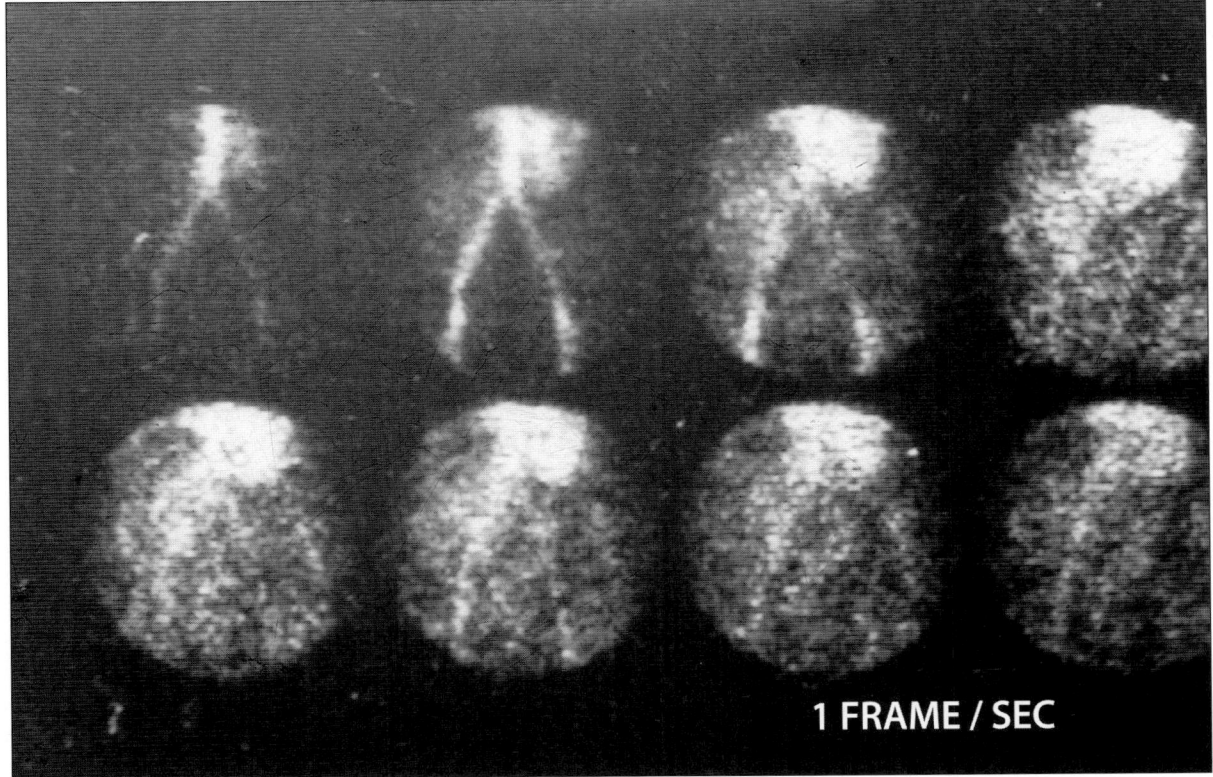

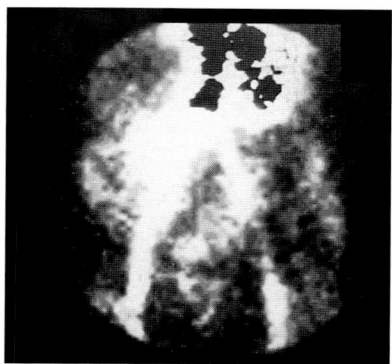

Fig. 3.116. Scan shows decreased, nonhomogeneous perfusion of the graft with activity in the lesser pelvis due to urinary extravasation. Impending rejection

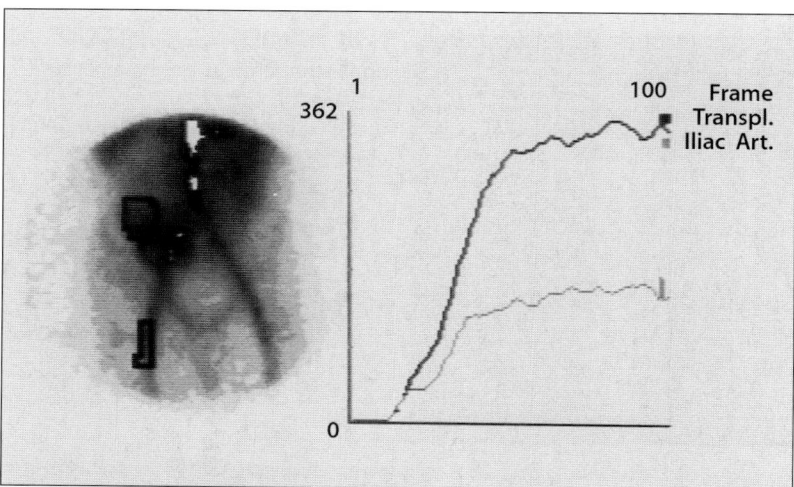

Fig. 3.117. Perfusion of this graft is delayed but still adequate. Diffuse nonhomogeneous uptake probably has a circulatory cause. No excretion was observed by the end of the examination. The scan findings are suspicious for interstitial nephritis

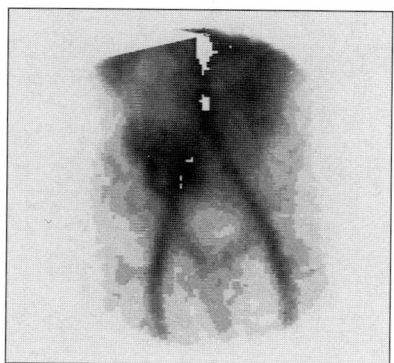

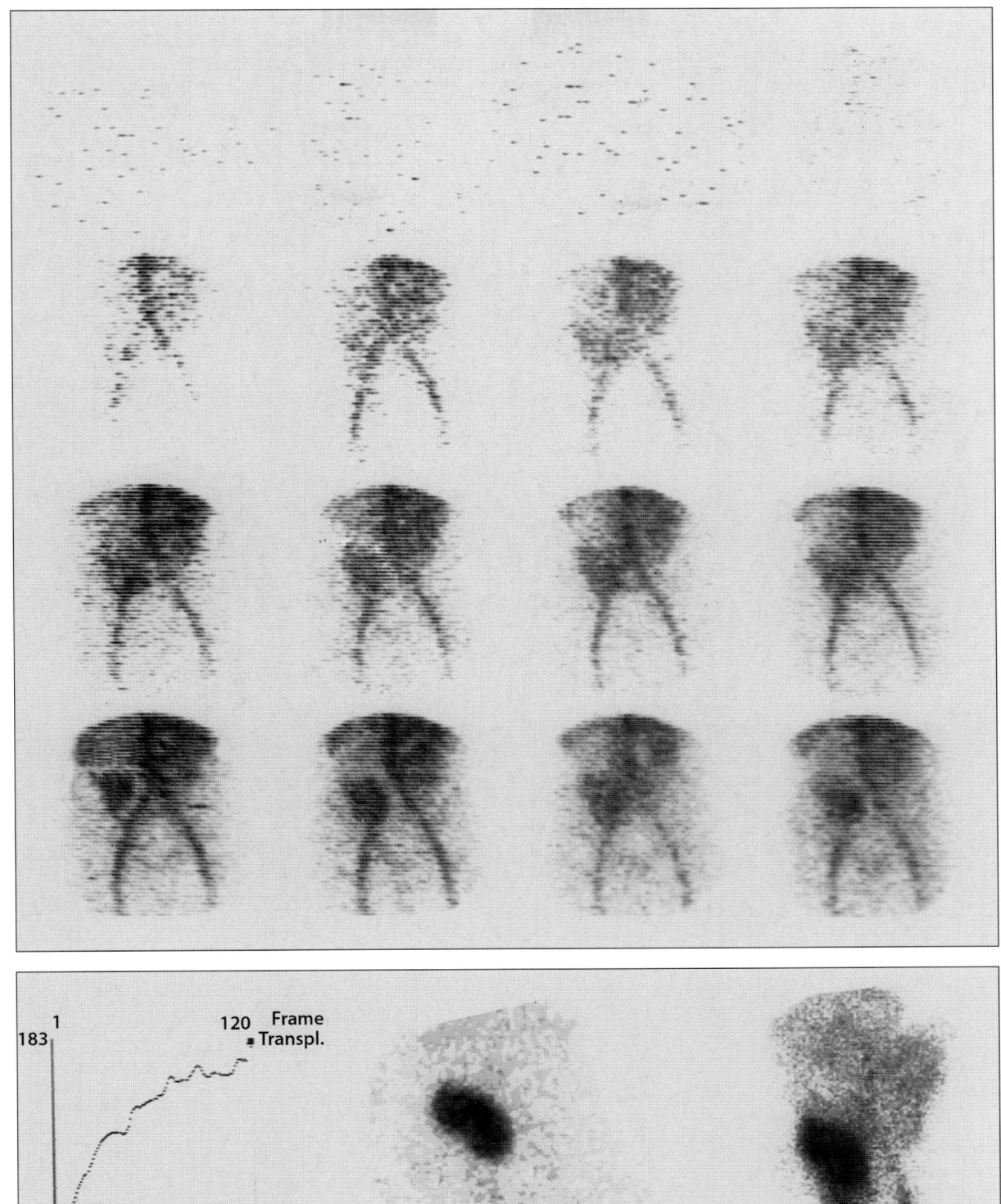

Fig. 3.117. *Continued*

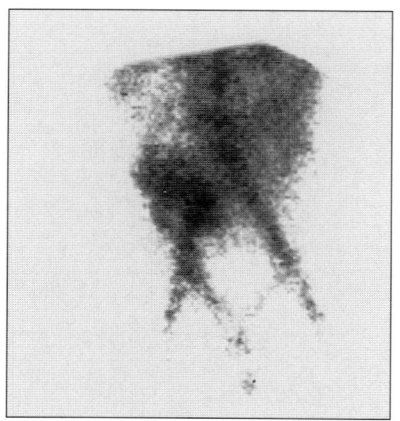

Fig. 3.117. Perfusion of this graft is delayed but still adequate. Diffuse nonhomogeneous uptake probably has a circulatory cause. No excretion was observed by the end of the examination. The scan findings are suspicious for interstitial nephritis

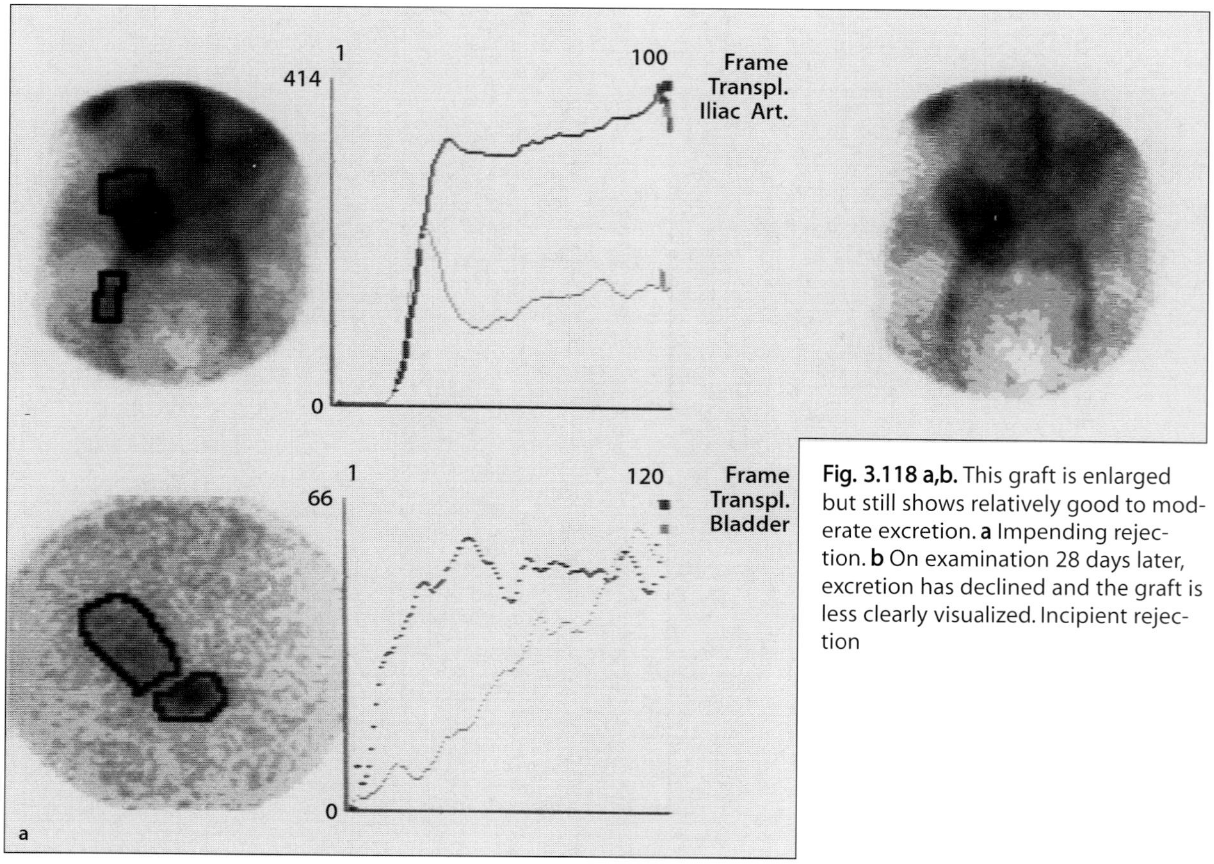

1

414

100   Frame
Transpl.
Iliac Art.

0

1

66

120   Frame
Transpl.
Bladder

Fig. 3.118 a,b. This graft is enlarged but still shows relatively good to moderate excretion. **a** Impending rejection. **b** On examination 28 days later, excretion has declined and the graft is less clearly visualized. Incipient rejection

0

a

Fig. 3.118 b

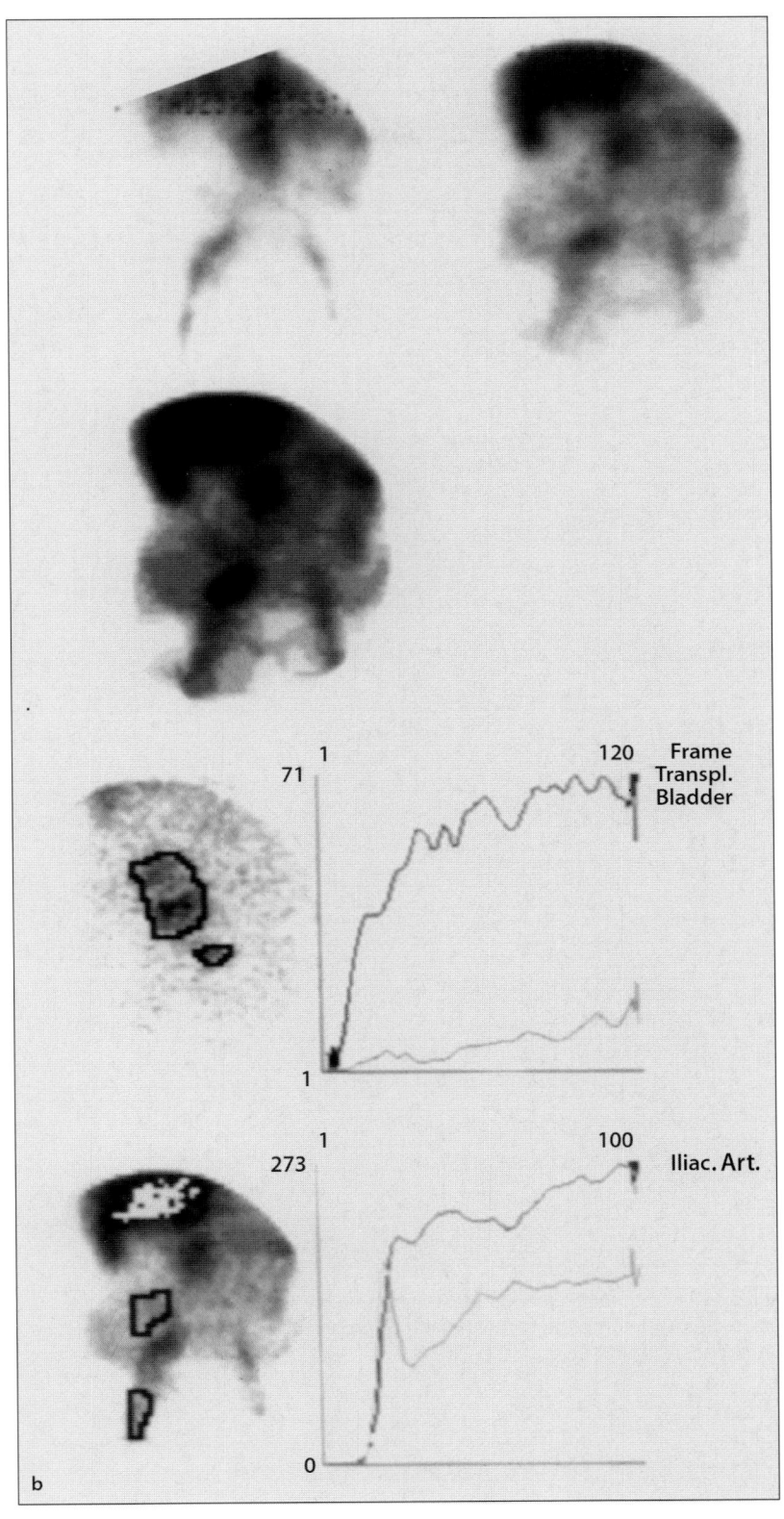

b

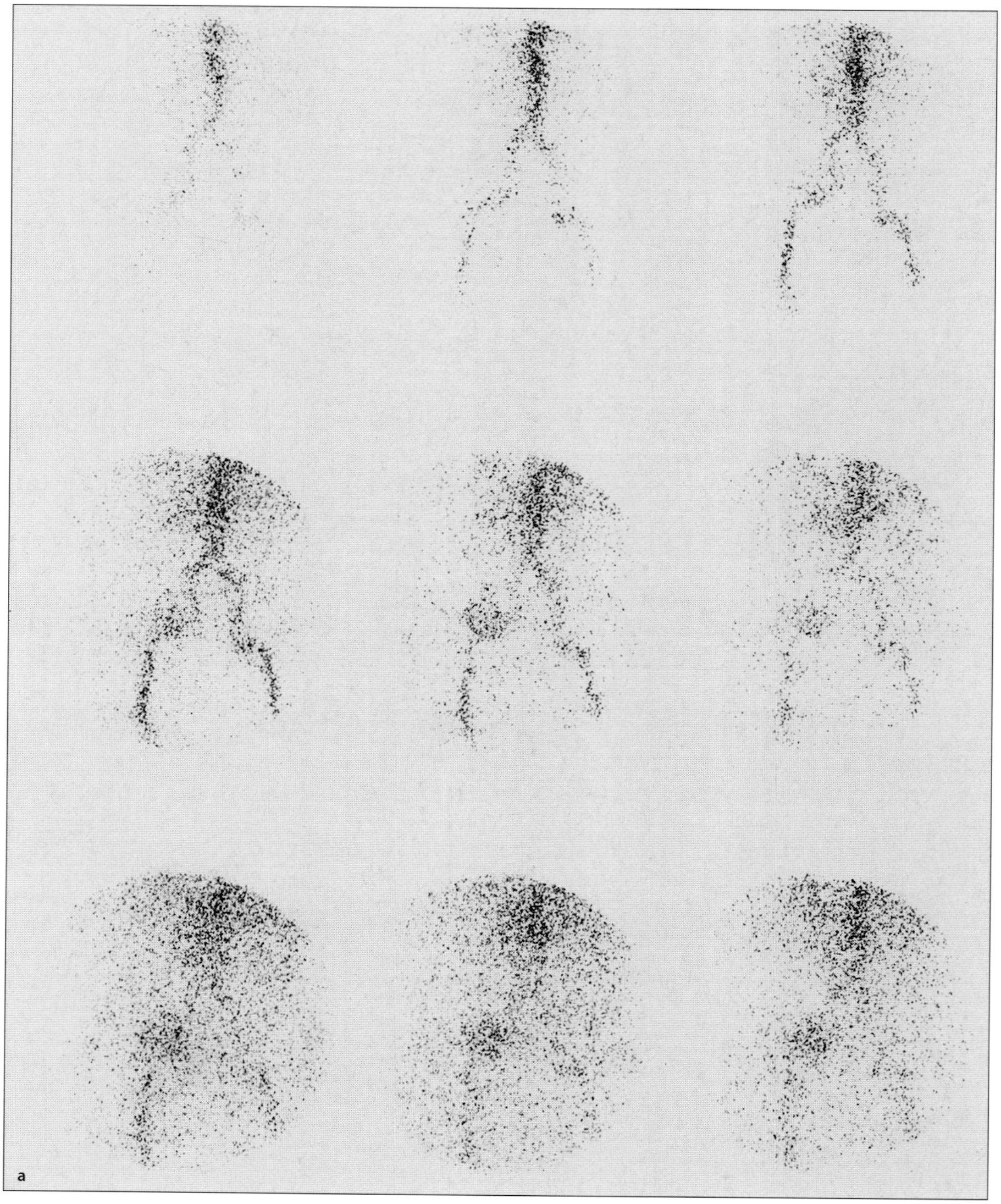

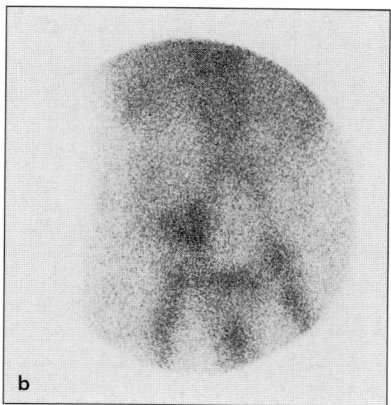

Fig. 3.119 a. Incipient rejection of a renal graft. b,c Incipient recovery. d–f Almost complete recovery with good perfusion, excretion, and opacification

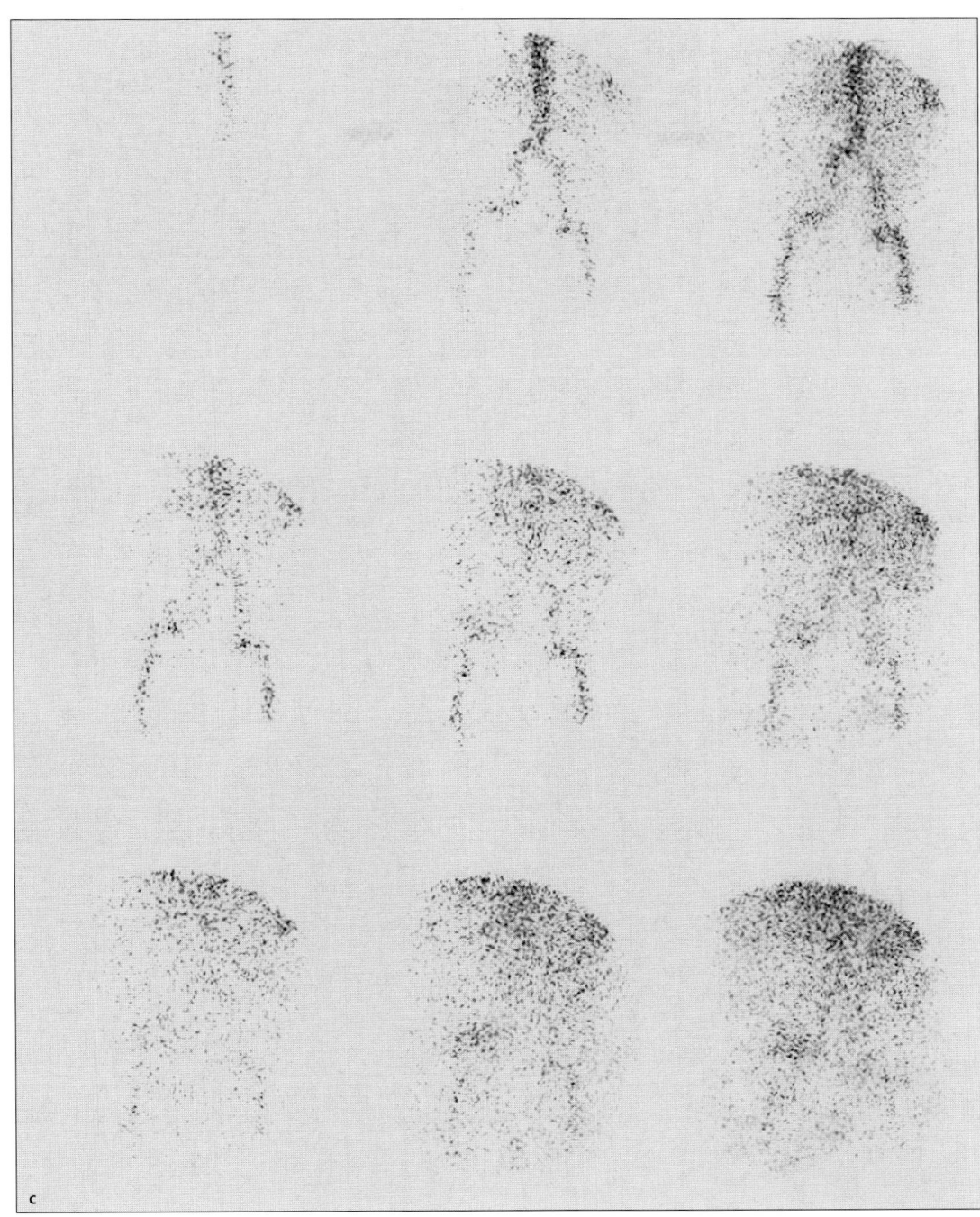

Fig. 3.119 c

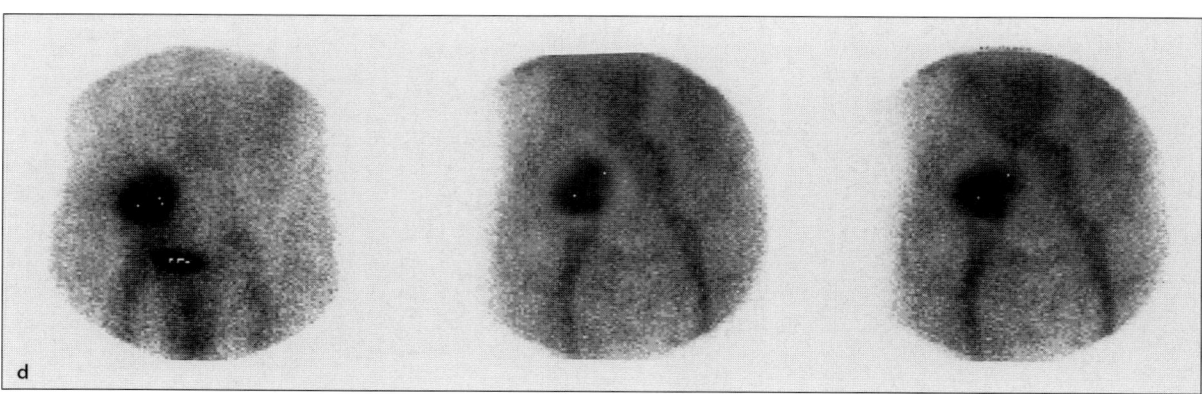

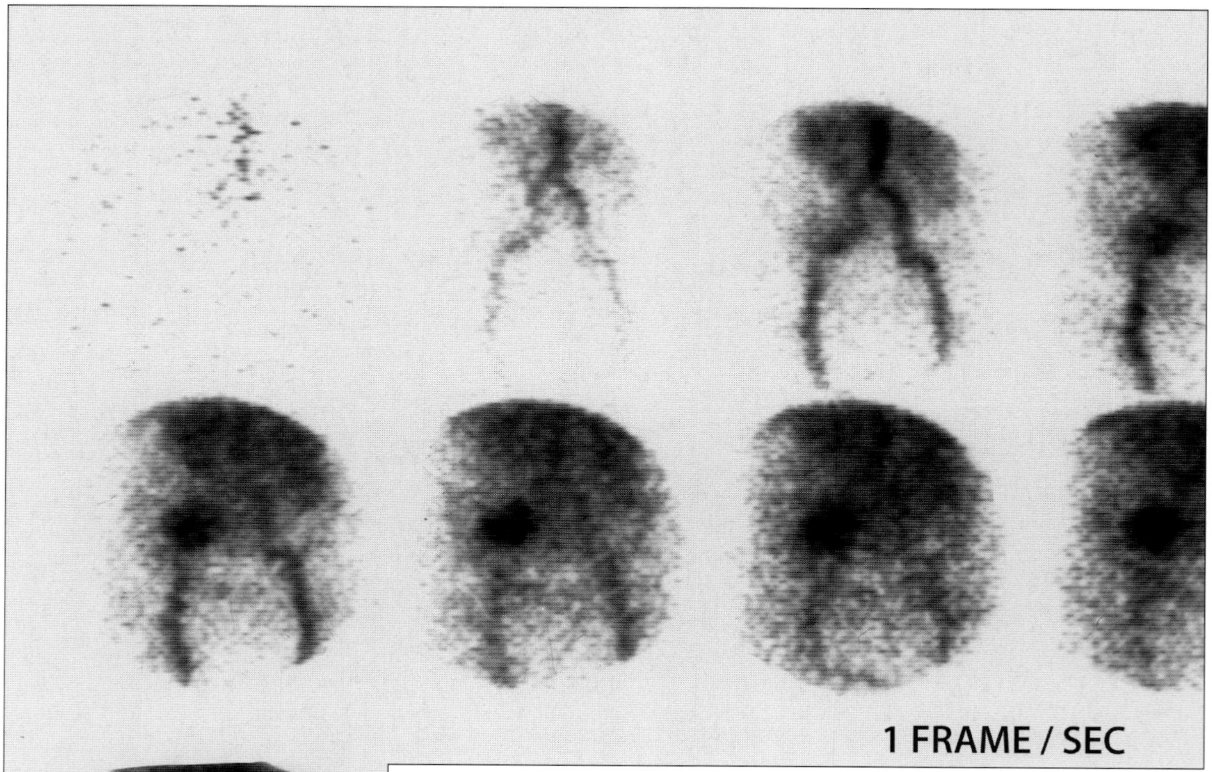

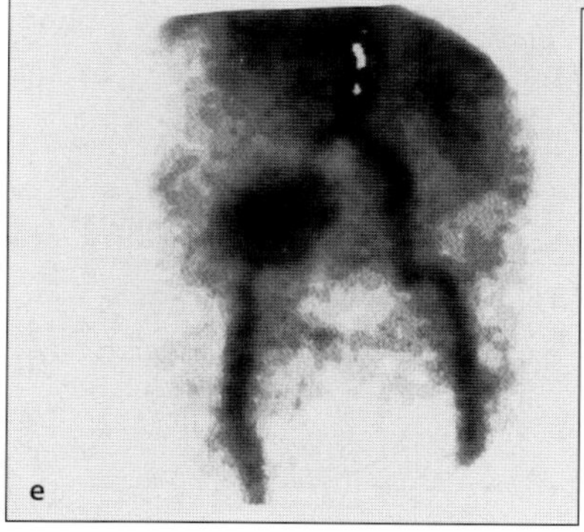

1 FRAME / SEC

Fig. 3.119. a Incipient rejection of a renal graft. **b,c** Incipient recovery.
d–f Almost complete recovery with good perfusion, excretion, and opacification

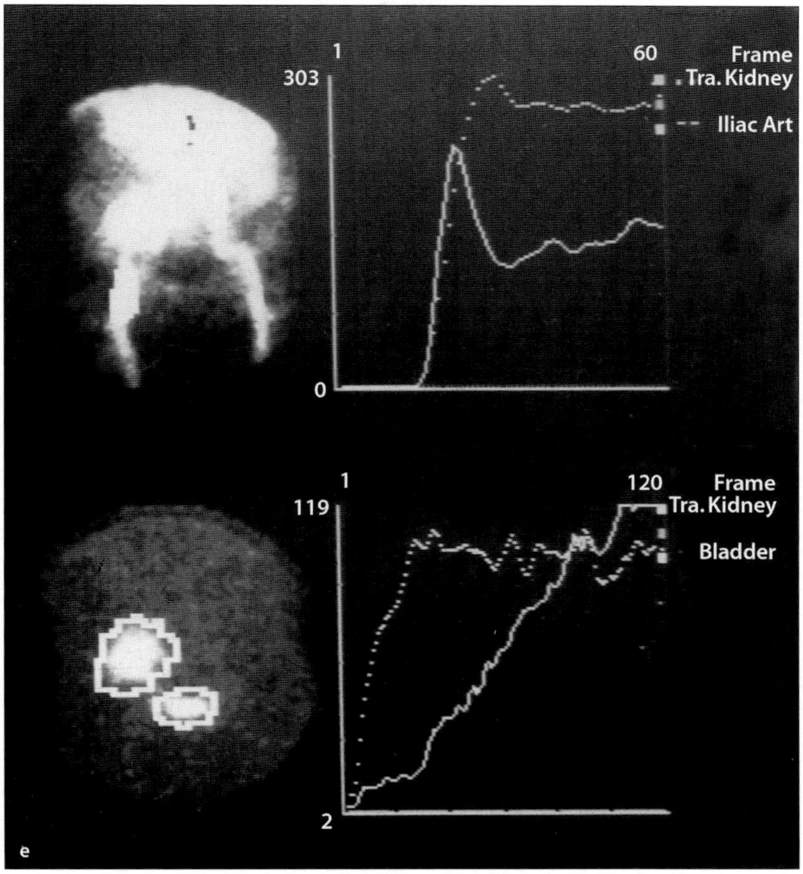

Fig. 3.119. e. *Continued*

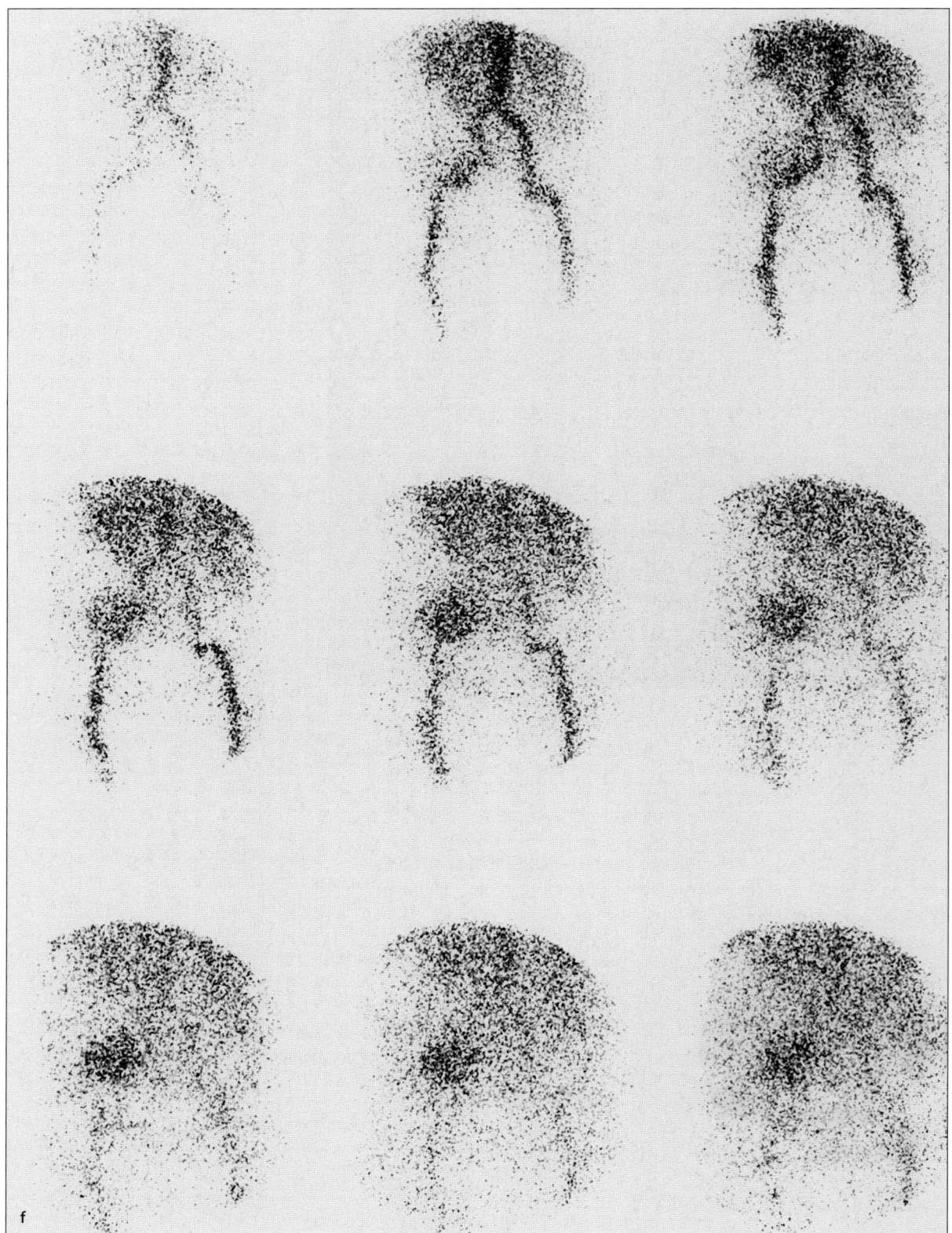

Fig. 3.119. a Incipient rejection of a renal graft. **b,c** Incipient recovery. **d–f** Almost complete recovery with good perfusion, excretion, and opacification

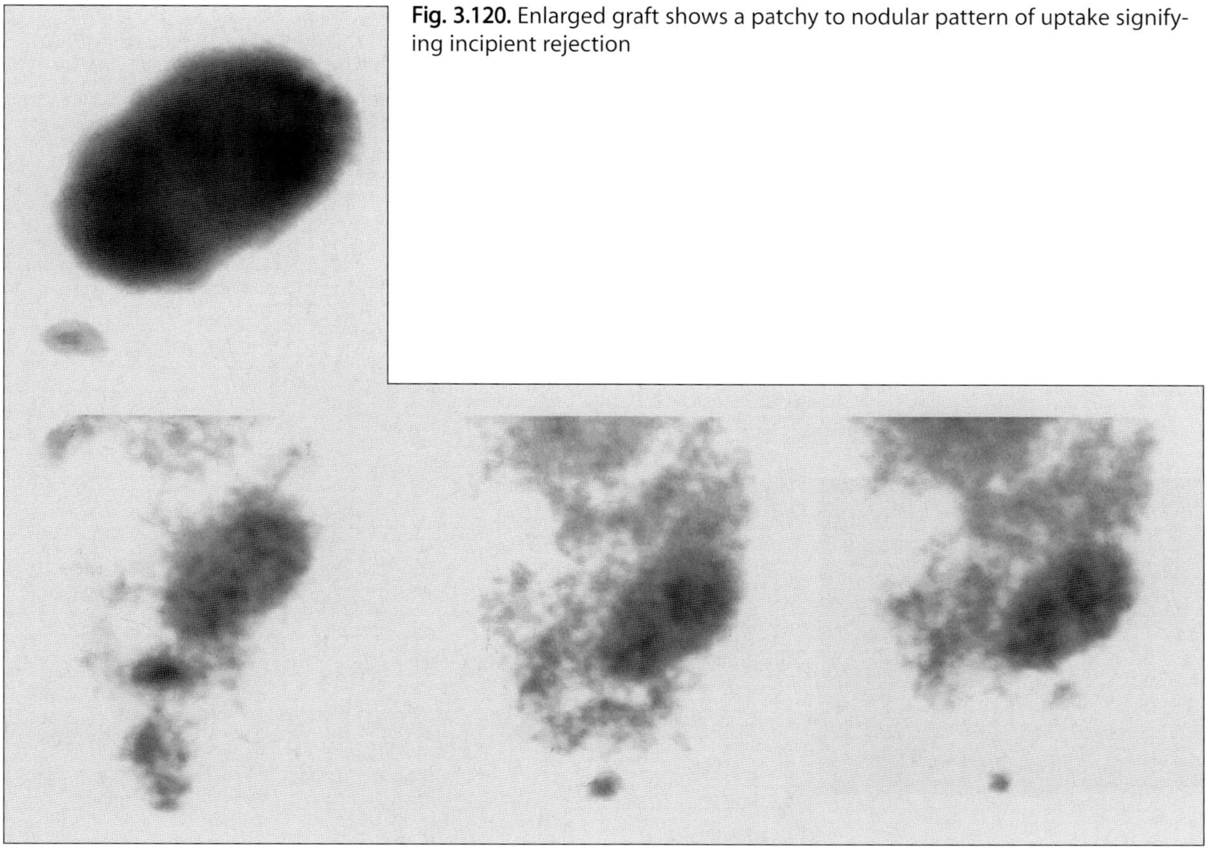

Fig. 3.120. Enlarged graft shows a patchy to nodular pattern of uptake signifying incipient rejection

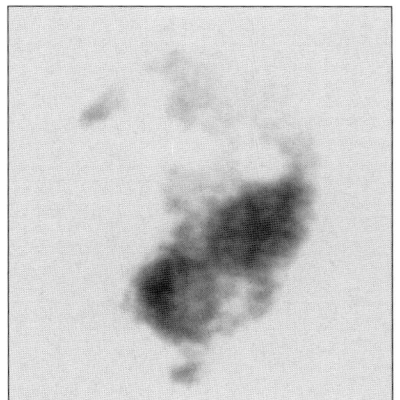

Fig. 3.121. Encapsulated hematoma located in the angle between the renal graft and bladder

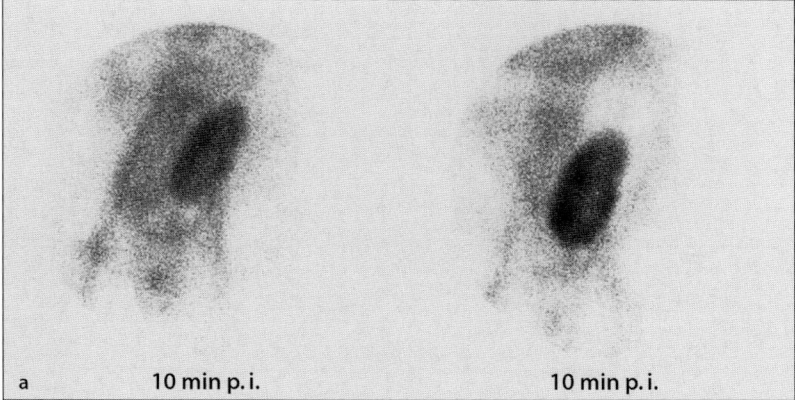

a   10 min p. i.   10 min p. i.

Fig. 3.122 a,b. Postsurgical hematoma in the upper portion of the graft (*a1, b1*). At follow-up 13 days later (*a2, b2*) the hematoma has become encapsulated, but seroma formation has occurred

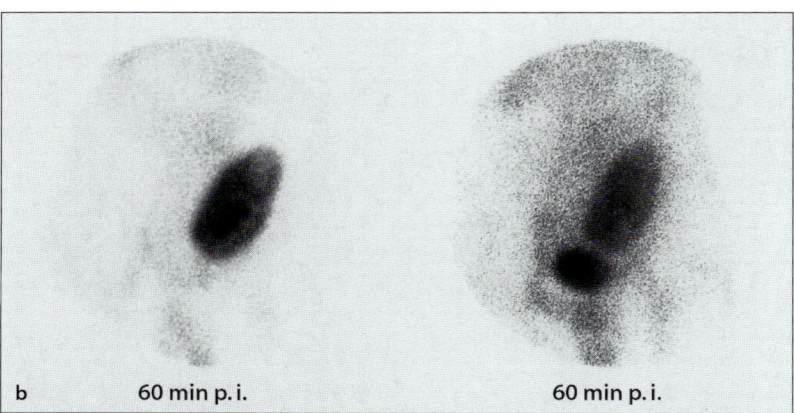

Fig. 3.122 a,b. Postsurgical hematoma in the upper portion of the graft (*a1, b1*). At follow-up 13 days later (*a2, b2*) the hematoma has become encapsulated, but seroma formation has occurred

b   60 min p.i.   60 min p.i.

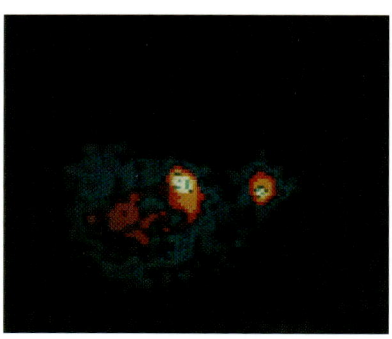

Fig. 3.123. Hyperplasia of the right adrenal gland

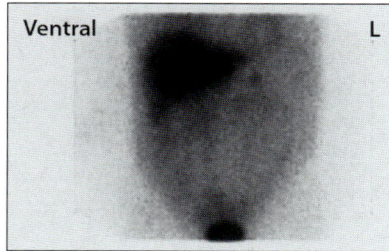

Ventral   L

Fig. 3.124. Adrenal pheochromocytoma imaged with meta-iodobenzylguanidine (MIBG)

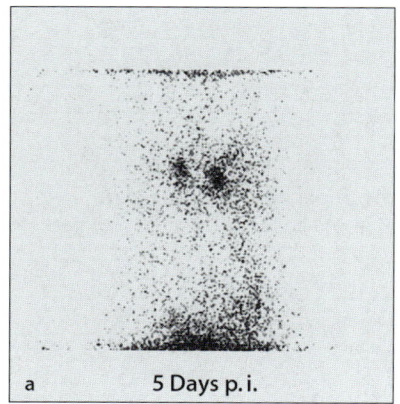

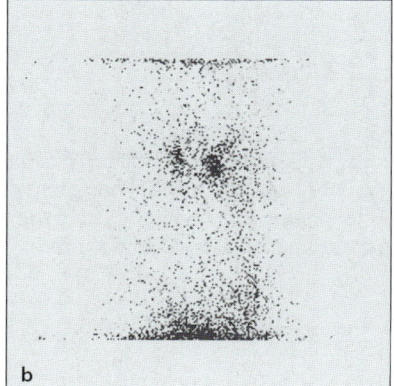

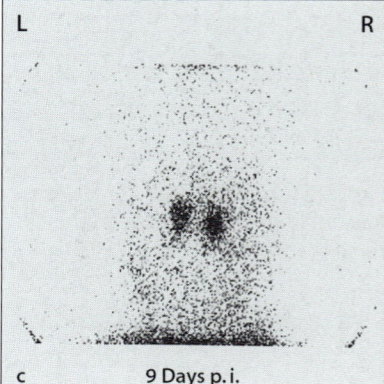

a   5 Days p.i.   b   L   R

c   9 Days p.i.

Fig. 3.125 a,b. Findings suspicious for adrenal hyperplasia

4 Bone

The human skeleton performs a dual function, providing mechanical support for the soft tissues while also serving as a mineral reservoir. The morphologic structure of the bone ensures a static load-bearing capacity that is appropriate for ordinary demands.

As a reservoir organ, the bone is subject to constant remodeling and intense metabolic activity, and therefore information on the morphologic and metabolic state of the organ is of particular relevance. The high radiation absorption of calcium is ideal for classic skeletal radiography, which can provide detailed structural images of bone. Skeletal pathology can be inferred from morphologic changes in the bone, but radiographs do not provide direct information on metabolic processes. In virtually all inquiries that are primarily morphologic in nature, nuclear medicine imaging is considered less informative than other techniques (ultrasound, CT, MRI). But in cases where the function of an organ is of primary interest, nuclear medicine is unequaled and continues to take precedence over the other modalities.

4.1 Sources of Error in Scan Interpretation

▌ Failure to obtain an adequate or accurate history (Figs. 4.1–4.3)
▌ Incomplete knowledge of topographic anatomy
▌ Omission of clinical inspection (Fig. 4.4 a, b)
▌ Acquiring static images in only one plane (Fig. 4.5 a, b)
▌ Misinterpretation of artifacts such as external contaminants or technical faults
  Classification of bone radiopharmaceuticals:
▌ Osteotropic agents: agents that are taken up by bone (bone tracers).
▌ Nonosteotropic agents: agents such as ^{67}Ga, which are not taken up by healthy bone tissue.

4.2 Benign and Malignant Bone Lesions, Fractures, Systemic Diseases

Radionuclide bone scans are unable to furnish a specific tissue diagnosis (this requires histologic evaluation). They can, however, narrow the differential diagnosis when the scan findings are correlated with clinical findings.

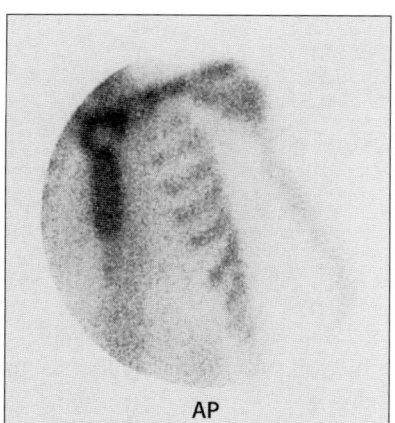

Fig. 4.1. Patient with a known plasmacytoma was evaluated for skeletal involvement. The bone scan shows a defect in the manubrium sterni. This should not be interpreted as sternal involvement by the underlying disease. A bone biopsy is required

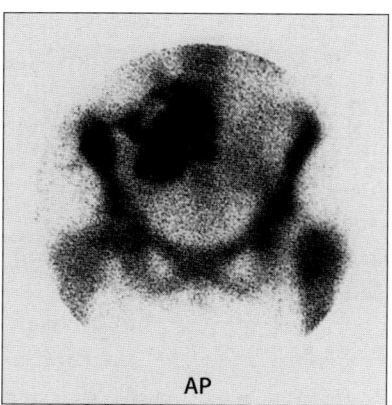

Fig. 4.2. Patient with known malignant lymphoma was evaluated for metastases. Bone scan shows an area of increased uptake projected over the iliosacral region and lower lumbar spine. This should not be interpreted as lymphomatous involvement. The cause is a Bricker bladder

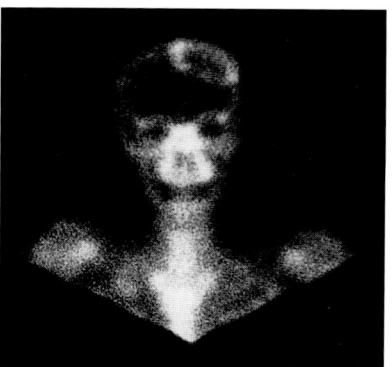

Fig. 4.3. Patient with breast carcinoma was evaluated for metastases. Bone scan shows a ringlike area of increased uptake in the skull with a cold center. This should not be interpreted as a metastasis with central necrosis. The patient's history identifies it as an old craniotomy site used to evacuate a posttraumatic hematoma

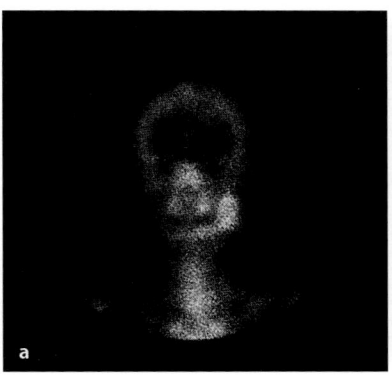
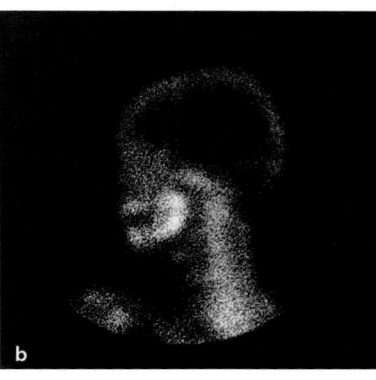

Fig. 4.4 a,b. Bone scan shows increased uptake throughout the mandible in a carcinoma patient. This is not caused by metastasis but by granulomas associated with dental disease

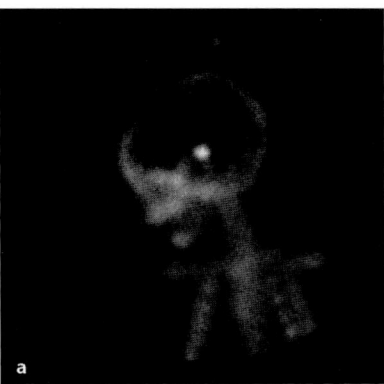
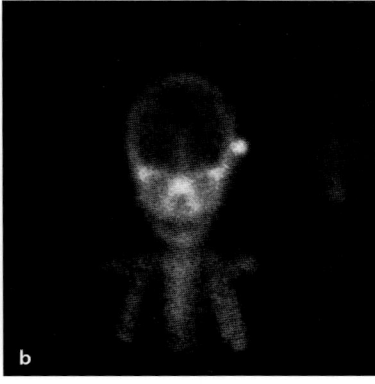

Fig. 4.5 a,b. Bone scan shows a temporal hot spot in a 1-year-old child screened for metastases. The AP image (**b**) identifies the spot as a contamination artifact

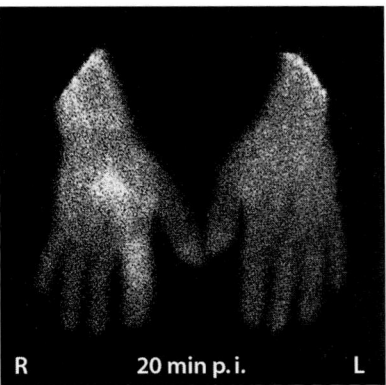

Fig. 4.6. A 44-year-old man presented with swelling on the radial side of the palm and at the distal end of the index finger with intermittent painful motion. The early static images (20 min after injection of 15 mCi ^{99m}Tc MDP) show areas of intense uptake in the second and third metacarpals and in the metacarpophalangeal joint of the index finger. This finding is not seen on the delayed static images (2 hours postinjection). The hypervascular lesion is a hemangioma

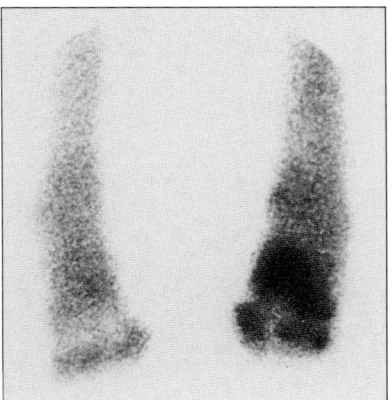

Fig. 4.7. A 42-year-old diabetic woman presented with swelling in the metatarsal region. Image at 2 hours postinjection shows intense uptake in the region, consistent with diabetic osteomyelitis

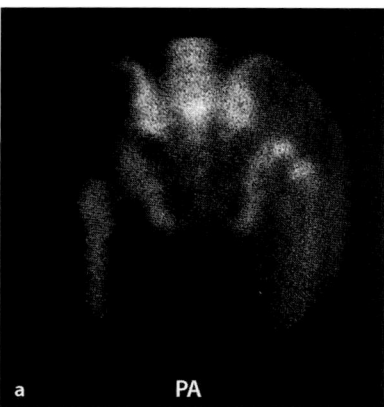

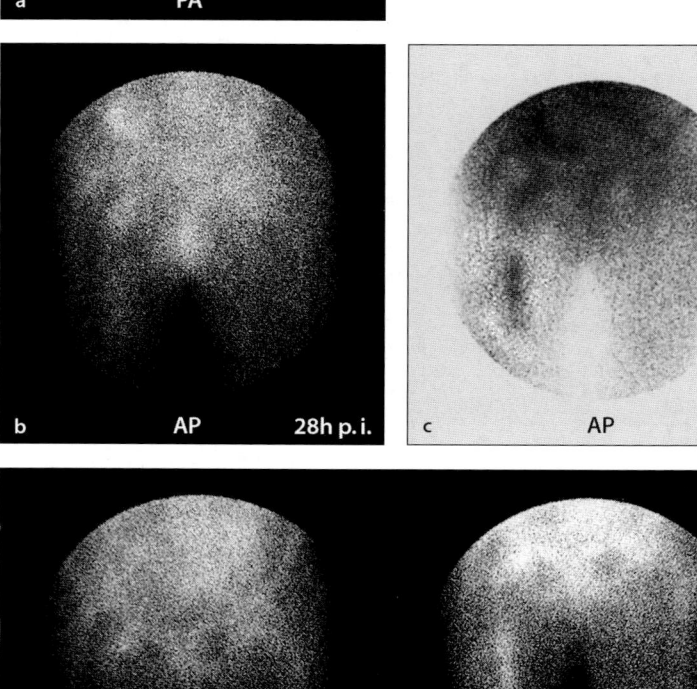

Fig. 4.8 a–d. A 50-year-old man with a prosthetic hip replacement presented with painful motion of the operated hip. **a** Bone scan 2 hours after injection of 15 mCi ^{99m}Tc MDP shows a hot spot in the lateral portion of the right acetabulum and in the right greater trochanter. Side-to-side comparison shows slightly increased uptake around the stem of the femoral component. **b–d** The findings are even more conspicuous on ^{67}Ga citrate scans acquired at 6, 28 and 48 hours and confirm prosthetic loosening with a local inflammatory response. It is noteworthy that radiographs did not yet show any abnormalities

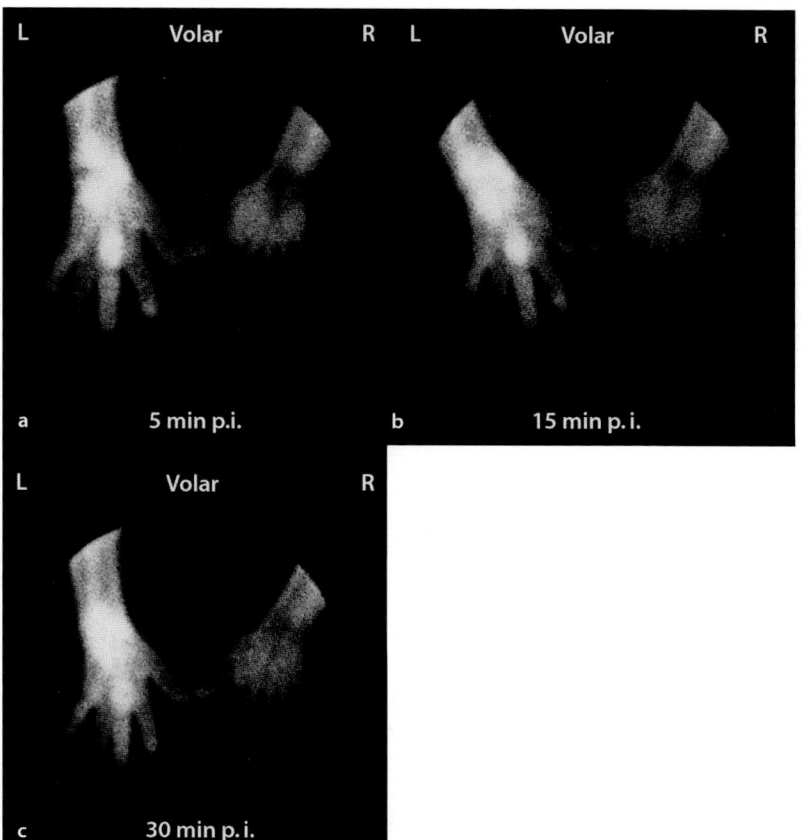

Fig. 4.9 a–c. A 39-year-old woman had her wrist immobilized for a suspected navicular fracture. Early static images acquired at 5 min, 15 min, and 30 min after injection of 15 mCi ^{99m}Tc MDP show markedly increased uptake, visible also on the delayed statics. 264,858 counts were obtained over the wrist compared with 9462 on the contralateral side. The scan findings are consistent with reflex sympathetic dystrophy

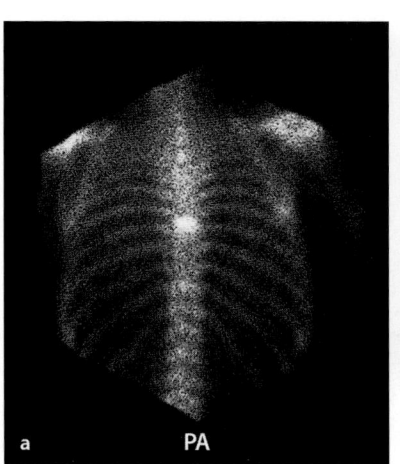

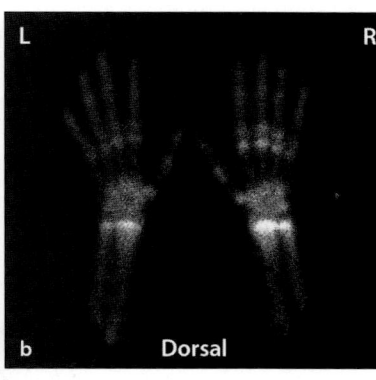

Fig. 4.10 a,b. An 18-year-old uremic patient on dialysis complained of pain in his chest and both wrists (right > left). Scan 2 hours after injection of ^{99m}Tc MDP shows increased uptake in the T7 vertebra (**a**) and distal end of the right radius (**b**). Osteoporosis-related compression fractures of the T7 vertebra and right radius

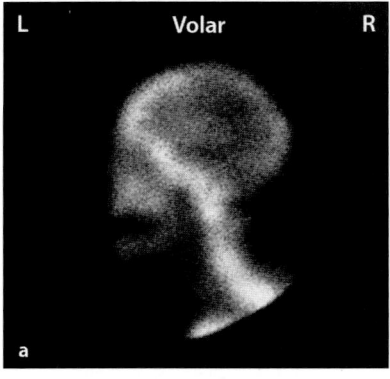

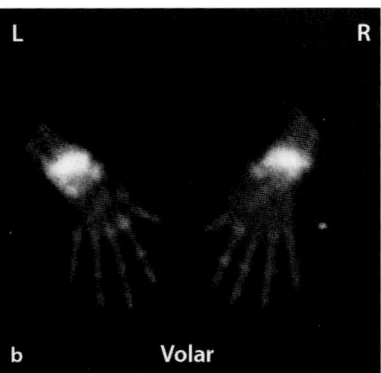

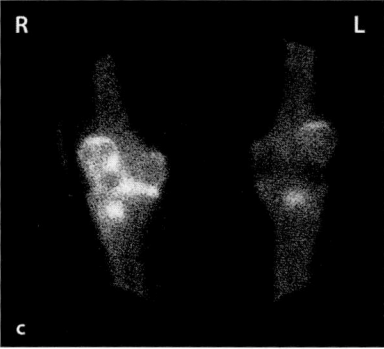

Fig. 4.11 a–c. A 20-year-old woman with psoriasis presented with bilateral wrist pain. Scan 2 hours after injection of ^{99m}Tc MDP shows intense uptake in all metacarpophalangeal and proximal interphalangeal joints of both hands (b) as a manifestation of extracutaneous involvement by the underlying disease

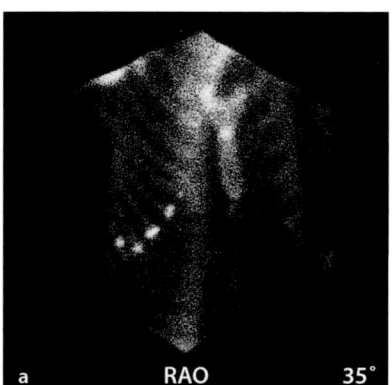

Fig. 4.12 a,b. Woman 41 years of age with back pain. a Scan 2 hours after injection of ^{99m}Tc MDP shows hot spots in the 5th through 9th ribs on the right side with otherwise normal skeletal findings. The scan findings, plus the patient's recollection of a household accident, establish the diagnosis of serial rib fractures. b Incidental note is made of urinary stasis in the right kidney, which could account for the back pain

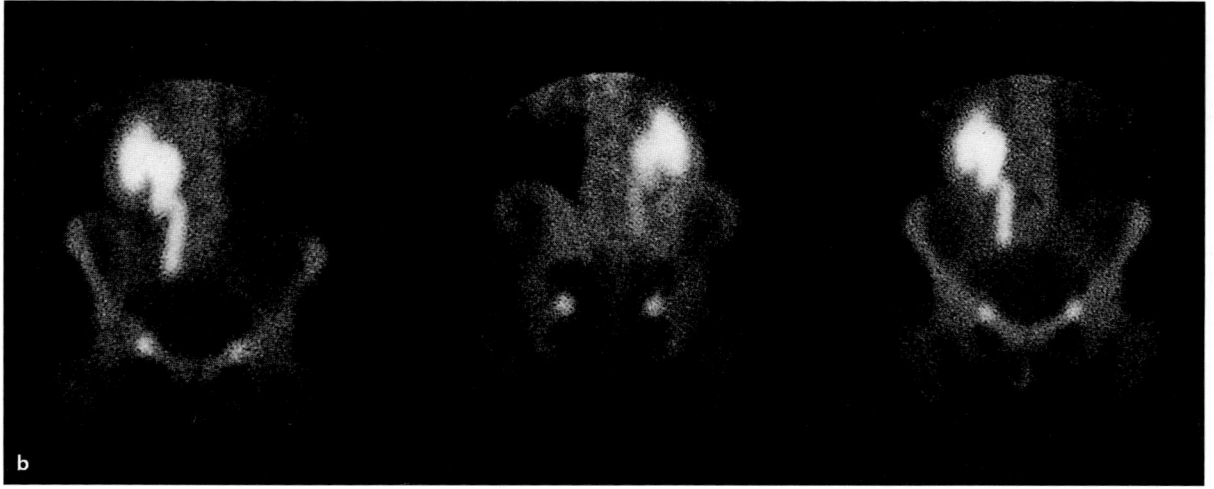

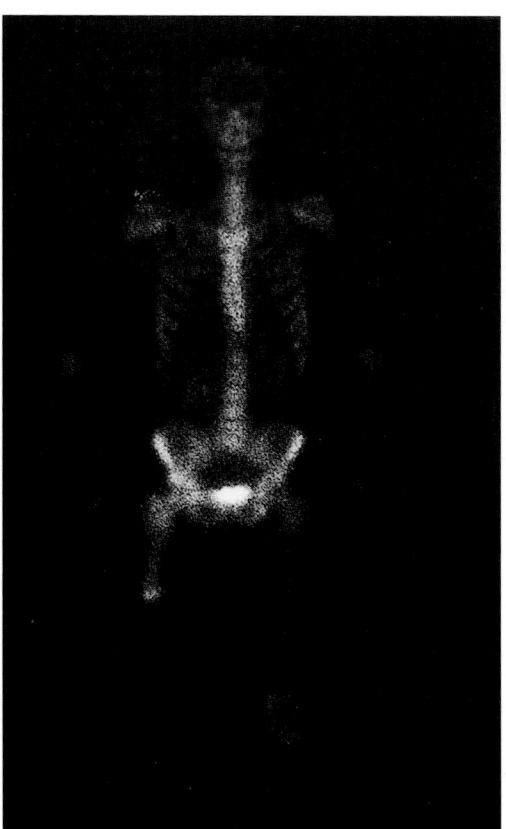

Fig. 4.13. Man 50 years of age had a midthigh leg amputation 30 years ago. He presented now with pain, redness, and slight swelling of the stump. Scan 2 hours after injection of bone tracer shows a hot spot in the distal end of the stump, signifying inflammation due to irritation

Fig. 4.14 a–c. A 60-year-old man with cachexia and low back pain was evaluated for suspected vertebral metastases. The bone scan shows no skeletal abnormalities but does show enlargement of the right kidney, which appears as a scalloped mass. Angiography and surgery disclosed hypernephroid carcinoma

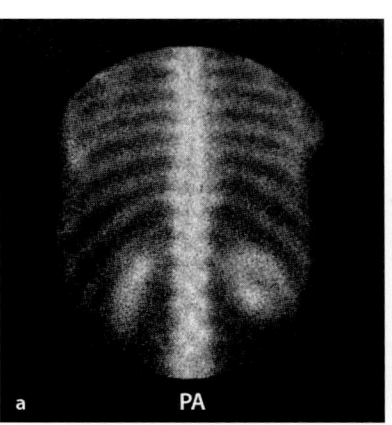

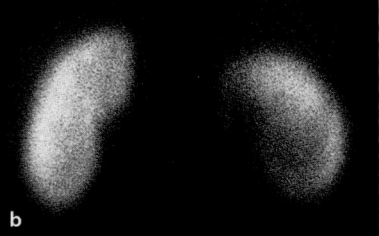

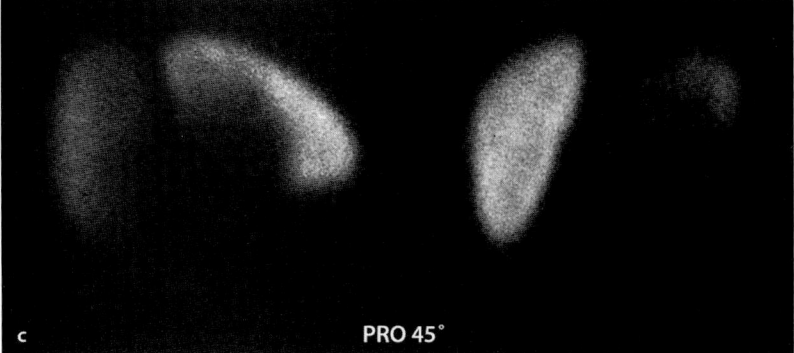

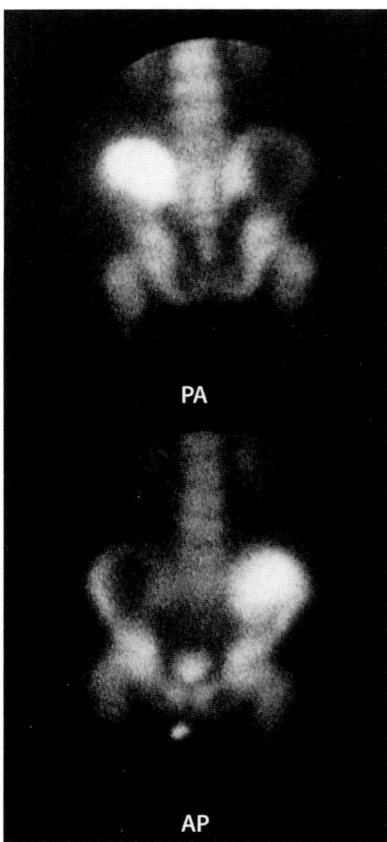

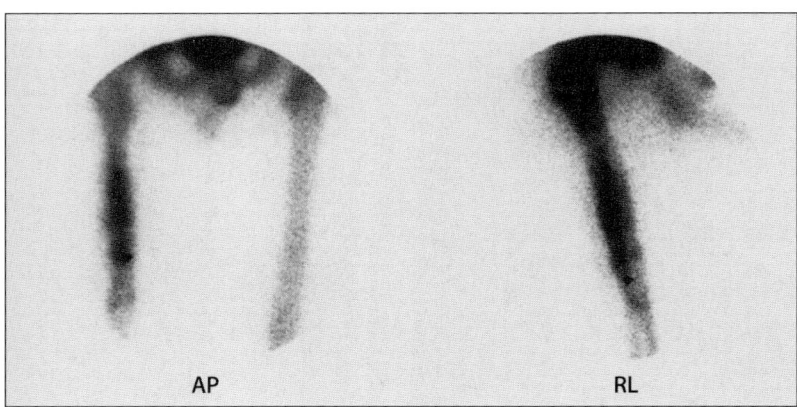

Fig. 4.16. This patient underwent surgical treatment of a juvenile bone cyst of the right femur that included plating of the bone. He presented now with walking difficulties. Bone scan shows intense but nonhomogeneous uptake in the plate bed, signifying a rejection response. Surgical removal of the plate confirmed the diagnosis

Fig. 4.15. A 40-year-old man with a known hydatid liver cyst complained of walking difficulties. Scan 2 hours after injection of bone tracer shows an area of intense uptake with a spongy structure, indicating pelvic involvement by echinococcal cysts

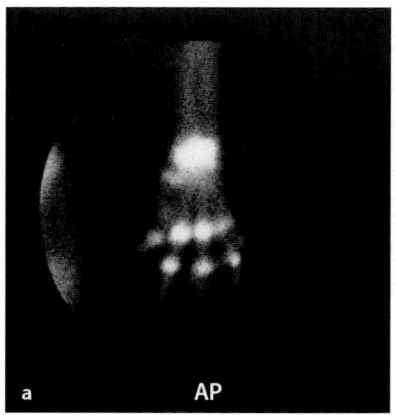

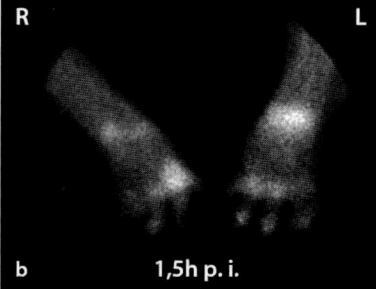

Fig. 4.17 a,b. Woman 55 years of age was evaluated for possible exacerbation of rheumatoid arthritis (RA). **a** Early static images show increased uptake in the right wrist and in the metacarpophalangeal joints of the second and third fingers of both hands, indicating a local flare-up. **b** Delayed static images show intense uptake in both wrists and all the hand joints due to RA

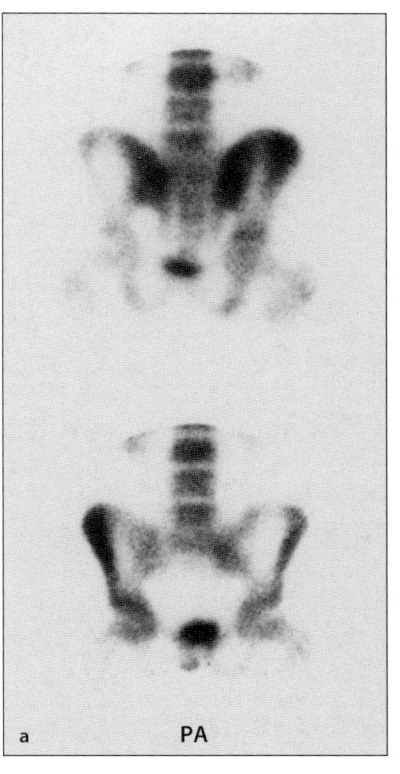

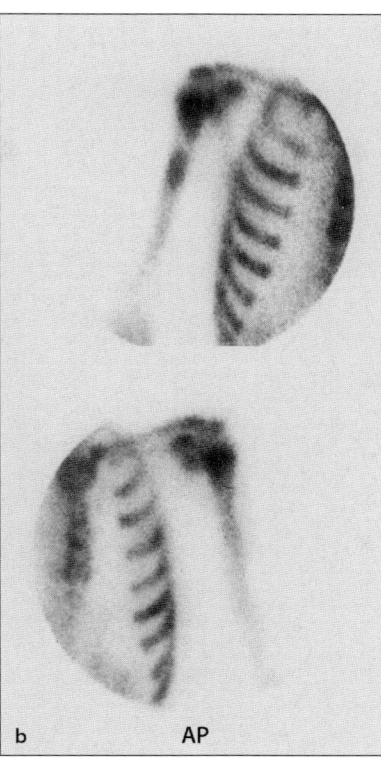

Fig. 4.18 a,b. A 14-year-old boy experienced back pain while playing soccer three days before. Radiographs showed slight rarefaction in the iliac wing with no other apparent abnormalities in the lumbar region. Bone scanning was performed to exclude osteomyelitis. The scan shows multiple hot spots in the pelvis (**a**, corresponding to the radiograph) and in the L3 to L5 vertebrae, ribs, and right humerus (**b**). A complete workup at a pediatric hospital revealed stage IV neuroblastoma with skeletal metastases

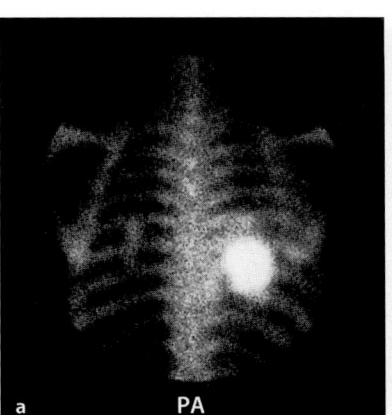

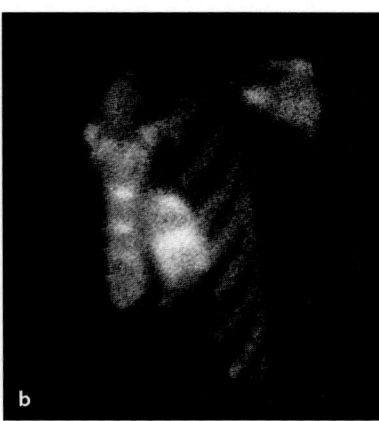

Fig. 4.19 a,b. Follow-up examination was performed in a 19-year-old boy whose left leg had been disarticulated for osteosarcoma. Scan 2 hours after injection of bone tracer shows no signs of skeletal metastases but does show an elliptical area of paravertebral increased uptake on the right side and a vertical band of activity on the left side. The right-sided lesion is a calcified necrotic metastasis, and the left lesion represents pleural calcification

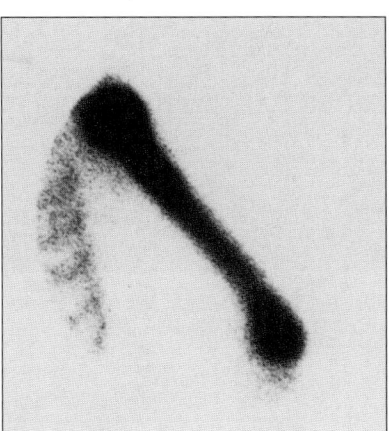

Fig. 4.20. A 76-year-old woman was examined for unexplained swelling of the upper arm. The bone scan shows very intense uptake throughout the humerus that does not transgress joint lines. This pattern is characteristic of Paget's disease

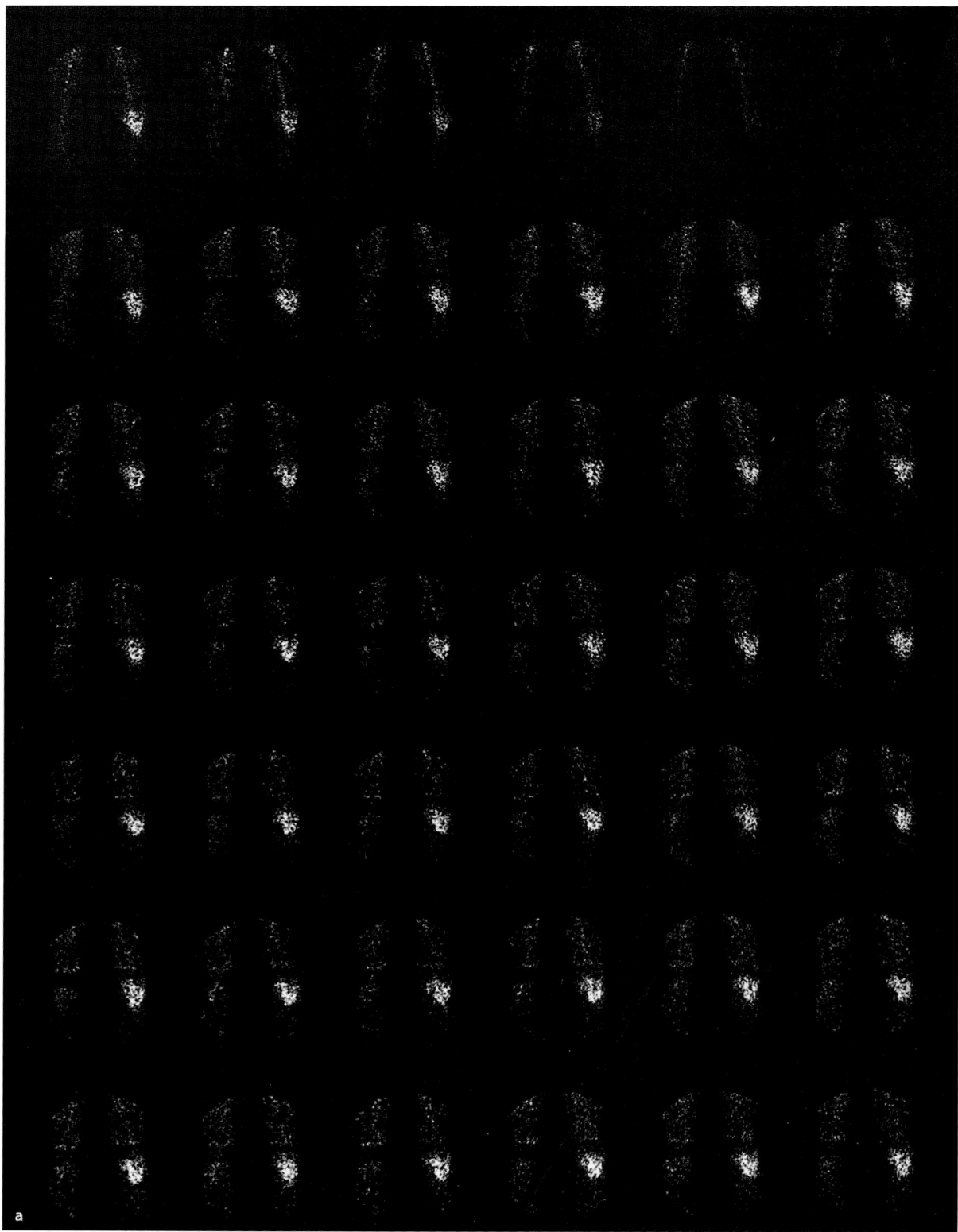

Fig. 4.21 a–c. While playing sports, a 17-year-old boy experienced knee pain that persisted for one week. The early static images (42 serial images acquired at 2-second intervals) show a hypervascular area in the proximal tibia that is still clearly visible in the 2-hour image. Histology confirmed osteosarcoma

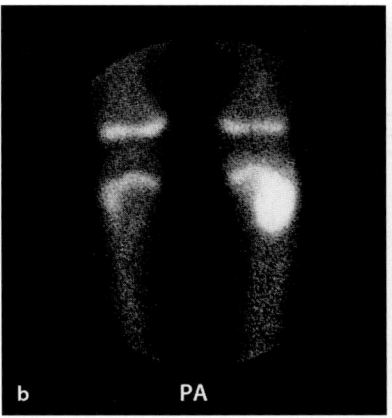

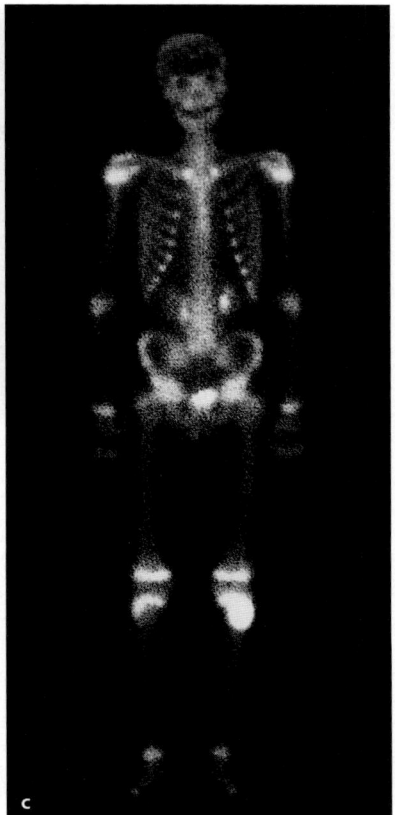

Fig. 4.21 b, c

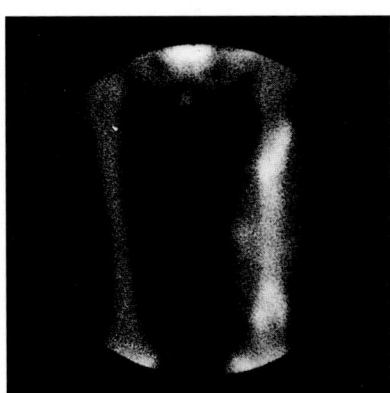

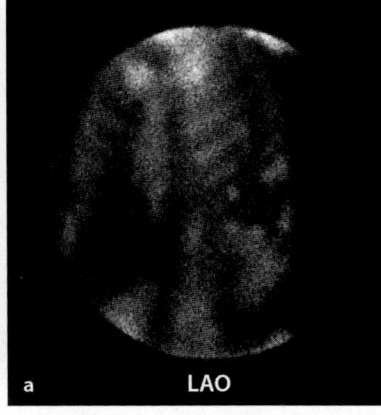

Fig. 4.23 a,b. Follow-up bone scan in a 39-year-old woman with Hodgkin's sarcoma. The 2-hour image shows focal areas of intense uptake, some with cold centers, in the skull and ribs. The scan findings are consistent with metastases from the primary sarcoma. The cold spots represent necrotic foci in some of the metastases

Fig. 4.22. A 13-year-old girl presented with a painful swelling of the thigh. Bone scan 2 hours after injection of bone tracer shows very intense uptake throughout the femur with irregular margins. Biopsy identified the lesion as chondrosarcoma

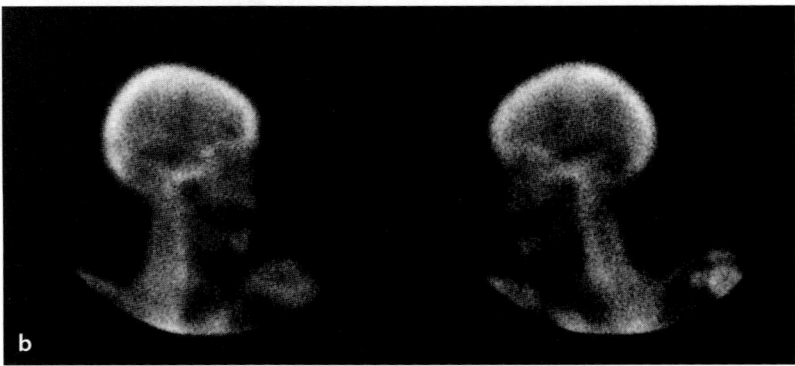

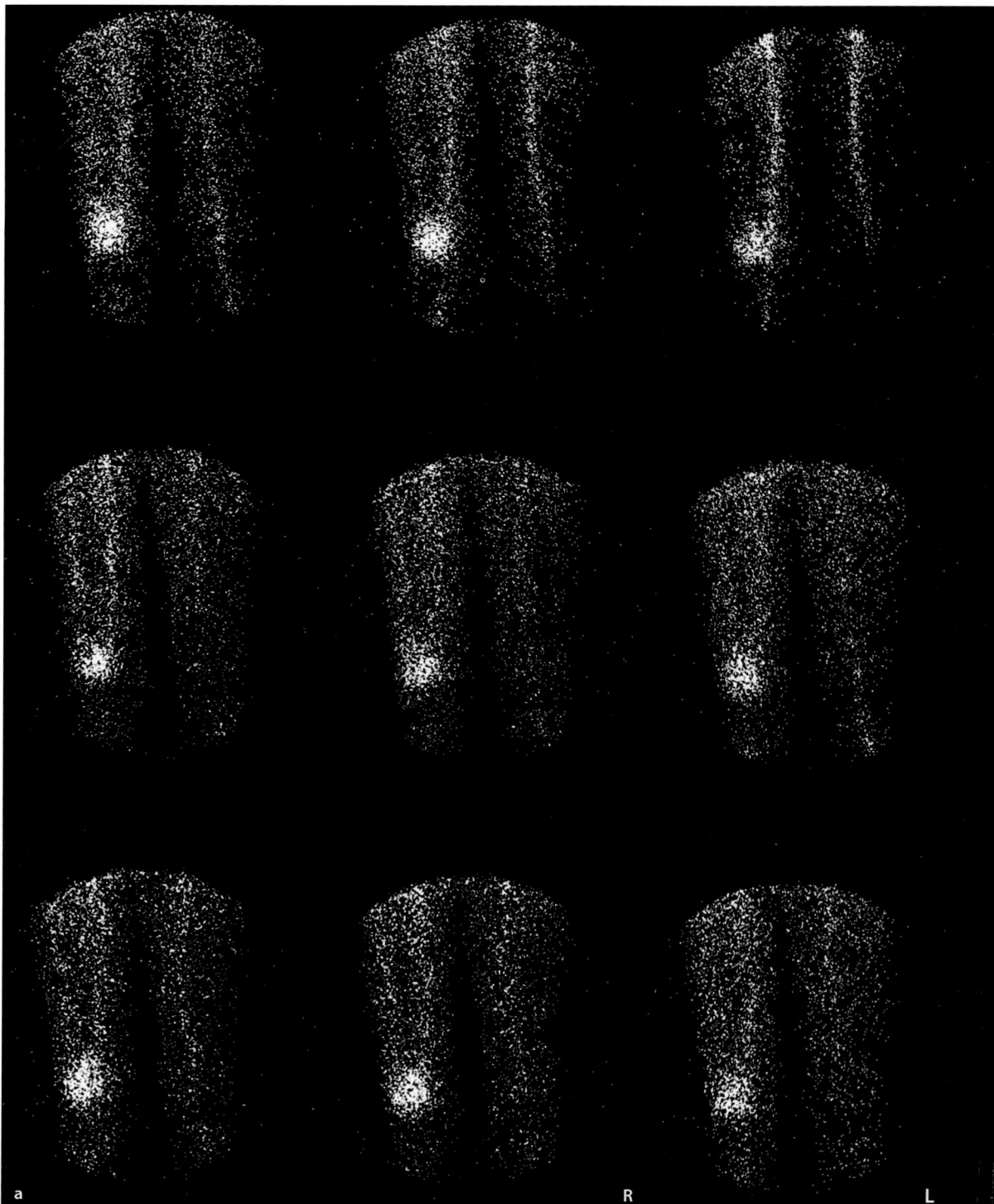

Fig. 4.24 a–c. A 12-year-old boy presented with a four-week history of knee pain. An immediate postinjection image sequence was acquired at 6-second intervals for 54 seconds, and a whole-body scan was performed at 2 hours. A hypervascular lesion is seen in the distal, periarticular portion of the femur and is still visible in the 2-hour image. The lesion is located in the distal femoral metaphysis with extension to the epiphyseal plate. Histology revealed pleomorphic cell osteosarcoma

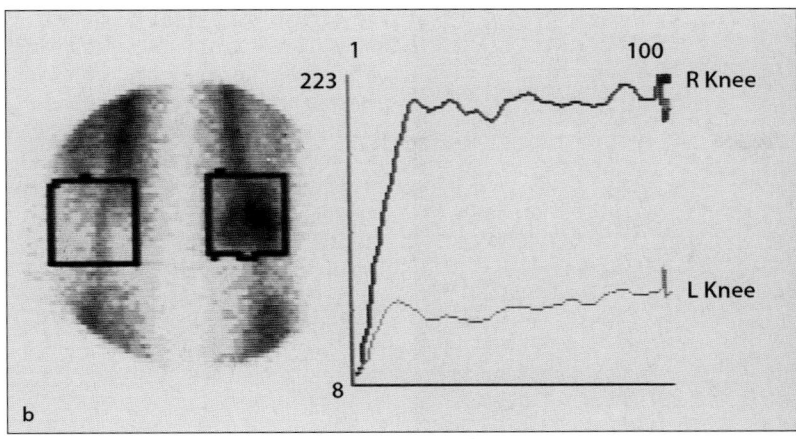

Fig. 4.24 b, c

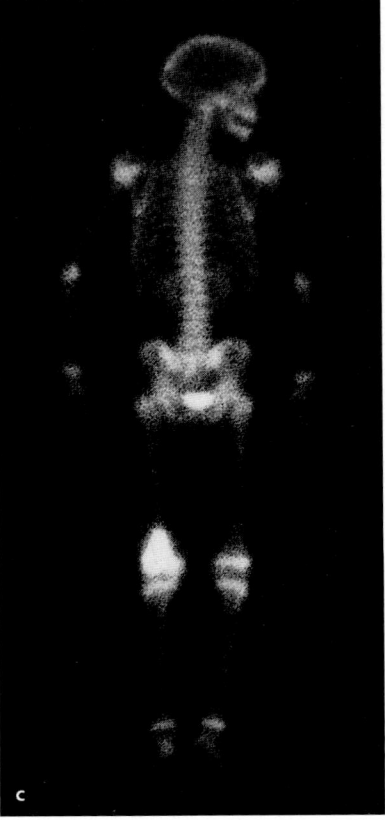

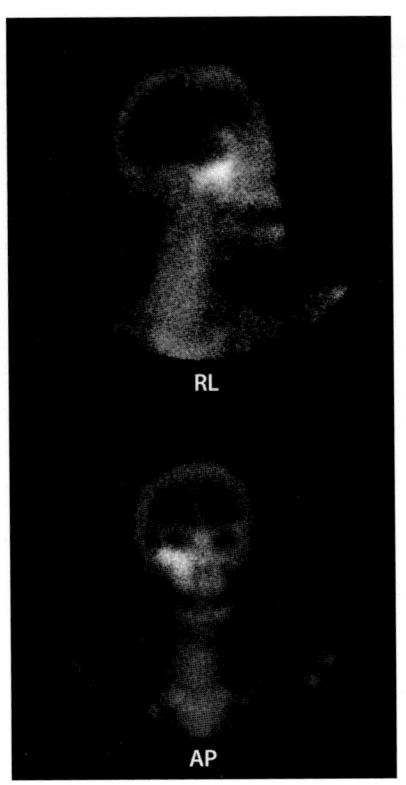

Fig. 4.25. A 60-year-old man with known plasmacytoma complained of pain in the right half of the face. Bone scan 2 hours postinjection shows intense uptake in the area of the right clinoid process and dorsum sellae. Metastatic plasmacytoma

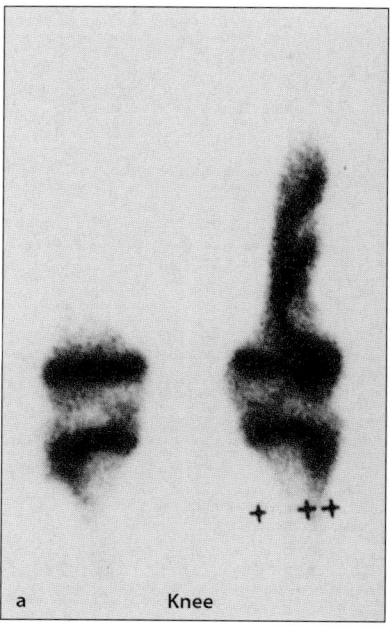

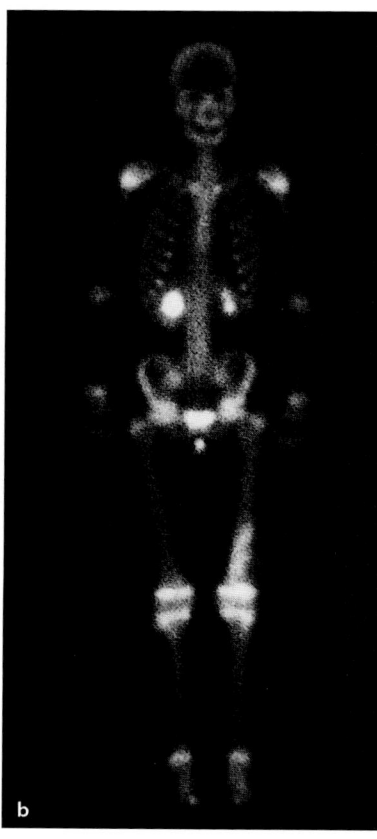

Fig. 4.26 a,b. A 13-year-old girl with known osteosarcoma presented with diffuse thigh and back pain while on cytostatic therapy (in preparation for surgery). A whole-body scan was performed to exclude lumbar vertebral metastases and determine tumor extent in the thigh. The scan shows intense uptake at the tumor site and also in both kidneys. The back pain is attributable to cytostatic-induced nephropathy

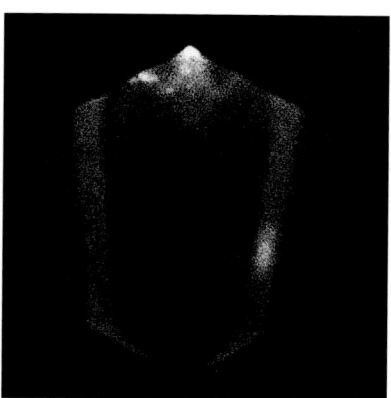

Fig. 4.27. An asymptomatic 42-year-old woman with known malignant lymphoma underwent a whole-body scan to screen for metastases. The hot spot in the femur is a solitary metastasis

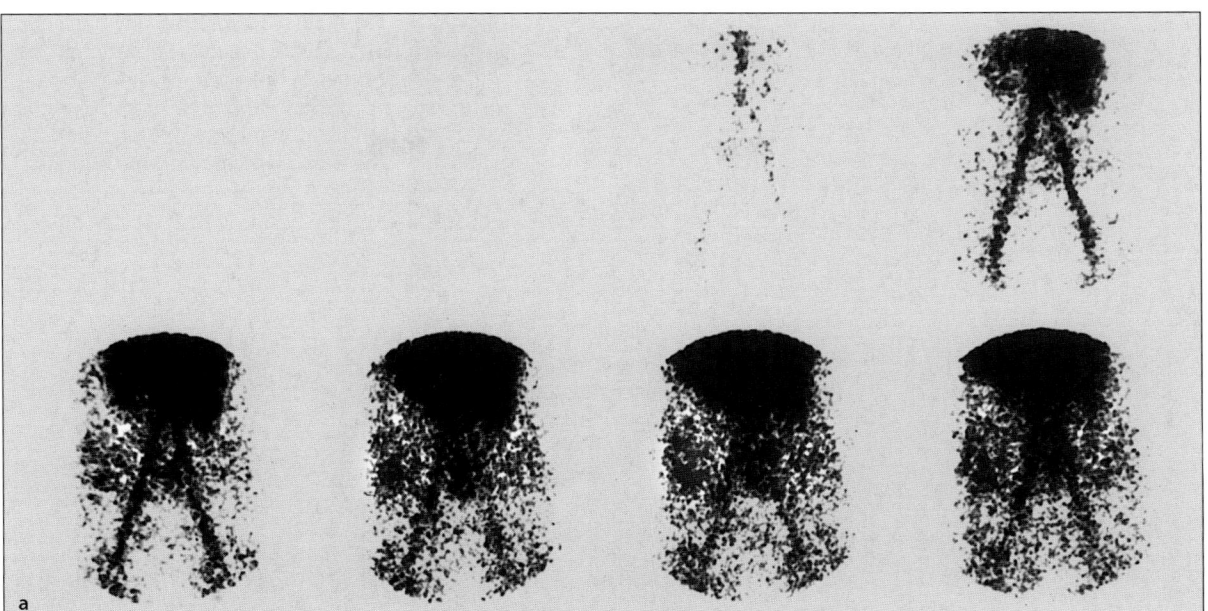

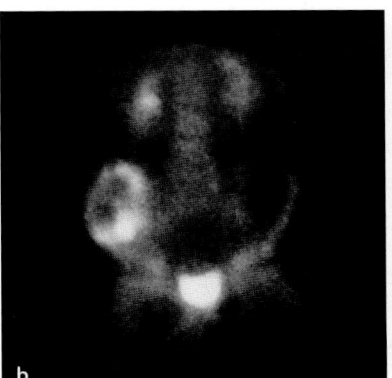

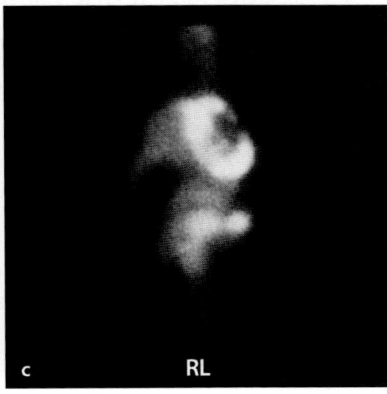

Fig. 4.28 a–c. A 15-year-old boy had been treated for suspected coxitis for several weeks. Bone scan shows an area of very intense uptake with a cold center in the iliac wing. Histology confirmed Ewing sarcoma with central necrosis

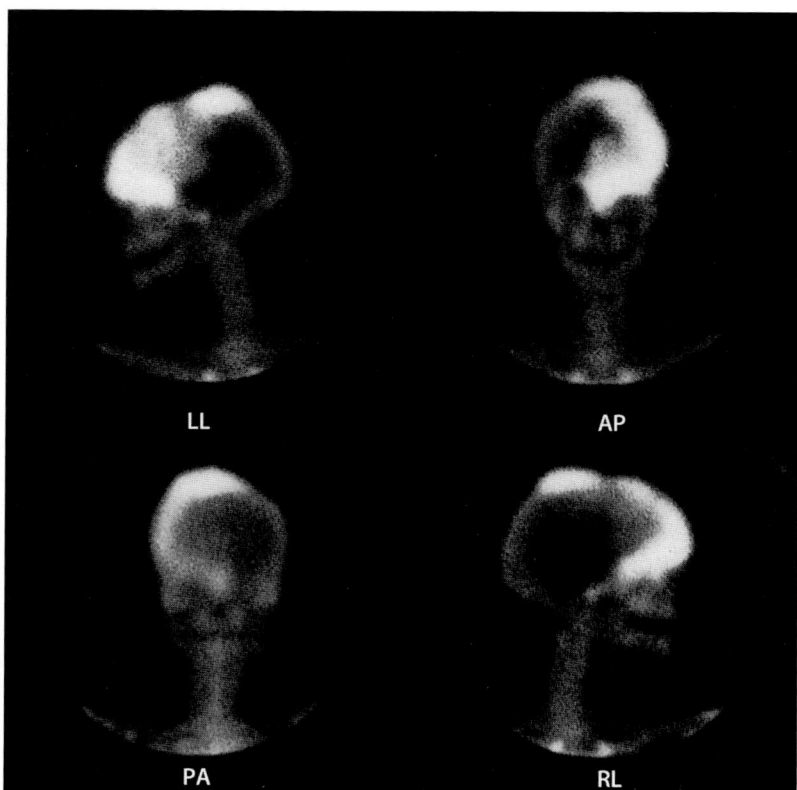

Fig. 4.29. A 14-year-old boy presented with severe headaches, predominantly frontal, of unknown cause. The bone scan show very intense uptake in the left frontoparietotemporal region of the skull. Ossifying fibroma of bone

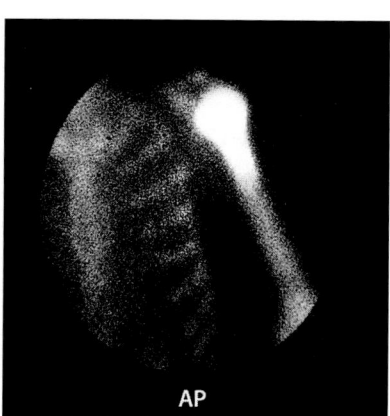

Fig. 4.30. A 19-year-old boy was examined for unexplained complaints in the upper arm. The bone scan shows very intense uptake in the proximal portion of the humerus. Histology confirmed osteoplastic osteosarcoma

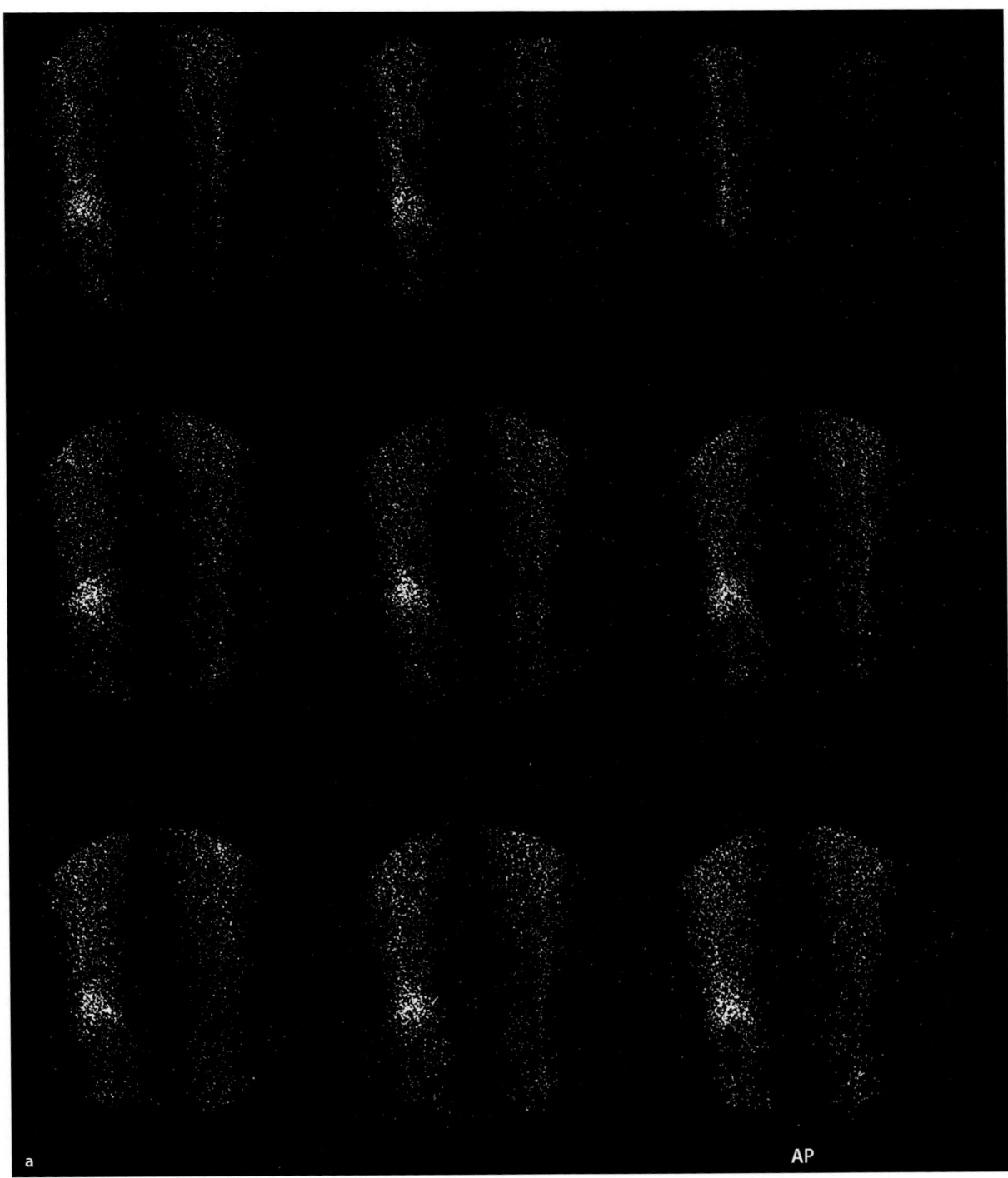

Fig. 4.31 a–c. A 58-year-old woman complained of pain in the right ankle joint for several months. Sequential images were acquired at 6-second intervals immediately after injection of bone tracer (**a**), and early and delayed static images were also obtained (**b, c**). All the images show increased uptake, which is most intense in the distal tibia. Histology confirmed a giant cell tumor of the tibia

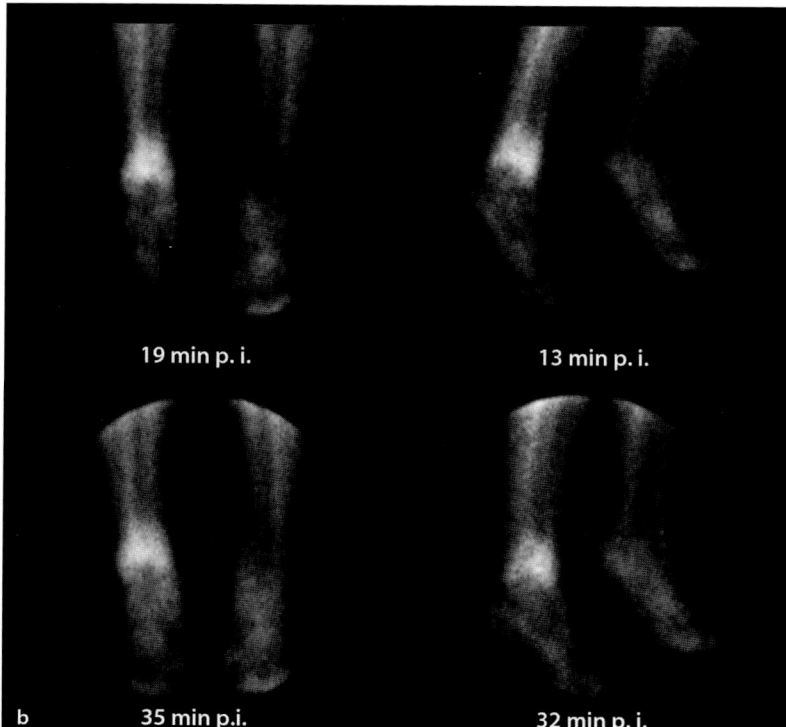

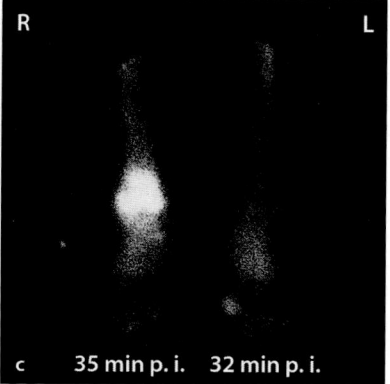

19 min p. i.

13 min p. i.

35 min p.i.

32 min p. i.

b

c   35 min p. i.   32 min p. i.

Fig. 4.31 a–c. A 58-year-old woman complained of pain in the right ankle joint for several months. Sequential images were acquired at 6-second intervals immediately after injection of bone tracer (**a**), and early and delayed static images were also obtained (**b, c**). All the images show increased uptake, which is most intense in the distal tibia. Histology confirmed a giant cell tumor of the tibia

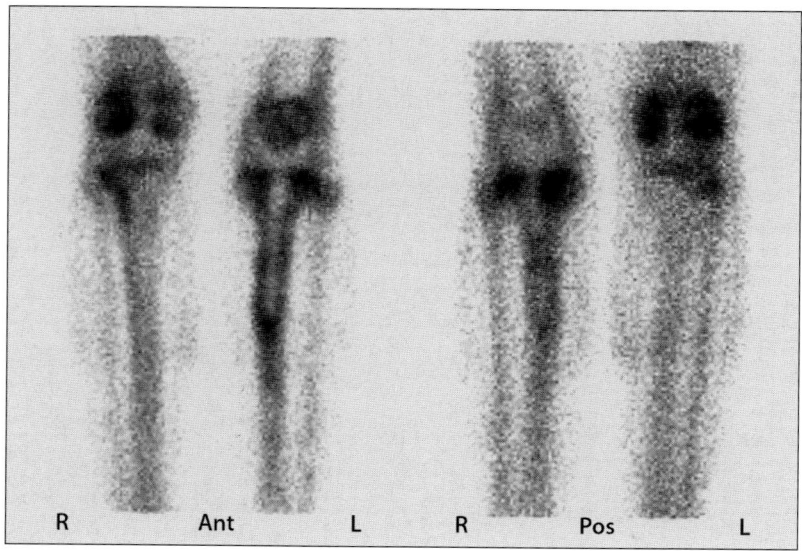

R   Ant   L   R   Pos   L

Fig. 4.32. A 9-year-old boy who had been previously operated for Ewing sarcoma of the tibia presented again with walking difficulties. The increased uptake around the prosthesis is characteristic of rejection

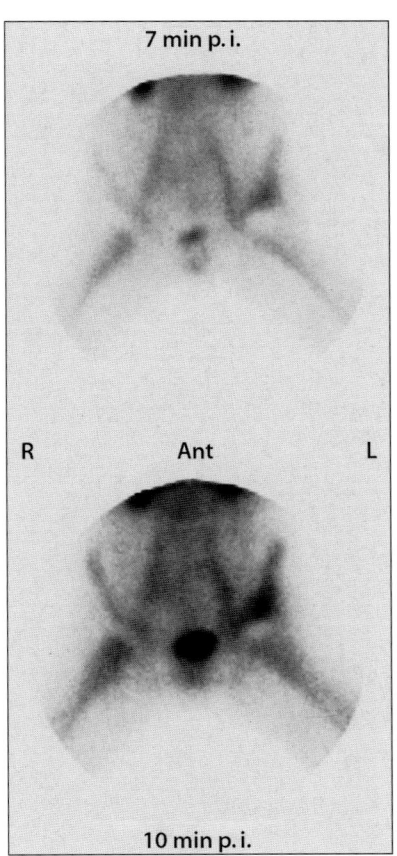

7 min p.i.

R   Ant   L

10 min p.i.

Fig. 4.33. A 9-month-old infant was favoring one leg and screamed when the leg was passively moved. The bone scan shows decreased activity in the hip region with a hot spot projected over the acetabular roof. Perthes' disease

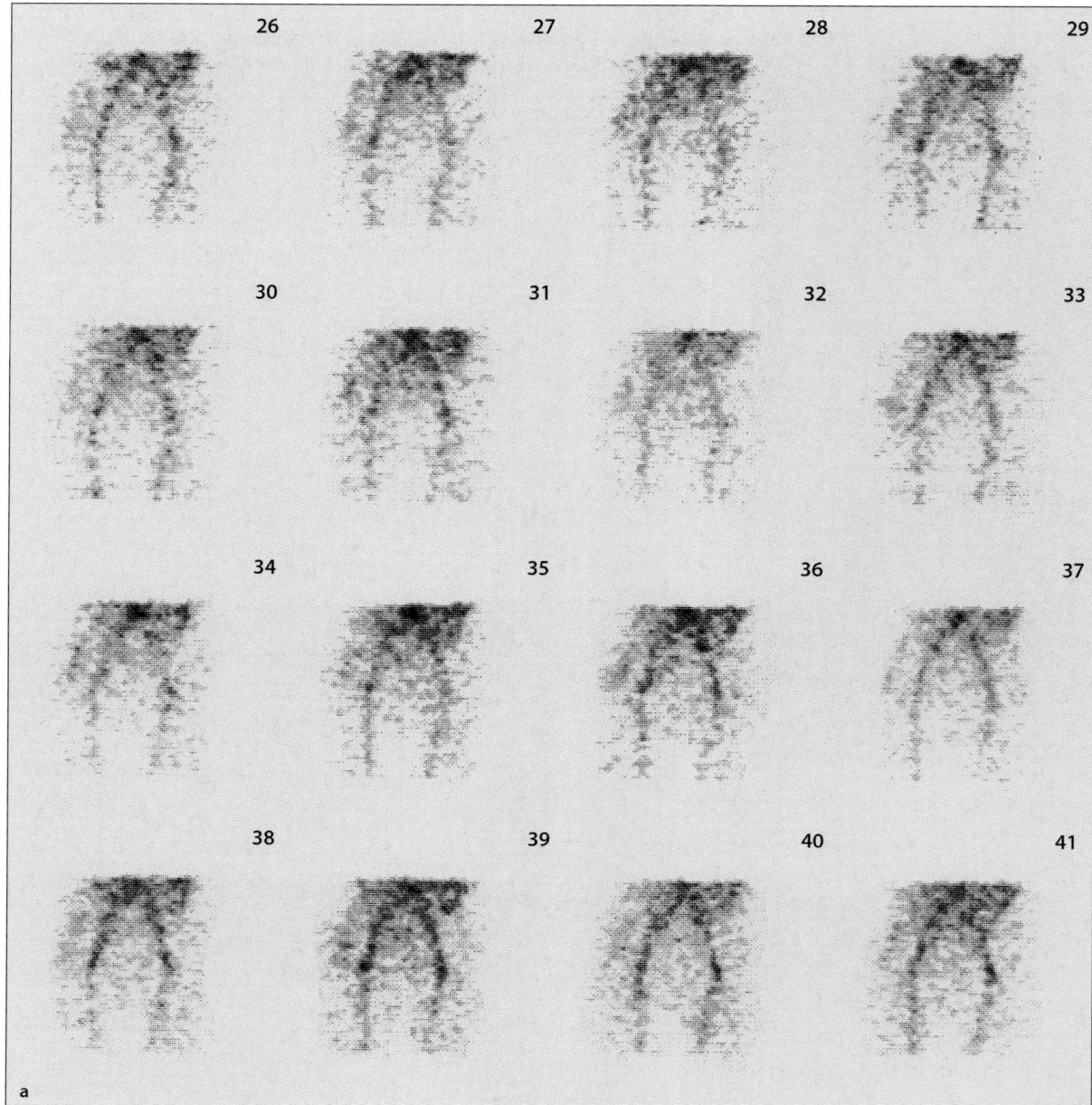

Fig. 4.34 a,b. A 70-year-old woman with bilateral hip replacements complained of increasing pain and limited motion in the right hip. A bone scan was performed to exclude rejection. Both the perfusion-phase scan and the early static images are negative, but the delayed statics (2 hours postinjection) show a focal area of increased uptake in the soft tissues bordering on the prosthesis. A calcified hematoma was found at explantation

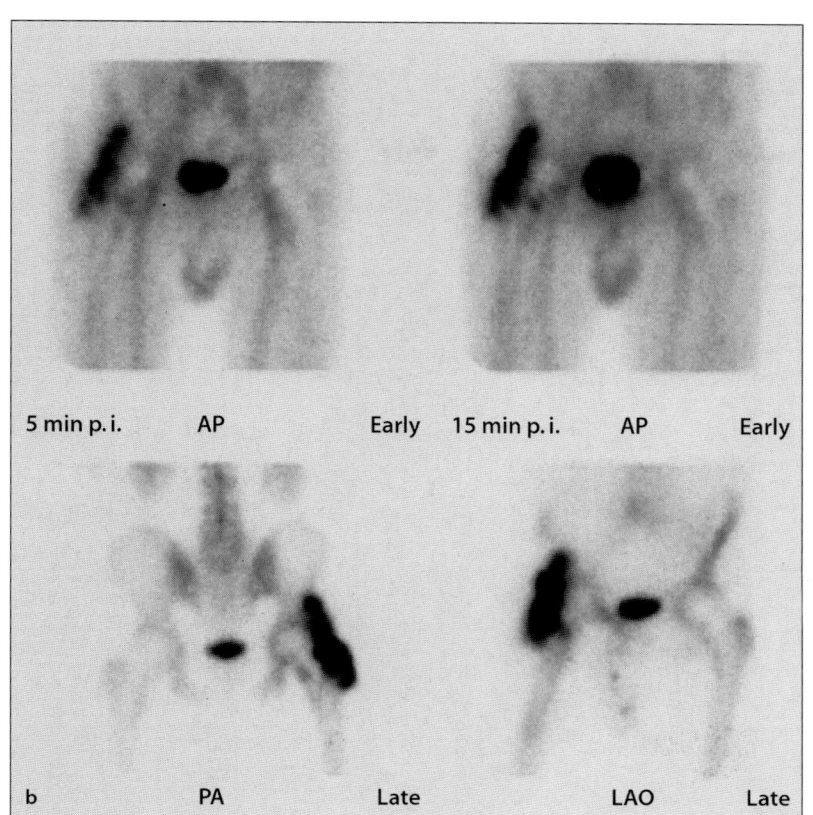

Fig. 4.34 b

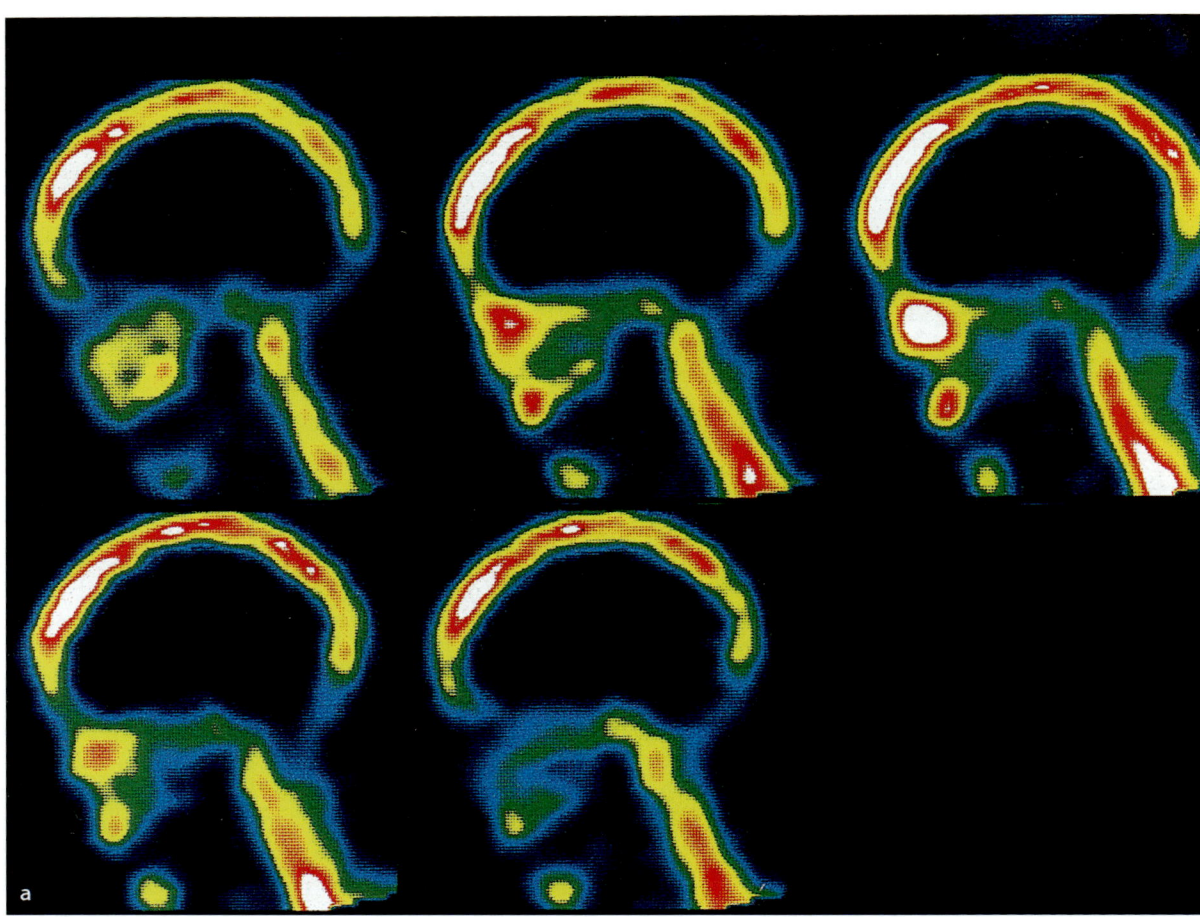

Fig. 4.35 a–c. A 58-year-old woman presented with facial pain and intermittent purulent nasal discharge. Scan 2 hours postinjection shows increased uptake in the right nasal cavity. Histology established malignant melanoma

Fig. 4.35 b, c

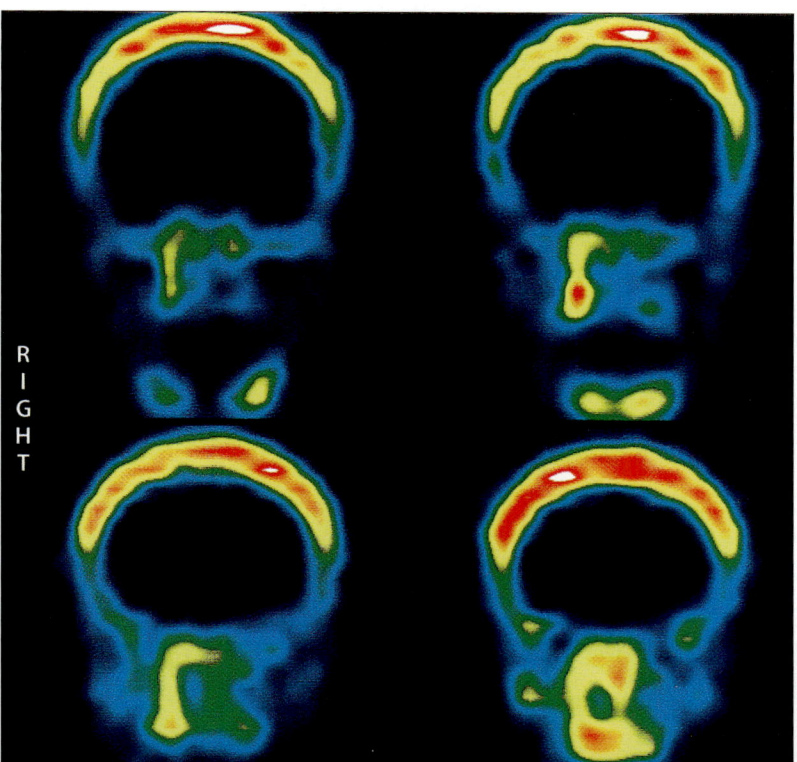

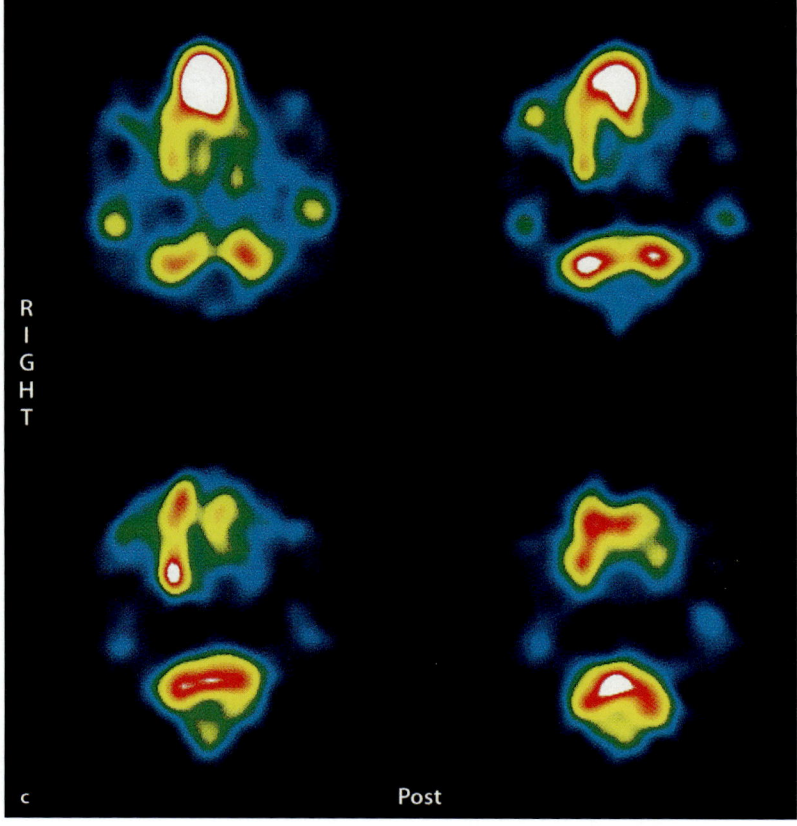

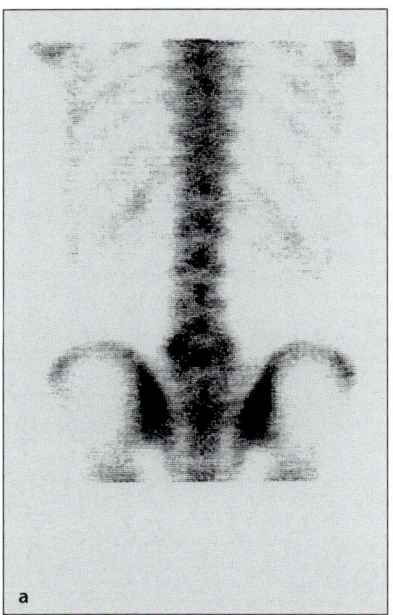

Fig. 4.36 a,b. Bone scan in a 12-year-old boy with back pain shows a circular area of increased uptake in the L5 vertebra that persists on the 2-hour image (projections in various planes). MRI confirmed the diagnosis of a florid inflammation

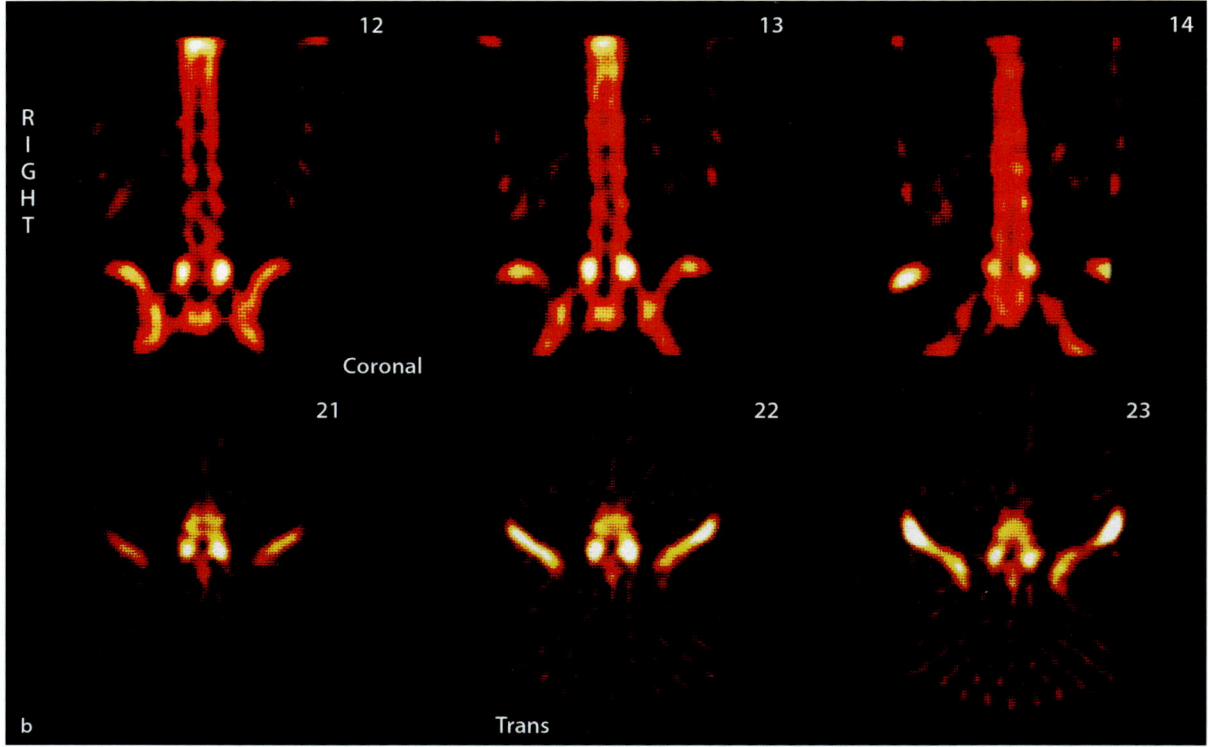

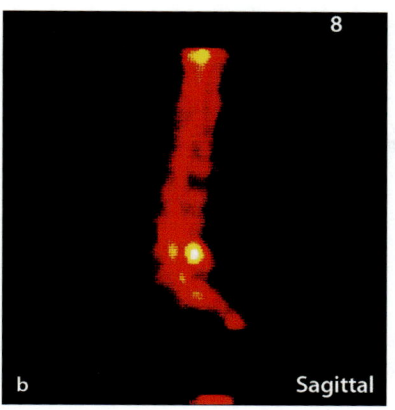

Fig. 4.36 b. *Continued*

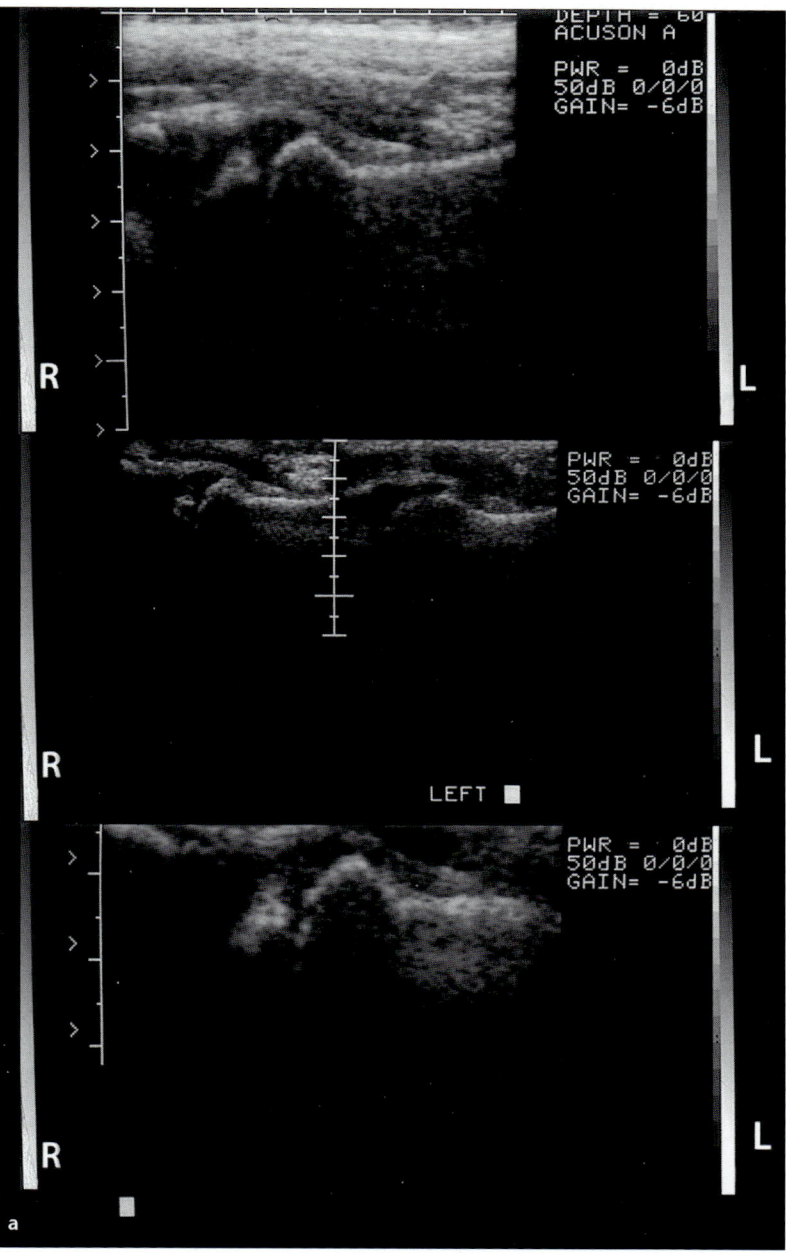

Fig. 4.37 a–c. Postural guarding of the left leg was noticed in a 1-year-old infant, and the left hip felt warmer than the right. **a** Ultrasound demonstrates widening of the hip joint space. **b** Bone scan sequence at 4-second intervals and the early static images show diffuse slightly increased uptake throughout the left hip region, which persisted until the end of the examination (with ^{99m}Tc MDP). Synovitis of the left hip joint

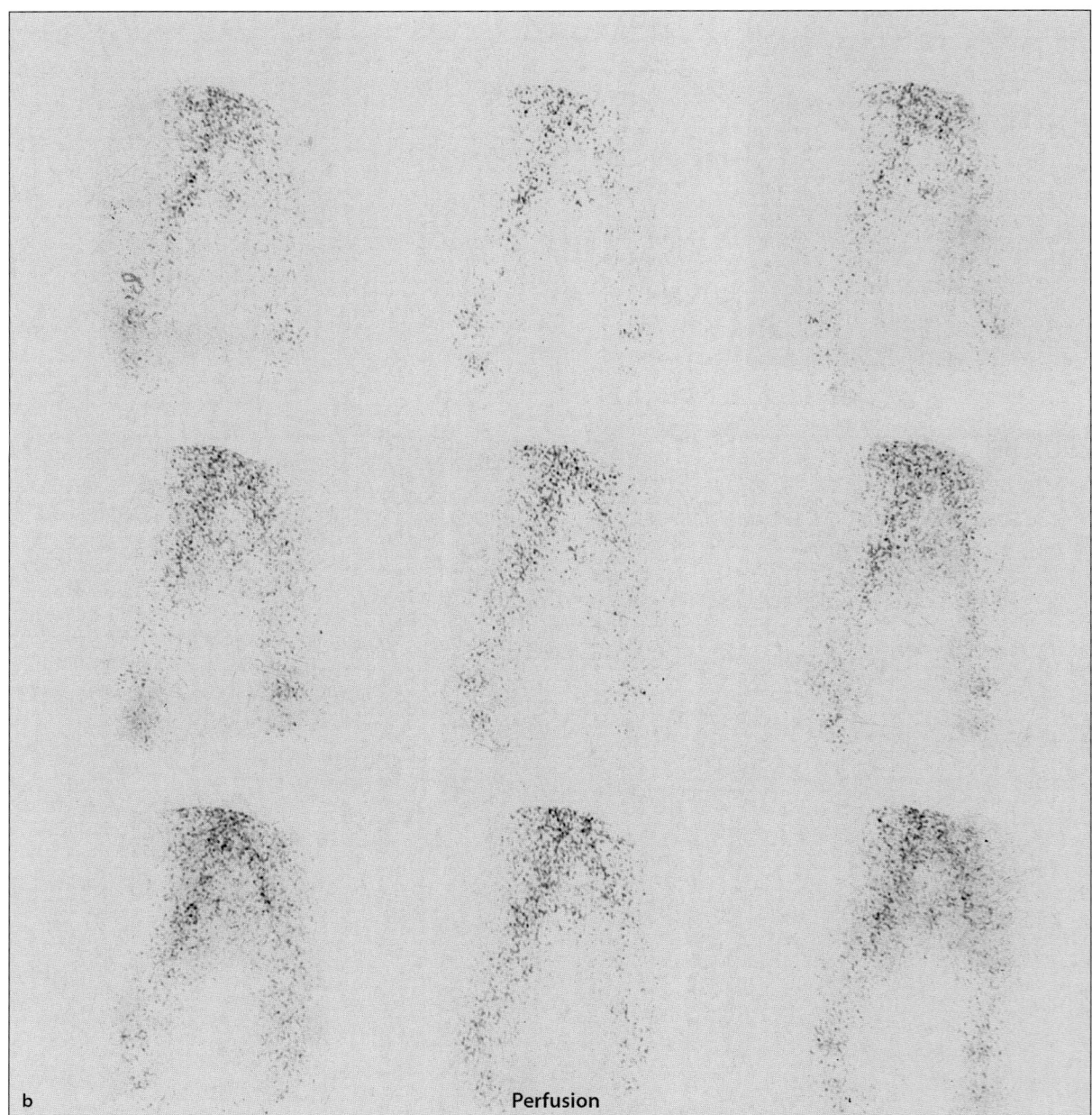

b   Perfusion

Fig. 4.37 a–c. Postural guarding of the left leg was noticed in a 1-year-old infant, and the left hip felt warmer than the right. **a** Ultrasound demonstrates widening of the hip joint space. **b** Bone scan sequence at 4-second intervals and the early static images show diffuse slightly increased uptake throughout the left hip region, which persisted until the end of the examination (with ^{99m}Tc MDP). Synovitis of the left hip joint

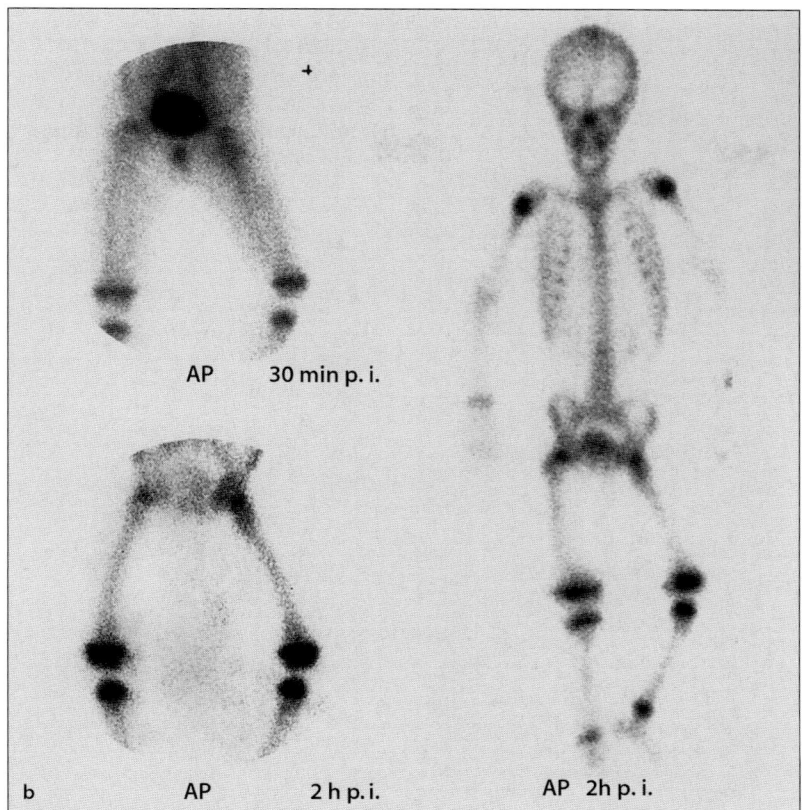

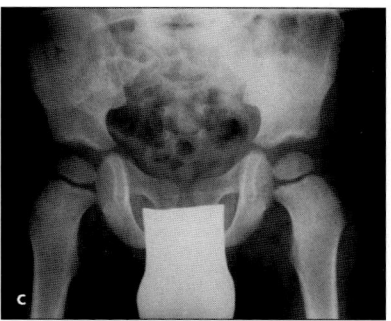

Fig. 4.37 b, c

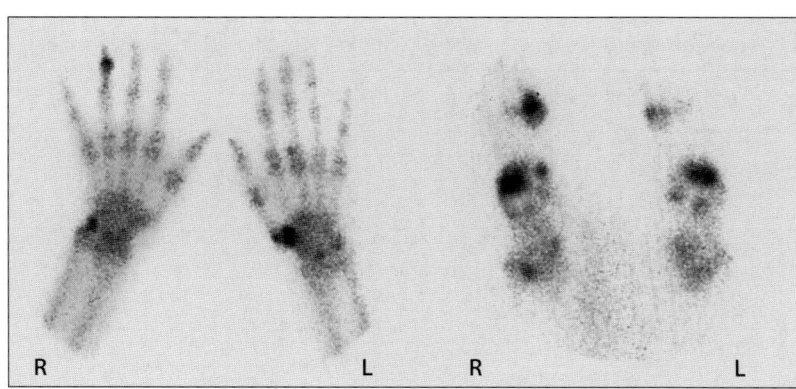

Fig. 4.38. A 40-year-old man presented with swelling and redness of the metacarpophalangeal joint of the thumb and the metatarsophalangeal joint of the big toe, accompanied by painful limitation of motion. Bone scan shows intense tracer uptake in both joints caused by an attack of gout. Laboratory tests confirmed the radionuclide diagnosis

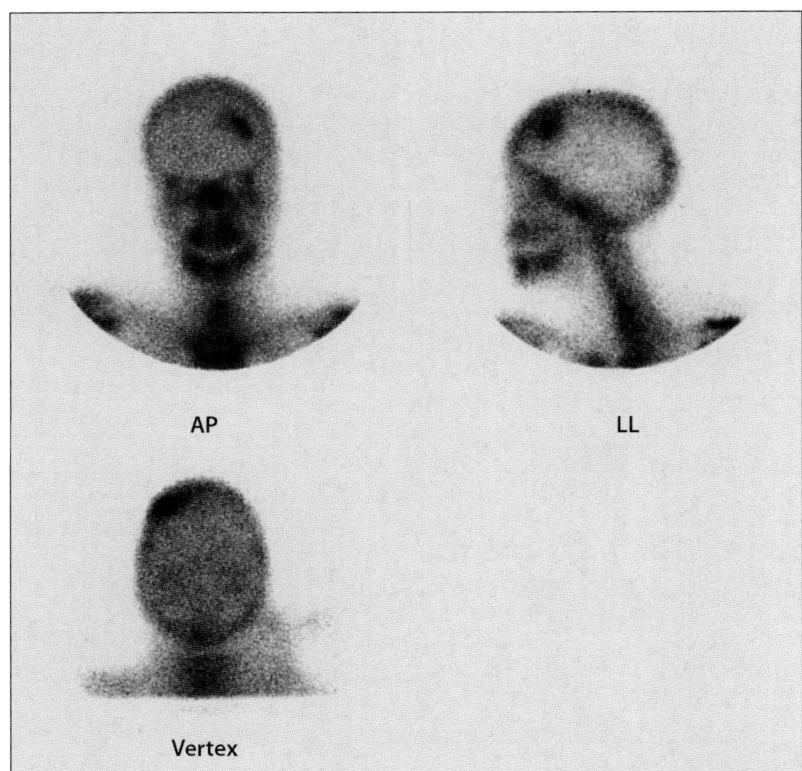

Fig. 4.39. A 30-year-old baker was evaluated for recurrent headaches. Bone scan 2 hours postinjection shows a well-defined hot spot in the left frontal area. Eosinophilic granuloma in a setting of histiocytosis

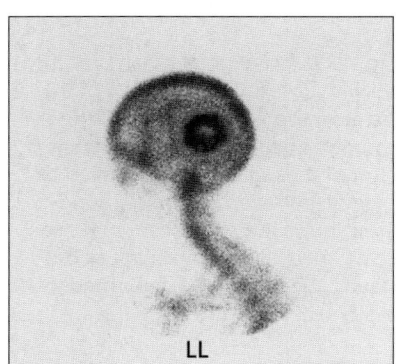

Fig. 4.40. A 60-year-old woman who was post-mastectomy for breast cancer presented for radionuclide follow-up. The bone scan shows an area of increased uptake with a colder center in the left temporal area. Breast cancer metastasis with central necrosis

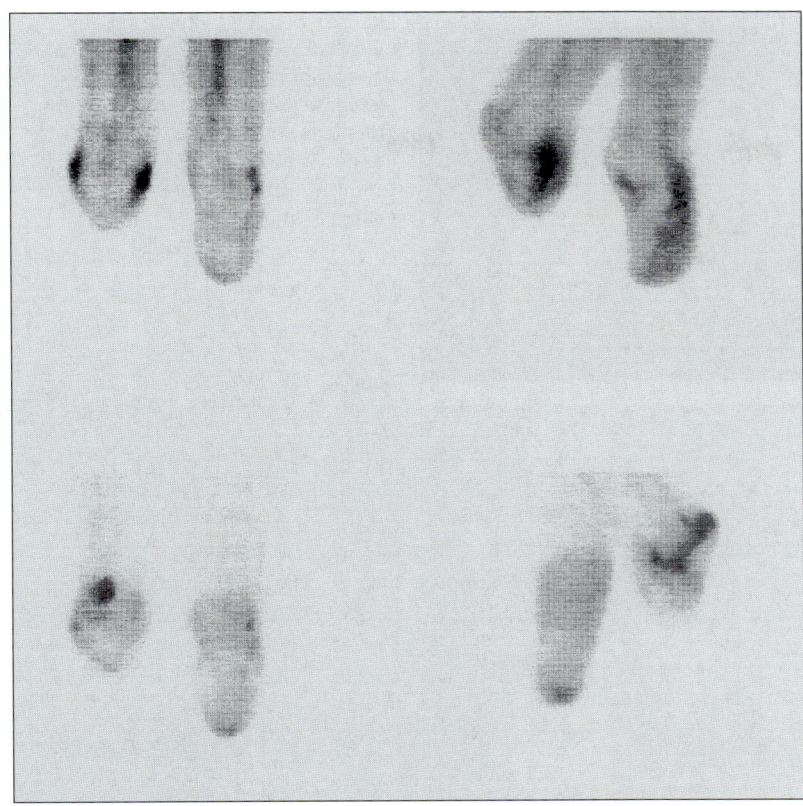

Fig. 4.41. An 80-year-old man who had both lower legs amputated for wartime injuries presented with pain in both stumps (right > left). At bone scanning, the early static images (15 minutes postinjection) show medial and lateral areas of increased uptake on the right side and a lateral band of increased activity on the left side. The delayed statics show only right lateral increased uptake. The prostheses have caused bilateral stump irritation with incipient soft-tissue inflammation on the lateral side of the right stump

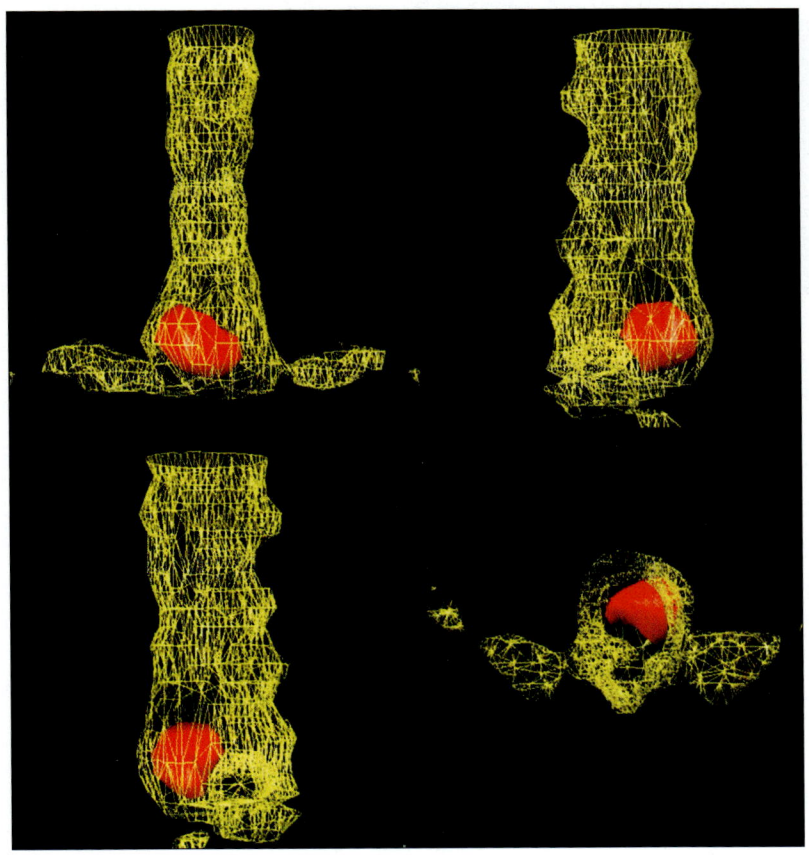

Fig. 4.42. A 55-year-old woman who was post-mastectomy for breast cancer presented with lower back pain. Radiographs were negative. The bone scan could not definitely exclude metastasis by visual interpretation, but special processing demonstrated a metastasis in the body of the L5 vertebra. No additional signs of metastasis were found anywhere in the skeleton

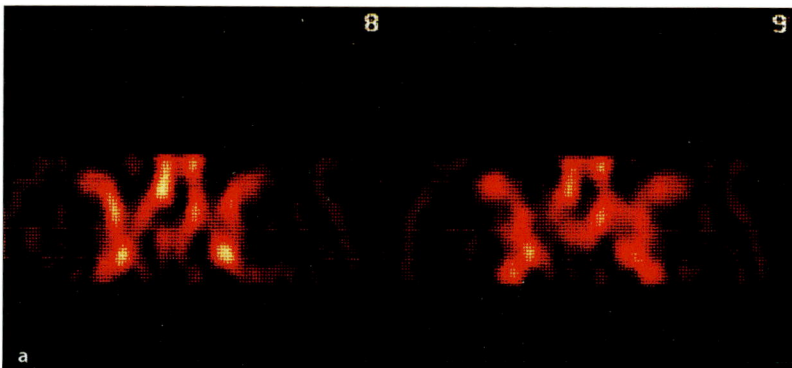

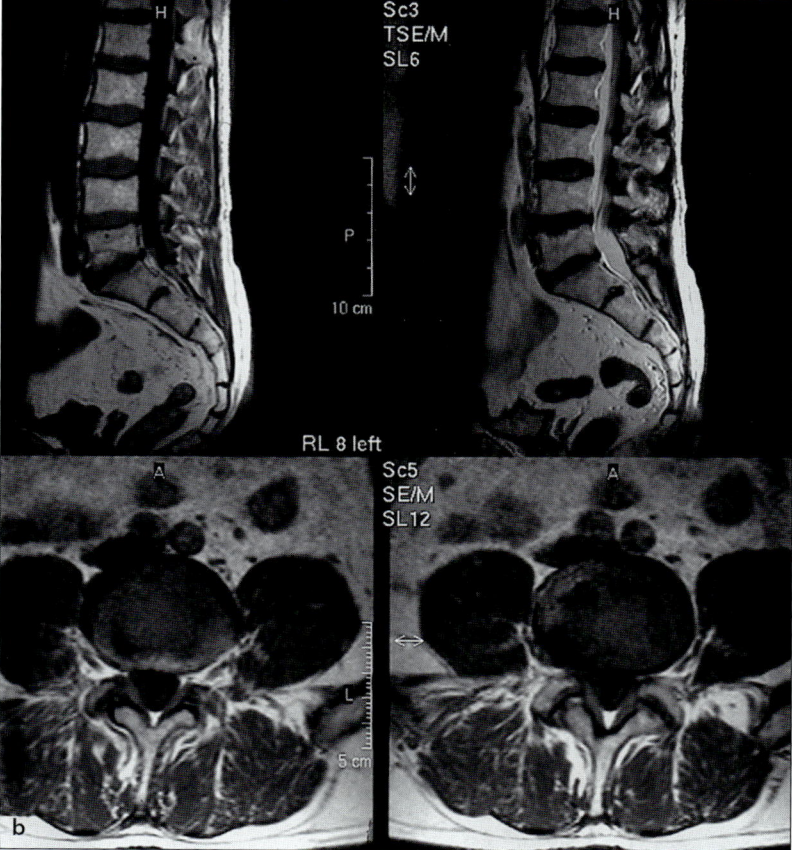

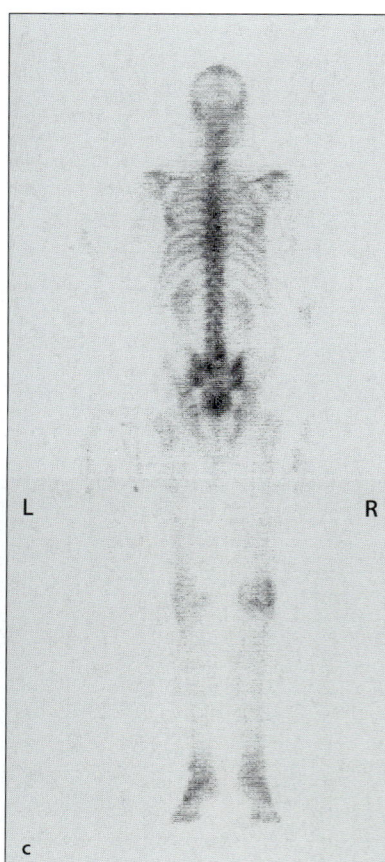

Fig. 4.43 a–c. A 64-year-old man with whiplash injury complained of significant pain on motion of the lower lumbar spine and lumbosacral junction. The planar bone scans and SPECT images show no evidence of a fracture. MRI supported the diagnosis of whiplash injury

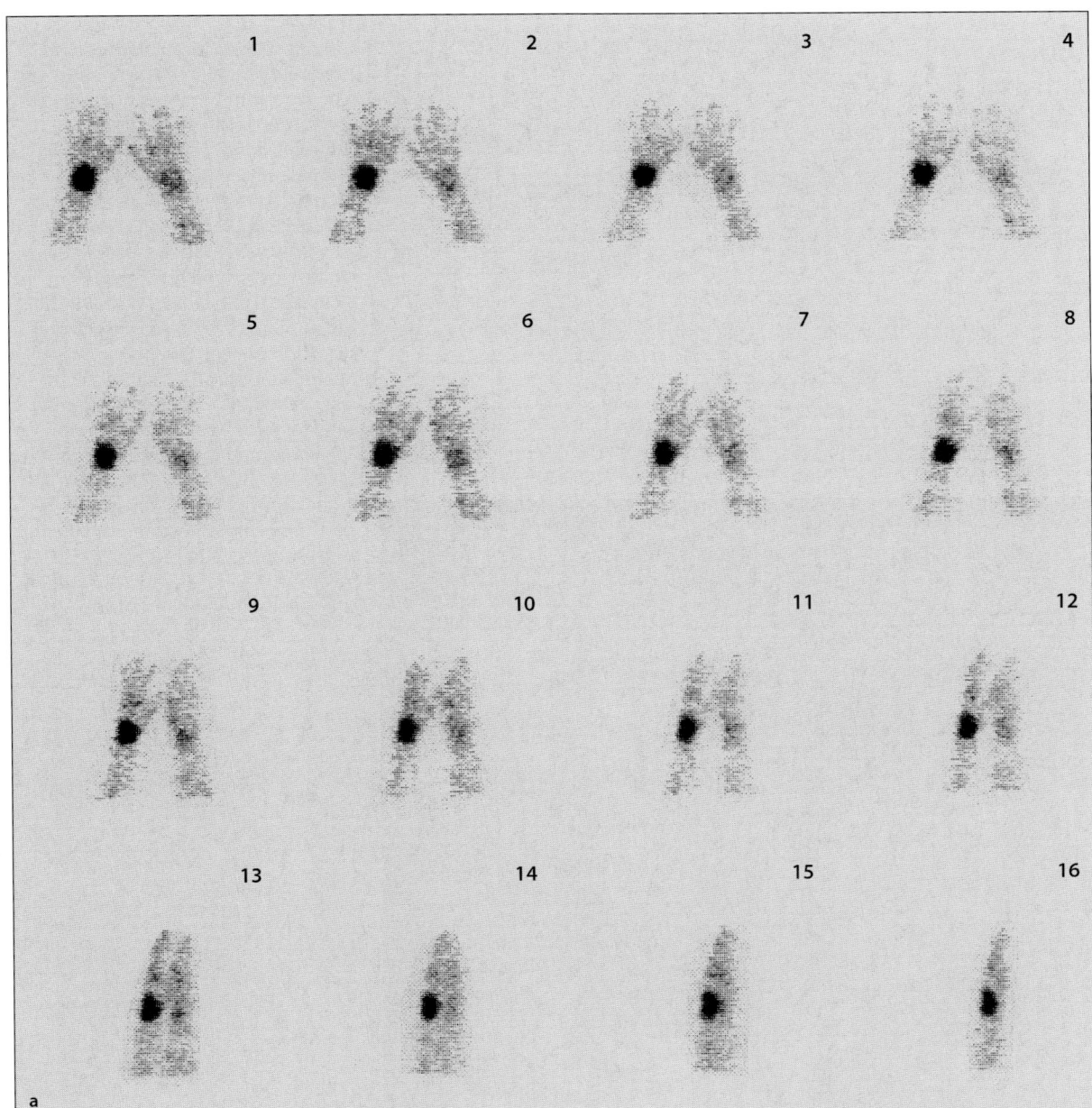

Fig. 4.44 a–d. A 33-year-old man experienced sudden, severe wrist pain. His family doctor treated the pain conservative-ly (ointment dressings), and the pain abated slightly but then returned. Bone scanning was performed one week later. The perfusion-phase scan, early and delayed static images, and SPECT images all show markedly increased turnover in the lunate bone and moderately increased turnover in the rest of the carpal bones. This raised very strong suspicion of necrosis and malacia of the lunate bone. The changes in the rest of the carpal bones may signify early reflex sympathet-ic dystrophy. MRI confirmed the lunate diagnosis but could not confirm reflex sympathetic dystrophy, which may have been simulated by scattered radiation in the radionuclide study. Nuclear medicine is a more sensitive modality, as it reflects metabolic activity

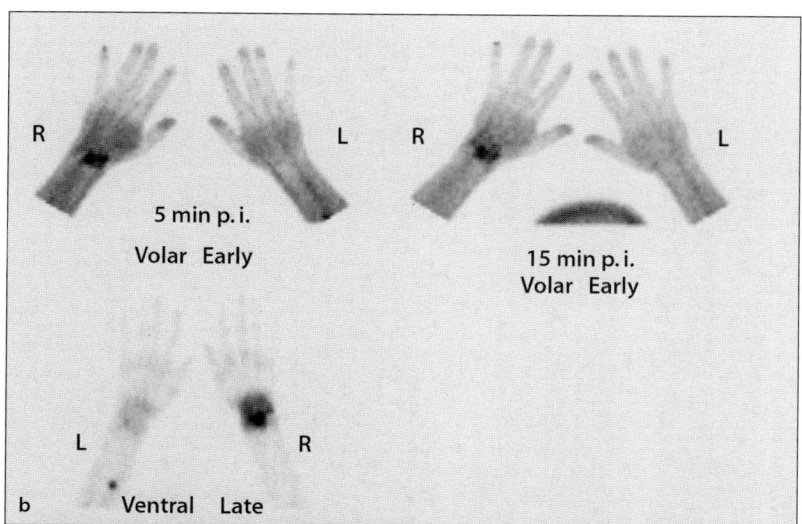

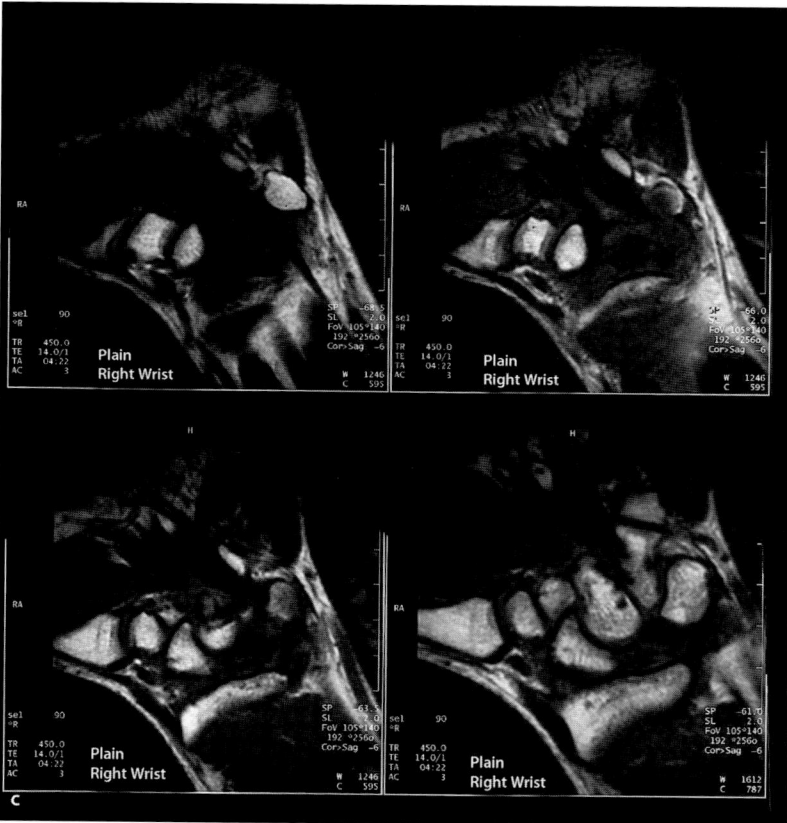

Fig. 4.44 a–d. A 33-year-old man experienced sudden, severe wrist pain. His family doctor treated the pain conservatively (ointment dressings), and the pain abated slightly but then returned. Bone scanning was performed one week later. The perfusion-phase scan, early and delayed static images, and SPECT images all show markedly increased turnover in the lunate bone and moderately increased turnover in the rest of the carpal bones. This raised very strong suspicion of necrosis and malacia of the lunate bone. The changes in the rest of the carpal bones may signify early reflex sympathetic dystrophy. MRI confirmed the lunate diagnosis but could not confirm reflex sympathetic dystrophy, which may have been simulated by scattered radiation in the radionuclide study. Nuclear medicine is a more sensitive modality, as it reflects metabolic activity

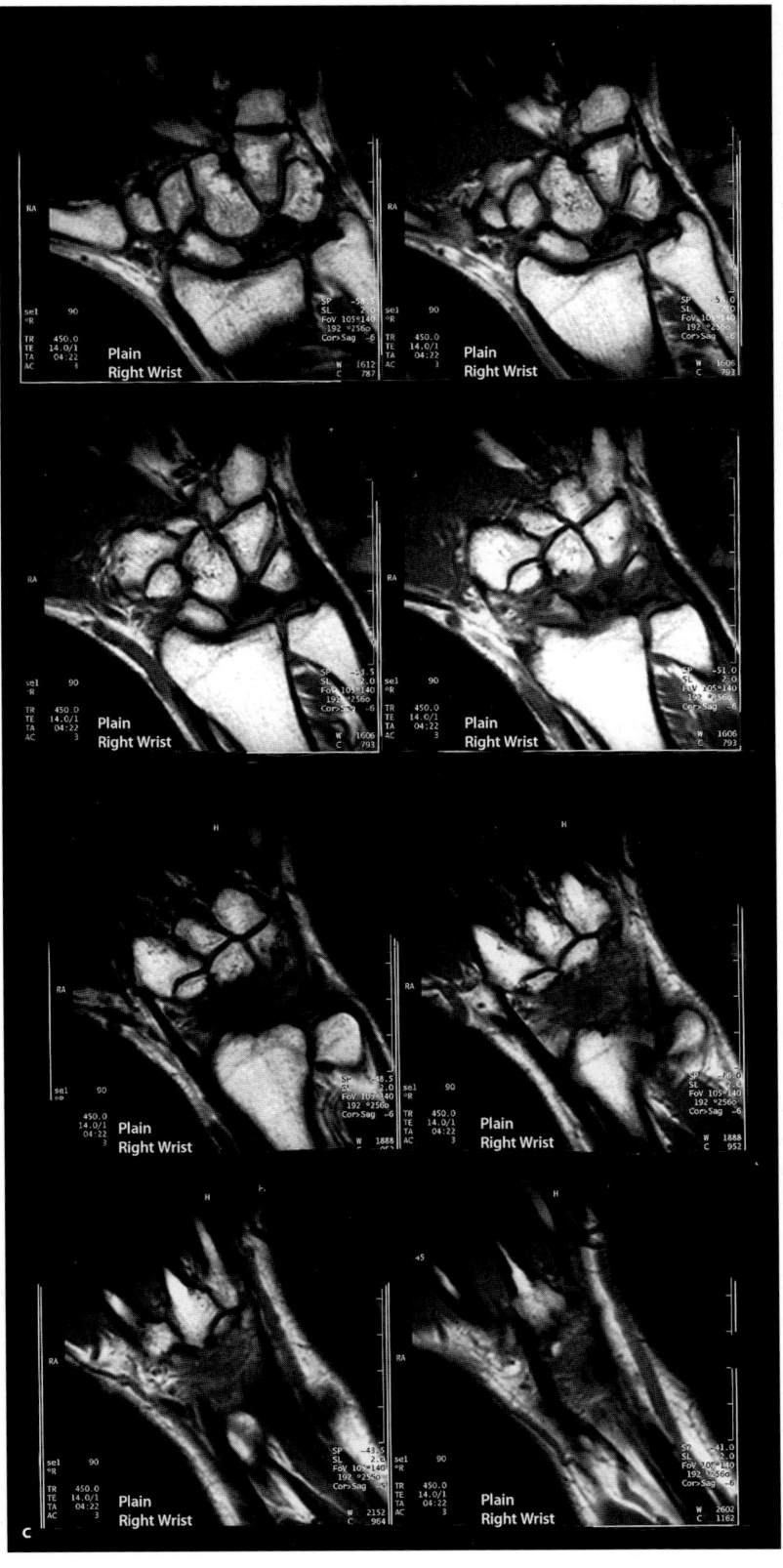

Fig. 4.44 c. *Continued*

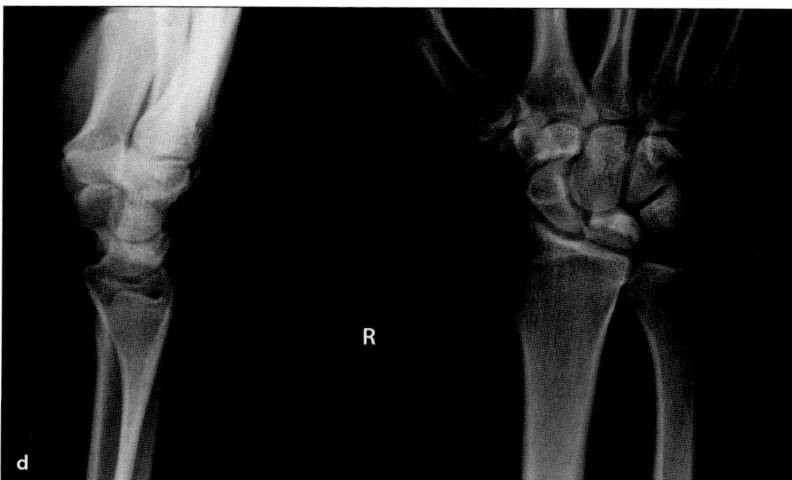

Fig. 4.44 a–d. A 33-year-old man experienced sudden, severe wrist pain. His family doctor treated the pain conservatively (ointment dressings), and the pain abated slightly but then returned. Bone scanning was performed one week later. The perfusion-phase scan, early and delayed static images, and SPECT images all show markedly increased turnover in the lunate bone and moderately increased turnover in the rest of the carpal bones. This raised very strong suspicion of necrosis and malacia of the lunate bone. The changes in the rest of the carpal bones may signify early reflex sympathetic dystrophy. MRI confirmed the lunate diagnosis but could not confirm reflex sympathetic dystrophy, which may have been simulated by scattered radiation in the radionuclide study. Nuclear medicine is a more sensitive modality, as it reflects metabolic activity

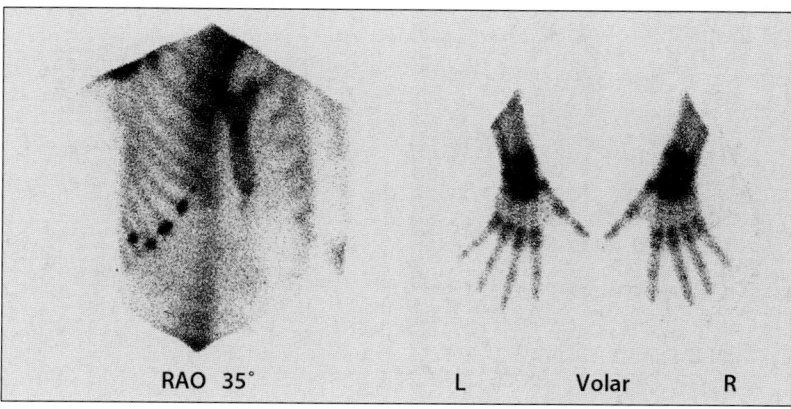

Fig. 4.45. A 54-year-old stenotypist sustained a blow to the chest. She also complained of pain in all the joints of her hands. The bone scan shows hot spots at the osteochondral junction of the 6th through 9th ribs, consistent with serial fractures of those ribs. Intense uptake is also seen in all the joints of the hands. Scan findings indicate an overuse response to repetitive occupational stresses

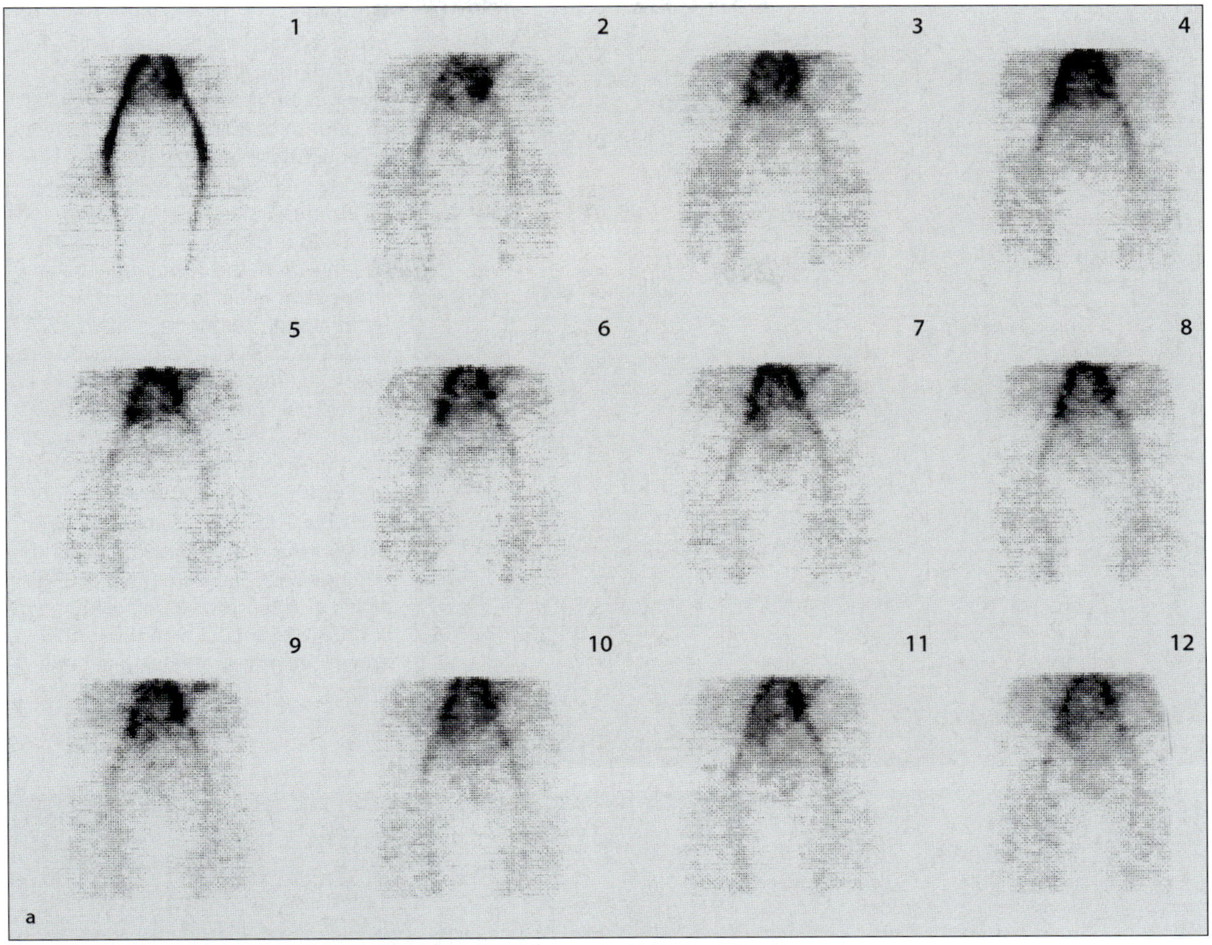

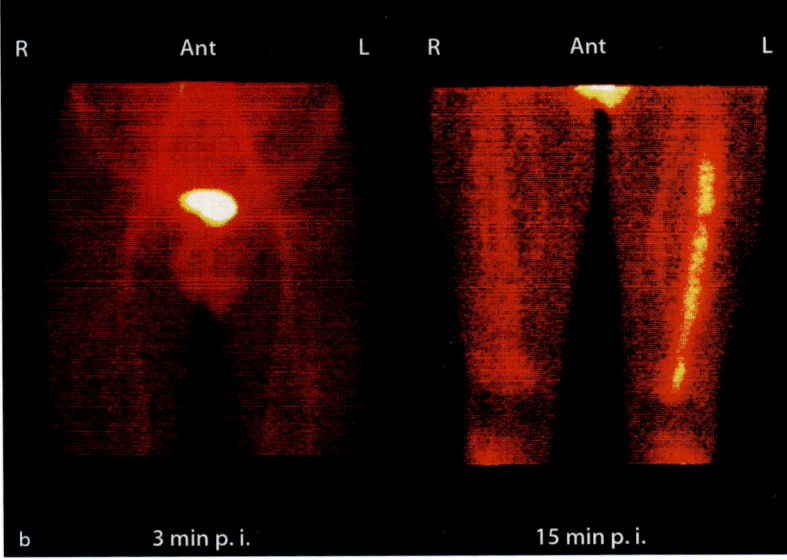

Fig. 4.46 a–c. A 23-year-old man complained of generalized pain in the left leg. Radiographs showed cystic changes. Bone scanning was requested prior to operative treatment. **a** Sequential images acquired at 30-second intervals for 4 minutes show no abnormalities. **b** Early static images were acquired at 3 and 15 minutes postinjection. The 15-minute image shows faint initial uptake in the femoral shaft but none in the cystic areas. The delayed statics showed pronounced areas of increased uptake in the left tibia and bands of increased activity in the left femur and femoral head, indicating a normally vascularized process involving the left femur and tibia. The findings are consistent with fibrous dysplasia. **c** Radionuclide findings were supplemented by MRI, which also suggests a polyostotic type of fibrous dysplasia with the formation of secondary aneurysmal bone cysts

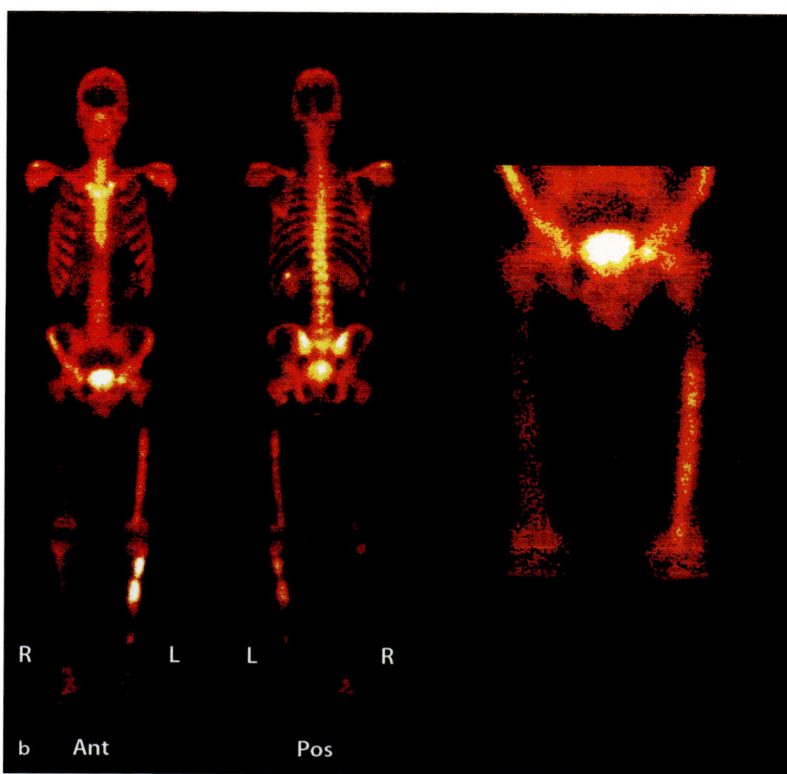

b   Ant   Pos

Fig. 4.46 a–c. A 23-year-old man complained of generalized pain in the left leg. Radiographs showed cystic changes. Bone scanning was requested prior to operative treatment.
a Sequential images acquired at 30-second intervals for 4 minutes show no abnormalities. **b** Early static images were acquired at 3 and 15 minutes postinjection. The 15-minute image shows faint initial uptake in the femoral shaft but none in the cystic areas. The delayed statics showed pronounced areas of increased uptake in the left tibia and bands of increased activity in the left femur and femoral head, indicating a normally vascularized process involving the left femur and tibia. The findings are consistent with fibrous dysplasia. **c** Radionuclide findings were supplemented by MRI, which also suggests a polyostotic type of fibrous dysplasia with the formation of secondary aneurysmal bone cysts

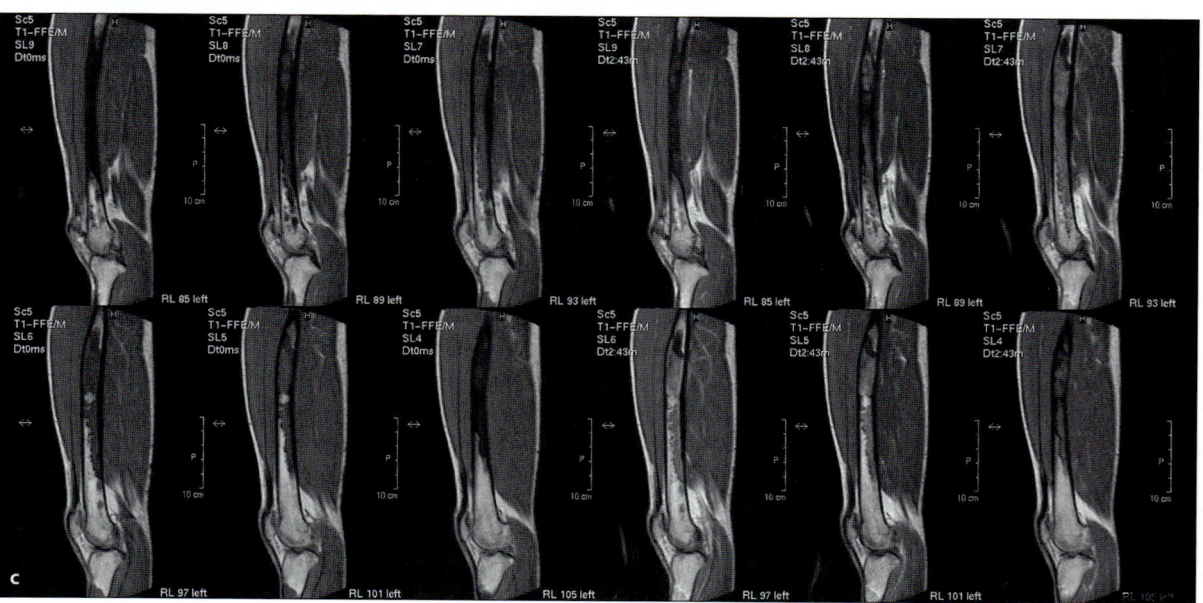

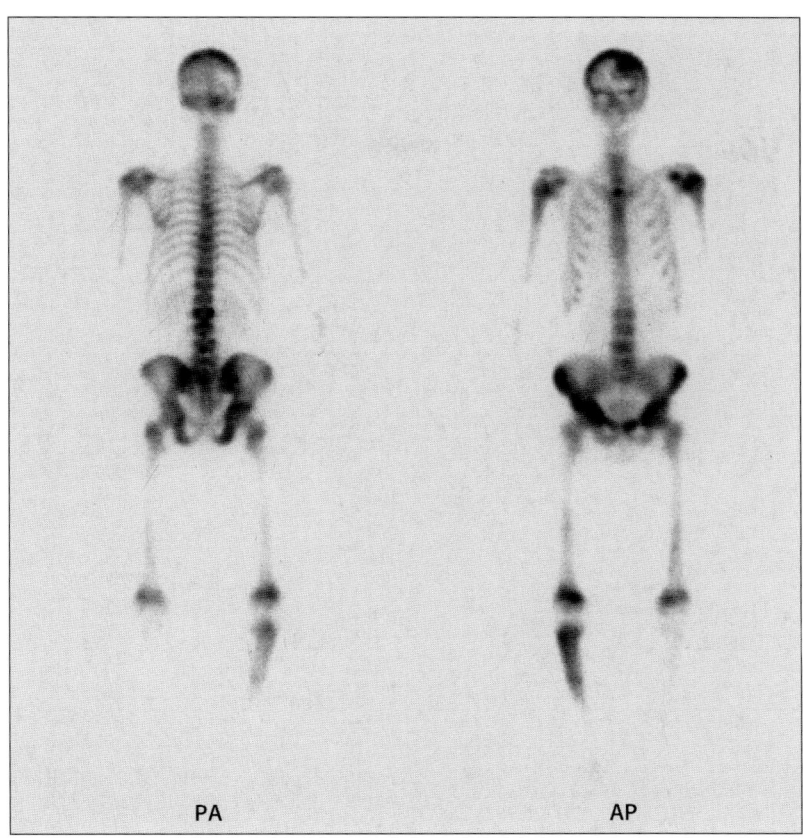

PA   AP

Fig. 4.47. A 55-year-old man was evaluated for suspected progression of Albers-Schoenberg disease. Scan 2 hours after injection of bone tracer shows involvement of the following regions: skull and skull base, upper arm and shoulder (periarticular on the right, incipient on the left), multiple vertebral bodies, pelvis, right tibia, and early involvement of both femurs

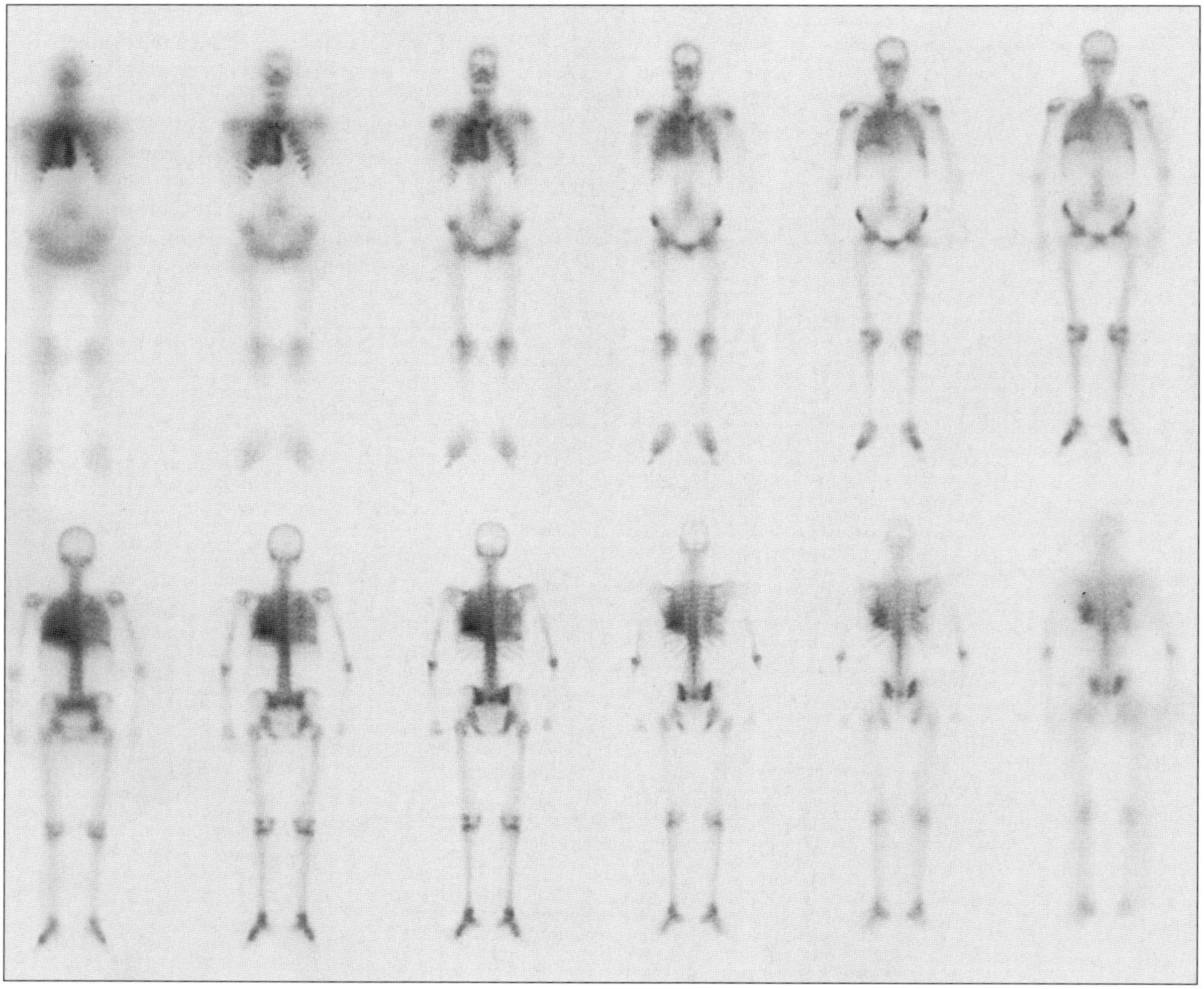

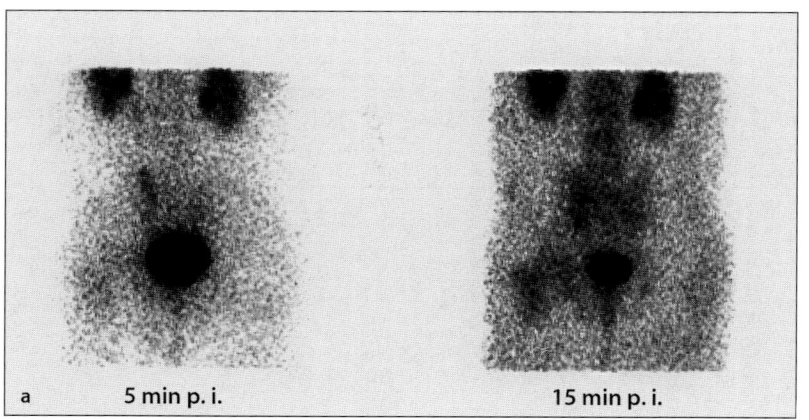

Fig. 4.48. A 44-year-old man with cachexia of unknown cause was screened for metastatic disease. Bone scan (Phocon technique) 2 hours after injection of bone tracer shows generally low skeletal uptake with rarefaction of bone and diffuse uptake in both lungs. Laboratory tests showed significant hypercalcemia

Fig. 4.49 a,b. A 50-year-old man complained of pain during walking. Bone scans at 5 minutes, 15 minutes (**a**) and 2 hours postinjection (**b**) show increased tracer uptake in the hip joint. Coxitis was confirmed by CT, and an effusion was percutaneously aspirated

a   5 min p. i.   15 min p. i.

Fig. 4.49 b

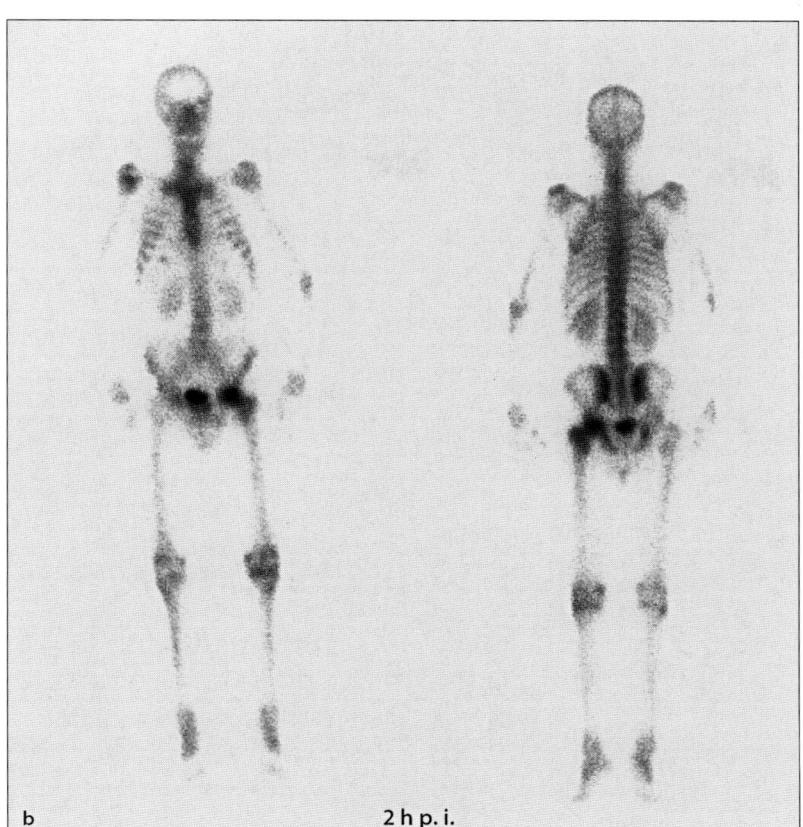

b   2 h p. i.

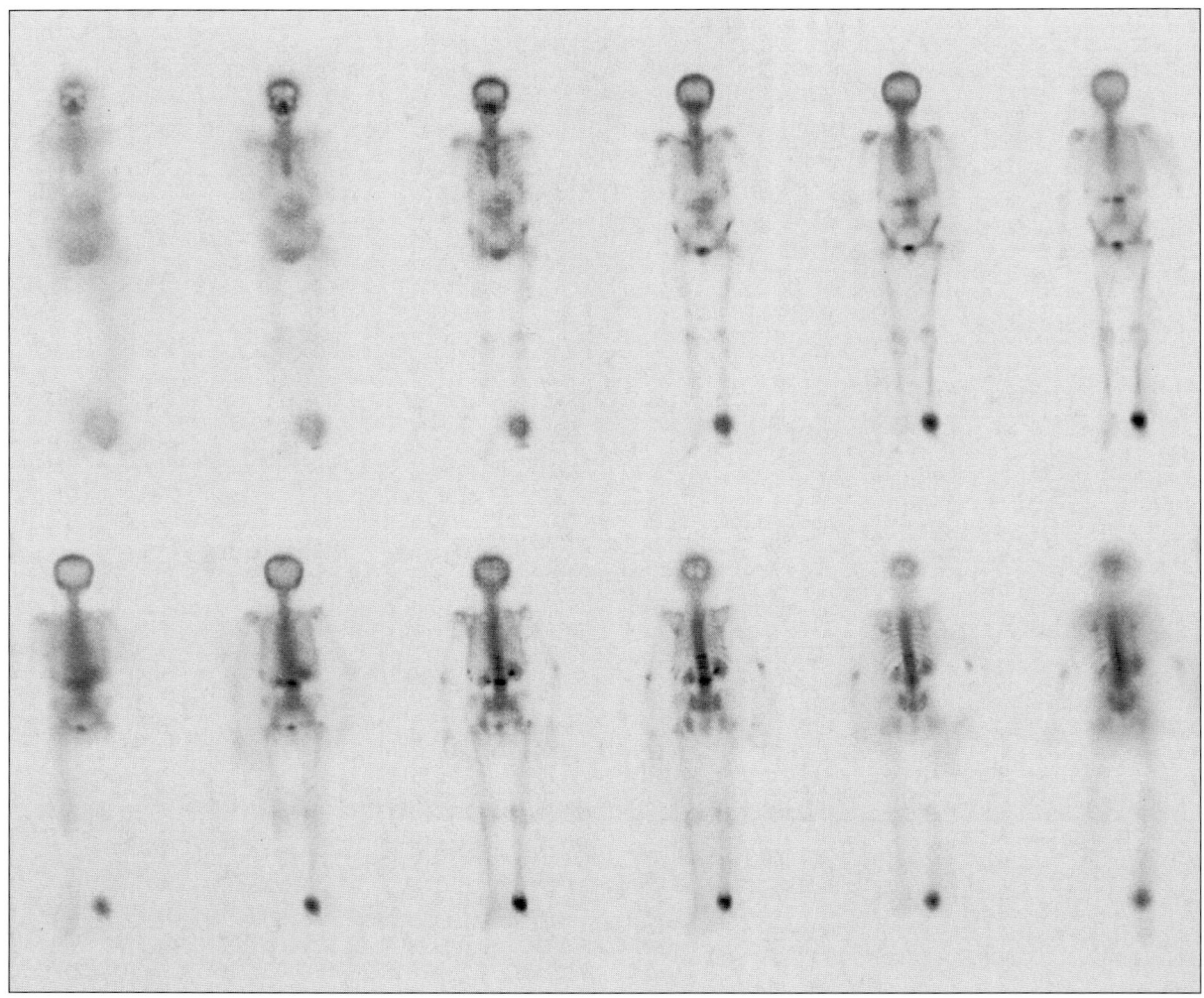

Fig. 4.50. A 71-year-old woman presented with pain in her back and left ankle. Whole-body scan 2 hours after injection of bone tracer shows a generally low degree of skeletal uptake except in several vertebrae at the thoracolumbar junction and in the left ankle region. The patient has osteoporosis with compression fractures in the vertebral column and left ankle joint

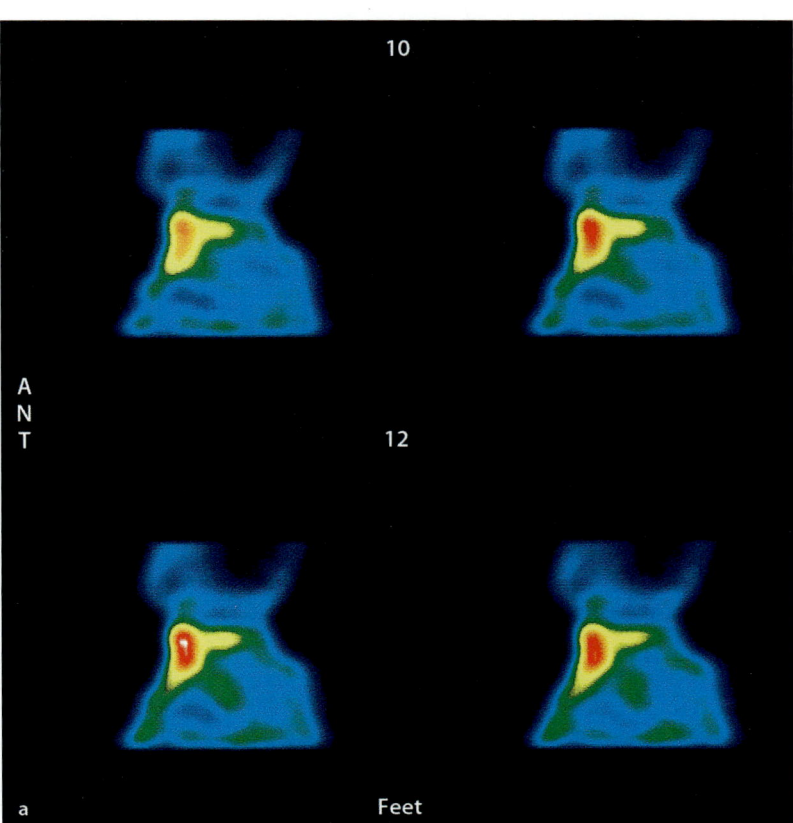

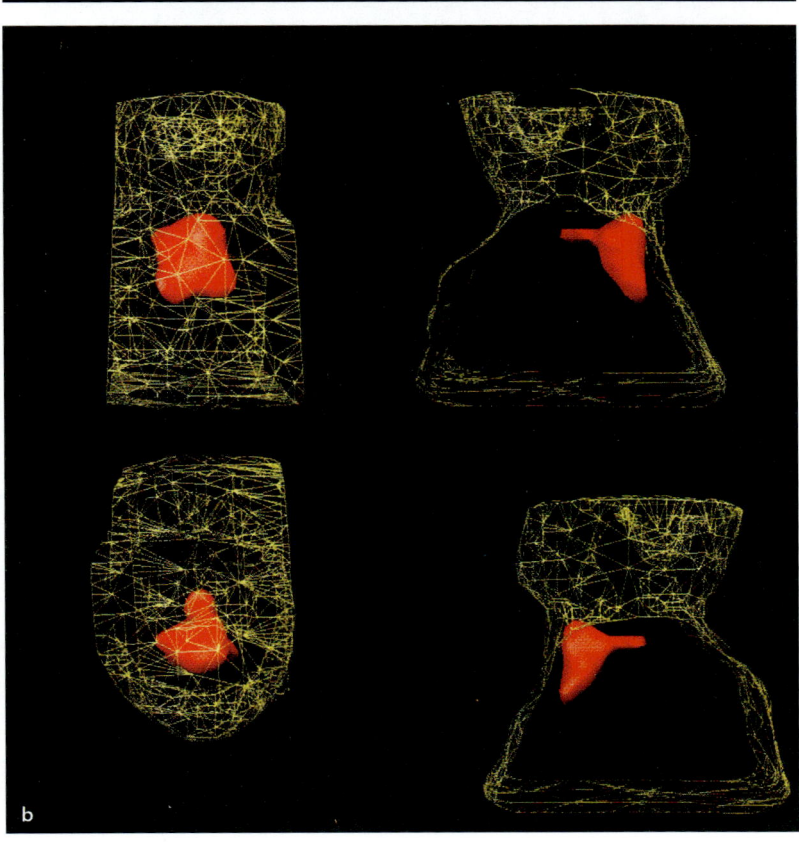

Fig. 4.51 a,b. A 65-year-old man presented with hoarseness and severe throat pain. Image acquired 78 hours after injection of ^{67}Ga citrate shows increased uptake in the arytenoid cartilage. Suspicion of malignant transformation of the cartilage was confirmed histologically

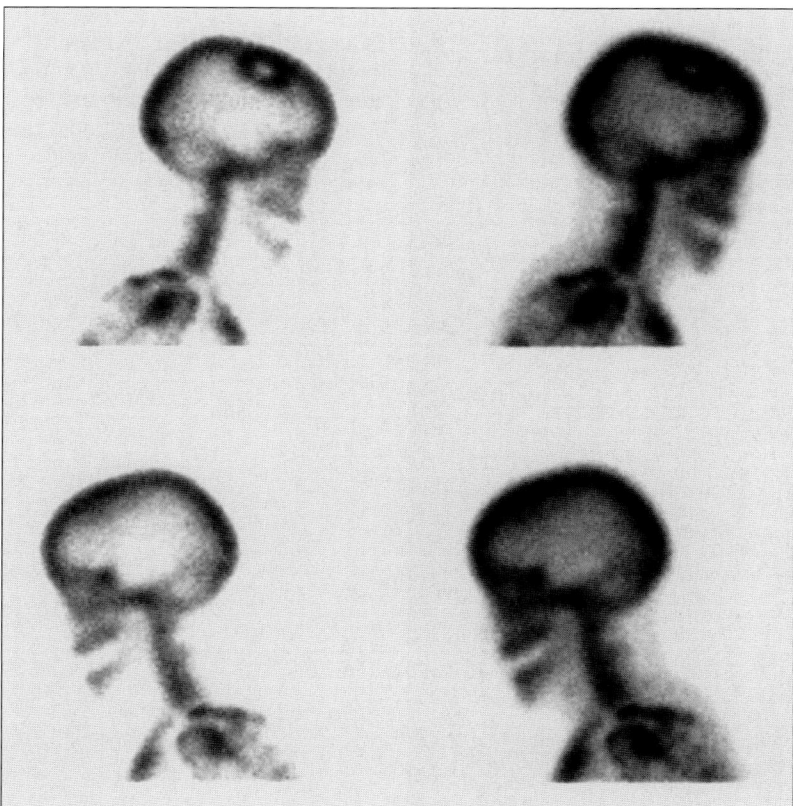

Fig. 4.52. Follow-up in a 53-year-old woman who underwent local excision of breast carcinoma. Scan acquired 2 hours after injection of bone tracer shows no skeletal abnormalities except in the skull, where there is a ringlike area of increased uptake with a cold center. Solitary bone metastasis with central necrosis

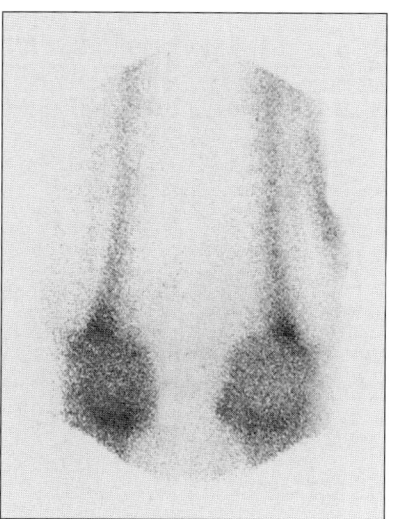

Fig. 4.53. A 40-year-old woman complained of pain in the lower leg. At bone scanning, the 20-second sequential perfusion-phase images and early static images show no abnormalities. Image acquired 2 hours after bone tracer injection shows a bandlike area of diffuse increased uptake. Myositis ossificans

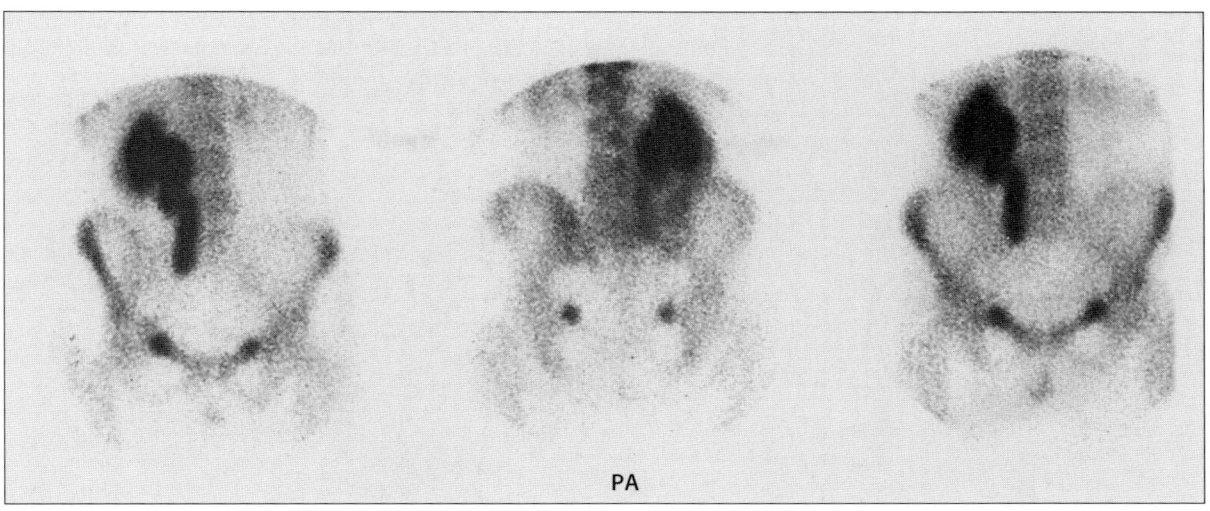

Fig. 4.54. A 45-year-old woman who had undergone lower abdominal surgery complained of severe back pain. Scan acquired 2 hours after bone tracer injection shows no abnormalities anywhere in the skeleton. Incidental note is made of tracer retention in the renal pyelocaliceal system, suggesting hydronephrosis as the cause of the pain

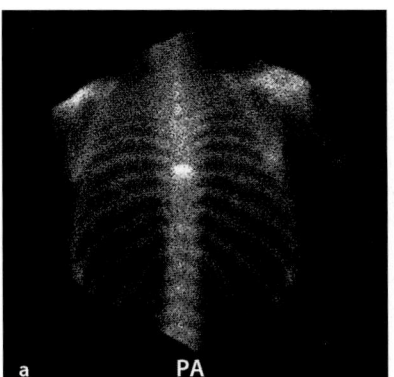
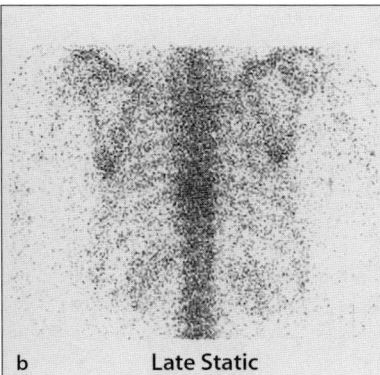

Fig. 4.55 a,b. A 39-year-old man from Eastern Europe had been treated conservatively for thoracic back pain for one year. The early static views (sequential images were omitted due to the lesion location) and the 2-hour image show increased uptake in the T7 vertebra. Tuberculin skin test was positive, and tuberculosis of the thoracic spine was confirmed histologically. Follow-up scan after one year's treatment showed complete regression of disease

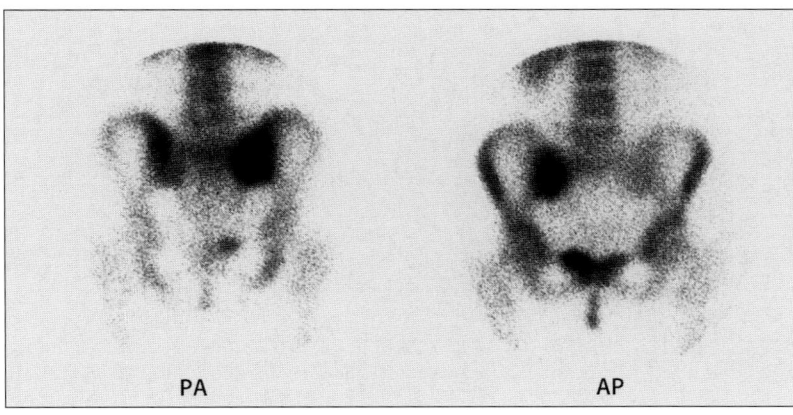

Fig. 4.56. A 28-year-old man presented with severe low back pain. In a scan acquired 2 hours after injection of bone tracer, side-to-side comparison shows increased uptake on the right side of the iliosacral joint. Tuberculin skin test was positive. Tuberculous ileitis

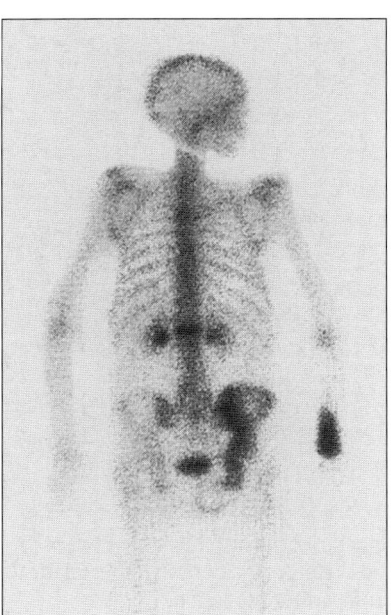

Fig. 4.57. This patient was hospitalized with multiple, nonspecific complaints. Scan 2 hours after injection of bone tracer shows intense uptake in the left iliac wing, left radius, and L2 vertebra. Paget's disease

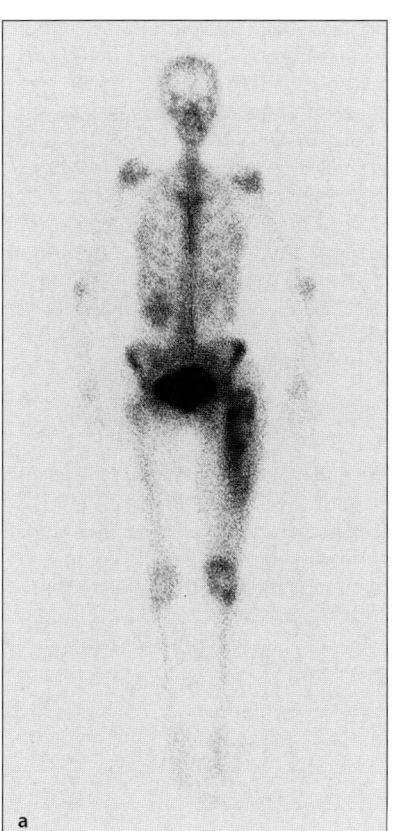

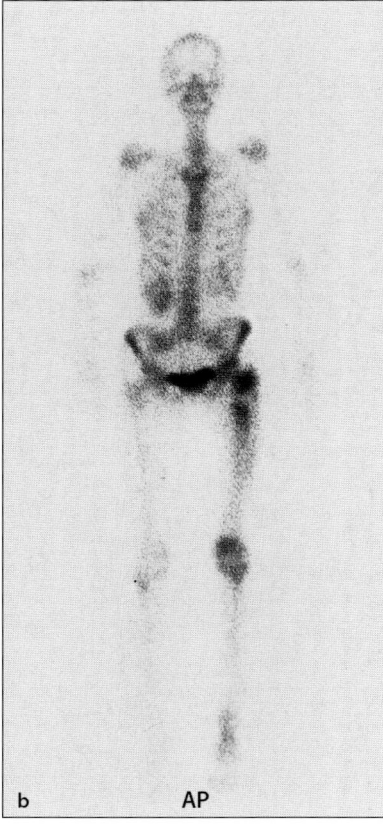

Fig. 4.58 a,b. A 21-year-old woman was diagnosed with a malignant tumor of the upper leg (**a**). Follow-up after one year of radiotherapy (the patient wanted to keep the leg) shows a successful result indicated by a regression of tracer uptake at the tumor site (**b**)

a

b   AP

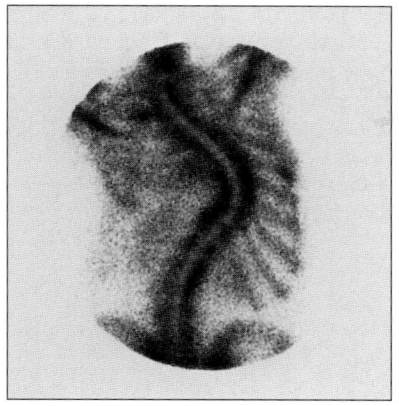

Fig. 4.59. A 50-year-old woman with kyphoscoliosis and chest pain was examined for an active spinal inflammatory process. Bone scan 2 hours after tracer injection shows no evidence of spinal inflammation. Subsequent cardiac study revealed CHD

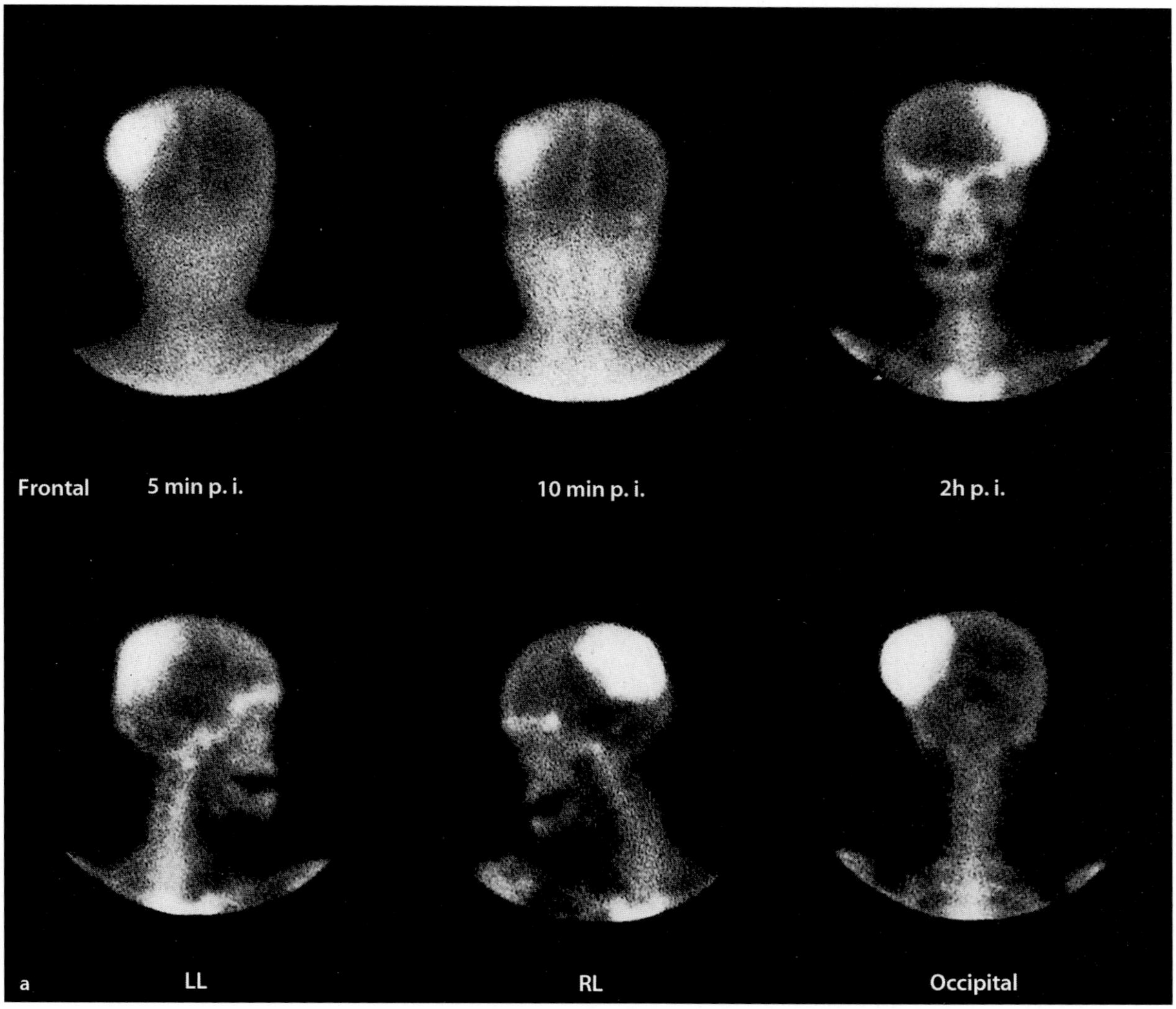

Frontal 5 min p. i.	10 min p. i.	2h p. i.
a LL	RL	Occipital

Fig. 4.60 a,b. A 50-year-old man was evaluated for nonspecific complaints. Bone scan 2 hours after tracer injection shows multiple site of increased bone uptake, most notably in the skull (**a**) and in the lower limbs (**b**), which show some osseous deformity. Multifocal involvement by Paget's disease

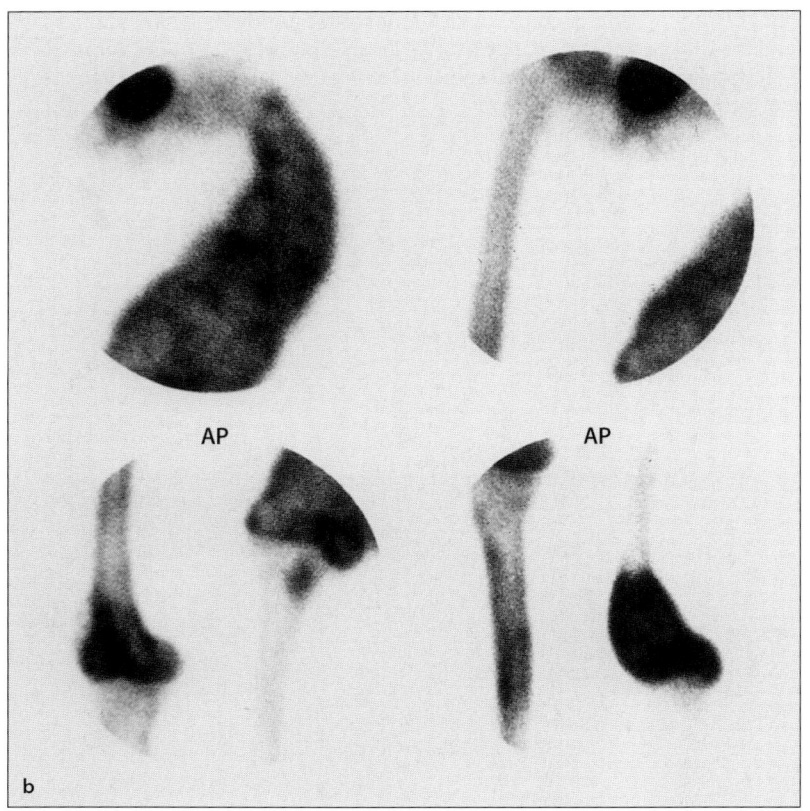

Fig. 4.60 a,b. A 50-year-old man was evaluated for nonspecific complaints. Bone scan 2 hours after tracer injection shows multiple site of increased bone uptake, most notably in the skull (**a**) and in the lower limbs (**b**), which show some osseous deformity. Multifocal involvement by Paget's disease

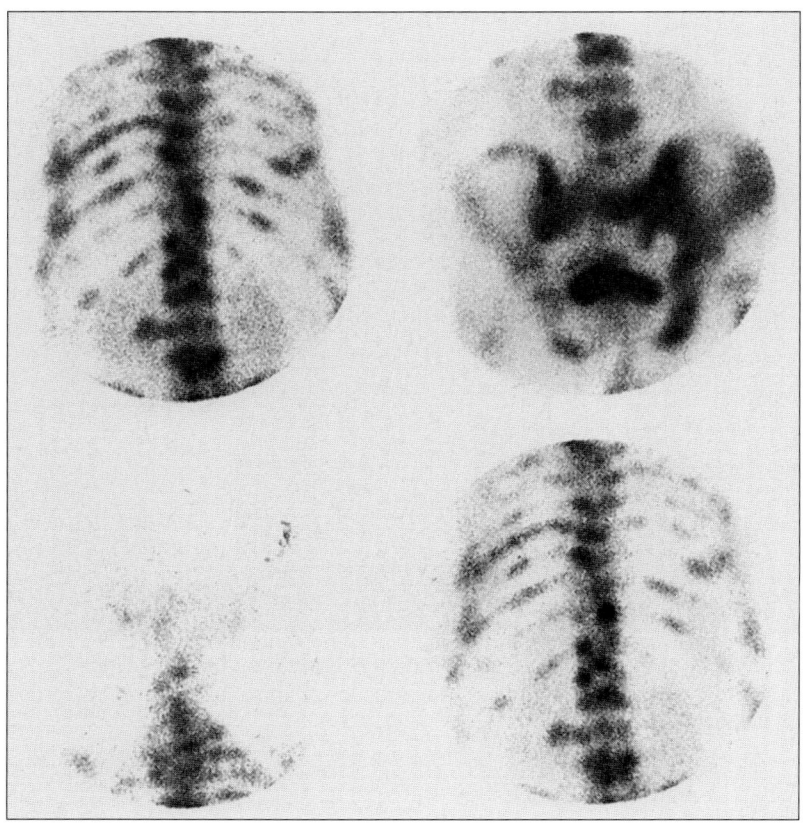

Fig. 4.61. A 60-year-old man who had undergone prostatic surgery presented for follow-up examination. Bone scan 2 hours after injection of ^{99m}Tc-labeled pyrophosphate shows multiple hot spots throughout the skeleton. Metastases from prostatic carcinoma

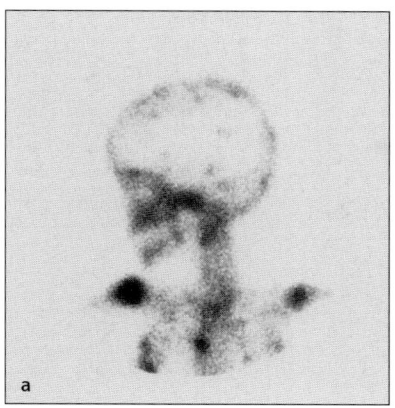

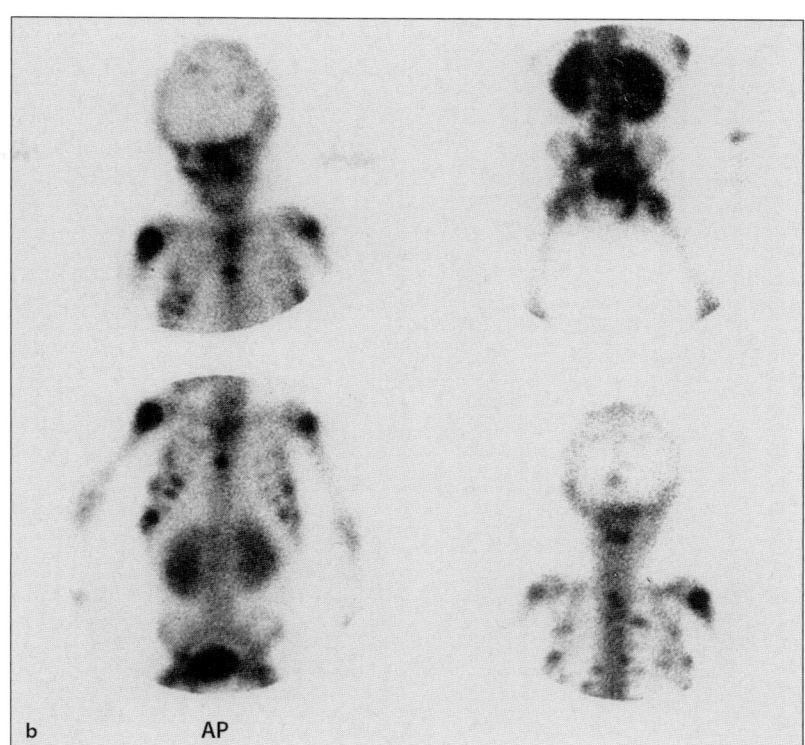

Fig. 4.62 a,b. A 2-year-old child with a malignant tumor was screened for metastatic disease. Scan 2 hours after injection of bone tracer shows widely disseminated hot spots representing skeletal metastases

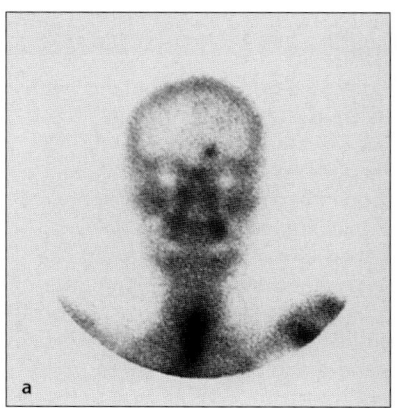

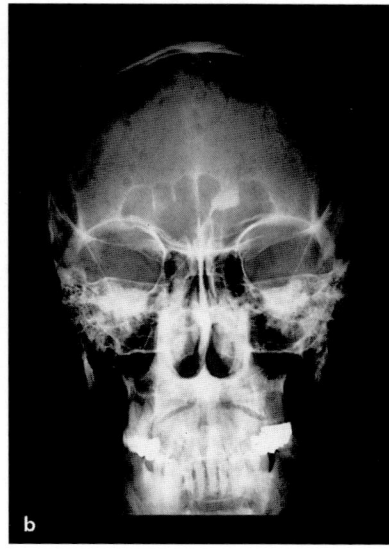

Fig. 4.63 a,b. A 60-year-old man complained of pressure in the frontal skull region. Scan 2 hours after tracer injection shows a hot spot directly above the nasal root. Radiographs also showed a definite lesion. Histology identified the lesion as a fibroma

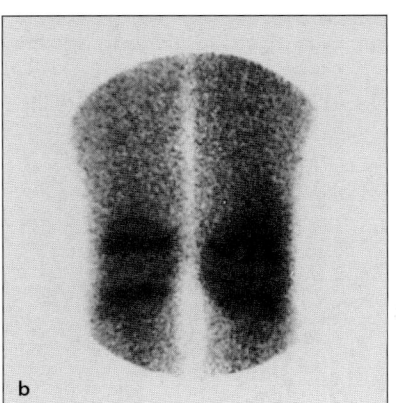

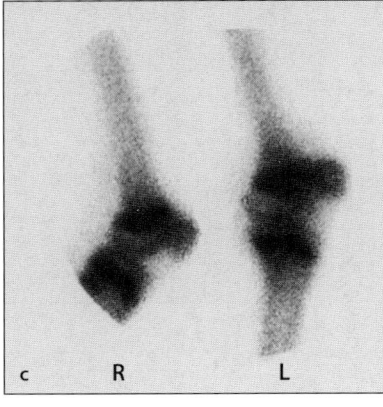

Fig. 4.64 a–c. A 38-year-old man with swelling and limited motion in the knee was evaluated for osseous changes. Sequential images were acquired immediately after bone tracer injection, and early and delayed static views were also obtained. The sequential images and early statics show diffuse, slightly increased uptake projected over the knee joint. The late static images show a relatively wide joint space but no abnormal uptake. Knee effusion without osseous involvement

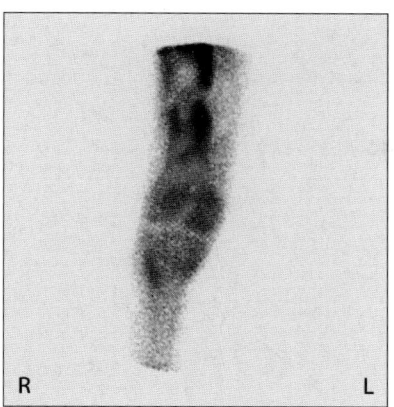

Fig. 4.65. A 20-year-old man with a femoral fracture was scanned under traction to evaluate fracture reduction. The gaping fracture site appears as a linear defect on the bone scan. Traction was adjusted accordingly

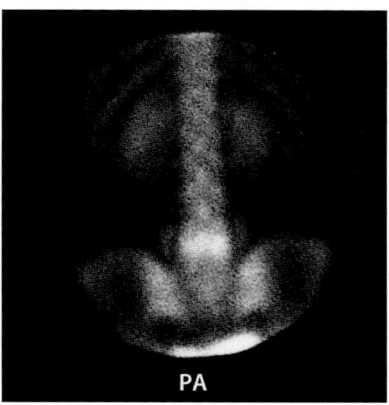

Fig. 4.66. A 35-year-old woman with a surgically drained abscess presented with sepsis and severe pain in the distal lumbar spine. Scan with bone tracer shows an area of increased activity in L4 with curvilinear boundaries. Osseous involvement of the L4 vertebra

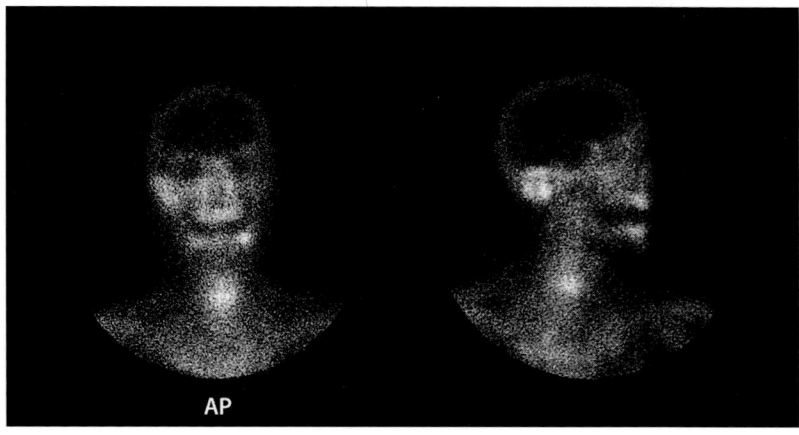

Fig. 4.67. A young patient presented with low-grade fever and headaches of undetermined cause. Scan 2 hours after injection of bone tracer shows increased uptake in the left mastoid process. Suppurative mastoiditis, treated by open drainage. Incidental note is made of a dental granuloma on the right side

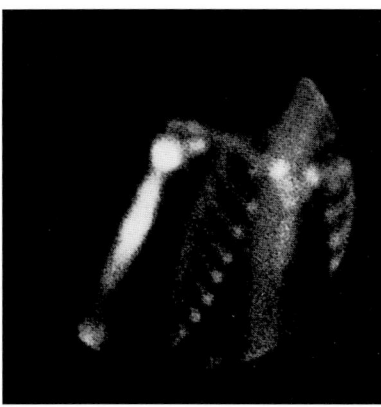

Fig. 4.68. An 8-year-old boy was evaluated for pain and tenderness in the right upper arm. Scan 2 hours after injection of bone tracer shows increased uptake in the proximal part of the humerus. Histology identified the lesion as fibrous bone dysplasia

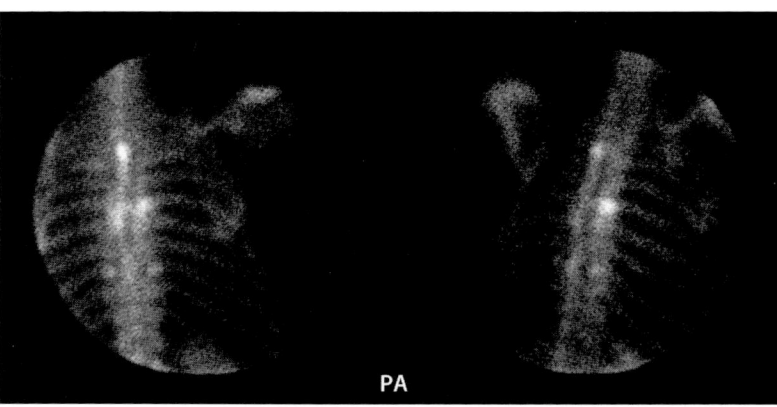

Fig. 4.69. A young woman who had undergone a spinal interbody fusion at the thoracic level presented with a recurrence of pain at the fusion site. Scan 2 hours after injection of bone tracer (sequential images were omitted due to lesion location) shows scattered areas of increased uptake around the arthrodesis plate, signifying incipient rejection. This was confirmed surgically

5 Miscellaneous

5.1
Arteries, Veins, and Lymphatics

Nuclear medicine studies of vascular structures are based on the visualization of blood vessels and lymphatics on sequential or static images acquired after the intravenous or intradermal injection of a radiopharmaceutical agent.

Normal tracer-responsive lymph nodes will not take up radiotracer if their connection to the distal lymph channels has been interrupted. With a partial or complete obstruction, the lymph drains around the lymph nodes through collateral pathways. The retroperitoneal lymphatic system is bounded above and below by the sternum and symphysis and laterally by the inguinal lymph nodes. The impairment of lymphatic drainage is characterized by the retention of radiotracer along the distal afferent lymphatics. As a functional examination, lymphoscintigraphy makes it possible to determine both the intensity of lymphatic drainage and the velocity of the lymph flow.

5.2
Bone Marrow

Bone marrow scanning has gained a place in clinical diagnosis by demonstrating the uptake pattern and distribution of agents that are taken up by functional red marrow

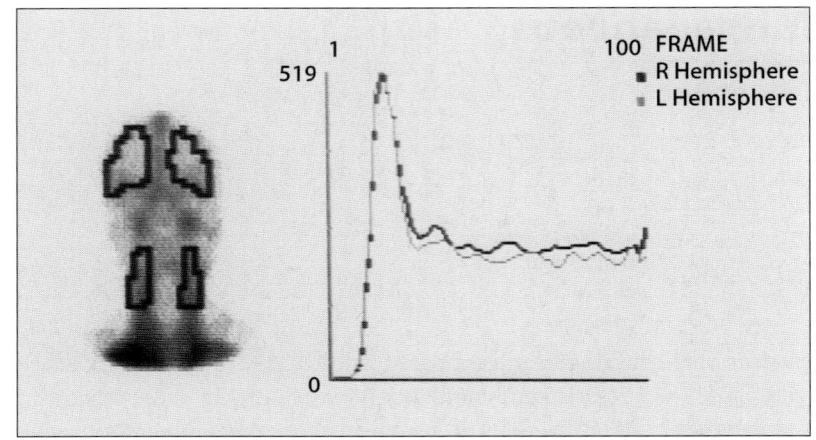

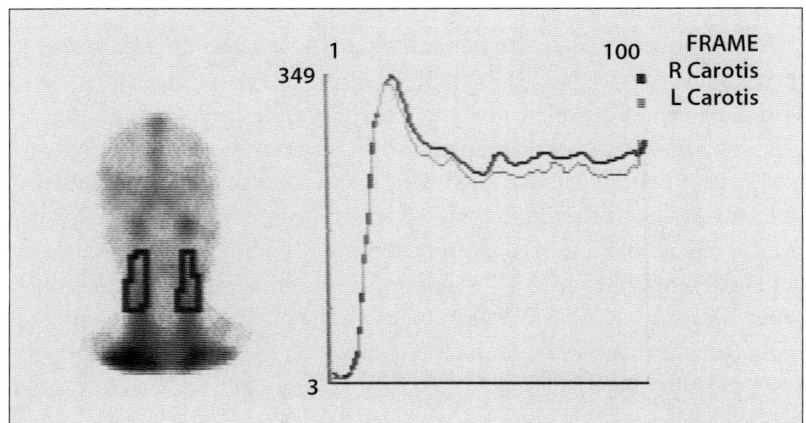

Fig. 5.1. ROI image demonstrates normal flow velocity in both carotid arteries and in the middle cerebral artery

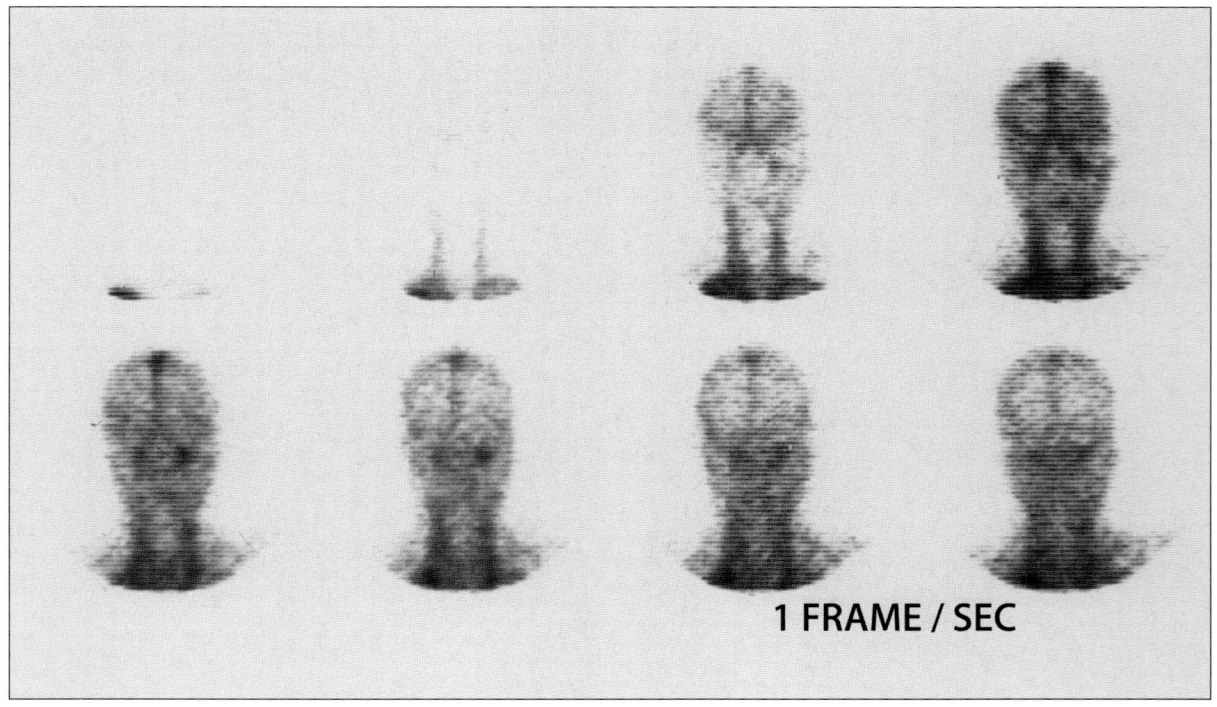

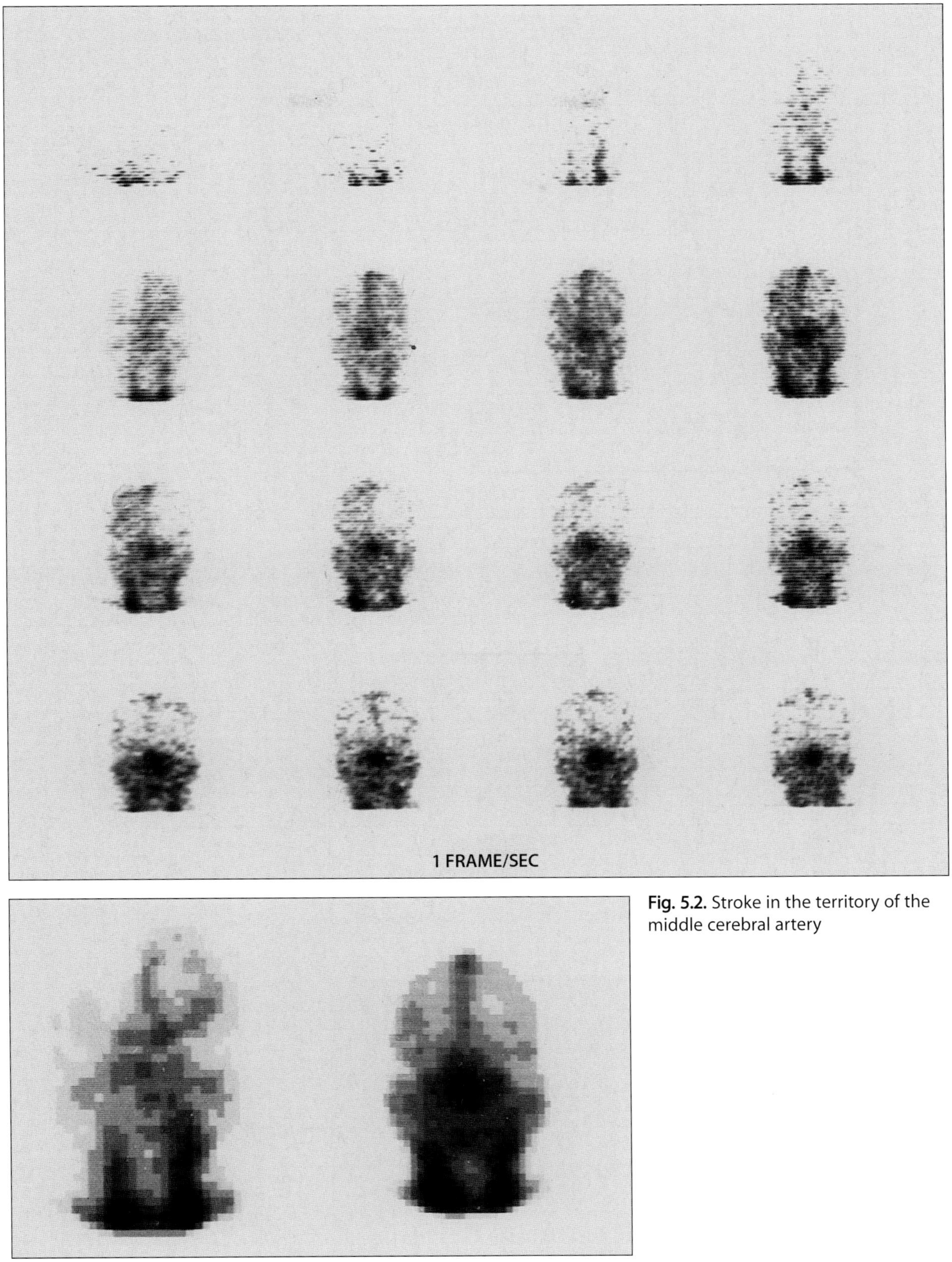

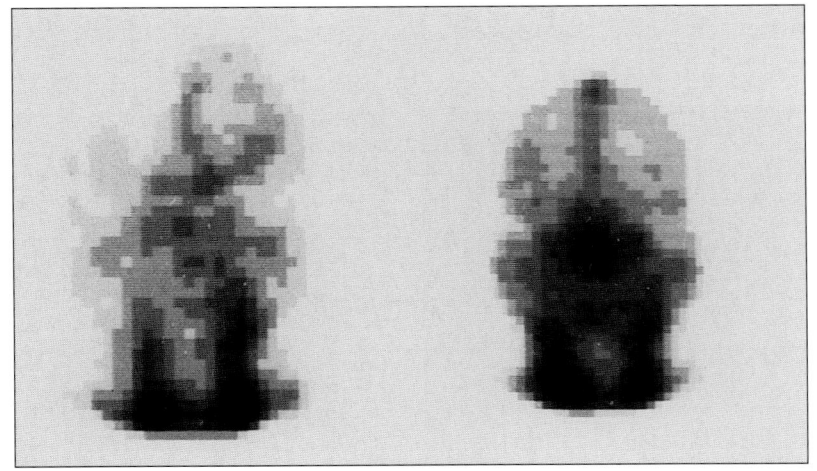

1 FRAME/SEC

Fig. 5.2. Stroke in the territory of the middle cerebral artery

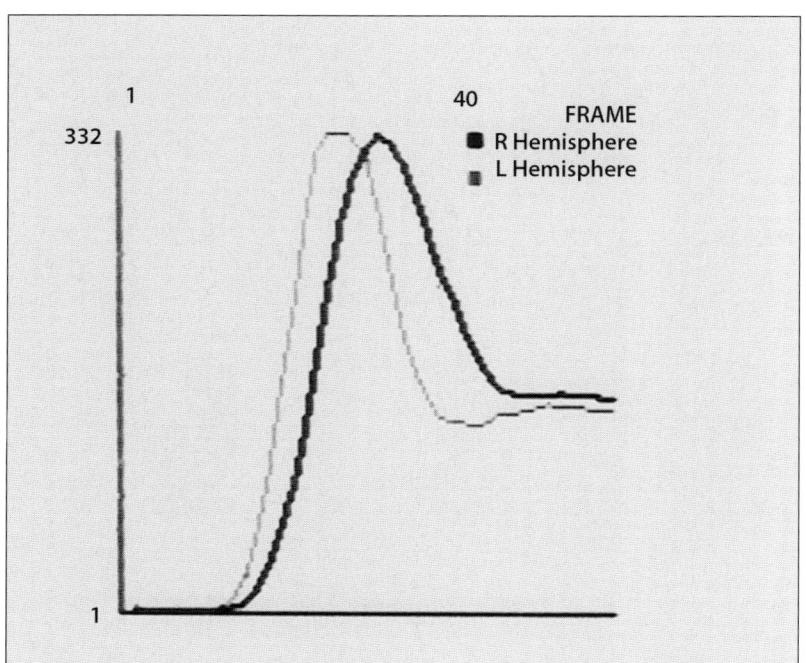

Fig. 5.2. Stroke in the territory of the middle cerebral artery

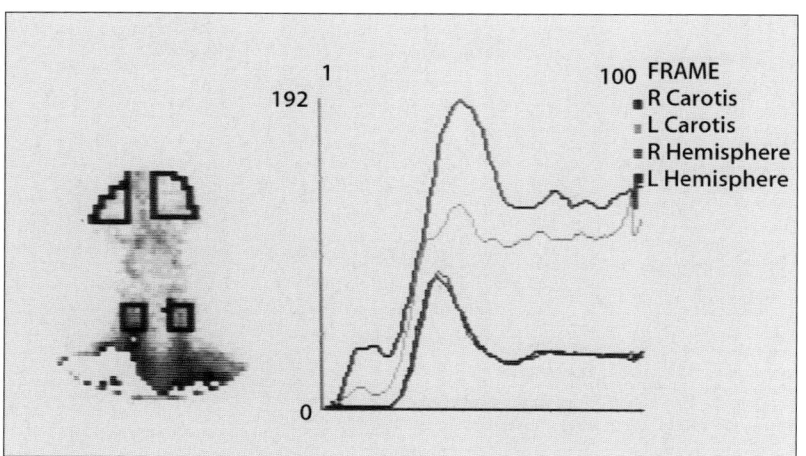

Fig. 5.3. Flow obstruction by plaque in the left common carotid artery does not affect cerebral blood flow velocity in the territory of the middle cerebral artery

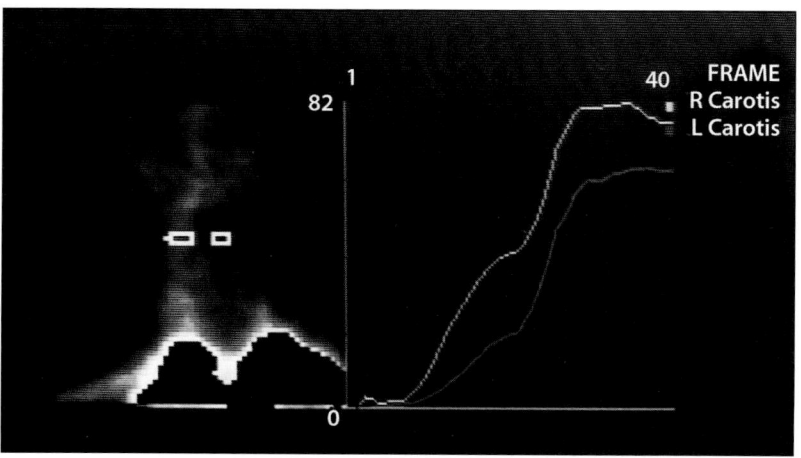

Fig. 5.4. Abnormal flow velocity caused by plaque in both carotid arteries (more severe on the left side)

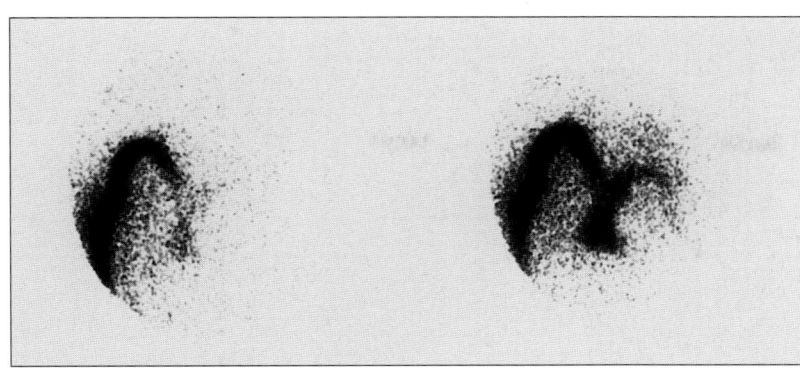

Fig. 5.5. Good visualization of the superior vena cava

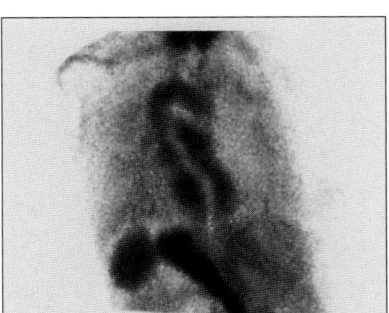

Fig. 5.6. Visualization of the aortic arch

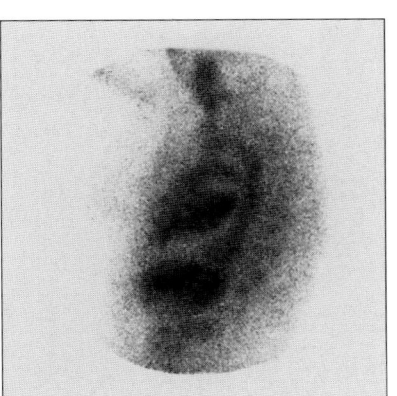

Fig. 5.7. Visualization of the thoracic duct

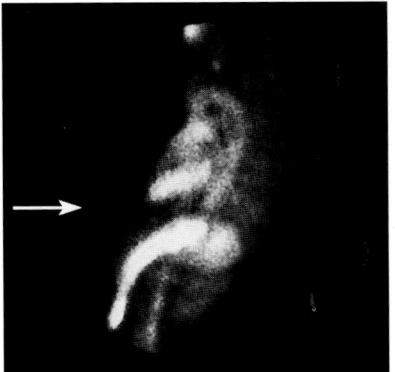

Fig. 5.8. Radionuclide investigation of mediastinal widening (*arrow*) demonstrates an aneurysm in the upper portion of the thoracic aorta

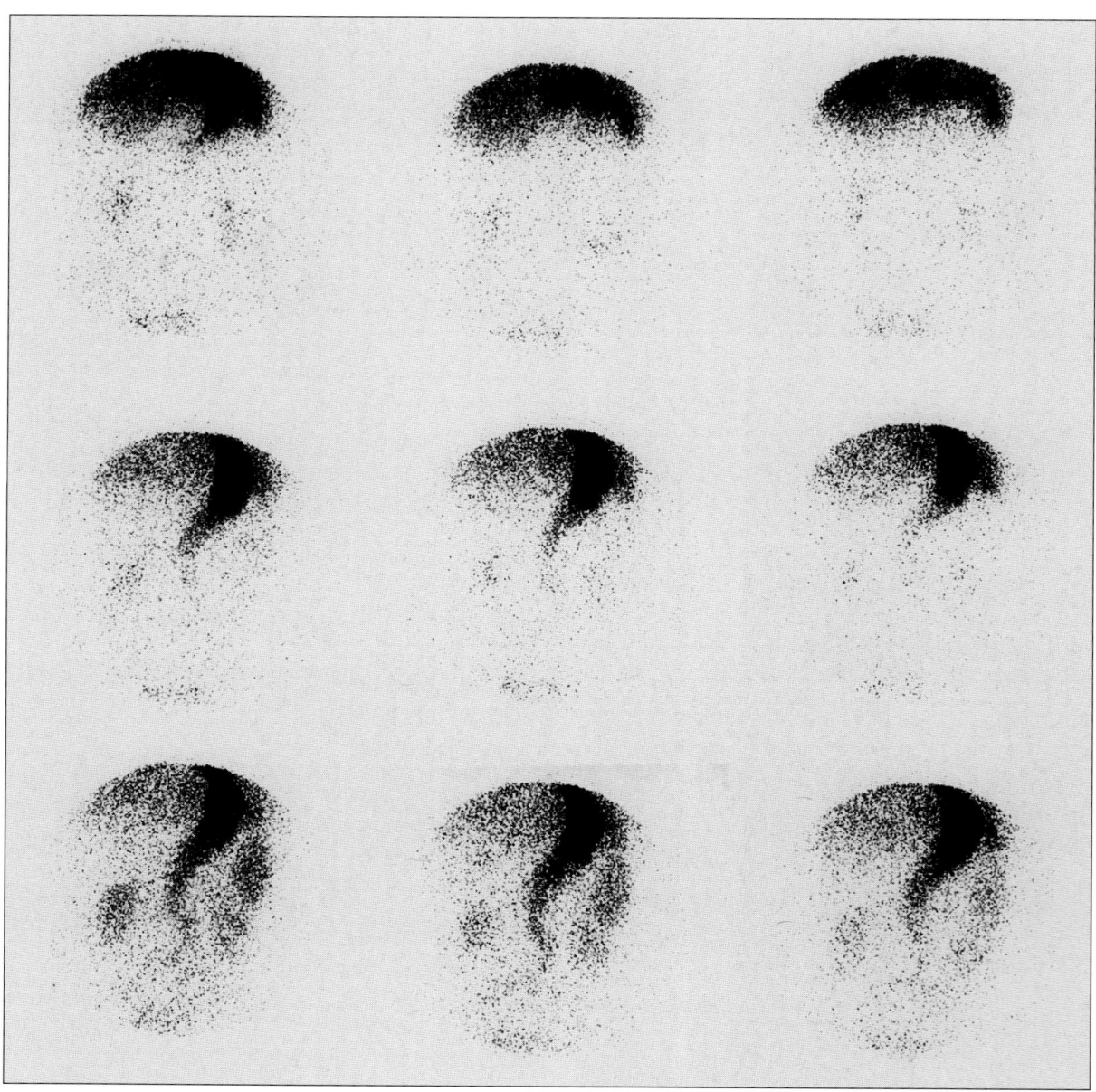

Fig. 5.9. Radionuclide investigation of circulatory impairment in both legs shows conical expansion of the abdominal aorta at the renal level due to obstruction by a tumor or embolus. The specific nature of the obstructive lesion is indeterminate by radionuclide imaging

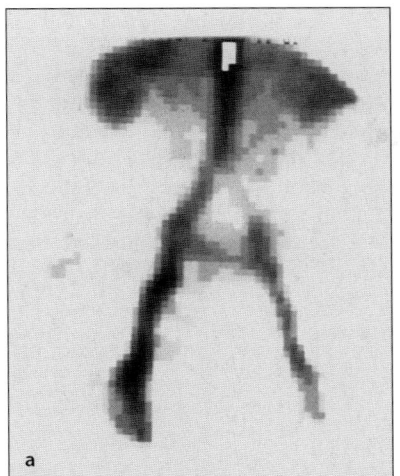

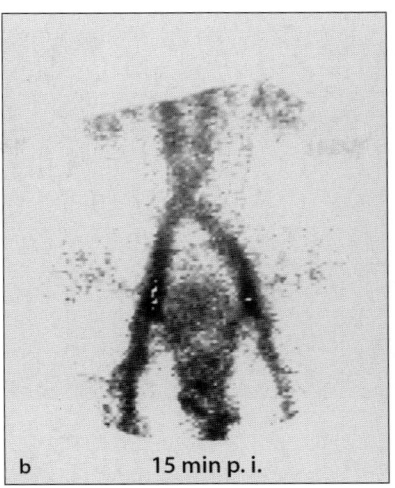

15 min p. i.

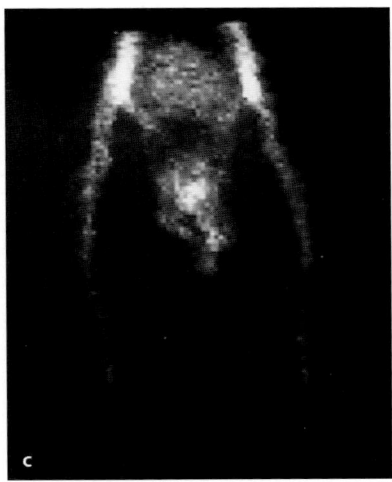

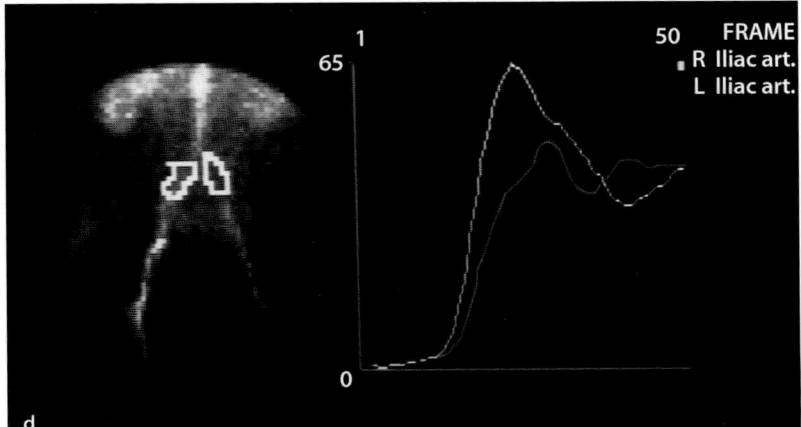

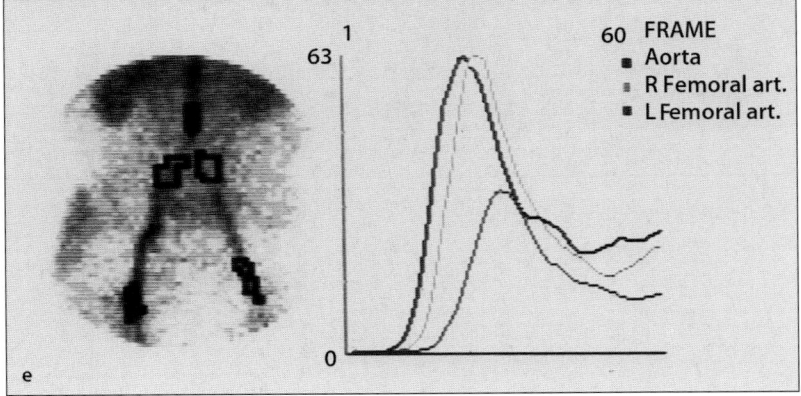

Fig. 5.10 a–g. Radionuclide blood flow study in the left leg demonstrates occlusion of the left common iliac artery. Delayed visualization of the artery is a result of retrograde flow through collateral vessels. The occlusion also affects the territory of the femoral artery, and multiple obstructions are seen in both femoral arteries (left > right) with associated collateralization

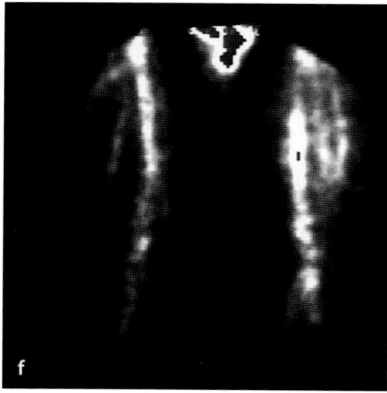
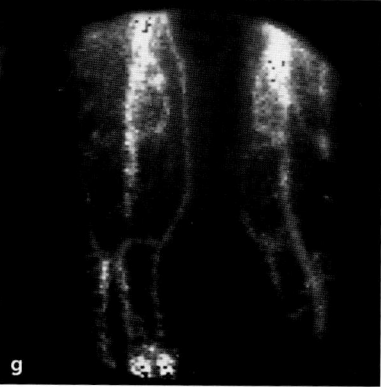

Fig. 5.10 a–g. Radionuclide blood flow study in the left leg demonstrates occlusion of the left common iliac artery. Delayed visualization of the artery is a result of retrograde flow through collateral vessels. The occlusion also affects the territory of the femoral artery, and multiple obstructions are seen in both femoral arteries (left > right) with associated collateralization

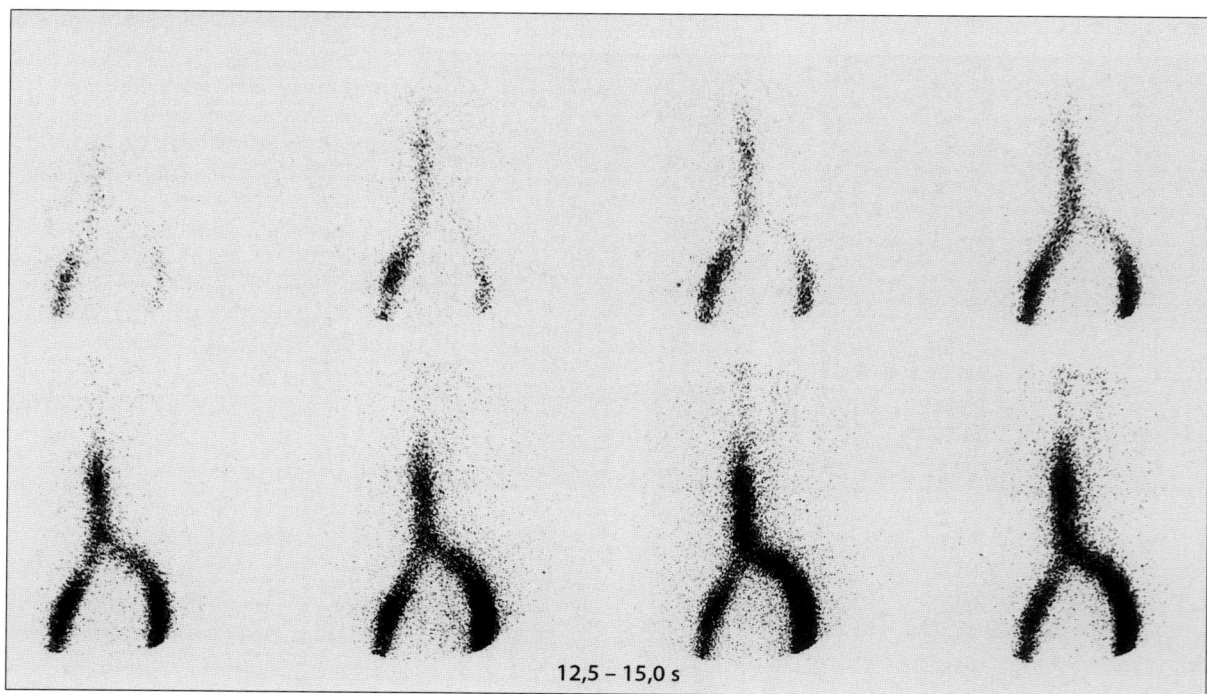

12,5 – 15,0 s

Fig. 5.11. This scan demonstrates encasement of the inferior vena cava by tumor

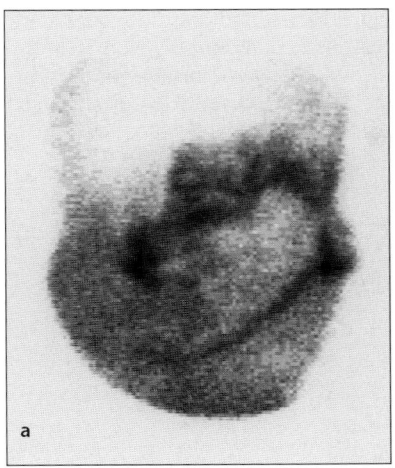

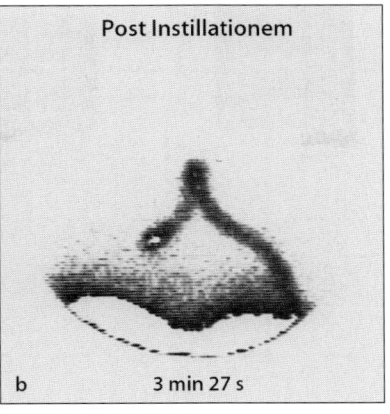

Post Instillationem

b   3 min 27 s

Fig. 5.12 a–d. Evaluation of a LeVeen shunt implanted for drainage of ascites in hepatic cirrhosis. The scan confirms a well-functioning shunt

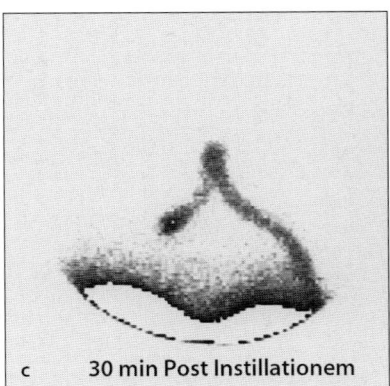

c   30 min Post Instillationem

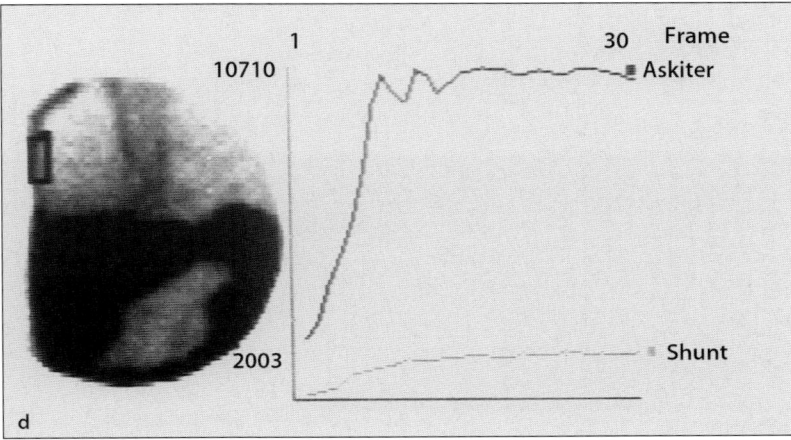

d

Fig. 5.13 a–c. Radionuclide evaluation of hepatic blood supply. Normal findings (**a**), incipient portal hypertension (**b**), established portal hypertension (**c**)

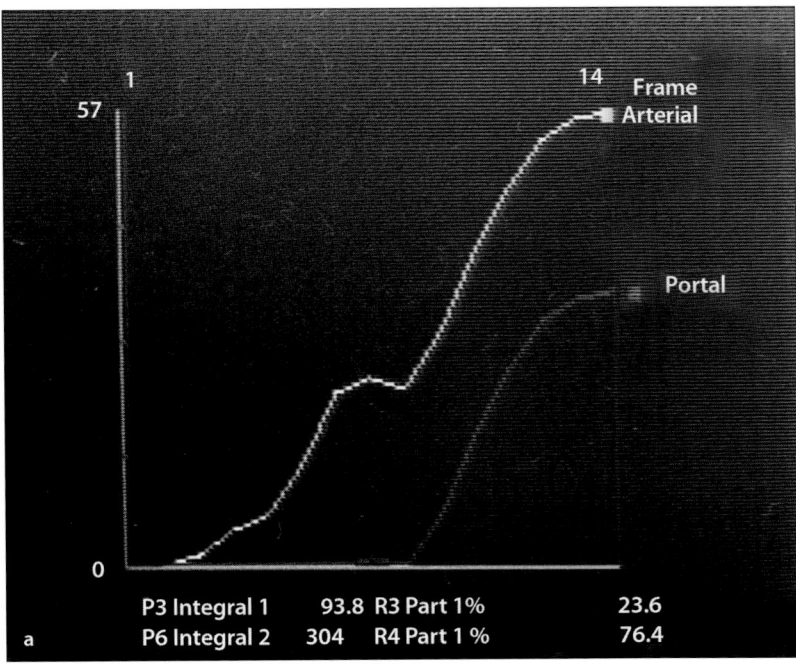

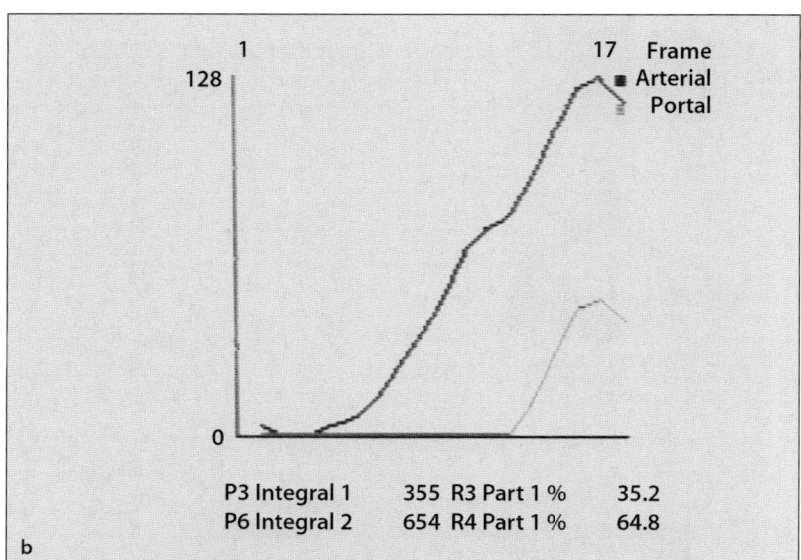

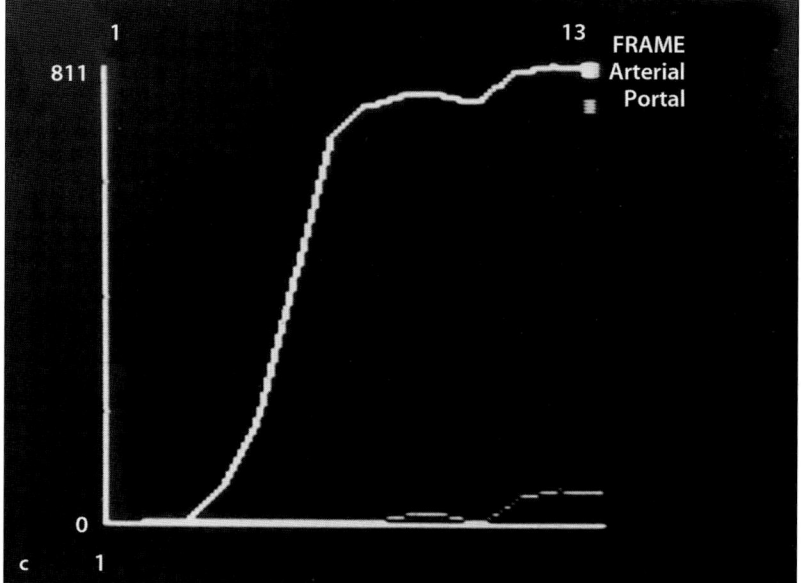

Fig. 5.13 a–c. Radionuclide evaluation of hepatic blood supply. Normal findings (a), incipient portal hypertension (b), established portal hypertension (c)

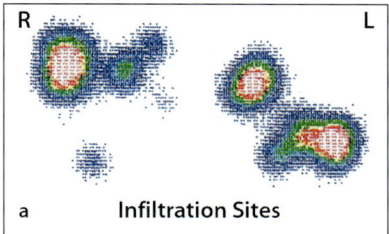

Infiltration Sites

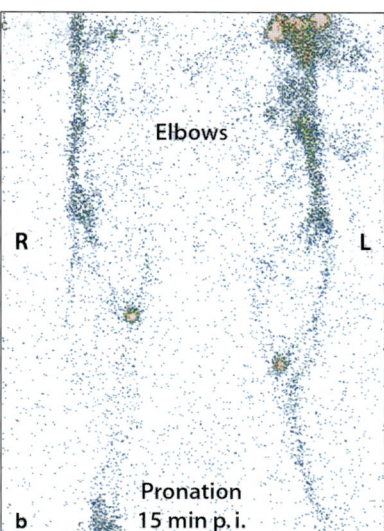

Elbows

R   L

Pronation
15 min p.i.

Fig. 5.14 a–d. A 32-year-old woman presented with swelling of both arms (right > left) and chronic fungal infection of the nails. Scan of the right arm shows narrowed vascular calibers and collateral formation at the level of the elbow. In the upper arm, tracer is delivered to the axilla almost entirely by collaterals and diffusion. Radionuclide transport in the left arm is better but still impaired. The axillary lymph nodes are particularly enlarged on the right side, which is consistent with the clinical presentation. Mixed chronic and florid lymphadenitis, predominantly right-sided, with segmental obliteration of some lymph channels

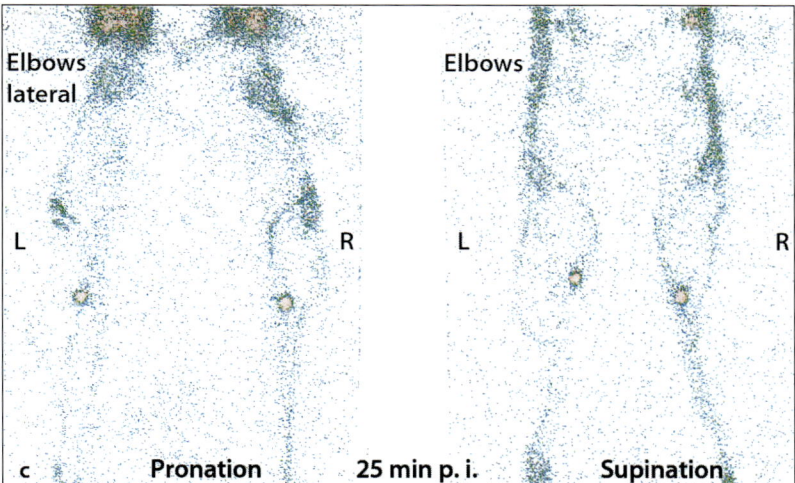

Elbows lateral   Elbows

L   R   L   R

Pronation   25 min p.i.   Supination

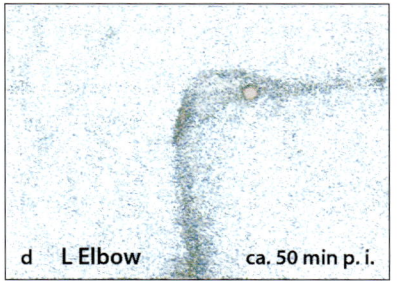

d L Elbow   ca. 50 min p.i.

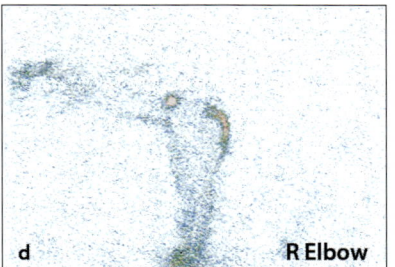

d   R Elbow

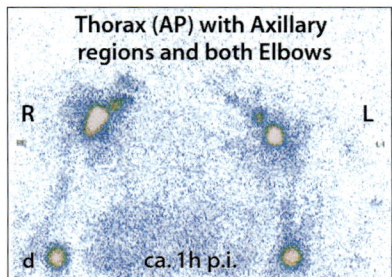

Thorax (AP) with Axillary regions and both Elbows

R   L

d   ca. 1h p.i.

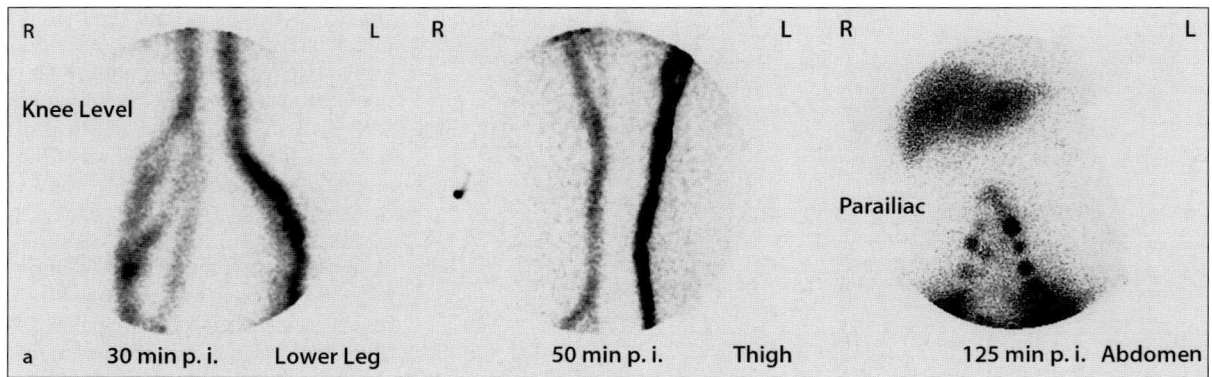

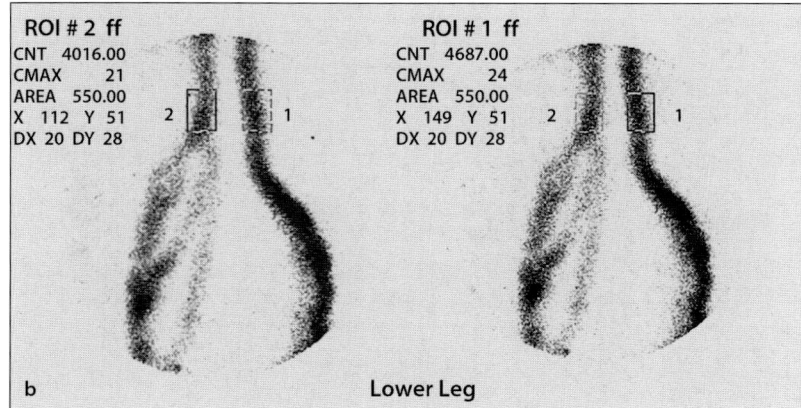

Fig. 5.15 a,b. This woman complained of intermittent ankle edema. Lymphoscintigraphy shows no abnormalities. An apparent difference between the sides was noted during position changes. Physiologic variant

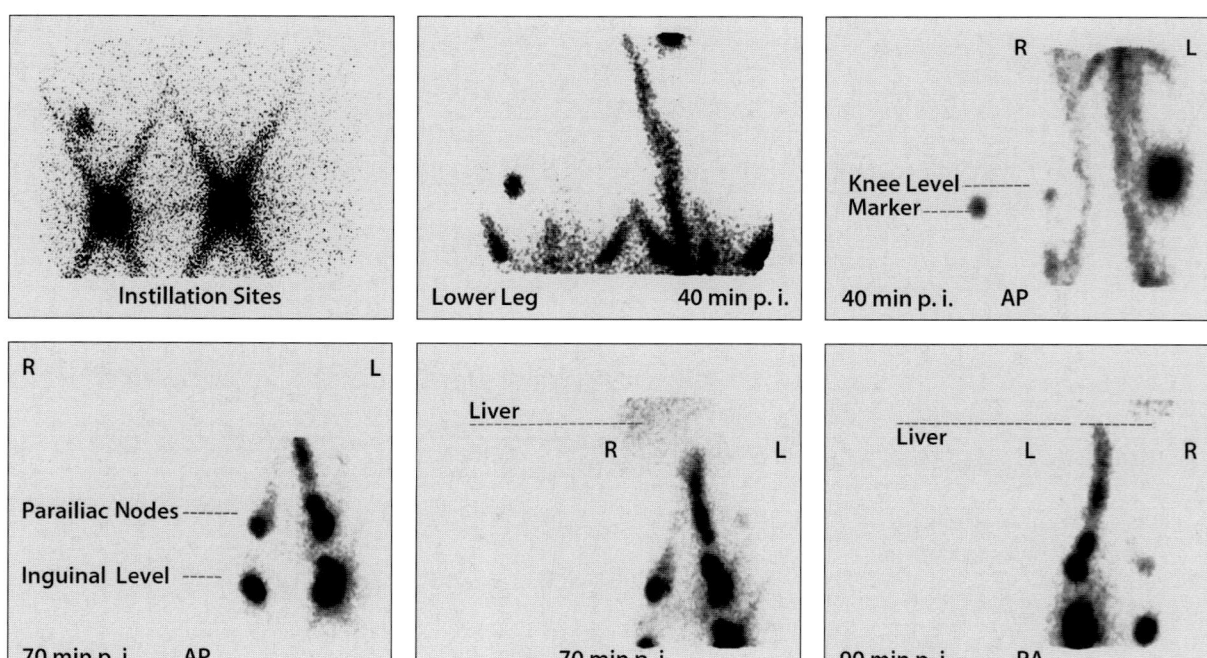

Fig. 5.16. A 30-year-old woman weighing 116 kg presented with significant, bilateral nodular lipomatosis that was most pronounced in the right thigh. Radionuclide transport is delayed on both sides and almost absent on the right side. Tracer does not reach the porta hepatis by the end of the examination

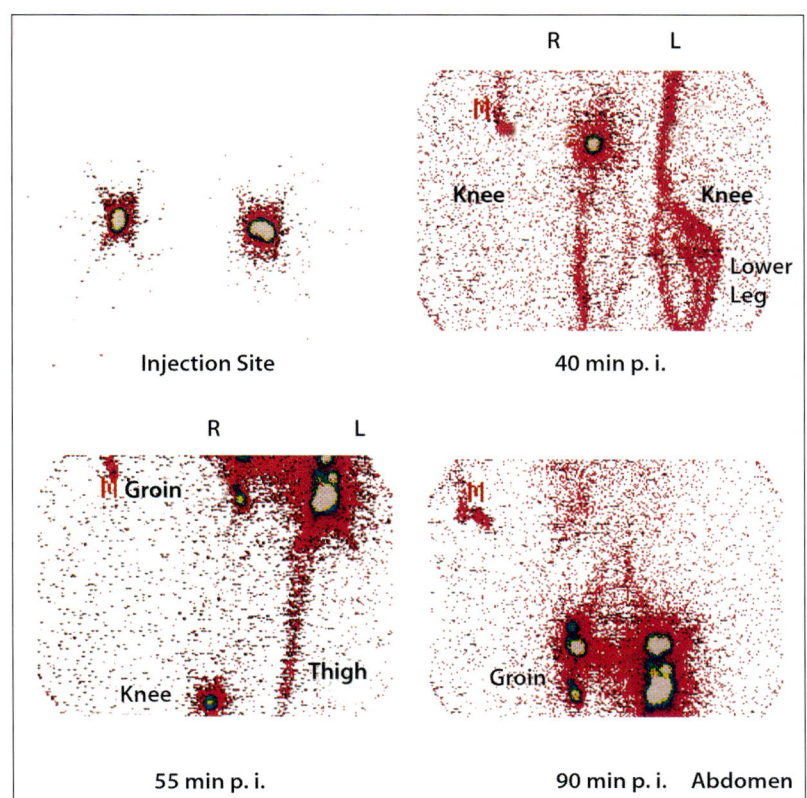

Fig. 5.17. The right leg has been swollen for several years. Side-to-side comparison shows a decreased number and size of vessels in the right lower leg, with diffusion accounting for transport on the right side. Probably a congenital condition

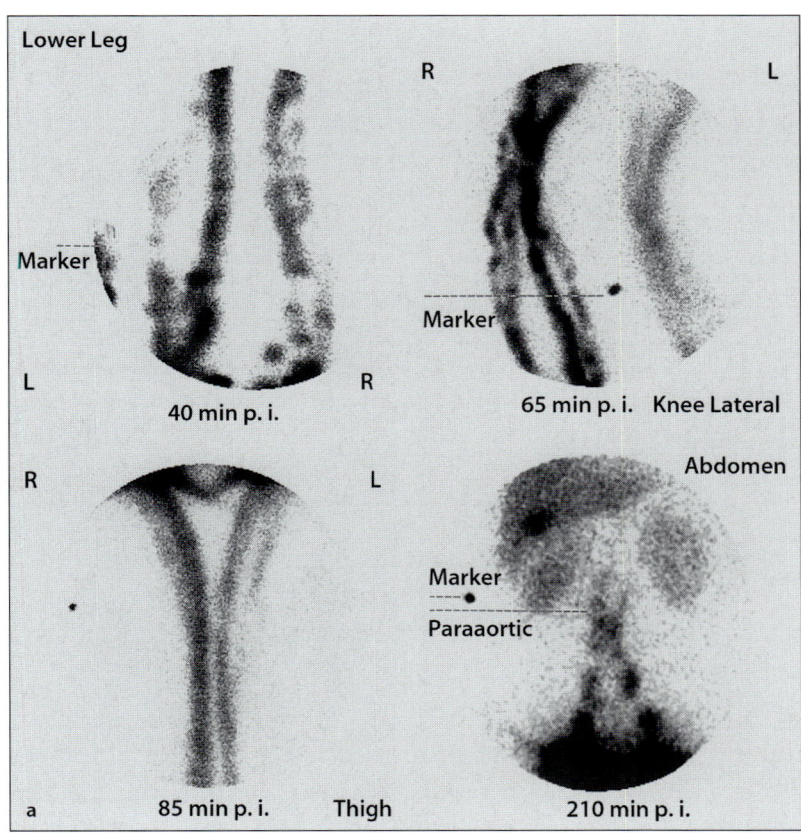

Fig. 5.18 a–c. This patient had pain in both legs, more pronounced on the left side. Physical examination showed tenderness and generalized redness of the left leg with interdigital mycosis. Radionuclide scan shows a well-developed lymphatic system with multiple sites of obstruction. Side-to-side comparison shows decreased radionuclide transport in the left leg. Acute lymphadenitis with digital mycosis

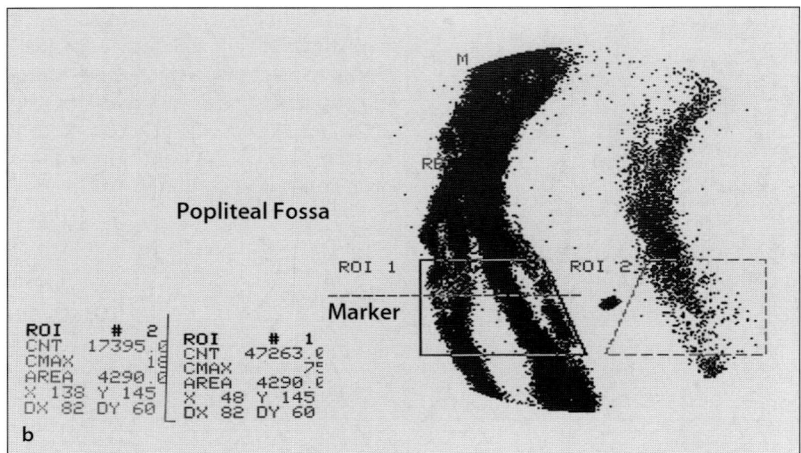

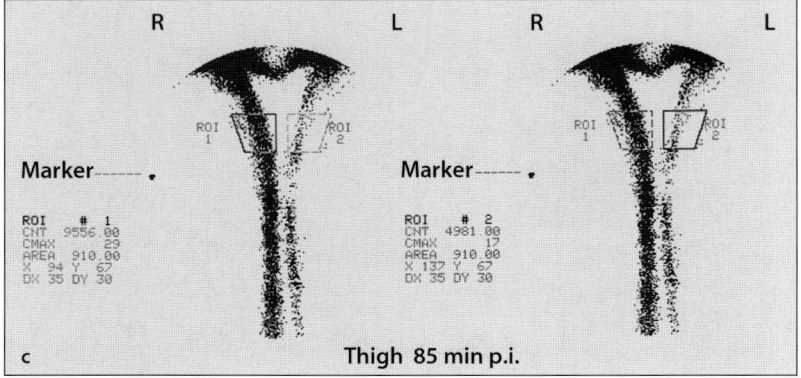

Fig. 5.18 a–c. This patient had pain in both legs, more pronounced on the left side. Physical examination showed tenderness and generalized redness of the left leg with interdigital mycosis. Radionuclide scan shows a well-developed lymphatic system with multiple sites of obstruction. Side-to-side comparison shows decreased radionuclide transport in the left leg. Acute lymphadenitis with digital mycosis

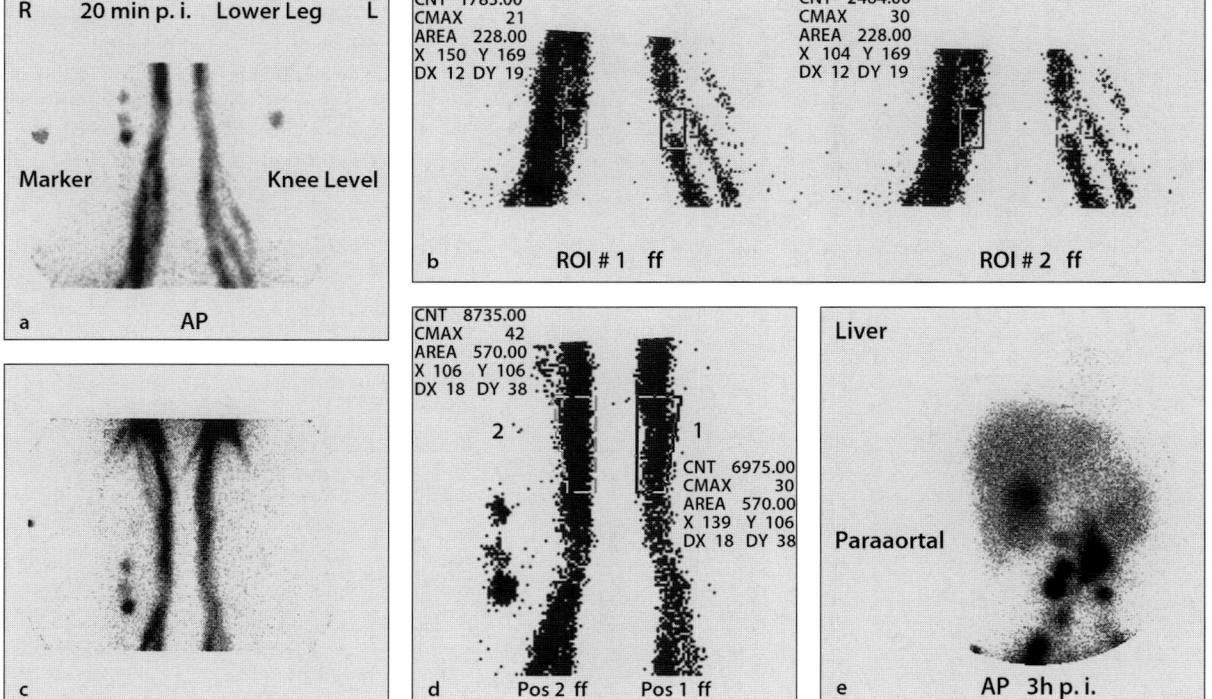

Fig. 5.19 a–e. This patient presented with unexplained leg edema and weight gain. Radionuclide scan shows delivery of the tracer almost to the porta hepatis, where further transit is blocked by an obstructing tumor

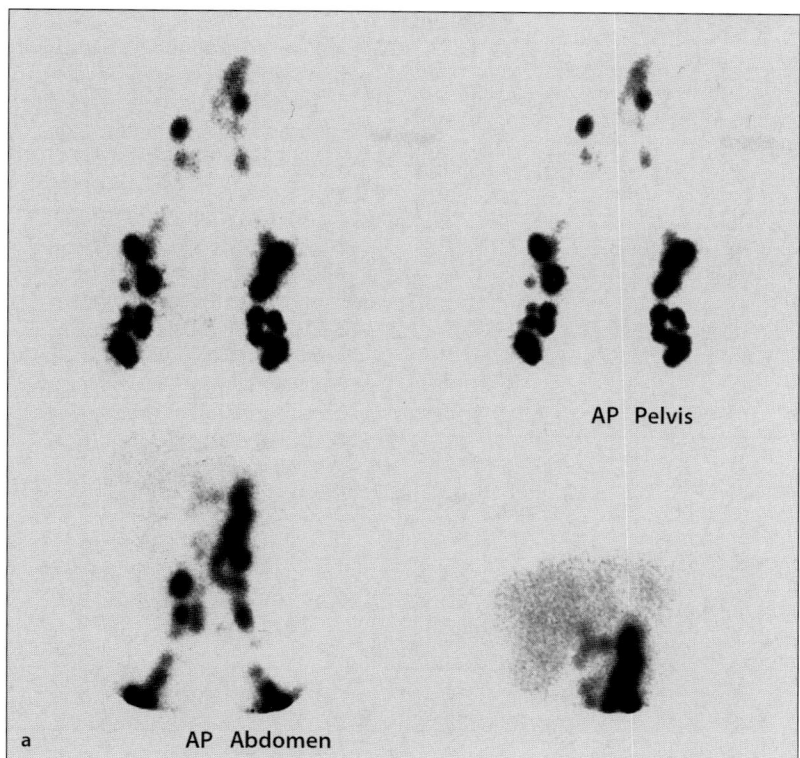

AP Pelvis

AP Abdomen

Fig. 5.20 a–c. Scan in a patient with upper abdominal complaints and bilateral leg edema demonstrates good bilateral transport approximately to the porta hepatis. The scan also shows a right-sided obstruction that is bypassed by collateral lymph vessels and a complete obstruction in the diaphragmatic compartment. Extensive upper abdominal tumor

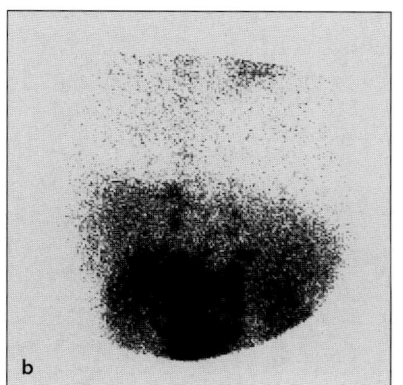

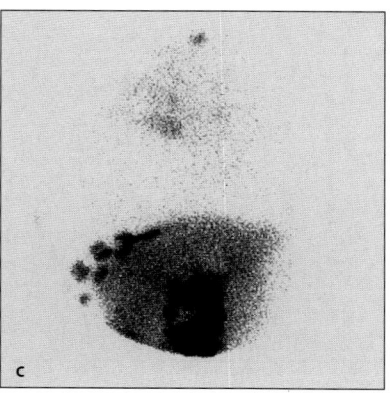

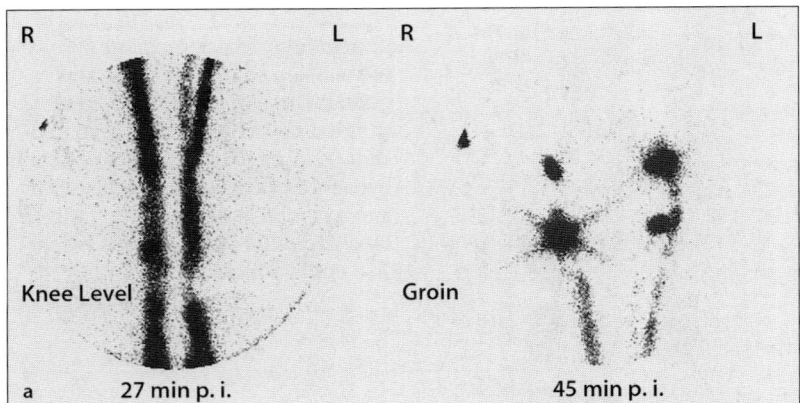

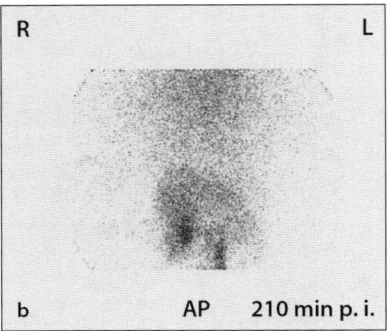

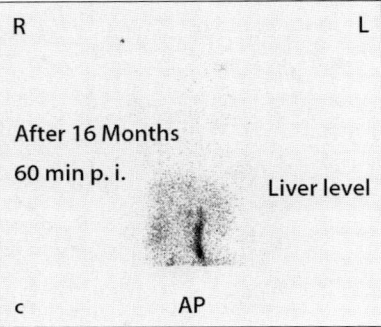

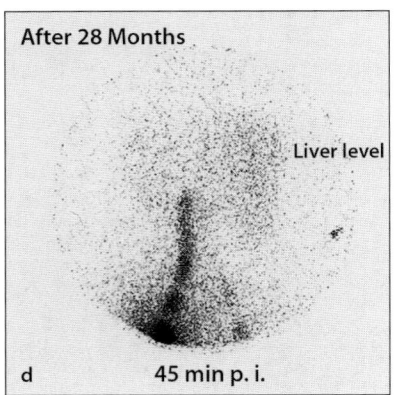

Fig. 5.21 a–d. A 20-year-old woman claimed a history of nephritis in childhood. She presented now with leg edema, which had been attributed to the childhood illness. Radionuclide renal scan demonstrates normal glomerular filtration, tubular function, and excretion. Lymphoscintigraphy shows an almost complete obstruction of lymphatic drainage in the lesser pelvis. Further investigation revealed endometriosis, for which treatment was provided. Follow-ups at 2 years (**c**) and 3 years (**d**) show considerable regression of the obstruction and a decrease in transit time from 210 to 45 minutes

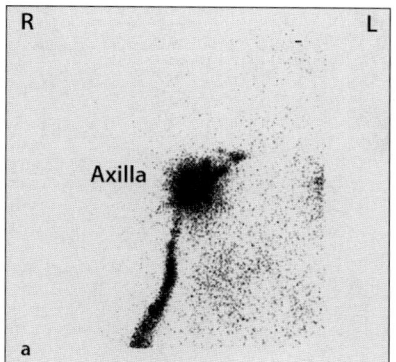

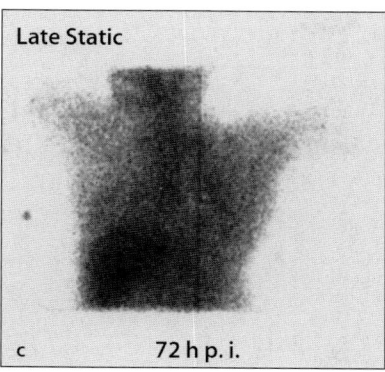

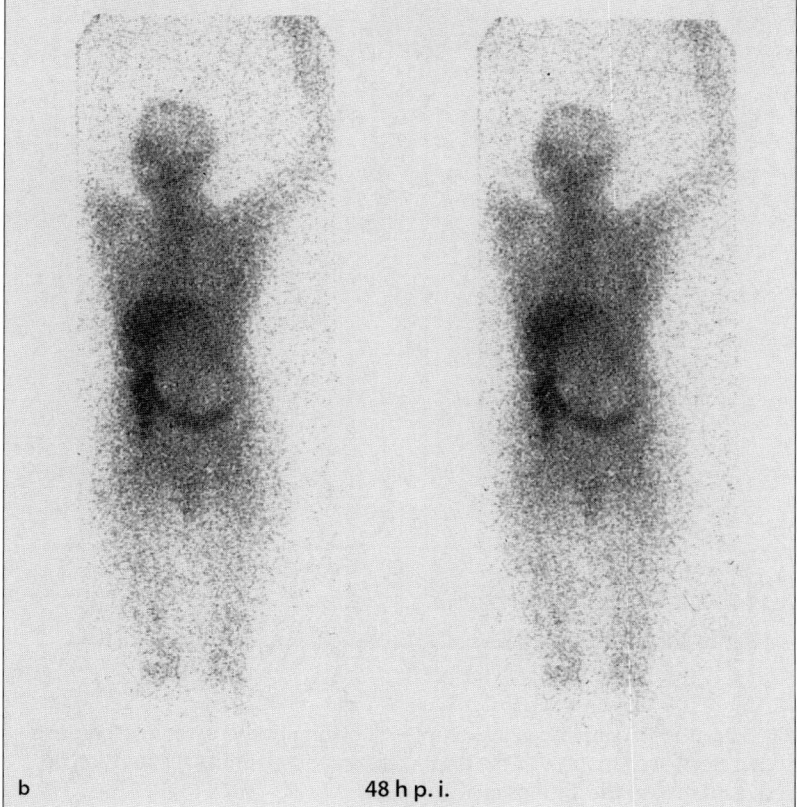

Fig. 5.22 a–c. A 55-year-old woman complained of pain and fullness in the upper left quadrant of the chest. Cardiologic studies were negative. On physical examination of the slightly obese patient, a large soft-tissue mass was palpated in the left axilla. Lymphoscintigraphy demonstrates a conglomerate mass at the axillary level, which was surgically removed and identified histologically as a lymph node metastasis from signet-ring cell carcinoma. Gastroenterologic examination confirmed the diagnosis and established that the tumor was inoperable. It is noteworthy that the mass did not take up ^{67}Ga (**b, c**)

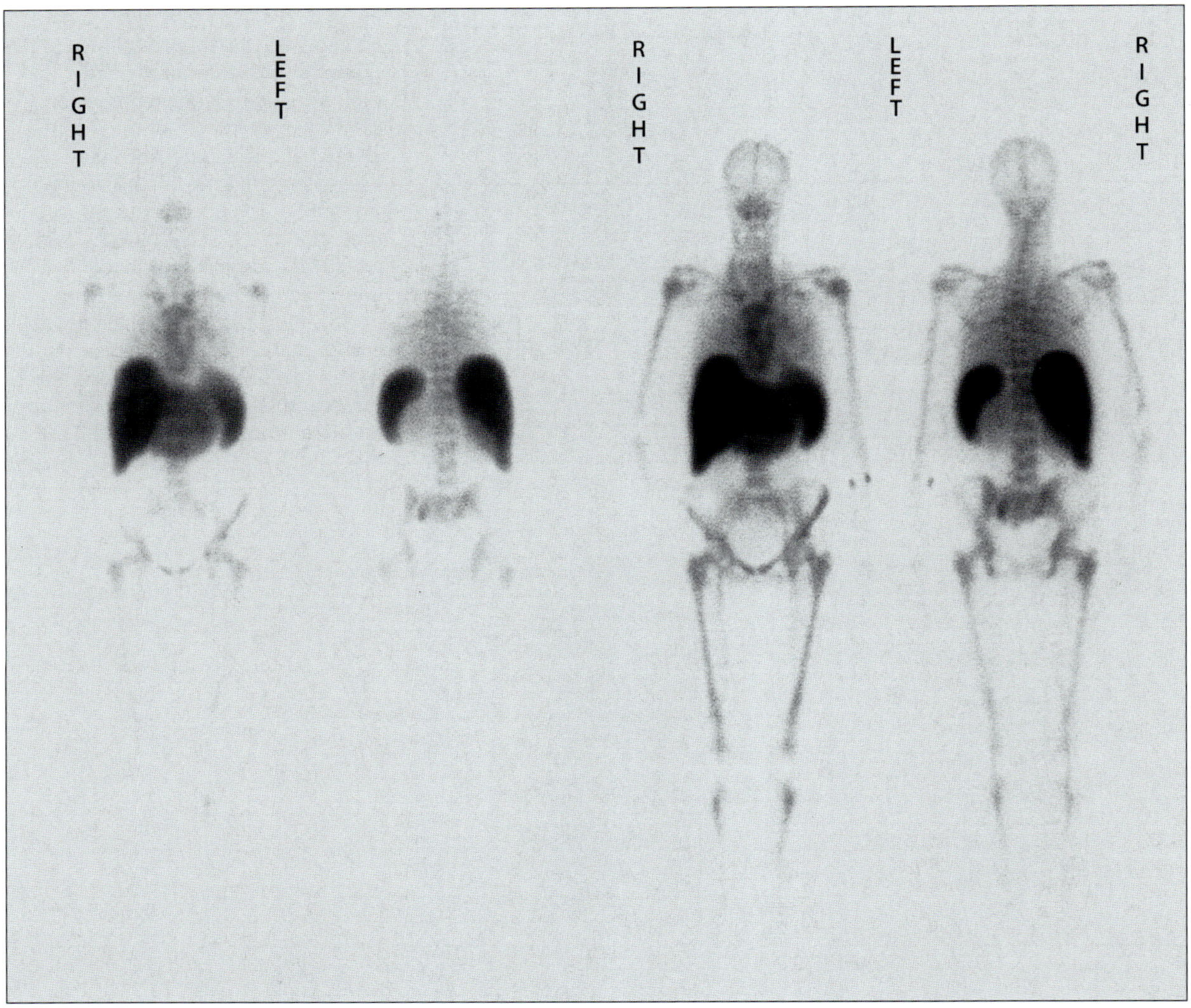

RIGHT   LEFT   RIGHT   LEFT   RIGHT

Fig. 5.23. Bone marrow scan demonstrates extramedullary hematopoiesis in a 70-year-old immunocytoma patient

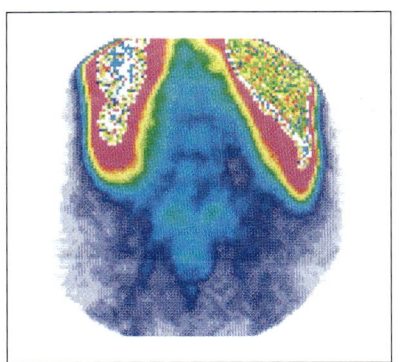

Fig. 5.24. Bone marrow scan in a 65-year-old woman with osteomyelofibrosis shows decreased marrow in the axial skeleton and an unusual extension of active marrow at the lumbosacral junction

Appendix

A
Historical Development

A1
Head and Neck

Brain

Nuclear medicine owes its existence to the pioneering work of Marie Curie, who discovered radioactivity in 1898; to scientists such as Planck (1901), Einstein (1905), Rutherford (1911), and Bohr (1913), who worked out the physical and mathematical principles; and to Hevesy (1923), who developed the radiotracer principle. Blumgart and Weiss (1927) were the first to use radioactive materials in medical diagnosis. The development of artificial radioactive materials by Curie and Juliot (1934) was an important milestone in the development of nuclear medicine.

Building on the observations of Wassermann et al. (1911) on the affinity of certain dyes for tumors, the discovery of the blood-brain barrier by Goldmann (1913), and the discovery by Scraby et al. (1942) that brain tumors cause a breakdown of the blood-brain barrier, Moore (1948) was the first to use a radioactive compound for the detection of brain tumors. He used a chemical exchange reaction to label the traditional tumor-seeking dye fluorescein with radioactive iodine. The historical development of nuclear medicine radiopharmaceuticals is outlined in Tables A-1 and A-2.

Table A-1. Historical development of radiopharmaceuticals (after Di Chiro et al. 1967)

Radionuclide	Chemical compound	Year	Researchers
I-131	Diiodofluorescein	1948	Moore
P-32	Ion	1948	Erickson et al.
			Selverstone et al.
K-42	Ion	1950	Susen et al.
			Selverstone et al.
I-131	Human serum albumin (HSA)	1951	Chou et al.
B-10	Borax	1951	Sweet et al.
I-131	Iodide	1952	Chou et al.
Rb-86	Carbonate	1952	Zipser et al.
As-76	Arsenate (ammonium)	1953	Benda et al.
As-74	Ion	1953	Brownell et al.
Bi-206	Bismuth nitrate	1957	Mundinger
	Bismuth carbonate lecithin		
Cu-64	EDTA	1958	Babnall et al.
Zr-89	Zirconium ion	1958	Mealy
Cr-51	Chromium ion	1959	Edström
Hg-203	Chlormerodrine	1960	Blau and Bender
I-131	Iodothyronine	1960	Bender
As-72	Arsenate	1961	Mallard et al.
I-131	Octaiodofluorescein (OIF)	1962	Tocus et al.
	Polyvinylpyrrolidone (PVP)	1962	Tauxe et al.
F-18	Fluoroborate	1962	Askenasy et al.
Hg-197	Ion	1963	Sodee
	Chlormerodrin	1963	Sodee
I-131	Antifibrinogen	1963	Di Chiro et al.
	Iododeoxycytidine (ICDR)	1963	Kriss et al.
Ga-68	Chelate	1963	Anger et al.
	Phthalocyanate	1964	Shealy et al.
	Protoporphyrin		
	Ion		
	Arsenate, sodium		
	Gallate, sodium		
	Versenate		
Tc-99m	Pertechnetate, sodium	1964	Harper et al.
Co-57	Porphyrin	1964	McAffee et al.
Sr-85	Nitrate	1964	Charkes et al.
I-131	Fibrinogen (human)	1964	Monasterio
	Iodopamide	1964	Nordyke et al.
			McAffee et al.

Radionuclide	Chemical compound	Year	Researchers
I-125	Antitumor antibody, human brain	1964	Day et al.
I-124	Globulin (human)	1964	Lippincott et al.
Se-57	Selenite	1965	Cavalierie et al.
I-131	Albumin (colloidal), human serum	1965	Morrison et al.
	Albumin (macroaggregated), human serum	1965	Rosenthal
Tc-99m	Iron complex	1966	Ciric et al.
I-131	Albumin as oleic acid complex	1966	Tator et al.
Tc-99m	Human serum albumin (HSA)	1967	Di Chiro et al.
	Iron-ascorbic acid complex	1967	Stapleton et al.
In-113m	DTPA	1967	Stern et al.
	EDTA		
Sr-87m	Chloride	1967	Tox et al.
Yb-169	DTPA	1968	Hosain et al.
Tc-99m	DTPA	1970	Hausser et al.
			Brookemann et al.
Co-57	Bleomycin	1972	Nouel et al.
			Mamo et al.
Ga-67	Citrate	1972	Jones et al.
In-111	Transferrin	1972	Zeidler et al.
Tc-99m	Bleomycin	1973	Toru Mori et al.
		1977	Akerman et al.
	Polyphosphate	1973	Grames et al.
	Tetracycline	1974	Holman et al.
	Diphosphonate	1974	Fischer et al.
In-111	Bleomycin	1974	Yeh et al.
		1975	Merrick et al.
Tc-99m	Glucohepatonate	1975	Waxman et al.
	Gluconate	1975	Mussa
	Citrate	1975	Ectors et al.
	Pyrophosphate	1975	Kengo et al.
Br-77	Dimethoxyphenylisopropylamine	1975	Sargent et al.
C-11	Carbon monoxide	1975	Coleman et al.
Tc-99m	Ethylhydroxydiphosphonate (EHDP)	1976	Ell et al.
Ga-68	ATP	1976	Hopp et al.
H-3	Digoxin	1976	Williams et al.
Tl-201	Thallium	1978	Ancri et al.
Tc-99m	Methyldiphosphonate	1979	Frusian et al.

Table A-2. Radionuclide compounds for evaluation of cerebral blood flow

Radionuclide	Chemical compound	Year	Researchers
Kr-85	Krypton	1955	Lassen et al.
Th-B	Thorium-B, concentrated red blood cells (RBC)	1955	Nylin et al.
P-32	Phosphorus	1959	Eichhorn
Kr-79	Krypton	1960	Lewis et al.
I-131	Human serum albumin (HSA)	1960	Love et al.
	Diodrast	1960	Oldendorf et al.
	Hippuran	1961	Oldendorf et al.
Cr-51	Concentrated RBC	1961	Ljunggren et al.
I-131	Antipyrine	1962	Sapirstein et al.
			Steiner et al.
Xe-133	Xenon, gas	1963	Mallett and Veall
	Xenon, in salt solution	1963	Glass and Harper
O-15	Oxyhemoglobin	1969	Ter-Pogossian et al.
C^+	Carboxyhemoglobin		
H^{2+}			
Xe-127	Xenon	1970	Arnot et al.
Tc-99m	Concentrated RBC	1973	Atkins et al.
C-11	Carbon monoxide	1975	Coleman et al.
N-13	Ammonia		
I-123	Antipyrine	1975	Uszler et al.
Kr-81m	Krypton	1976	Faszio et al.
Kr-77	Krypton	1978	Yamamato et al.
N-13	Nitrogen	1978	Madsen et al.
N-13	Nitrogen oxide	1978	
C-11	Acetylene		
$O-H_2O-14$			

References

Acnari D, Basset JY, Lonchampt MF, Etavard C (1978) Diagnosis of cerebral lesions by thallium 201. Radiology 128:417

Akerman M, De Tovar G, Chorny DB (1977) Comparative study of technetium-99m gluconate and four other technetium complexes (pertechnetate, DTPA, citrate and bleomycin) in the diagnosis of metastatic brain tumors. J Nucl Med 18:630

Anger HO, Gottschalk A (1993) Localization of brain tumors with the positron scintillation camera. J Nucl Med 4:326

Arnot RN, Clark JC, Glass HJ (1970) Investigation of 127xenon as a tracer for measurement of regional cerebral blood flows. In: Ross Russell RW (ed) Proceedings of the 6th International Symposium on the regulation of cerebral blood flow (Cords). Pitman, London

Askenasy HM, Anbar M, Laor Y, Lewitus Z, Kosary IZ, Guttmann S (1962) The localization of intracranial space-occupying lesions by fluoroborate ions labeled with flourine-19. Am J Roentgenol 88:350

Atkins HL, Eckelmann WC, Klopper JF, Richards P (1973) Vascular imaging with 99mTc-red blood cells. Radiology 106:357

Bagnall HJ, Benda P, Brownell GL, Sweet WH (1958) Position-scanning with copper-64 versenate in the diagnosis of intracranial lesions. Partition of copper-64 versenate in, and excretion from, the body. J Neurosurg 15:411

Bell RL (1960) Concentration of labeled tri-iodothyronine and radioactive albumine in human cerebral neoplasma. J Nucl Med 1:180

Benda P, David M, Constans J (1953) Arsenic radioactif 76 As et detection peroperatoire des tumeurs cerebrales. Rev Neurol (Paris) 89:101

Blau M, Bender MA (1960) Clinical evaluation of Hg 203 neohydrin and 131 I albumin and brain tumor localization. J Nucl Med 1:106

Blumgart HL, Weiss S (1927) Studies on the velocity of blood flow. VII. The pulmonary circulation time in normal resting individuals. J Clin Invest 4:399

Brookeman VA, Williams CM (1970) Evaluation of 99mTc-DTPA acid as a brain scanning agent. J Nucl Med 11:733

Brownell GL, Sweet WH (1953) Localization of brain tumors with positron emitters. Nucleonics 11:40

Cavalieri RR, Scott KG, Sairenji PDE (1966) Selenite (75 Se) as a tumor-localizing agent in man. J Nucl Med 7:197

Charkes ND, Sklaroff DM (1964) Early diagnosis of metastatic bone cancer by photoscanning with strontium-85. J Nucl Med 5:168

Chou SN, Aust JB, Moore GE, Peyton WT (1951) Radioactive iodinated human serum albumin as tracer agent for diagnosing and localizing intracranial lesions. Proc Soc Exp Biol (NY) 77:193

Chou SN, Moore GE, Marvin JF (1952) Localization of brain tumors with radioiodine 131. Science 115:119

Ciric I, Quinn JL III., Bucy PC (1966) Radioactive brain scans in the diagnosis of non-neoplastic intracranial lesions. Presented at the thirty-fourth Annual Meeting of The Harvey Cushing Society, St. Louis, MO, 18 April 1966

Coleman RE, Hoffmann EJ, Phelps ME, Welch MJ, Terpogossian MM (1975) Application of computerized radionuclide transaxial tomography with positron emitting radio-pharmaceuticals. J Nucl Med 16:521

Day ED, Mahaley MS, Woodhall B, Pircher F (1964) Localization of purified I125-anti-tumor radioantibodies in human brain tumors. J Nucl Med 5:357

Di Chiro G, Spar IL, Bale WF, Laskowski EJ, Doodland RL, Matthews WB (1963) "RIAF" – Radioiodinated anti-fibrogen encephalography. Preliminary experiences. Acta Radiol (Stockh) 1:967

Di Chiro G, Ashburn WL, Grove AS (1968) Which radioisotopes for brain scanning? Neurology (Minneap) 18:225

Ectors M, Abramovici J, Jonckheer MH (1975) Comparative study of Tc-99m-citrate, Tc-99m-diphosphonate, and Tc-99m-pertechnetate in brain scintigraphy. J Nucl Med 16:526

Edström R (1959) Distribution of trivalent 51 Cr in the human body; its possible use for brain tumor localization. Acta Psychiatr Scand 34:33

Ehrlich P (1985) Das Sauerstoffbedürfnis des Organismus. Eine farbanalytische Studie. Hirschwald, Berlin

Eichhorn O (1959) Die Radiocirculographie, eine klinische Methode zur Messung der Hirndurchblutung. Wien Klin Wochenschr 71:499

Ell PJ, Lotritsch KH, Hilbrand E, Meixner M, Barolin G, Scholz H (1976) Specific diagnosis of brain disease with double isotope brain scanning. J Nucl Med 15:32

Erickson TC, Larson FC, Gordon ES (1948) Uptake of radioactive phosphorus by glioblastoma multiforme and therapeutic applications. Am Neurol Ass 73:112

Faszio F, Nardini M, Fieschi C (1976) Assessment of regional cerebral blood flow by continuous infusion of krypton-81m. 8th Salzburg Conference on Cerebral Vascular Disease, Salzburg, Sept. 1976

Firusian N, Schmidt CG (1979) 99mTc-MDP-Verbindungen in der Diagnostik von Hirntumoren. Nucl Med (Suppl) 16:269

Fischer KC, Pendergrass HP, Kusick KA, Potsaid MS (1975) Increased brain scan specificity utilizing 99mTc-pertechnetate and 99mTc-(SN)-diphosphonate. J Nucl Med 16:705

Glass HJ, Harper AM (1963) Measurement of regional blood flow in cerebral cortex of man through intact skull. BMJ p 593

Grames MG, Jansen C (1973) The abnormal bone scan in cerebral infarction. J Nucl Med 14:941

Harper PV, Beck R, Charlestn D, Lathrop KA (1964) Optimization of a scanning method using Tc-99m. Nucleonics 22:50

Hauser W, Atkins HL, Nelson KG, Richards P (1970) Technetium-99m DTPA a new radiopharmaceutical for brain and kidney scanning. Radiology 94:679

Holman BL, Kaplan WD, Dewanjee MK et al. (1974) Tumor detection and localisation with 99mTc-tetracycline. Radiology 112:147

Hopp B, Hnatowich GL, Brownell GL et al. (1976) Techniques for positron scintigraphy of the brain. J Nucl Med 17:473

Hosain F, Reba RC, Wagner HN Jr (1968) Ytterbium-169 diethylenetriaminepentaacetic acid complex. Radiology 91:1199

Jones AE, Koslow M, Johnston GS, Ommaya AK (1972) 67 GA-citrate scintigraphy of brain tumors. Radiology 105:693

Kengo Matus, Iio Masahide, Chiba Kazzuo, Yamada Hidea, Abe Masahide, Murata Hajime (1975) Diagnostic aids for the differential diagnosis of brain tumor and CVD by using Tc-99m pyrophosphate. J Nucl Med 16:549

Kriss JP, Maruyama Y, Tung LA, Bond SB, Revesz L (1963) The fate of 5-bromodeoxyuridine, 5-bromodeoxycytidine, and 5-iodoeoxycytidine in man. Cancer 23:263

Lassen NA, Munck O (1955) The cerebral blood flow in man determined by the use of radioactive krypton. Acta Physiol Scand 33:30

Lewis BM, Sokoloff L, Wechsler L, Wentz WB, Kety SS (1960) A method for the continouus measurement of cerebral blood flow in man by means of radioactive krypton (Kr 79). J Clin Invest 39:707

Lippincott SW, Corcoran C, Jansen CR et al. (1964) Labeling of human globulin with I 124 for positron scanning of neoplasma. J Nucl Med 5:193

Ljunggren K, Nylin G, Berggreen B, Hedlund S, Regnström O (1961) Observations on the determination of blood passage times in the brain by means of radioactive erythrocytes and externally placed detectors. Int J Appl Radiat 12:53

Love WD, Meallie LP, Burch GE (1960) Assessment of cerebral circulation by an external isotope technique. Clin Res 8:74

Madsen MT, Nickleers R, Gatley SJ, Hichwa RD, Simpkin DJ, Martin JL (1978) The use of positron emitting anaesthetic compounds for regional cerebral blood flow studies. J Nucl Med 19:700

Mallard JR, Fowler JF, Sutton M (1961) Brain tumor detetion using radioactive arsenic. Br J Radiol 34:562

Mallet BL, Veall N (1963) Investigation of cerebral blood-flow in hypertension, using radioactive-xenon inhalation and extracranial recording. Lancet 1:1081

Mamo L, Houdart R, Rey A (1972) Intérét de l'exploration à la bléomycine marquée dans le détection des processus expansifs malins intracraniens. Rev Neurol (Paris) 120:577

Mc Affee JG, Fueger GF (1964) The value and limitations of scintillation scanning in the diagnosis of intracranial tumors. In: Quinn JL III (ed) Scintillation scanning in clinical medicine. Saunders, Philadelphia, p 183

Mealy J Jr (1958) Application of positron-emitting zirconium-89 for potentional use in brain tumor localization. Surg Forum 9:718

Merrick MV, Chauer B, Clay B, Lavender JP, Mc Cready VR, Thakur ML, Walter LH (1975) Indium (111 In)-labelled bleomycin for the detection of intracranial lesions. J Nucl Med 14:263

Monasterio G (1964) Radioactive fibrinogen for the diagnosis of tumors. Bull Soc Int Chir 23:233

Moore GE (1947) Fluorescein as an agent in the differentiation of normal and malignant tissue. Science 106:130

Moore GE (1948) The use of radioactive diiodoflurescein in the diagnosis and localization of brain tumors. Science 107:569

Morrison RT, Evans TC (1965) 131 I colloidal albumin – A new brain tumor localizing agent. J Nucl Med 6:340

Mundinger F (1957) Un nouvo radioisotop per la localizzazione diagnostica di affezioni cerebrali. Prima communicazione. Minerva Med 48:4478

Mussa GC (1975) Results with TC-99m gluconat as a positive indicator in the diagnosis of brain and lung cancers in children. J Nucl Med 16:552

Myers WG, Wagner HN Jr (1974) Nuclear medicine: how it began. Hosp Pract 9:103

Nordyke RA, Goebert HW Jr (1964) Use of I 131 iodipamide for brain tumor detection. J Nucl Med 5:377

Nouel JP, Renault H, Robert J, Jeanne C, Wicarty L (1972) La bléomycine marquée au Co 57. Nouv Press Med 1:95

Nylin G, Blömer HB (1955) Studies on distribution of cerebral blood flow with thorium B-labeled erythrocytes (preliminary report). Circ Res 3:79

Nylin G, Silfverskiöld BP, Löfstedt S, Regnström O, Hedlund S (1960) Studies on cerebral blood flow in man using radioactive-labeled erythrocytes. Brain 83:293

Oldendorf WH, Crandall PH (1961) Bilateral cerebral circulation curves obtained by intravenous injection of radioisotopes. J Neurosurg 18:195

Oldendorf WH, Crandall PH, Nordyke RA, Rose AS (1960) A comparison of the arrival in the cerebral hemispheres of intravenously injected radioisotope. Neurology (Minneap) 10:223

Rosenthall L (1965) Human brain scanning with radioiodinated macroaggregates of human serum albumin. A preliminary report. Radiology 85:110

Sapirstein LA (1962) Measurement of the cephalic and cerebral blood flow fractions of the cardiac output in man. J Clin Invest:1429

Sargent T III., Kalben A, Shulgin T, Stauffer H, Kusubov N (1975) A potential new brain-scanning agent: 4-77Br-2,5-dimethoxyphenylisoprophylamine (4-Br-DPIA). J Nucl Med 16:243

Selverstone B, Solomon AK (1948) Radioactive isotopes in study of intracranial tumors; preliminary report of methods and results. Trans Am Neurol Ass 73:115

Selverstone B, Sweet WG, Ireton RJ (1950) Radioactive potassium, a new isotope for brain tumor localization. Surg Forum 1:37176. Stapleton JE, Odell RW, Mc Kamey MR (1967) Technetium/iron/ascorbic acid complex. Am J Roentgenol 101:152

Shealy CN, Aronow S, Brownell GL (1964) Gallium-68 as a scanning agent for intracranial lesions. J Nucl Med 5:161

Sodee DB (1963) A new scanning isotope, Mercury-197. A preliminary report. J Nucl Med 4:335

Sodee DB (1963) The results of 350 brain scans with radioactive mercurial diuretics. J Nucl Med 4:185

Sorsby A, Wright AD, Elkeles A (1942) Vital scanning in brain surgery. Proc R Soc Med 36:137

Stapleton JE, Odell RW, Mc Kamey MR (1967) Technetium iron ascorbic acid complex. Am J Roentgenol 101:152

Steiner SH, Kwan HSU, Oliner L, Behnke RH (1962) The measurement of cerebral blood flow by external isotope counting. J Clin Invest:2221

Stern HS, Goodwin DA, Heffel US, Wagner HN Jr, Kramer HH (1967) In 113m for blood-pool and brain scanning. Nucleonics 25:62

Sullivan MP, Viett TJ, Fernbach DJ (1969) Clinical investigations in the treatment of meningeal leukemia: radiation therapy regimes vs. conventional intrathecal methotrexate. Blood 34:301

Susen AF, Snall WT, Moore FS (1950) Studies on the external diagnosis localization of brain lesions using radiocative potassium. Surg Forum 1:362

Sweet WH, Javid M (1952) The possible use of neutron-capturing isotopes such as boron-10 in the treatment of neoplasms. 1. Intracranial tumors. J Neurosurg 9:200

Tator CH, Evans JR, Olszewski J (1966) Tracers for the detection of brain tumors. Evaluation of radioiodinated human serum albumin and radioiodinated fatty acid. Neurology (Minneap) 16:650

Tauxe WN, Sedlack RE, Pitlyk PJ, Kerr FWL (1962) Preliminary report on the localization of brain tumors with I 131 labeled polyvinylpyrrolidone. Proc Mayo Clin 37:109

Ter-Pogossian MM, Eichling JJO, Davis DO, Welch M, Metzger JM (1969) The determination of regional cerebral blood flow by means of water labeled with radioactive oxygen 15. Radiology 93:31

Tocus EC, Okita GT, Evans JP, Mullan S (1962) The localization of octoiodofluorescein-I 131 in human brain tumors. Cancer 15:153

Toru Mori, Ken Hamamoto, Kanji Torizuka (1973) Studies of the usefullness of 99m Tc-labeled bleomycin for tumor imaging. J Nucl Med 14:431

Uszler JM, Bennet LR, Mena I, Oldendorf WH (1975) Human CNS perfusion scanning with 123I-iodoantipyrine. Radiology 115:197

Wassermann A, Keysser F, Wassermann M (1911) Beiträge zum Problem, Geschwülste von der Blutbahn aus therapeutisch zu beeinflussen. Dtsch Med Wochenschr 37:2389

Waxman AD, Tanasescu D, Siemsen JK, Wolfstein RS (1975) Technetium-99m gluco-heptonate as a brain scanning agent: a critical comparison with pertechnetate. J Nucl Med 16:580

Williams R, Flanigan S, Bissett J, Doherty J (1976) Differential uptake of tritiated digoxin in benign and malignant central nervous system neoplasma. Am J Med Sci 272:132

Yamamoti YL, Little J, Meyer E, Thompson C, Feindel W (1978) Krypton-77 positron emission tomopgraphy for evaluation of medical and surgical treatment in stroke patients. J Nucl Med 19:701

Yeh SDJ, Grando RE, Young CW, Benua RS (1974) Metabolic and scintigraphic studies of 111 indium bleomycin in man and tumor bearing animals. J Nucl Med 15:546

Zeidler U, Weinrich W, Brunngraber V, Eckhardt W, Junker D, Bettletts G, Kalden J (1973) Indium-111 as a brain scanning agent. Proceedings of a symposium, Monte Carlo 1972, IAEA, Wien

Zipser A, Freedberg AS (1952) The distribution of administered radioactive rubidium (Rb86) in normal and neoplastic tissues of mice and humans. Cancer Res 12:867

A2
Chest

Lungs

The history of perfusion lung scanning dates back to 1947, when Müller and Rossier injected radiogold-labeled carbon particles through a cardiac catheter into the branches of the pulmonary artery for therapeutic purposes. Ernst et al. (1958) continued this work in laboratory animals, prompting Gibel et al. (1962) to conduct animal experiments on the usefulness of these particles for pulmonary scintigraphy. Ya et al. (1961), Ariel (1963), and Haynie et al. (1963) injected radiolabeled ceramic microspheres 5 μm in diameter, which became trapped in the pulmonary capillary bed. Altenbrunn and Stober (1963) tested ^{131}I-labeled starch granules for perfusion lung scanning. Quinn (1963) tested soluble radiopharmaceuticals ([203]Hg-chlormerodrin, ^{131}I-labeled human serum albumin, ^{51}Cr-labeled red blood cells) for the scintigraphic detection of pulmonary infarction, but these experiments were unsuccessful.

The decisive breakthrough came in 1963, when Taplin et al. produced an ^{131}I-labeled macroaggregate from human serum albumin and tested it in experimental animals. This radiopharmaceutical was immediately adopted for clinical use by Wagner et al. (1964a) and then by other groups of authors (Quinn and Whitley 1964; Dworkin et al. 1964; Taplin et al. 1964).

With regard to ventilation lung scanning, the distribution of inhaled radioactive particles in the lung was already known from experimental studies on radiation biohazards (Kornberg et al. 1961). The discovery that particles approximately 1 μm in size are partially deposited in the alveoli (Morrow 1964) suggested the idea of using inhaled radioactive aerosols for ventilation imaging. In 1965, Altenbrunn reported on the methodology and results of lung scanning with an inhaled [198]Au-colloid aerosol. In the same year, Pircher et al. presented their results in experimental animals and clinical patients. Taplin and Poe (1965) tested various radioactive substances for their suitability as ventilation scanning agents and obtained good results with [125]I-, [131]I- and ^{99m}Tc-labeled human serum albumin, [197]Hg chlormerodrin, and [198]Au colloid.

References

Altenbrunn HJ, Stober D (1963) Untersuchungen zur 131-J-Markierung von Stärkekörnern und ihre Anwendbarkeit zur Darstellung der Lungendurchblutung. Fortschr Röntgenstr 98:757

Ariel JM (1963) Referiert in "Highlights of the Society of Nuclear Medicine Meeting". JAMA 183:32–33

Dworkin HJ, Hamilton C, Simeck CM, Beierwalters WH (1964) Lung scanning with colloidal RISA. J Nucl Med 5:48

Ernst H, Iglauer E, Kronschwitz H, Spode E (1958) Tierexperimentelle Untersuchungen zur Frage der Therapie von Lungentumoren mit Hilfe radioaktiver Gold-Kohle-Suspensionen. Strahlentherapie 107:382

Gibel WH, Matthes TH, Ernst H, Spode E (1962) Tierexperimentelle Untersuchungen zur Diagnostik von Gefäßverschlüssen der A. pulmonalis durch radioaktive Gold-Kohle-Suspension. Fortschr Röntgenst 96:350

Haynie TP, Calhoon JH, Nasjleti CE, Nofal MM, Beierwalters WH (1963) Visualization of pulmonary artery occlusion by photoscanning. JAMA 185:306–308

Kornberg HA, Bair WJ, Cohn SH et al. (1961) Effects of inhaled radioactive particles. Pub. 848, Report of Subcommittee on inhalation hazards. Committee on Pathological Effects of Atomic Radiation, NAS, NRC, Washington/DC

Morrow PE (1964) Evaluation of inhalation hazards based upon the respirable dust concept and the philosophy and application of selective sampling. Am Ind Hyg Assoc J 25:213

Müller JH, Rossier PH (1947) De l'emploi d'isotopes radioactifs artificiels, dans le but d'exercer un effet radio-biologique localise. Experientia 3:75

Pöircher FJ, Temple JR, Kirsch WJ, Reeves RJ (1965) Distribution of pulmonary ventilation determined by radioisotope scanning. Am J Roentgenol 94:807–814

Quinn JL, Whitley JE (1964) Lung scintiscanning. Radiology 83:937–943

Quinn JL, Whitley JE, Hudspeth AS, Watts FC (1963) An approach to the scanning of pulmonary infarct. Presented at the Tenth Annual Meeting, Society of Nuclear Medicine, June

Taplin GV, Poe ND (1965) Dual lung-scanning technic for evaluation of pulmonary function. Radiology 85:365–368

Taplin GV, Dore EK, Johnson DE, Kaplan HS (1963) Scientific exhibit on colloidal radioalbumin aggregates for organ scanning. Tenth Annual Meeting, Society of Nuclear Medicine, Montreal, Canada

Taplin GV, Johnson DE, Dore EK, Kaplan HS (1964) Lung photoscans with macroaggregates of human serum radioalbumin. Health Phys 10:1219–1228

Wagner HN, Sabiston DC, Iio M, Mc Affee Jg, Meyer JK, Langan JK (1964) Regional pulmonary blood flow in man by radioisotope scanning. JAMA 187:601–603

Ya PM, Guzman T, Loken MK, Perry JF (1961) Isotope localization with tagged microspheres. Surgery 49:644

Cardiovascular System

After Blumgart and Weis published the first studies on the hemodynamics of the pulmonary circulation in 1927, efforts first centered on technically simple techniques in which counting tubes were used to record the passage of a radionuclide-tagged tracer through the heart and lung and generate a time-activity curve. Prinzmetal (1948) called this procedure radiocardiography. In 1950, Waser et al. published a method for the quantitation of blood flow using radiolabeled saline. The nuclear medicine determination of cardiac output is based on the Stewart-Hamilton procedure (Hamilton et al. 1932; Thompson et al. 1964; Yoder et al. 1971) as modified by Huff et al. (1955) and Veal et al. (1955). The mean transit time is the time-weighted mean value of the transit times of a large number of tracer particles through a designated compartment. The relationship of this parameter to tracer distribution and flow rate, which was established empirically by Stewart (1894) and theoretically by Meier and Zierler (1954), emphasizes its practical importance for clinical investigations. Hegglin et al. (1962) proved that circulation times are a measure of blood flow velocity. The methodologic approach to radionuclide ventriculography was first described by Hoffmann and Kleine in 1968. Count-rate statistics were improved by determining the time-activity curves for several cardiac cycles after equilibrium distribution of the radiotracer. In 1972, Strauss et al. applied this method to gamma camera scintigraphy by producing ECG-triggered radionuclide ventriculograms at end diastole and end systole and displaying the images in a cine-angiogram format that permitted a qualitative assessment of regional wall motion. In 1975, Geffers applied Fourier analysis to time-activity curves. Fourier analysis was continually improved in subsequent years, becoming a powerful and essential tool for cardiovascular investigations (Adam et al. 1975; Sharma et al. 1976; Hör et al. 1980; Kaltenbach et al. 1981).

References

Adam WE (1975) Scintigraphie, Sequenz-, Funktionsszintigraphie. In: Pabst HW, Deff K (Hrsg) Nuclearmedizin und Kinetik. Medico, Berlin, S 497

Adam WE, Tarkowska A, Bitter F, Strauch M, Geffers H (1979) Equilibrium (gated) radionuclide ventriculography. Cardiovasc Radiol 2:161

Bonte FJ, Parkey RW, Grahan KD et al. (1974) A new method for radionuclide imaging of myocardial infarcts. Radiology 110:473

Carr EA Jr, Beierwaltes WH, Patno ME et al. (1962) The detection of experimental myocardial infarcts by photoscanning. Am Heart J 64:650

Freundlieb CH, Höck A, Vyska K, Machulla HJ, Stöcklin G, Feinendegen LE Nuklearmedizinische Analyse des Fettsäurenumsatzes im Myokard. In: Oeff K, Schmidt HAE (Hrsg) Nuklearmedizin und Biokinetik, Bd I. Schattauer, Stuttgart New York, S 415

Geffers H, Meyer G, Bitter F, Adam WE (1975) Analysis of heart function by gated blood pool investigation-camera cinematography. 4th Conference on Information Processing in Scintigraphy. Orsay, France., p 462

Gorten RJ, Hardy LB, McCraw BH et al. (1966) The selective uptake of Hg-203 chlormerodrin in experimentally produced myocardial infarcts. Am Heart J 72:71

Hamilton WF, Moore JW, Kinsman JM, Spurling RG (1932) Studies on the circulation IV. Further analysis of the injection method and of changes in hemodynamics under physiological and pathological conditions Am J Physiol 99:534

Hegglin R, Rutishausen W, Kaufmann G, Lüthy E, Scheu H (1962) Kreislaufdiagnostik mit der Farbstoffverdünnungsmethode. Kreislaufzeiten, Herzminutenvolumen, Blutvolumen, Klappeninsuffizienz., Stuttgart

Hoffmann G, Kleine N (1968) Die Methode der radiocardiographischen Funktionsanalyse. Nuklearmedizin 7:350

Holman BL, Dowanjee MK, Idoine J et al. (1973) Detection and localization of experimental myocardial infarction with 99mTc-tetracycline. J Nucl Med 14:595

Hör G, Kanamoto N, Standke R, Maul FD, Klepzig H, Kober G, Kaltenbach M (1980) Transluminale Angioplastie: Erfolgskontrolle durch Verfahren der Nuklearmedizin nach nicht-operativer Dilatation kritischer Koronararterienstenose. Herz 5:168

Hubner PJB (1970) Radioisotopic detection of experimental myocardial infarction using mercury derivatives of fluorescein. Cardiovasc Res 4:509

Huff RL, Feller DD, Jodd OS, Bogardus GM (1955) Cardiac output of men and dogs measured by in vivo analysis of iodinated (J131) human serum albumin. Circ Res 3:564

Kaltenbach M, Kober G, Schere D et al. (1981) Ergebnisse der transluminalen Koronarangioplastik. In: Breddin K (ed) Thrombose und Atherogenese. Witzstrock, Baden-Baden, S 173

Kramer RJ, Goldstein RE, Hirshfeld JW et al. (1974) Accumulation of gallium-67 in regions of acute myocardial infarction. Am J Cardiol 33:861

Malck P, Vavrejn B, Ratusky J et al. (1967) Detection of myocardial infarction by in vivo scanning. Cardiology 51:22

McKusik K (1981) Comparison of three Tc.99m isonitriles for detection of ischemic heart disease in humans. J Nucl Med (Abstract) 27:878

Meier P, Zierler KL (1954) On the theory of the indicator dilution method for measurement of blood flow and volume. J Appl Physiol 6:731

Prinzmetal M, Corday E, Bergman HC, Schwartz L, Spritzler RJ (1948) Radiocardiography: a new method for studying the blood flow through the chambers of the heart in human beings. Science 108:340

Sharma B, Goodwin JF, Raffael MJ, Steiner RE, Reinbow RG, Taylor SH (1976) Left ventricular angiography on exercise: a new method of assessing left ventricular function in ischaemic heart disease. Br Heart J 38:59

Stauss HW, Zaret BL, Hurley PJ, Natarajan TK, Pitt B (1972) A scintiphotographic method for measuring left ventricular ejection fraction in man without cardiac cathetherisation. Am J Cardiol 28:575

Strauß HW, Harrison K, Langan JK, Lebowitz E, Pitt B (1975) Thallium-201 for myocardial perfusion. Circulation 51:641

Stewart GN (1894) Researches on the circulation time in organs and on the influences which affect it. Preliminary report. J Physiol 15:1

Thompson HK, Starmer CF, Wahlen RE, McIntosh HD (1964) Indicator transit time considered as a gamma variate. Circ Res 14:502

Veall N, Pearson JD, Hanley T, Lowe AE (1954) A method for the determination of cardiac output. Proc Sec Radioisotope Conference, Oxford

Waser PG, Hunzinger W (1950) Bestimmung von Kreislaufgrößen mit radioaktivem Kochsalz. Cardiologica 15:219

Willerson JT, Parkey RW, Bonte FJ et al. (1975) Technetium stannous pyrophosphate myocardial scintigrams in patients with chest pain of varying etiology. Circulation 51:1046

Yoder RD, Swan EM (1971) Cardiac output: comparison of Stewart-Hamilton and gamma-function techniques. J Appl Physiol 31:318

A3
Abdomen

Gastrointestinal Tract

Pancreas

Progress in nuclear medicine imaging of the pancreas has been relatively modest compared with other areas. Nevertheless, radionuclide imaging of the pancreas is performed with considerable frequency, as indicated by these reports on the numbers of examinations done yearly in various countries:

- United States: 35,000 (Bennett and Fleischer 1974)
- Japan: 18,900 (Kaheki and Saegusa 1974)
- England/Wales: 1791 (Potter and Rogers 1974)

The prevalence of pancreatic disease is reflected in the table below, which is based on the findings of Kuhnen (1969) in 1000 autopsies.

Pancreatic findings	No. of instances
General diffuse fibrosis	395
Lipomatosis	320
Edema	103
Infarction	89
Interlobular fibrosis	69
Periductular fibrosis	43
Terminal tryptic necrosis	36
Fat necrosis	29
Ductectasia	28
Carcinoma	166
Acute pancreatitis	14
Pancreatic cyst	13
Advanced autolysis	318
Normal findings	108

The following radiopharmaceuticals have been used for pancreatic imaging:

- ^{75}Se methionine (Blau 1961)
- ^{131}I erythrosin b (Ledoux-Lebhard et al. 1967)
- ^{99m}Tc cystine, ^{99m}Tc methionine, ^{99m}Tc polypeptides (Tobis and Endow 1968)
- ^{131}I toluidine blue (Normann et al. 1969)
- ^{131}I acetyltryptophan, ^{131}I tyrosine, ^{131}I phenylalanine (Kato et al. 1970)
- ^{18}F phenylalanine (Hoyte et al. 1971)
- ^{13}N alanine (Cohen et al. 1974)
- ^{99m}Tc acetylmethionine (Holan et al. 1974)
- ^{99m}Tc thyrosylsulfate (Colombetti and Pinsky 1974)

References

Bennett LR, Fleischer A (1974). 1st. World Congress of Nuclear Medicine, Tokyo, p 401

Blau M (1961). Biochim Biophys Acta 49:381

Cohen MB, Spolter L, MacDonald N (1974). 1st. World Congress of Nuclear Medicine, Tokyo 1974, p 907

Colombetti L, Pinsky S (1974). 1st. World Congress of Nuclear medicine, Tokyo 1974, p 55

Holan D, Micludia L, Bushwald I (1974). 1st. World Congress of Nuclear Medicine, Tokyo 1974, p 860

Hoyte EM, Lin SS, Christman DR (1971). General Nucl Medicine 12:280

Kaheki A, Saegusa K (1974). 1st. World Congress of Nuclear Medicine, Tokyo, p 292

Kato S, Kurata K, Sugisawa Y (1970). Yakugaku Zasshi 90:1499

Kuhnen K (1969). Med Dissertation, University of Heidelberg

Ledoux-Lebhard G, Heitz F, Behar A, General G (1964). Radiol Electrol 48:373

Normann I, Seljelid R, Lakken K (1969). Scand J Clin Lab Invest 24 (Suppl 110):118

Potter DC, Rogers RT (1974). 1st. World Congress of Nuclear Medicine, Tokyo, p 1399

Tobis M, Endow GS (1968). Int J Appl Radiat Isot 19:835

Liver

The constant search for noninvasive techniques for diagnosing hepatobiliary disease began with Abel and Rowntree in 1909, who discovered that tetrachlorphenolphthalein is selectively eliminated in the bile. In 1923, Delprat reported on liver function testing with dyes. Rosenthal and White (1925) recognized the sulfonate of tetrabromophenolphthalein (bromsulfphthalein) as the clinically most important dye. Initially it was thought that dye excretion was a function of the Kupffer cells. Sprinson and Rittenberg (1949), Mendeloff (1949), and Williams (1950) disproved this by showing that bromsulfpthlhalein was taken up chiefly by hepatocytes. Sheppard et al. (1951) showed that certain particle sizes of a labeled colloid gold were phagocytized and stored by Kupffer cells. Wieland (1951) was then able to image the liver by administering colloids labeled with short-lived radiotracers. Dobson and Jones (1952) proposed using the behavior and disappearance rate of ^{32}P chromium phosphate colloid as a measure of hepatic blood flow. In 1954, Vetter et al. described the use of ^{198}Au colloid to determine hepatic blood flow. By using external scintillation probe measurements and assuming that colloid uptake was proportional to blood flow in the reticuloendothelial system (RES) of the liver, these authors were able to estimate the volume flow of hepatic perfusion. In 1955, Taplin et al. used the radiolabeled hepatocyte-specific dye ^{131}I rose bengal for liver examinations, but Moertel and Owen questioned the suitability of this agent for liver function testing in 1958. In the same year, Nordyke and Blahd used externally applied scintillation probes to record the time course of intravenously administered ^{131}I rose bengal over the temporal region, liver, and bowel while simultaneously determining blood clearance.

A key advance was the introduction of the scintillation camera by Anger in 1958. This made it possible to detect tracer passage at short intervals over multiple areas of clinical concern, such as the liver, gallbladder, bowel, and heart. As early as 1961, Tubis et al. produced a stable compound of ^{131}I with bromsulfphthalein for radionuclide imaging of the liver.

Another advance was the introduction of short-lived radiopharmaceuticals for hepatic imaging. Harper et al. first used ^{99m}Tc-labeled fat emulsion in 1963, which is sequestered in the RES, and Yeh et al. described ^{99m}Tc toluidine blue for hepatobiliary imaging. The diverse biologic functions of the liver and the resulting clinical inquiries account for the broad spectrum of technetium-labeled radiopharmaceuticals that have an affinity for the RES:

- Sulfur colloid (Harper et al. 1964)
- Antimony sulfide colloid (Degrossi et al. 1965; Akhtar 1969)
- HSA colloid (Kort 1969)
- Gelatin (Pollahne et al. 1970)
- Dioxide (Johnson and Gollan 1970)
- Sodium phytate (Subramanian et al. 1973)
- ^{113m}Indium colloid-labeled agents: gelatin (Goodwin et al. 1969), mannitol (Sewatkar et al. 1970), Fe particles (Colombetti et al. 1969), and acetonyl acetate (Sinn et al. 1974)

Various technetium-labeled hepatobiliary agents with affinity for polygonal cells and bile have also been described:

- Penicillamine (Krishnamurthy 1972)
- Dihydrothioctic acid (Tonkin and De Land 1974)
- Mercaptide complexes (Jackson et al. 1973)
- Protamine complex (Spencer et al. 1974)
- Tetracycline (Fliegel et al. 1974)
- Iminodiacetic acid (IDA) compounds (Harvey et al. 1975)
- Pyridoxal amino acid complexes (Baker et al. 1974, 1975; Fotopoulos et al. 1977)

Various other compounds have also been tested as hepatobiliary agents: ^{123}I bromsulfphthalein (Goris 1973; Britton et al. 1975), indocyanine green (Ansari 1975), iodotetrinic acid (Buttermann et al. 1975), and rose bengal (Serafini et al. 1975). Winstead et al. (1975) described the marked accumulation of activity in the liver and excretion in bile observed with ^{11}C-labeled aminonitriles.

Of the various hepatobiliary radiopharmaceuticals that are available, ^{99m}Tc HIDA derivatives have shown the most favorable characteristics (Wistow et al. 1977; Subramanian et al.) and have yielded the most satisfactory clinical results (Pauwels et al. 1977, 1978; Weissmann et al. 1979). An evaluation of hepatobiliary agents by Wistow et al. (1977) in healthy baboons showed that ^{99m}Tc HIDA derivatives (diethyl and dimethyl HIDA) provided more rapid biliary accumulation and excretion than ^{131}I rose bengal and other ^{99m}Tc-labeled compounds. These derivatives were similar with regard to cumulative biliary excretion, but when blood clearance and urinary excretion were also considered, diethyl HIDA was found to be clearly superior (Wistow et al. 1977). This was subsequently confirmed by tests in human subjects (Pors Nielsen et al. 1978).

References

Abel JJ, Rowntree LG (1909) Pharm Ther 1:23

Akhtar M (1969) Ein einfaches Verfahren zur Herstellung von 99m Tc-Sulfurkolloid für die Leberszintigraphie. Fortschr Geb Röntgenstr 110:271

Anger HO (1958) Scintillation camera. Rev Sci Instrument 29:27

Ansari AN, Atkins HL, Lambrecht RM, Redvanly CS, Wolf AP (1975) 123 I-indocyanine green (123 I-ICG) as an agent for dynamic studies of the hepatobiliary system. In: Dynamic studies with radioisotopes in medicine. Wien. IAEA 1975 Vol. I, p 111

Baker RJ, Bellen JC, Ronai PM (1974) 99m Tc-pyridoxylidene glutamate: a new rapid cholescintigraphic agents. J Nucl Med 15:476a

Baker RJ, Bellen JC, Ronai PM (1975) 99m Tc-pyridoxylidene glutamate: a new hepatobiliary radiopharmaceutical. J Nucl Med 16:720

Britton KE, Suwanik R, Tuntawiroon C et al. (1975) Computerassisted blood background subtraction (CABBS) hepatography with 131-J and 123 I-brom-sulph-thalein (BSP). In: Dynamic studies with radioisotopes in medicine. Wien, IAEA, Vol. I, p 175

Buttermann G, Wolf I, Paest HW, Hör G, Schulze PE (1975) Quantitative analysis of hepatograms using a gamma camera and labeled contrast media. In: Dynamic studies with radioisotopes in medicine. Wien, IAEA, Vol. I, p 137

Colombetti LG, Goodwin DA, Hermanson R (1969) 113m In-labeled compound for liver and spleen studies. J Nucl Med 10:597

Degrossi OK, Martinez JS, Gotta H (1965) A new 99m Tc-labeled colloid for liver scanning. Minerva Nucl 9:424

Delprat GD Jr. (1923) Studies on liver function: rose bengal elimination from the blood as influenced by liver injury. Arch Int Med 32:401

Dobson EL, Jones HB (1952) The behavior of intravenously injected particulate material: its rate of disappearance from the blood stream as a measure of liver blood flow. Acta Med Scand 144:71

Fliegel CP, Dewanjee MK, Holman LB, Davis MA, Treves S (1974) 99m Tc-tetracycline as a kidney and gallbladder imaging agent. Radiologie 110:407

Fotopoulos A, Chiotelis E, Koutoulidis C, Dassiou A, Papadimitriou J (1977) Evaluation of 99m Tc-pyridoxal-phenylalanine as a hepatobiliary agent, part I, experimental studies. J Nucl Med 18:1189

Goodwin DA, Stern HS, Wagner HN, Kramer HH Jr. (1966) Indium-113m: a new radiopharmaceutical for liver scanning. Nucleonics 24:65

Goris ML (1973) 123 I-iodobromsulphalein as a liver and biliary scanning agent. J Nucl Med 14:820

Harper PV, Lathrop KA, McCardley RJ (1963) Improved liver scanning with 6-hour 99mTc in fat emulsion. J Nucl Med 4:189

Harper PV, Lathrop KH, Richards P (1964) 99m Tc as a radiocolloid. J Nucl Med 5:382b

Harwey E, Loberg M, Cooper M (1975) 99m tc-HIDA: a new radiopharmaceutical for hepatobiliary imaging. J Nucl Med 16:533d

Jacksen RA, Bolles TF, Kubiatowicz DO, Krejcarek GE (1973) 99m Tc- mercaptide complexes and their potential application as a liver specific agent. J Nucl Med 14:411c

Johnson AE, Gollan F (1970) 99m tc-Dioxide for liver scanning. J Nucl Med 11:564

Kort W (1969) 99m Tc-Humanserumalbumin in kolloidaler Form für die Leberszintigraphie. Strahlentherapie 137:420

Krishnamurthy GT, Tubis M, Endow JS, Blahd WH (1972) 99m Tc-penicillamine – a new radiopharmaceutical for cholescintigraphy. J Nucl Med 13:447

Lin TH, Khentigan A, Winchell HS (1974) A 99m Tc-labeled replacement for 131 I-rose bengal in liver and biliary tract studies. J Nucl Med 15:613

Mendeloff AJ (1949) Fluorescence of intravenously administered rose bengal appears only in hepatic polygonal cells. Proc Soc Exp Biol (NY) 70:556

Moertel CG, Owen CA (1958) Evaluation of the radioactive (131 I-tagged) rose bengal liver function test in non-jaundiced patients. J Lab Clin Med 52:902

Nordyke RA, Blahd WH (1958) The differential diagnosis of biliary tract obstruction with radioactive rose bengal. J Lab Clin Med 51:565

Pollahne W, Deckart H, Romer J (1970) 99m Tc-Gelatine. Ein Radiopharmakon für die Leberszintigraphie. Radiol Biol Radiother (Berlin) 11:541

Pauwels S, Steels M, Piret L, Beckers C (1977) Diethyl-IDA: a promising hepatobiliary radiopharmaceutical. J Nucl Med 18:1141

Pauwels S, Steels M, Piret L, Beckers C (1978) Clinical evaluation of 99m tc-Diethyl-IDA in hepatobiliary disorders. J Nucl Med 19:783

Pors Nielsen S, Trap-Jensen J, Lindenberg J, Lykkegard Nielsen M (1978) Hepato-biliary scintigraphy and hepatography with 99m Tc-diethyl-acetanilido-iminodiac-etate in obstructive jaundice. J Nucl Med 19:452

Rosenthal SM, White EC (1925) Clinical application of the bromsulphalein test for hepatic function. J Am Med Ass 84:1112

Rosenthall L, Shaffer EA, Lisbona R, Pare P (1978) Diagnosis of hepatobiliary disease by 99m Tc-HIDA cholescintigraphy. Radiologie 126:467

Serafini AN, Hupf HB, Lindberg D, Smoak WM, Gilson AJ (1975) Iodine-123 rose bengal in the evaluation of the jaundiced patient. J Nucl Med 16:567D

Sewatkar AB, Patel MC, Sharma SM (1970) A simple and safer 113m In-colloid preparation for scanning the liver. Int J Appl Radiat 21:36

Sheppard CW, Jordan G, Hahn PF (1951) Disappearance of isotopically labeled gold colloids from the circulation of the dog. Am J Physiol 164:345

Sinn H, Selmair H, Georgi P, Maier-Borst W (1974) Experimentelle Untersuchungen über die Verwendung des 113m In-(pentandion 2,4,3)-komplexes zur Leberszintigraphie. J Nucl Med (Suppl) 12:514

Spencer RP, Miller RE, Aantar MA (1974) 99m Tc-protamine complexe with biliary excretion. J Nucl Med 15:535a

Sprinson DB, Rittenberg D (1949) The rate of interaction of the amino acids of the diet with the tissue proteins. J Biol Chem 180:715

Subramanian G, McAffee JG, Henderson RW, Rosenstreich M, Krokenberger L The influence of structural changes on biodistribution of Tc-99m labeled and N-substituted IDA derivates. In. (ed) Nuclear medicine, state of the art and future. Schattauer, Stuttgart New York, p 136

Subramanian G, McAffee JG, Mehtor A, Blair J, Thomas FD (1973) 99m Tc-stannous-phytate – a new in vivo colloid for imaging the reticuloendothelial system. J Nucl Med 14:459

Taplin GV, Meredith OM, Kade H (1955) The radioactive (131 I-tagged) rose bengal uptake-excretion test for liver function using external gamma-ray scintillation counting techniques. J Lab Clin Med 45:665

Tjen MSLM (1979) The clinical pharmalogy of technetium diethyl-IDA. Elsevier, Amsterdam, p 225

Tonkin AL, De Land FH (1974) Dihydrothioctacid: a new polygonal cell imaging agent. J Nucl Med 15:539

Tubis M, Nordyke RA, Posnick E, Blahde WH (1961) The preparation and use of 131 J-labeled sulfobromphthaleien in liver function testing. J Nucl Med 2:282

Vetter H, Falkner R, Neumayer R (1954) The disappearance rate of colloidal radiogold from the circulation and its application to the estimation of liver-blood flow in normal and cirrhotic subjects. J Clin Invest 33:1594

Weissmann HS, Frank M, Rosenblatt R, Goldman M, Freeman LM (1979) Cholescintigraphy, ultrasonography and computerised tomography in the evaluation of biliary tract disorder. Semin Nucl Med 9:22

Wieland RL (1951). In: Radioisotope therapy. Academic Press, London New York

Williams WL (1950) Intravital staining of damaged liver cells. Anat Rec 107:1

Winstead MB, Widner PJ, Means JL et al. (1975) Carbon-11 aminonitriles. J Nucl Med 16:582C

Wistow BW, Subramanian G, Heertum RL van, Henderson RW, Cagne GM, Hall RC, McAffee JG (1977) The evaluation of 99m Tc-labeled hepatobiliary agent. J Nucl Med 18:455

Yeh SH, Delahay JE, Kriss JP (1968) 99m Tc-labeled toluidine blue for liver-scintillography. Int J Appl Radiat Isot 19:885

Choledochoduodenal Function

Galen (139–200 A.D.) stated that the liver functioned as a processor of the blood and described two waste products: the black bile, which is absorbed and processed by the spleen, and the yellow bile, which is secreted into the gallbladder.

Research during the first half of the 19th century greatly advanced our understanding of biliary physiology. Biliary transport and its response to various agents are reviewed in Table A-3, which summarizes the results of animal experiments and various test protocols that have appeared in the world literature since 1926.

For many years experts have argued whether the sphincter of Oddi can function autonomously, independent of the duodenal pressure.

Table A-3. Biliary tract response to various agents based on animal experiments and a variety of test protocols

Agent	Gallbladder muscle	Cholecysto-cystic sphincter	Pressure in the bile duct	Choledocho-duodenal sphincter	Duodenal wall muscle	Bile secretion into the duodenum
Cholecysto-kinin (CCK)	Contraction			Relaxation	Contraction[b]	Increase
Low doses			Increase[a]	Relaxation		
Very high doses		Contraction		Contraction		
Secretin	Slight contraction		Increase			
Low doses						Increased response to CCK
High dose				Contraction		Inhibition
Gastrin	Contraction					
Vagal stimulation	Contraction	Contraction	No response to mild stimulus	No response to electrical stimulus		Decrease
Parasympathomimetics	Contraction		Increase	Contraction	Contraction	
Vagotomy	Relaxation	Relaxation	No response	Relaxation	Increased response to CCK (initial phase) / Decreased response to CCK (late phase)	Delay
Parasympatholytics	Relaxation		Decrease	Relaxation		
Epinephrine	Relaxation		Increase	Variable	Relaxation	Inhibition
α-Sympatho-mimetics	Weak contraction			Contraction	Relaxation	
β-Sympatho-mimetics	Relaxation	Relaxation		Relaxation	Relaxation	
Splanchnic nerve stimulation	Relaxation	Contraction		Variable	Relaxation	Inhibition
Fats	Contraction	Contraction		Relaxation[c]		
Acid				Contraction		Inhibition

[a] Pressure is decreased in some experiments, perhaps due to an increase in secretion.
[b] Experiments in cats show that CCK relaxes the area around the sphincter and stimulates contraction of the distal duodenum.
[c] Relaxation occurs in dogs immediately after a fatty meal, followed by contraction (10–30 L).

In 1957, Boyden showed in meticulous dissections that the sphincter muscle is derived structurally and embryologically from fibers of the muscularis mucosae.

Besides a longitudinal fascicle that extends to the papillary opening and is believed to straighten the papilla during the expulsion of bile, duodenal motor function plays an essential role by "actively milking" the bile duct (Hallenbeck 1967) or even by acting as a "cocktail shaker" during digestion (Hand 1973).

The duodenal papilla was first inspected endoscopically in 1965, but it was not until 1969 that endoscopic retrograde cholangiopancreatography (ERCP) assumed clinical importance (Ol 1970; Takagi 1970). Geenen and Hogan reported on manometric studies of the duodenal papilla in 1980.

The statement by Frerichs (1858) that "clinical practice must bring to a focus the results from various research fields while reconciling and completing the biases that result from the division of labor," plus the fact that ERCP is fraught with complications, prompted us to investigate the functional interaction of the duodenal papilla and common bile duct under physiologic conditions using radionuclide techniques.

A study conducted under physiologic conditions in healthy subjects and patients with various types of biliary tract disease showed that, regardless of underlying disease, gender, and age, the time-activity curves obtained by radionuclide scanning display the same shape over the common bile duct and over the horizontal part of the duodenum (el Helou and Hör 1979). This can be explained by the assumption of Hallenbeck (1967). We cannot explain the unchanged time-activity curve patterns seen over both organs in the presence of prepapillary outflow obstruction or papillary sclerosis. The explanation probably has a hormonal or neurologic basis. So far there has been no proof that a relationship exists between choledochoduodenal function and hepatobiliary disease.

References

Adler RD, Metzger AL, Grundy SM (1974) Biliary lipid secretion before and after cholecystectomy in American Indians with cholesterol gall stones. Gastroenterology 66:1212

Agosti A, Matovani P, Mori L (1971) Action of caerulein and related substances on the sphincter of Oddi. Arch Pharmakol 268:114

Agren G, Lagerlöf H (1937) The biliary response in the secretin test. Acta Med Scand 92:359

Amer MS (1969a) Mechanism of action of cholecystokinin. Clin Res 17:520

Amer MS (1969b) Studies with cholecystokinin. II. Cholecystokinetic potency of porcine gastrins I and II and related peptides in three systems. Endocrinology 84:1277

Amer MS (1972) Studies with cholecystokinin in vitro. III. Mechanism of the effect on the isolated rabbit gallbladder strips. J Pharmacol Exp Ther 183:527

Amer MS, Becvar WE (1969) A sensitive in-vitro method for the assay of cholecystokinin. J Endocrinol 43:637

Andersson KE, Andersson R, Hedner P (1972) Cholecystokinetic effect and concentration of cyclic AMP in gall-bladder muscle in vitro. Acta Physiol Scand 85:511

Andersson KE, Hedner P, Hedner CGA (1974) Differentiation of the contractile effects of prostaglandin E2 and the C-terminal octapeptide of the cholecystokinin in isolated guineapig gall-bladder. Acta Physiol Scand 90:657

Bainbridge FA, Dale HH (1905) The contractile mechanism of the gall-bladder and its extrinsic nervous control. J Physiol 33:138

Bayliss WM, Starling EH (1899) The movements and innervaton of the small intestine. J Physiol 24:99

Bergh GS (1942a) The sphincteric mechanism of the common bile duct in human subjects. Surgery 11:299

Bergh GS (1942b) The effect of food upon the sphincter of Oddi in human subjects. Am J Digest Dis 9:40

Bergh GS, Layne JA (1940) A demonstration of the independent contraction of the sphincter of the common bile duct in human subjects. Am J Physiol 128:690

Boyden EA (1957a) The choledochoduodenal junction in the cat. Surgery 41:773

Boyden EA (1957b) Anatomy of the choledochoduodenal junction in man. Surg Gynec Obstet 104:641

Burget GE (1926) The regulation of the flow of bile. II. Effect of eliminating the sphincter of Oddi. Am J Physiol 79:130

Caroli J, Varay A, Gilles E (1945) Le fonctionnement du sphincter vesiculaire chez l'homme. Observations d'une double intubation. Arch Mal App Dig 34:352

Copher GH, Kodoma S (1926) The regulation of the flow of bile and pancreatiac juice into the duodenum. Arch Intern Med 38:647

Cotton PB (1977) Progress report. Gut 18:316

Cox HT, Doherty JF, Kerr DF (1958) Changes in the gall-bladder after elective gastric surgery. Lancet 1:764

Crema A, Berte F, Benzi G, Frigo GM (1963) Action of sympathomimetic agents on the choledochoduodenal junction "in vitro". Arch Int Pharmacodyn 146:586

Crema A, Berte F, Benzi G, Frigo GM (1964) The responses of the sphincterial areas of the extrahepatic biliary tract to the stimulation of sympathetic and parasympathetic nerves. Acta Physiol Pharmacol Ther Latinoam 14:24

Crema A, Benzi G, Frigo GM, Berte F (1965) Occurrence of alpha- and beta-receptore in the bile duct. Proc Soc Exp Biol Med 120:158

Crispin JS, Choi YW, Wiseman DGH, Gillespie DJ, Lind JF (1970) A direct manometric study of the canine choledochoduodenal junction. The effect of atropine. Arch Surg 101:215

Chushieri A, Hughes JH, Cohen M (1972) Biliary pressure studies during cholecystectomy. Br J Surg 59:267

Dahlgren S (1967) The effect of cholecystokin on duodenal motility. Acta Chir Scand 133:403

Dardik H, Schein CJ, Warren A, Gliedmann MS (1969) Adrenergic receptors in the canine biliary tract. Surg Gynec Obstet 128:823

Dardik H, Gliedman ML, Christ R, Koslow A, Schein CJ (1970) Neuroendocrine influences on the dynamics of the choledochal sphincter. Surg Gynec Obstet 131:675

Diamond JS, Siegel SA, Myerson S (1940) II. The biliary pigment curve during the secretin test. Its diagnostic significance in the non-functioning gall-bladder. Am J Digest Dis 7:133

Doubilet H, Colp R (1937) Resistance of the sphincter of Oddi in the human. Surg Gynecol Obstet 64:622

Doyle JS (1968) Dynamics of the common duct. Lancet 1:531

Dubois FS, Kistler GH (1933) Concerning the mechanism of contraction of the gall-bladder in the guinea pig. Proc Soc Exp Biol Med 30:1178

El Helou A, Hör G (1979) Nuklearmedizinische Nierendiagnostik. Therapiewoche 29:7785–7795

Elman R, McMaster PD (1926) The physiological variations in resistance to bile flow to the intestine. J Exp Med 44:151

Geenen, Hogan (1980) Monometische Untersuchungen der Papilla Vateri. In: Classen, Hennig, Seifert (eds) Gastrointestinal Endoscopy Thieme, Stuttgart

Gilsdorf RB, Urdaneta LF, Leonhard AS (1970) Neuroeffector drug influences on pancreatic and biliary sphincter resistances in the awake cat. Curr Top Surg 2:41

Hallenbeck GA (1967) Biliary and pancreatic intraductal pressures. In: Code CF (ed) Handbook of physiology, Section 6, Alimentary canal, vol. secretion. American Physiological Society, Washington/DC

Halpert B, Lewis JH (1930) Experiments on the isolated whole gall-bladder of the dog. Am J Physiol 93:506

Hand BH (1973) Anatomy and function of the extrahepatic biliary system. Clin Gastroenterol 2:3

Larvey RF, Mathur MS, Dowsett L, Read AE (1974) Measurement of cholecystokinin-pancreozymin levels in peripheral venous blood in man. Gastroenterology 66:707

Hedner P, Rorsman G (1969) On the mechanism of action for the effect of cholecystokinin on the choledochoduodenal junction in the cat. Acta Physiol Scand 76:248

Hong SS, Magee DF, Crewdson F (1956) The physiologic regulation of gall-bladder evacuation. Gastroenterology 30:625

Hopton DS (1973) The influence of the vagus nerves on the biliary system. Br J Surg 60:216

Howat HT (1965) Tests of human gall-bladder function. In: Taylor (ed) The biliary system. Blackwells, Oxford, p 249

Inberg MV, Ahonen PJ, Scheinin TM (1970) Gall-bladder function and bile composition after selective gastric and truncal vagotomy in the dog. Scand J Clin Lab Invest 25 (Suppl 113):55

Inberg MV, Vuorio M (1969) Human gall-bladder function after selective gastric and total abdominal vagotomy. Acta Chir Scand 135:625

Isaza J, Jones DT, Dragstedt LR, Woodward ER (1971) The effect of vagotomy on motor function of the gall-bladder. Surgery 70:616

Ivy AC, Oldberg E (1928) A hormone mechanism for gall-bladder contraction and evacuation. Am J Physiol 86:599

Ivy AC, Goldman L (1939) Physiology of the biliary tract. JAMA 113:2413

Johnson FE, Boyden EA (1943) The effect of sectioning various autonomic nerves upon the rate of emptying of the biliary tract in the cat. Surg Gynecol Obstet 76:395

Johnson FE, Boyden EA (1952) The effect of double vagotomy on the motor activity of the human gall-bladder. Surgery 32:591

Jung FT, Greengard H (1933) Response of the isolated gall-bladder to cholecystokinin. Am J Physiol 103:275

Kozoll DD, Necheles H (1942a) A study of the mechanics of bile flow. I. Response to physiological intra-venous solutions. Surg Gynecol Obstet 74:27

Kozoll DD, Necheles H (1942b) A study of the mechanics of bile flow. II. Responses to intraduodenal solutions. Surg Gynecol Obstet 74:692

Kozoll DD, Necheles H (1942c) A study of the mechanics of bile flow. III. Responses to pharmacological stimuli. Surg Gynecol Obstet 74:961

Levy B, Ahlquist RP (1967) Adrenergic receptors in intestinal smooth muscle. Ann NY Acad Sci 139:781

Lieb CC, McWorther JE (1914) The innervaton of the gall-bladder. Proc Soc Exp Biol Med 12:102

Liedberg G, Halabi M (1970) The effect of vagotomy on flow resistance at the choledocho-duodenal junction. Acta Chir Scand 136:208

Liedberg G, Persson CGA (1970) Adrenoceptors in the cat choledochoduodenal junction studied in situ. Br J Pharmacol 39:619

Lin TM, Spray GF (1969) Effect of pentagastrin, cholecystokinin, caerulein and glucagon on the choledochal resistance and bile flow of conscious dog. Gastroenterology 56:1178

Lin TJ, Spray GF (1971) Choledochal, hepatic and cholecystokinetic actions of secretin (S); potentiation by cholecystokinin (CCK). Gastroenterology 60:783

Long H (1942) Observations on the choledocho-duodenal mechanism and their bearing on the physiology and pathology of the biliary tract. Br J Surg 29:422

Lueth HC (1931) Studies on the flow of bile into the duodenum and the existence of a sphincter of Oddi. Am J Physiol 99:237

Mack AJ, Todd JK (1968) A study of human gall-bladder muscle in vitro. Gut 9:546

McMaster PD, Elman R (1926) On the expulsion of bile by the gall-bladder; and a reciprocal relationship with the sphincteric activity. J Exp Med 44:173

Magee DF (1965) Physiology of gall-bladder emptying. In: Taylor (ed) The biliary system. Blackwell, Oxford, p 233

Marks IN (1959) Changes in the icteric index of the duodenal aspirate after the injection of secretin and pancreozymin. Gastroenterology 37:73

Menguy RB, Hallenbeck GA, Bollman JL, Grindlay JH (1958) Intraductal pressures and sphincteric resistance in canine pancreatic and biliary ducts after various stimuli. Surg Gynec Obstet 106:306

Mori J, Azuma H, Fujiwara M (1971) Adrenergic innervation and receptors in the sphincter of Oddi. Eur J Pharmacol 14:365

Nakayama S (1973) The effects of secretin and cholecystokinin on the sphincter muscles. In: Fujita T (ed) Gastro-entero-pancreatic endocrine system. Igaku Shoin, Tokyo, p 145

Nechels H, Kozoll DD (1942) A study of the sphincter of Oddi in the human and in the dog. Am J Digest Dis 9:36

Nora PF, McCarthy W, Sanez N (1974) Cholecystokinin cholecystography in acalculous gall-bladder disease. Arch Surg 108:507

Ottennyan R, Classen M In: Gastroenterologische Endoskopie, S 102

Persson CGA (1972) Adrenoceptors in the gall-bladder. Acta Pharmacol Toxicol 31:177

Persson CGA (1972) Effect of morphine, cholecystokinin and sympathomimetics on the sphincter of Oddi and intramural pressure in cat duodenum. Scand J Gastroenterol 7:345

Persson CGA Adrenergic, cholecystokinetic and morphine-induced effects on extra-hepatic biliary motility. Acta Physiol Scand (Suppl 383)

Persson CGA (1973) Dual effects on the sphincter of Oddi and gall-bladder inducted by stimulation of the right great splanchnic nerve. Acta Physiol Scand 87:334

Raih TJ, Ashmore CS, Wilson SD, DeCosse JJ, Mogan WJ, Dodds WJ, Sstef JJ (1973) Effect of enteric hormones on the canine choledochal sphincter. Gastroenterology 64:787

Ravdin IS, Morrison JL (1913) Gall-bladder function. I. The contractile of the gall-bladder. Arch Surg 22:710

Rost F (1913) Die funktionelle Bedeutung der Gallenblase. Experimentelle und anatomische Untersuchungen nach Cholecystektomie. Mitt Med Chir 26:710

Ryan JD, Doubilet H, Mulholland JH (1949) Observations on biliary-pancreatic dynamics in a normal human. Gastroenterology 13:1

Sandblom P, Voegtlin WL, Ivy AC (1935) The effect of cholecystokinin on the choledochoduodenal mechanism (sphincter of Oddi). Am J Physiol 113:175

Schein CJ, Gliedman ML (1970) The influence of vagotomy on the normal and diseased gall-bladder. Digstion 3.243

Shingleton WW, Anlyan WG, Hart D (1952) Effects of vagotomy, splanchiectomy and celiac ganglienectomy on experimentally produced spasm of sphincter of Oddi in animals. Ann Surg 135:721

Shore JM, Silverman A, Siegel M, Bakal M (1971) Direct observations of the canine sphincter of Oddi. Ann Surg 174:264

Siegel CI, Mendeloff AI, Salik JO (1964) The emptying mechanism of the common bile duct. Gastroenterology 52:1119

Smith JL, Walters, Beal JM (1952) A study of choledochal sphincter action. Gastroenterology 20:129

Snape WJ (1948) Studies on the gall-bladder in unanesthetized dogs before and after vagotomy. Gastroenterology 10:129

Stasiewicz J, Szalaj W, Gabryelewicz A (1973) In vitro studies on adrenergic receptor within gall-bladder. Przegl Lek 30:244

Tansy MF, Mackowiak RC, Chaffee RB (1968) Reflex control of release of bile into the small intestine. Clin Res 16:532

Tansy MF, Mackowiak RC, Chaffee RB (1971) A vagosympathetic pathway capable of influencing common bile duct motility in the dog. Surg Gynec Obstet 133:225

Toouli J, Watts JM (1972) Actions of cholecystokinin/pancreozymin, secretin and gastrin on extra-hepatic biliary tract motility in vitro. Ann Surg 175:439

Torsoli A, Ramorino ML, Alessandrini A (1970) Motility of the biliary tract. Rendic Gastroent 2:67

Torsoli A, Corazziari E, Habib FI, Melchiorri P, Fave GD, Improta G (1973) Effects of some gastrointestinal hormones and related polypeptides on upper small intestinal motility in man. Rendic Gastroent 5:18

Watts JM, Dunphy JE (1966) The role of the common bile duct in biliary dynamics. Surg Gynec Obstet 122:1207

Wenz W (1973) Perkutane transhepatische Cholangiographie. Radiologie 13:41

Williams RD, Huang TT (1969) The effect of vagotomy on biliary pressure. Surgery 66:353

Wormsley KG (1969) Response to duodenal acidification in man. I. Electrolyte changes in the duodenal aspirate. Scand J Gastroenterol 4:717

Wormsley KG (1970) Response to duodenal acidification in man. III. Comparison with the effects of secretin and pancreozymin. Scand J Gastroenterol 5:353

Wyatt AP (1969) Effect of gastrectomy on biliary dynamics. Gut 10:91

Yau WM, Makhlouf n, Edwards LE, Farrar JT (1973) Mode of action of cholecystokinin and related peptides on gall-bladder muscle. Gastroenterology 65:451

Kidney

Efforts to evaluate renal function with radionuclides can be traced back to the early days of nuclear medicine imaging (Zum Winkel 1964; Pabst and Hör 1978; Deckart 1976; Hör and Pabst 1979) (Table A-4). Important milestones in the historical development of radionuclide renal imaging are listed below:

- Radioisotope renography with ^{131}I hippurate (Taplin et al. 1956; Zum Winkel 1964)
- Renal imaging (McAffee and Wagner 1960)
- Determination of the total clearance of renally excreted radiopharmaceuticals by the classic clearance principle (Burbank et al. 1961)
- Determination of total clearance by the slope method (Gott et al. 1961; Bianchi et al. 1961; Blaufox 1972)
- Utilization of ^{99m}Tc for radionuclide imaging (Harper et al. 1962)
- Differential determination of renal clearance by combining the slope method and the renogram (Taplin et al. 1963)
- Clearance determination using a partially shielded whole-body counter or a partial-body-shielded measuring set (Oberhausen and Romahn 1968)
- First clinical use of sequential renal scanning with ^{131}I hippuran and ^{99m}Tc O$_4$ in the perfusion phase (radionuclide aortography, perfusion scanning) (Myers 1964; Zum Winkel et al. 1965; Burke et al. 1966; Powell and Anger 1968)
- Renal computed scintigraphy (Loken et al. 1969; Winkler et al. 1969)

Table A-4. Development of radiopharmaceuticals for renal imaging

Procedure	Radiopharmaceuticals	Authors
Radioisotope renography	^{131}I orthoiodohippurate (OIH) ^{125}I hippurate ^{123}I hippurate	Tubis et al. (1960)
Static renal scintigraphy	Labeled Hg compounds (should be avoided due to radiation hazard)	
	^{99m}Tc penicillinamine complex	Halpern et al. (1972)
	^{99m}Tc iron-ascorbic acid complex	Lichte and Hör (1975) Hennig and Woller (1969)
	^{99m}Tc Sn gluconate	Charamza and Budikova (1969) Boyd et al. (1973)
	^{99m}Tc heptonate	Arnold et al. (1975)
	^{99m}Tc dimercaptosuccinic acid (DMSA)	Enlander et al. (1974)
		Lin et al. (1974) Handmaker et al. (1975)
	^{99m}Tc Sn thioglucose	Deckart et al. (1976)
Renal function scanning (RFS)	^{131}I hippurate ^{123}I hippurate	Atkins et al. (1971) Hauser et al. (1970) Holroyd et al. (1970) Butterman et al. (1976, 1977)
	^{99m}Tc DTPA	Hauser et al. (1970)
	^{99m}Tc O$_4$	Powell (1965)
	^{99m}Tc DMSA	Lin et al. (1974) Enlander et al. (1974) Handmaker et al. (1975)
Selective serial perfusion scanning (quantitative renal blood flow)	Intraarterial injection: ^{133}Xe or ^{99m}Tc O$_4$ Inhalation of ^{133}Xe Microsphere technique:	Zum Winkel et al. (1965) Steinhoff and Pabst (1968) Schmitz-Feuerhake et al. (1976)
	^{131}I albumin ^{99m}Tc albumin	Rudolph and Heymann (1967) Seifert (1971) Haas et al. (1972) Hör et al. (1972)
	Indicator dilution: ^{32}P-, ^{51}Cr- or ^{99m}Tc-labeled red blood cells	Grängsjö et al. (1966)
	^{51}Cr EDTA	Reubi et al. (1973)
	^{99m}Tc O$_4$	Pabst (1972)
Intravenous serial perfusion scanning	Perfusion phase of sequential imaging ^{99m}Tc O$_4$	Keim et al. (1979) Hör and Pabst (1979 b) Hecking et al. (1975)
Radionuclide aortography, qualitative or semiquantitative renal perfusion	^{99m}Tc DMSA	Powell (1965) Freemann et al. (1968)

References

Arnold RW, Subramanian G, McAffee RJ, Thomas FD (1975) Comparison of Tc complexes for renal imaging. J Nucl Med 16:357

Atkins HL, Eckelmann WC, Hauser W (1971) Evaluation of glomerular filtration rate with 99mTc-DTPA. J Nucl Med 12:338

Bianchi C, Zampieri A (1961) Sulla clearance renale del radiohypaque 131J. Bull Soc Ital Biol Sper 37:260

Blaufox MD, Funck-Brentano JL (eds) (1972) Radionuclides in Nephrology. Proc Int Symp, New York London

Boyd RE, Robson I, Hunt FC, Sorby PJ, Murray JPC, McKay WI (1973) ^{99m}Tc-gluconate complexes for renal scintigraphy. Br J Radiol 46:604

Burbank MK, Tauxe WN, Maher FT, Hunt JC (1961) Evaluation of radioiodinated hippuran for the estimation of renal plasma flow. Proc Mayo Clin 36:372

Burke G, Halko A, Coe FL (1966) Dynamic clinical studies with radioisotopes and the scintillation camera. I. Sodium iodohippurate I-131 renography. JAMA 197/1:85

Buttermann G, Wolf I, Hör G, Pabst HW (1976) Clinical experiences in studying liver and kidney diseases using ^{123}I-compounds. In: Qualm SM, Stöcker G, Weinreich R (eds) Iodine-123 in Western Europe (Proc. Panel Disc. KFA Jülich, Feb. 13, 1976. Jül-Conf. 20, Aug. 1976) S 19

Buttermann G, Wolf I, Hör G, Pabst HW, Kuhlmann H (1977) Verbesserung nuklearmedizinischer Nierendiagnostik durch Integration der dynamischen Szintigraphie mit statischem Nierenscan und Berechnung der integralen und regionalen, seitengetrennten Clearance unter Verwendung von ^{123}J-Hippuran. In: Schmidt HAE (Hrsg) Nuklearmedizin. Schattauer, Stuttgart New York S 361

Charamza O, Budikova M (1969) Herstellungsmethode eines ^{99m}Tc-Zinnkomplexes für die Nierenszintigraphie. Nuklearmedizin 8:301

Deckart H (1976) Nuklearmedizinische Nierendiagnostik. Schriftreihe Anwendung von Isotopen und Kernstrahlungen in Wissenschaft und Technik. Isocommerz, Berlin

Deckart H, Weiland I, Blottner A (1976) ^{99m}Tc-Thioglukose – ein neues Radiopharmakon für die Nierenszintigraphie. Radiobiol Radiother 17:674

Enlander D, Weber PM, Dos Remedios LV (1974) Renal cortical imaging in 35 patients: superior quality with ^{99m}Tc-DMSA. J Nucl Med 15:743

Freeman LM, Chien-Hsing M, Blaufox MD (1968) Diagnosis of arteriovenous fistula of the kidney with renal blood flow scintiphotography. Radiology 91:1189

Freeman LM, Johnson PM (1975) Clinical scintillation imaging, 2nd edn. Grune & Stratton, New York London San Francisco

Gott FS, Pritchard WH, Young WR, MacIntyre WJ (1961) Renal blood flow measurement from the blood clearance of a single injection of hipputope. Clin Res 9:201

Grängsjö GHR, Ulfendahl, Wolgast M (1966) Determination of regional blood flow by means of small semiconductor detectors and red cells tagged with Phosphorus 32. Nature 211:1411

Haas JP, Claus HG, Kutzner J (1972) Vergleichende Untersuchungen über die Aussagekraft von Angioszintigraphie, der Angiographie und der Szintigraphie der Nieren. In: Hug O (Hrsg) Deutscher Röntgenkongress 1970. Thieme, Stuttgart, S 106

Halpern SM, Tubis J, Endow C, Walsh J, Kunsa B, Zwikker N (1972) ^{99m}Tc-penicillamine-acetazolamide complex – a new renal scanning agent. J Nucl Med 13/45:723

Handmaker H, Young W, Lowenstein M (1975) Clinical experience with ^{99m}Tc-DMSA – a new imaging agent. J Nucl Med 16:28

Harper PV, Andross G, Lathrop KA (1962) Preliminary observations on the use of six hour 99mTc as a tracer in biology and medicine. Argonne Cancer Res. Hosp. Semiannual report to the Atomic Energy Commission. ACRH 18:76

Hauser W, Atkins L, Nelson KG, Richards P (1970) Technetium-99m-DTPA – a new radiopharmaceutical for brain and kidney scanning. Radiology 94:679

Hecking E, Pfannenstiel R, Pixberg HV et al. (1975) Klinischer Wert der Nierensequenzszintigraphie mit 131J-Hippuran und der Nierenperfusion mit 99mTc-Präparaten nach Computerverarbeitung. Fortschr Röntgenstr 123:103

Hennig K, Woller P (1969) Nierenszintigraphie mit ^{99m}Tc- Fe-Komplex. Radiobiol Radiother 10:75

Holroyd AM, Chrisholm GD, Glass HJ (1970) The quantitative analysis of renograms using the gamma-camera. Phys in Med Biol 15:483

Hör G, Pabst HW (1979a) Nephrologie. In: Emrich D (Hrsg) Nuklearmedizin – Funktionsdiagnostik und Therapie, 2. Aufl. Thieme, Stuttgart, S 332

Hör G, Pabst HW (1979b) Funktionsdiagnostik in der Urologie und Nephrologie. In: Emrich D (Hrsg) Nuklearmedizin – Funktionsdiagnostik und Therapie, 2. Aufl. Thieme, Stuttgart, S 332–380

Hör G, Buttermann G, Heinze HG, Klein U, Langhammer H, Müller-Fassbänder H, Pabst HW (1972) Selective angioscintigraphy – and angiography in kidney disease. In: Diethelm L (ed) Angiography/scintigraphy. Springer, Berlin Heidelberg New York, p 393

Keim JH, Johnson PM, Vaughan ED, Beg KH, Follett DA, Freemann LM, Laragh JH (1979) Computer-assisted study. Dynamic renal imaging: a screening test for renovascular hypertension. J Nucl Med 20:11

Lichte H, Hör G (1975) Nierenszintigraphie mit ^{99m}Tc-Penicillamin. Fortschr Röntgenstr 122:119

Lin TH, Khentigan A, Winchell HS (1974) 99mTc-Dimercaptosuccinic acid for renal imaging. J Nucl Med 15:512

Loken MK, Linnemann RE, Kush GS (1969) Evaluation of renal function using a scintillation camera and computer. Radiology 93:85

McAffee JG, Wagner HN (1960) Visualization of renal parenchyma by scintiscanning with 203 Hg-Neohydrin. Radiology 75:820

Myers WG (1964) Dynamic studies with a gamma-ray scintillation camera. Med Radioisot Scanning 1:377

Oberhausen E, Romahn A (1968) Bestimmung der Nierenclearance durch externe Gammastrahlenmessung. In: Radionuklide in Kreislaufforschung und Kreislaufdiagnostik 5. Jahrestagung d. Ges. f. Nuklearmedizin 1967, Schattauer, Stuttgart, S 324

Pabst HW (1972) Investigations of blood flow in the kidneys with radioisotopes. J Nucl Biol Med 16:158

Pabst HW, Hör G (1978) Nephrologie. In: Hundeshagen H (Hrsg) Nuklearmedizin, Handbuch der medizinischen Radiologie, Band XV/2. Springer, Berlin Heidelberg New York, S 509–678

Powell M (1965) Use of scintillation camera for evaluation of renal function. J Nucl Med 6:323

Powell MR, Anger HO (1966) Triple isotope renal evaluation with the scintillation camera. J Nucl Med 7/5:373

Reubi FC, Vorburger C, Tuckmann J (1973) Renal distribution volumes of indocyanine green, ^{51Cr}-EDTA and ^{24}NA in man during acute renal failure after shock. J Clin Invest 52:223

Rudolph AM, Heymann MA (1967) The circulation of the fetus in utero: methods for studing distribution of blood flow, cardiac output and organ blood flow. Circ Res 21:163

Schmitz, Feuerhake L, Fröhlich H, Hutzer-Meyer H (1976) Atraumatische Durchblutungsmessung mit radioaktiven Edelgasen. Huber, Bern

Seifert J (1971) Die renale Angioszintigraphie – ein Beitrag zur Differentialdiagnose raumfordernder, intrarenal gelegener Prozesse. In: Horst W (Hrsg) Aktuelle Nuklearmedizin. Springer, Berlin Heidelberg New York, S 59

Steinhoff H, Pabst HW (1968) Die 133Xenon-Clearance der Nieren. In: (Hrsg) Radionuklide in Kreislaufforschung und Kreislaufdiagnostik. Schattauer, Stuttgart New York, S 341

Taplin GV, Meredith OM Jr, Kade H, Winter CC (1956) The radioisotope renogram (an external test for individual kidney function and upper urinary tract patency). J Lab Clin Med 48:886

Taplin GV, Dore EK, Johnson DE (1963) Recent advances in the diagnosis of renal hypertension with radioisotope procedures. Proc 5th Japan Conference on Radioisotopes Special session No. 2, Tokyo, May 21–24

Tubis M, Posnick T, Nordyke RA (1960) Preparation and use of ^{131}J labeled sodium iodohippurate in kidney function tests. Proc Soc Exp Biol Med 103:497

Weinreich R, Schult O, Stöcklin C (1974) Production of ^{123}I via the ^{127}I(d,6) ^{123} Xe (Beta, EC) ^{123}I proc. Int J Appl Radiat 25:535

Winkler C, Knopp R, Schulte P (1969) Computer-Nephrographie. Ein Programm zur automatischen Auswertung und Befundausgabe von Isotopen-Nephrogrammen. Nucl Med 8:154

Zum Winkel K (1964) Nierendiagnostik mit Radioisotopen. Thieme, Stuttgart New York

Zum Winkel K, Jost H (1975) Intrarenal kinetics of radiopharmaceutical applied to the artery. In: Zum Winkel K et al. (ed) Radionuclides in nephrology. Thieme, Stuttgart, p 225

Zum Winkel K, Scheer KE, Schenk P, Gelinsky P, Prpic B, Adam WE (1965) Die funktionell-morphologische Diagnostik von Nierenkrankheiten mit der Kamera-Szintigraphie und der Isotopen-Nephrographie. Dtsch Med Wochenschr 90:2229

A4
Bone

In 1935, Chievitz and Hevesy were the first to perform radioisotope bone scans in humans. As early as 1942, Treadwell et al. observed that ^{89}Sr is taken up in primary bone malignancies, and Murley and Dudley made a similar observation with ^{72}Ga in 1951. Bauer et al. (1957) successfully calculated the accretion rate of new bone mineral based on measurements with ^{45}Ca.

Bauer and Wendeberg (1953) discovered that local radiotracer uptake occurs not just in malignant bone tumors but also in benign conditions such as fractures, Paget's disease, and osteomyelitis.

In 1963 and 1964, the first reports were published on positive radionuclide scans and negative radiographs in patients with skeletal metastases. Other authors reported on radiographically detectable metastases that were not visible on bone scans (Sklaroff and Charkes). In the years that followed, numerous works were published on radionuclide bone scans for the early detection of skeletal metastases. Nuclear medicine journals were brimming with reports on the results obtained with various radiotracers in orthopedic investigations and on the importance and diagnostic accuracy of various bone radiopharmaceuticals (Zum Winkel et al. 1971).

Subramanian and McAfee (1971) described ^{99m}Tc phosphorus compounds as the agents of choice for radionuclide bone scanning, but Charkes et al. (1973) pointed out the practical difficulties of scan interpretation. Some authors, such as Thrupkaew et al. (1974) and Georgi and Lorenz (1974), stated that radiofluorine was the best tracer for bone imaging owing to its biologic properties. Subramanian and McAfee used ^{99m}Tc diphosphonate in 1975, and this agent is still considered the best radiotracer for skeletal imaging.

References

Bauer GCH, Carlsson A, Lindquist B (1957) Bone salt metabolism in humans studied by means of radiocalcium. Acta Med Scand 158:143–150

Bauer GCH, Wendeberg B (1959) External counting of 47Ca and 85Sr in studies of localized skeletal lesions in man. J Bone Joint Surg 41(B):558–580

Charkes ND, Sklaroff DM (1964) Early diagnosis of metastatic bone cancer by photoscanning with strontium-85. J Nucl Med 5:168–179

Charkes ND, Sklaroff DM, Bierly J (1964) Detection of metastatic cancer to bone by scintiscanning with strontium-87m. Am J Roentgenol 91:1127

Charkes ND, Sklaroff DM, Young I (1966) a critical analysis of strontium bone scanning for detection of metastatic cancer. Am J Roentgenol 96:647–656

Charkes ND, Valentine G, Cravitz B (1973) Interpretation of the normal 99m Tc-polyphosphate rectilinear bone scan. Radiology 107:563–570

Chievitz O, Hevesy G (1935) Radioactive indicators in the study of phosphorus metabolism in rats. Nature 136:754–755

Georgi P, Lorenz JW (1974) Knochenszintigraphie mit digitaler Datenverarbeitung. Radiobiol Radiother (Berlin) 15:155–166

Murley WG, Dudley HC (1951) Studies of radiogallium in bone tumors. J Lab Clin Med 37:239–252

Sklaroff DM, Charkes ND (1963) Studies of metastatic bone lesions with strontium 85. Radiology 80:270–272

Subramanian G, McAffee JG (1971) A new complex of 99mTc skeletal imaging. Radiology 99:192–196

Subramanian G, McAffee JG, Blair RJ, Kallfelz FA, Thomas FD (1975) Technetium-99m-methylene diphosphonate – a superior agent for skeletal imaging: comparison with other technetium complexes. J Nucl Med 16:744–755

Thrupkaew AK, Henkin RE, Quinn JL (1974) False negative bone scans in disseminated metastatic disease. Radiology 113:383–386

Treadwell A, Low-Beer BV, Friedell HL, Lawrence JH (1942) Metabolic studies on neoplasm of bone with the aid of radioactive strontium. Am J Med Sci 204:251–530

Zum Winkel K, Dreyer H, Herb R, Harbst H, Georgi M, Maier-Borst W (1971) Szintigraphie von Knochen- und Gelenkaffektionen mit Fluor-18 im Vergleich zur Röntgendiagnostik. In: Glauner R (Hrsg) Angiologie und Szintigraphie bei Knochen- und Gelenkkrankheiten. Thieme, Stuttgart

B
Definitions and Units

1
Definitions of Terms in Nuclear Physics

▌ **Alpha particles.** Helium nuclei, consisting of two protons and two neutrons.

▌ **Atom.** The smallest complex structural unit of a molecule.

▌ **Electron shell.** Cloud of electrons orbiting an atomic nucleus.

▌ **Atomic nucleus.** Center of an atom, composed of protons and neutrons (except in the hydrogen nucleus) and containing 99.7% of the mass of the atom.

▌ **Deuteron (d).** Nucleus of deuterium (heavy hydrogen), consisting of one proton and one neutron.

▌ **Electron (e, e⁻, β⁻).** Elementary particle carrying a negative electric charge and having an extremely small mass (0.005 MU).

▌ **Isobars.** Nuclides that have the same mass number.

▌ **Isomers.** Metastable nuclides.

▌ **Isotopes.** Nuclei with the same number of protons but different number of neutrons. Isotopes of an element have identical chemical properties.

▌ **Isotones.** Nuclei with the same number of neutrons but different number or protons.

▌ **Mass number.** The sum of the number of protons and neutrons (old term: atomic weight).

▌ **Mass unit (MU).** Relative mass of an atom or elementary particle. MU of carbon = 12. One proton ≈ 1 MU ($1.67 \cdot 10^{-24}$ g).

▌ **Metastable (m).** Excited nuclear state of long duration. Metastable nuclei essentially emit only gamma rays.

▌ **Nuclide.** A species of atom characterized by the number of protons and neutrons contained in the nucleus.

▌ **Neutron (n).** An electrically neutral elementary particle that is a constituent of the nucleus. It has the same mass as a proton (1 MU).

▌ **Atomic number (Z).** The number of protons in a nucleus, also the number of electrons in a neutral atom.

▌ **Positron (e⁺, β⁺).** A short-lived particle, generated by nuclear reactions, that has a positive electric charge and the same mass as an electron (0.0005 MU).

▌ **Proton (p).** A positively charged elementary particle that is a constituent of the nucleus. It has the same mass as a neutron (1 MU).

▌ **Triton (t).** Nucleus of tritium, consisting of one proton and two neutrons.

2
Système Internationale Units

Système Internationale (SI) units comprise a self-consistent set of units that are used in all areas of science. The General Conference on Weights and Measures, acting on a recommendation from the International Commission on Radiation Units and Measurement (ICRU), has introduced special terms for SI units that are used in connection with radioactivity.

2.1 Radioactivity

The SI unit for radioactivity is the becquerel (Bq).

▌ 1 Bq = 1 disintegration per second
▌   = $2.7 \cdot 10^{-11}$ curie (Ci)
▌ 1 Ci = $3.7 \cdot 10^{10}$ Bq = 37 MBq

1 Bq	37 Bq	1 kBq	37 kBq	1 MBq
27 pCi	1 nCi	27 nCi	1 µCi	27 µCi

37 MBq	1 GBq	37 GBq	1 TBq	37 TBq
1 mCi	27 mCi	1 Ci	27 Ci	1 kCi

Examples:

▌ <u>Conversion of Bq to Ci</u>   <u>Conversion of Ci to Bq</u>
▌ 10 MBq   = 0.27 mCi   1 mCi =   37 MBq
▌ 20 MBq   = 0.54 mCi   2 mCi =   74 MBq
▌ 50 MBq   = 1.34 mCi   5 mCi = 185 MBq
▌ 100 MBq = 2.70 mCi
▌ 200 mBq = 5.41 mCi   10 mCi = 370 MBq
▌ 5 GBq   = 135 mCi   50 mCi = 1.80 GBq
▌ 100 mCi = 3.70 GBq
▌ 10 GBq   = 270 mCi   250 mCi =   9.25 GBq
▌ 1 Bq   =   1 disintegration/second
▌ 1 kBq   = 10^3 disintegrations/second
▌ 1 MBq   = 10^6 disintegrations/second
▌ 1 GBq   = 10^9 disintegrations/second

2.2 Prefixes

Prefixes are used to designate multiples or submultiples of units (e.g., 1 MV = 1 megavolt = 1 million volts). The standard prefixes for SI units are defined below.

Submultiple	Prefix	Symbol
10^{-3}	Milli	m
10^{-6}	Micro	µ
10^{-9}	Nano	n
10^{-12}	Pico	p

Multiple	Prefix	Symbol
10^3	Kilo	k
10^6	Mega	M
10^9	Giga	G
10^{12}	Tera	T

E	Exa-	=	10^{18}	=	1 quintillion
	Peta-	=	10^{15}	=	1 quadrillion
T	Tera-	=	10^{12}	=	1 trillion
G	Giga-	=	10^{9}	=	1 billion
M	Mega-	=	10^{6}	=	1 million
k	Kilo-	=	10^{3}	=	1000
h	Hecto-	=	10^{2}	=	100
da	Deca-	=	10^{1}	=	10
d	Deci-	=	10^{-1}	=	0.1
c	Centi-	=	10^{-2}	=	0.01
m	Milli-	=	10^{-3}	=	0.001
μ	Micro-	=	10^{-6}	=	0.000 001
n	Nano-	=	10^{-9}	=	0.000 000 001
p	Pico-	=	10^{-12}	=	0.000 000 000 001
f	Femto-	=	10^{-15}	=	0.000 000 000 000 001
a	Atto-	=	10^{-18}	=	0.000 000 000 000 000 001

2.3
Radiation Measurement and Radiation Safety

The standard SI unit of measurement for the *dose equivalent* (the absorbed dose multiplied by modifying factors) is the sievert (Sv).

- 1 Sv = 100 rem
- 1 rem = 0.01 Sv = 10 mSv

0.1 µSv	1 µSv	10 µSv	100 µSv
0.01 mrem	0.1 mrem	1 mrem	10 mrem

1 msV	10 mSv	100 mSv	1 Sv
100 mrem	1 rem	10 rem	100 rem

The standard SI unit for the *absorbed dose* (the amount of energy imparted to matter) is the gray (Gy).

- 1 Gy = 100 rd
- 1 rd = 0.01 Gy = 10 mGy

Relationship between SI units and non-SI units:

Physical measure	SI unit	Non-SI unit	Relationship
Radioactivity	Becquerel (Bq) 1 Bq = 1 disintegration/s	Curie (Ci)	1 Bq = 2.7·10^{-11} Ci = 27.0 pCi 1 Ci = 3.7·10^{10} Bq = 37 GBq
Absorbed dose	Gray (Gy) 1 Gy = 1 J/kg	rad (rd)	1 Gy = 100 rd 1 rd = 0.01 Gy = 10 mGy
Dose equivalent	Sievert (Sv)	rem	1 Sv = 100 rem 1 rem = 0.01 Sv = 10 mSv

3
Radionuclides

3.1
List of Isotopes

Nuclear medicine radioisotopes and their properties are reviewed in the table below.

Atomic number	Symbol	Element	Mass number	Half-life	Energy (MeV) β^+/β^-	γ
6	C	Carbon	11	20.3 m	+0.98	0.51
7	N	Nitrogen	13	10.0 m	+1.25	0.51
8	O	Oxygen	15	2.1 m	+1.68	0.51
9	F	Fluorine	18	109.7 m	+0.65	0.51
15	P	Phosphorus	32	14.0 d	1.71	–
24	Cr	Chromium	51	27.7 d	k	0.32
26	Fe	Iron	59	44.5 d	0.46	1.1/1.3
27	Co	Cobalt	57	272.0 d	k	0.12
			58	70.8 d	0.47	0.81
			60	5.27 a	0.31	1.33
29	Cu	Copper	67	2.50 d	0.395–0.577	0.51
31	Ga	Gallium	67	3.26 d	k	0.1/0.19/0.3
			68	1.13 h	+1.88	0.51
34	Se	Selenium	75	120 d	k	0.27
36	Kr	Krypton	81 m	13.0 s	–	0.19
37	Rb	Rubidium	81	4.57 h	-.99	0.95
			82	1.30 m	+3.15	0.51
38	Sr	Strontium	85	64.9 d	k	0.51
			89	50.5 d	1.46	–
			90	28.8 a	2.25	–
39	Y	Yttrium	90	64.0 h	2.27	–
42	Mo	Molybdenum	99	67.0 h	1.23	0.74
43	Tc	Technetium	99m	6.01 h	–	0.14
49	In	Indium	111	2.81 d	k	0.17/0.25
			113 m	1.66 h	–	0.39
53	I	Iodine	123	13.2 h	k	0.16
			125	59.3 d	k	0.03
			131	8.02 d	0.61	0.36
54	Xe	Xenon	133	5.24 d	0.34	0.08
62	Sm	Samarium	153	46.8 d	0.64–0.81	0.10
64	Gd	Gadolinium	159	18.6 h	1.0	0.36
68	Er	Erbium	169	9.50 d	0.34	0.11
75	Re	Rhenium	186	3.78 d	1.07	0.14
			188	17.0 h	2.1	–
77	Ir	Iridium	192	73.8 d	0.67	0.32
79	Au	Gold	198	2.70 d	0.96	0.41
81	Tl	Thallium	201	72.9 h	k	0.08
85	At	Astatium	211	7.22 h	5.8	0.51

Note:
κ = Electron capture
γ = energies (incomplete)
β = energies E-max

**3.2
Half-life of Radioisotopes**

The mathematical formulation of nuclear decay follows an exponential law:

$$N = N_0 \times e^{-\lambda(t)}$$

where:

- N_0 = number of radioactive atoms at (arbitrary) initial time zero
- N = number of radioactive atoms after time t
- λ = the decay constant (lambda)
- t = elapsed time measured from time zero
- e = 2.718... (basis of exponential function)

A fixed relationship exists between the decay constant λ and the half-life (HL) of an isotope:

$$\lambda = \ln 2/HL = 0.693/HL$$

(where ln 2 is the natural logarithm of 2). We can now write the decay law in its somewhat more familiar form:

$$N = N_0 \times e^{(-\ln 2/HL)t}$$

For practical purposes, it is often useful to be able to estimate the approximate rate of decay of radioactive emissions. This can be done by estimating how much activity is left after a given number of half-lives:

- 50% after 1 HL
- 26% after 2 HL
- 10% after 3.3 HL
- 1% after 6.7 HL
- 0.1% after 10 HL

4
Half-Value Layer (HVL)

The half-value layer (HVL) is the thickness of material that will attenuate the energy flux density of a given radiation by one-half.

Nuclide	Energy (MeV)	HVL (cm water)	HVL (cm lead)
^{201}Tl	0.075	3.6	0.022
	0.166	4.7	0.037
^{57}Co	0.122	4.3	0.013
	0.136	4.4	0.024
^{99m}Tc	0.141	4.5	0.028
^{111}In	0.171	4.8	0.045
	0.245	5.5	0.100
^{51}Cr	0.320	6.0	0.17
^{75}Se	0.121	4.3	0.018
	0.136	4.4	0.024
	0.265	5.6	0.120
	0.280	5.7	0.13
	0.401	6.8	0.27
^{131}I	0.364	6.3	0.23
	0.637	8.5	0.51
^{59}Fe	1.099	10.5	0.93
	1.292	11.4	1.05

5
Mo-99/Tc-99m Generator

5.1
Testing for Mo-99 Breakthrough

▌ Molybdenum breakthrough is defined as contamination of the ^{99m}Tc eluate by ^{99}Mo as a result of damage to the alumina column, faulty setup, or overuse of the generator.

▌ The equipment used for the measurement of ^{99m}Tc should include a device that tests for ^{99}Mo breakthrough using a specified thickness of lead shielding.

▌ Whenever a new generator is put into operation, ^{99}Mo breakthrough testing should be performed before the first eluate is used.

▌ Because the high-energy gamma emissions from ^{99}Mo would pose an excessive radiation risk to the patient, the eluate is acceptable for patient use only if the activity of ^{99}Mo does not exceed 0.1% of the activity of ^{99m}Tc.

▌ Testing for ^{99}Mo breakthrough is aided by the fact that approximately 13% of the ^{99}Mo decays directly to ^{99}Tc, accompanied by the release of gamma radiation at 739 keV. Thus when ^{99}Mo breakthrough occurs, the 739-keV emissions from the ^{99}Mo can be detected along with the 141-keV emissions from the ^{99m}Tc. Two measurements of the eluate are performed under identical conditions, one with and one without an approximately 4–6 cm thickness of lead shielding. Since the lead shielding absorbs almost all of the 141-keV emissions, only the 739-keV radiation from the ^{99}Mo is measured.

▌ When the results with and without lead shielding are compared, the measurement obtained with the shielding should not exceed 0.04% of the measurement without the shielding.

▌ In new generators, the molybdenum content of the eluate is automatically calculated and the result is displayed.

6
Recommendations of the European Association of Nuclear Medicine (EANM) Task Group

6.1
Adult Dose and Minimum Activities (MBq)

Radiopharmaceutical	Organ	Adult dose	Minimum
Tc-99m DTPA	Kidney	200	20
Tc-99m DMSA	Kidney	100	15
Tc-99m MAG3	Kidney	70	15
Tc-99m pertechnetate	Bladder	20	20
Tc-99m MDP	Bone	500	40
Tc-99m colloid	Liver-spleen	80	15
Tc-99m colloid	Bone marrow	300	20
Tc-99m RBCs	Spleen	40	20
Tc-99m RBCs	Blood pool	800	80
Tc-99m albumin	Heart	800	80
Tc-99m pertechnetate	First pass	500	80
Tc-99m MAA	Lung	80	10
Tc-99m pertechnetate	Stomach	150	20
Tc-99m colloid	Reflux	40	10
Tc-99m IDA	Hepatobiliary tract	150	20
Tc-99m pertechnetate	Thyroid	80	10
Tc-99m HMPAO	Brain	740	100
Tc-99m HMPAO	Leukocytes	500	40
I-123 hippuran	Kidney	75	10
I-123 sodium iodide	Thyroid	20	3
I-123 amphetamine	Brain	185	18
I-123 MIBG	Adrenal	200	35
I-123 MIBG	Adrenal	80	35
Ga-67	Whole body	80	10

6.2
EANM Pediatric Task Group

Conversion factors for dose adjustment by body weight, based on the fraction of the normal adult dose.

Body weight (kg)	Fraction of adult dose	Body weight (kg)	Fraction of adult dose
3	0.1	32	0.65
4	0.14	34	0.68
6	0.19	36	0.71
8	0.23	38	0.73
10	0.27	40	0.76
12	0.32	42	0.78
14	0.36	44	0.80
16	0.40	46	0.82
18	0.44	48	0.85
20	0.46	50	0.88
22	0.50	52–54	0.90
24	0.53	56–58	0.92
26	0.56	60–62	0.96
28	0.58	64–66	0.98
30	0.62	68	0.99

6.3
Formula for Calculating Radiation Dose by Body Surface Area

$$\text{Dose [child]} = \frac{\text{Dose [adult] (MBq} \times \text{Body surface area (m}^2)}{1.73\text{m}^2}$$

7
Collimators

Collimator designation	Type	Energy (keV)
LEAP	Low-energy all-purpose	140
HRP	High-resolution	140
HSR	High-sensitivity	140
HRC	High-resolution convergent	140
HSC	High-sensitivity convergent	140
ME	Medium-energy	360
HE	High-energy	510
Pinhole	4 mm	510

Subject Index

Printing and Binding: Stürtz AG, Würzburg